The Continuum of

Stroke Care

An Interprofessional Approach
to Evidence-Based Care

The Continuum of

Stroke Care
An Interprofessional Approach to Evidence-Based Care

Joanne V. Hickey, PhD, RN, APRN, ACNP-BC, FAAN, FCCM
Professor
Patricia L. Starck/PARTNERS Professor of Nursing
University of Texas Health Science Center at Houston School of Nursing
Houston, Texas

Sarah L. Livesay, DNP, RN, ACNP-BC, ACNS-BC, SCRN
Assistant Professor
Rush University College of Nursing
Chicago, Illinois

Wolters Kluwer

Philadelphia • Baltimore • New York • London
Buenos Aires • Hong Kong • Sydney • Tokyo

Acquisitions Editor: Shannon W. Magee
Product Development Editor: Maria M. McAvey
Senior Marketing Manager: Mark Wiragh
Editorial Assistant: Zachary Shapiro
Production Project Manager: Cynthia Rudy
Design Coordinator: Holly Reid McLaughlin
Manufacturing Coordinator: Kathleen Brown
Prepress Vendor: Absolute Service, Inc.

Copyright © 2016 Wolters Kluwer.

9 8 7 6 5 4 3 2 1

Printed in China

Library of Congress Cataloging-in-Publication Data

The continuum of stroke care : an interprofessional approach to evidence-based care / [edited by] Joanne V. Hickey, Sarah L. Livesay.
    p. ; cm.
  Includes bibliographical references and index.
  ISBN 978-1-4511-9346-6
  I. Hickey, Joanne V., editor. II. Livesay, Sarah L., editor.
  [DNLM: 1. Stroke—therapy. 2. Evidence-Based Practice—methods. 3. Patient Care Team. WL 356]
  RC388.5
  616.8'106—dc23
                    2015000750

LWW.com

Contributors

Cynthia Bautista, PhD, RN, CNRN, CCNS, ACNS-BC
Neuroscience Clinical Nurse Specialist
Yale-New Haven Hospital
New Haven, Connecticut

Terrie M. Black, DNP(c), MBA, BSN, RN, BC, CRRN, FAHA
Nurse Reviewer - Disease Specific Care
The Joint Commission
Oakbrook Terrace, Illinois

Kelly Blessing, MSN, FNP-C, RN
Nurse Practitioner
Division of Stroke and Vascular Neurology
Duke University Medical Center
Durham, North Carolina

Patricia A. Blissitt, RN, PhD, CCRN, CNRN, CCNS, CCM, ACNS-BC
Neuroscience Clinical Nurse Specialist
Harborview Medical Center
Assistant Professor, Clinical Faculty
University of Washington School of Nursing
Seattle, Washington

Christy L. Casper, MSN, ANP-BC
Neurocritical Care and Stroke
St. Anthony Hospital
Lakewood, Colorado

Susan M. Chioffi, MSN, ACNP-BC, RN
Nurse Practitioner
Division of Stroke and Vascular Neurology
Duke University Medical Center
Durham, North Carolina

Alexandra M. Graves, MS, ANP-BC, ANVP
Neurocritical Care and Stroke
St. Anthony Hospital
Lakewood, Colorado

Mary Guhwe, MSN, FNP-BC, SCRN
Nurse Practitioner
Division of Stroke and Vascular Neurology
Duke University Medical Center
Durham, North Carolina

Joanne V. Hickey, PhD, RN, APRN, ACNP-BC, FAAN, FCCM
Professor
Patricia L. Starck/PARTNERS Professor of Nursing
University of Texas Health Science Center at Houston School of Nursing
Houston, Texas

Mary L. King, MSN, RN, CNRN, CCRN, ACNS-BC
Clinical Nurse Specialist
Neurosurgical Intensive Care Unit
Barrow Neurological Institute
Phoenix, Arizona

Sarah L. Livesay, DNP, RN, ACNP-BC, ACNS-BC, SCRN
Assistant Professor
Rush University College of Nursing
Chicago, Illinois

Claranne Mathiesen, MSN, RN,
CNRN
Director Medical Operations Neurosciences
Lehigh Valley Hospital
Allentown, Pennsylvania
Assistant Professor Nursing
East Stroudsburg University
East Stroudsburg, Pennsylvania

Pamela S. Roberts, PhD, OTR/L,
SCFES, FAOTA, CPHQ
Program Director
Physical Medicine and Rehabilitation and
Neuropsychology
Cedars-Sinai Medical Center
Los Angeles, California

Karen B. Seagraves, MS, MPH,
ACNS-BC, ANP-BC
Marcus Stroke and Neuroscience Center
Grady Memorial Hospital
Atlanta, Georgia

Lindy Suarez, MSW, MHA, LCSW
Clinical Social Worker
Houston Methodist Hospital, Methodist
Neurological Institute
Houston, Texas

Preface

The idea to create *The Continuum of Stroke Care: An Interprofessional Approach to Evidence-Based Care* evolved over numerous discussions and a perceived need for a resource to integrate an evidence-based and an interprofessional team approach to stroke care. The fact that care provided by interprofessional teams achieves the best patient outcomes is well recognized based on cumulative evidence in which high-functioning interprofessional teams are considered critical for a safe health care system. The Institute of Medicine (IOM) issued recommendations and strategies for health care to become a more reliable and safe environment. One of the major recommendations of the report was strategies for engaging in more structured teamwork. Teamwork may take multiple forms in health care. The terms *interprofessional* and *interdisciplinary* are often used interchangeably in the literature to convey an integrative, collaborative approach to clinical practice. However, interprofessional suggests a high level of professional education, expertise, and collegiality between team members. Multidisciplinary, on the other hand, simply means several disciplines coming together without integration of their services. Therefore, we have chosen to use the term *interprofessional* rather than interdisciplinary or multidisciplinary to reflect the current imperatives for safe and effective care delivered by highly functional, collaborative, outcome-focused teams.

The intended audience for this book is health professionals who care for stroke patients, those interested in stroke care, and students from all health care disciplines. The purpose of the book is to provide a comprehensive, up-to-date, evidence-based resource to be used as a foundation for high-quality and safe care that results in optimal patient, population, and systems outcomes delivered by highly functional interprofessional teams. The scope of the book is comprehensive, addressing the various forms of stroke and the continuum of care from prevention through acute, rehabilitative, and community-based care as well as the individual and collaborative roles of the interprofessional team members. An icon ⊙ used throughout the chapters highlights important content about interprofessional team roles and responsibilities.

The many diverse health care systems around the globe are shaped by national demographic, social, political, technological, and economic values and resources. These factors are evidenced in the way stroke care is delivered in each country. Although the approach in this book is reflective of stroke care in the U.S. health care system, the standards of practice and care are based on evidence and best practice recommendations from the international stroke community. With the rapid development of new knowledge from the convergence of new research methodologies for bench and clinical investigations, coupled with unprecedented advances in biomedical technology and genetics, there will be continuing opportunities for translating new knowledge that will result in revisions and additions to the current knowledge and state of the science of stroke. This ongoing effort of building new knowledge and translating known stroke knowledge into practice to improve care for populations across the globe is the unending work of health professionals dedicated to quality stroke care, working together to achieve high-quality outcomes globally.

The contributors to this book represent health professionals at the cutting edge of practice, with extensive knowledge, expertise, and experience in caring for stroke patients. A common thread throughout all of the chapters is the focus on evidence-based practice and interprofessional team care. Within many chapters are clinical pearls, the sage pithy truisms shared by expert practitioners, and clinical vignettes and case studies to exemplify clinical encounters with stroke patients. The book is divided into three major sections. Section 1 provides an overview of stroke and interprofessional teams. Chapter 1 frames the scope of stroke as a global problem with recognition of the current and future burden around the globe. The greatest impact on changing the current stroke trajectory nationally and internationally is believed to be the implementation of comprehensive primary and secondary prevention strategies through the identification and successful management of risk factors. Chapter 2 explores stroke systems of care. Chapter 3 discusses the foundation for the structure, process, and science of interprofessional teams and their role in providing quality and safe care to stroke patients.

Section 2 examines stroke care across the continuum of care. Chapter 4 begins the discussion of the continuum of care with prehospital stroke care, followed by Chapter 5, which addresses the common diagnostics used in identifying stroke and its contributing risk factors. The major categories of stroke—ischemic, intracerebral hemorrhagic, and subarachnoid hemorrhage—are discussed in Chapters 6, 7, and 8, from prehospital through emergency department, critical care, and acute care, with an emphasis on evidence-based, patient- and family-centered, interprofessional team care. These chapters move the patient across the health–illness continuum from high acuity and postacute care into chronic illness management. In Chapter 9, stroke-related complications are addressed from a perspective of description, pathophysiology, assessment, treatment, and evaluation. This comprehensive chapter covers the complications from all types of stroke. Comprehensive rehabilitation of stroke patients is the focus of Chapter 10. The goal of all care is the integration of the poststroke patient back into the community, if possible, or offering other forms of long-term care and chronic illness management. This content is addressed in Chapter 11.

Section 3 considers quality, outcomes, and the future of stroke care. High-quality and safe care are the imperatives. Measurement and achievement of these goals are evident through quality indicators, patient and program outcomes, and criteria to evaluate stroke programs. This content is discussed in Chapter 12. Finally, the many social, scientific, and technological driving forces influencing the future of stroke are reviewed in Chapter 13 to round out a comprehensive deep dive into stroke care and practice.

Finally, we wish to acknowledge those who have assisted in making this book possible, including Shannon Magee, senior acquisitions editor, and Maria McAvey, product development editor, both at Wolters Kluwer, and our wonderful contributors. To our families and friends who have encouraged us and accepted our need to forgo other activities to work on the book, we are grateful. Our stroke patients and their families have inspired us to achieve the best in stroke care, and our superb colleagues who provide care to stroke patients on a daily basis motivated us to undertake this writing project as a tribute to their commitment to quality patient care and outcomes. It is you, our patients and their families, to whom we dedicate this book.

JVH and SLL

Contents

Overview of Stroke and Interprofessional Teams

CHAPTER 1

Stroke Epidemiology, Definition, Burden, and Prevention

Joanne V. Hickey

Every year, 15 million people around the globe have a stroke. Nearly 6 million die of stroke and another 5 million are left permanently disabled (World Heart Federation, 2014). Stroke is ranked second as the cause of disability after dementia worldwide. About three quarters of strokes are in persons 65 years of age and older. Hypertension contributes to more than 12.7 strokes worldwide. In developing countries, the incidence of stroke is declining largely due to improved methods to control hypertension and to success of smoking cessation programs. However, the overall rate of stroke remains high because of a global aging population (World Heart Federation, 2014). Stroke is a major cause of functional impairment, with 20% of survivors requiring institutional care after 3 months and 15% to 30% of stroke survivors left with permanent disabilities (Lloyd-Jones et al., 2010).

Multiple discoveries are rapidly changing our understanding of stroke, including the definition; diagnosis; treatment options; and approach to management, rehabilitation, and prevention of stroke. Basic science investigations into the pathophysiology of stroke, rigorous clinical studies for efficacy and effectiveness, improved registries for stroke-related data, rapidly advancing technology, and the integration of evidence-based care and practice models are changing the landscape of stroke. This chapter will address stroke epidemiology, definition of stroke, stroke burden, and prevention.

▮▮ INCIDENCE AND EPIDEMIOLOGY OF STROKE

In the United States, stroke is ranked as the fourth major cause of death after heart disease, cancer, and chronic lower respiratory disease (Centers for Disease Control and Prevention [CDC], 2014). A historical perspective provides a context for considering the rankings. Stroke moved from second to third as the major cause of mortality in 1937, although stroke mortality was stable from 1930 to 1960 at 175.0 per 100,000. A decline in mortality ensued from 1960 to the 2000s. By 2008, the age-adjusted annual death rate from stroke was 40.6 per 100,000, a clear three-fourths less than during the period of 1931 to 1960 (Towfighi & Saver, 2011). The total stroke mortality in the United States declined from a high of 214,000 in 1937 to 134,000 in 2008 (CDC, 2014). Concurrently, the National Center for Health Statistics revised their methodology for counting chronic lower respiratory disease (CLRD) deaths to include deaths due to pneumonia, influenza, and bronchitis in the CLRD category. This change resulted in a sharp increase in the number of deaths from 2007 to 2008 in the CLRD category. The increase in CLRD coupled with a decrease in stroke deaths resulted in the shifting of the rank of third to fourth for stroke mortality.

In a 2014 statement from the American Heart Association/American Stroke Association concerning factors influencing the decline in stroke mortality, the following conclusions were drawn.

> The decline in stroke mortality is real and represents a major public health and clinical medicine success story. The repositioning of stroke from third to fourth leading cause of death is the result of true mortality decline and not an increase in mortality from chronic lung disease, which is now the third leading cause of death in the United States. There is strong evidence that the decline can be attributed to a combination of interventions and programs based on scientific findings and implemented with the purpose of reducing stroke risks, the most likely being the improved control of hypertension. Thus, research studies and the application of their findings in developing intervention programs have improved the health of the population. The continued application of aggressive evidence-based public health programs and clinical interventions is expected to result in further declines in stroke mortality. (Lackland et al., 2014, p. 315)

Regardless of changes in the methods of counting deaths, the data show a decline in stroke that can be explained as result of improvement in the management of the risk factors of hypertension and smoking. Although this is encouraging, there are still almost 800,000 Americans who sustain a stroke each year; there is much left to be done in the primary and secondary prevention of stroke.

The American Heart Association Statistical Update for 2014 provides information about stroke, which is summarized as follows (Go et al., 2013).

- Each year in the United States, 795,000 people have a first or recurrent stroke. Approximately 610,000 of these are first strokes, and 185,000 are recurrent strokes.
- The classification of stroke includes 87% ischemic, 10% intercerebral hemorrhagic, and 3% subarachnoid hemorrhage.
- On a yearly basis, 55,000 more women than men have a stroke.
- Women have a higher lifetime risk of stroke than men among those 55 to 75 years of age, with a one in five chance for women as compared to one in six for men.
- About 6.8 million Americans 20 years of age and older have had a stroke.
- African Americans' risk of a first stroke is nearly twice that of Caucasians; African Americans are more likely to die following a stroke than Caucasians (Rogers et al., 2012).
- Risk of stroke in Hispanics falls between that of Caucasians and African Americans.

In summary, stroke is ranked the fourth cause of death in the United States. Stroke is both an acute and a chronic health problem that has a major impact on individuals, families, and the health care system. Although much progress has been made in understanding the pathophysiology, diagnosis, and treatment of stroke, there is still much to be learned. The high incidence of stroke in African Americans and Hispanics is still to be elucidated to better prevent and treat stroke in the future.

▓ EVOLVING DEFINITIONS OF STROKE

Although the global impact of stroke is well recognized, and the science in elucidating the pathophysiology of cerebrovascular disease has made remarkable progress, the term *stroke* is not defined consistently in clinical practice, in research, and in the population assessment and surveillance of stroke nor is it reflective of 21st century knowledge. With this background in mind, the American Heart Association (AHA) and the American Stroke Association (ASA) convened an expert panel to update the definition of stroke for the 21st century (Sacco et al., 2013). Both the definition and terms used to define and describe stroke have evolved over time. Recent advancements in imaging technology enhance the basic understanding of the pathophysiology of stroke, and other scientific advancements have warranted a critical review for relevance to the 21st century.

First called *apoplexy* by Hippocrates about 400 BC, the term *stroke* was introduced in 1689 by William Cole. Along the way, the term *cerebrovascular accident* (CVA) emerged, although in the last few decades, *stroke* has become the accepted term. An understanding that the acute nontraumatic brain injury called *stroke* was a heterogeneous presentation of signs and symptoms perhaps added to the confusion around a definition. The addition of the term *transient ischemic attack* in the late 1950s was a response to the work of C. Miller Fisher, which described the temporary episodes of brain and eye ischemia (Fisher, 1958; Mohr, 2004). In 1975, an Ad Hoc Committee on Cerebrovascular Disease published the following definition: "Transient ischemic attacks are episodes of temporary and focal dysfunction of vascular origin, which are variable in duration, commonly lasting from 2 to 15 minutes, but occasionally lasting as long as a day (24 hours). They leave no persistent neurological deficit" (p. 567). Of particular interest was that the 24-hour time frame was arbitrarily chosen based on consensus rather than scientific data. As noted by Sacco et al. (2013), when this definition of transient ischemic attack (TIA) was formulated, neither diagnostic procedures that could determine the presence of brain infarction were available nor were effective treatments for brain ischemia established. This definition of TIA was universally used until the beginning of the 21st century when accumulating data from scientific discoveries and diagnostic imaging prompted interest in revising definitions.

In 2002, an expert committee (Albers et al., 2002) proposed a new definition: "A TIA is a brief episode of neurologic dysfunction caused by focal brain or retinal ischemia, with clinical symptoms typically lasting less than one hour, and without evidence of acute infarction" (p. 1715). Easton et al. (2009) chaired an expert committee of the AHA/ASA, which published a scientific statement defining TIA and recommending evaluation. The definition proposed was "transient ischemic attack (TIA) is a transient episode of neurological dysfunction caused by focal brain, spinal cord, or retinal ischemia, without acute infarction" (p. 2276). Of note is that the duration of the event was removed. The *International Classification of Diseases* (ICD) system, owned by the World Health Organization (WHO), aims to standardize diagnostic classification for most diseases. The most current version is the ICD-10; it is the foundation for ICD-10-Clinical Modification (CM) or ICD-10-CM. According the preface to the ICD-10-CM for FY 2015, the ICD-10-CM is the United States' clinical modification of the WHO's ICD-10. The term "clinical" is used to emphasize the modification's intent which is to serve as a useful tool in the area of classification of morbidity data for indexing of health records, medical care review, and ambulatory and other health care programs, as well as for basic health statistics (CDC, 2015). The 11th revision of the ICD, along with its clinical modification (*ICD-11-CM*), is scheduled for release in 2017. The current ICD-1-CM classifies cerebrovascular disorders chiefly as TIA, cerebral ischemic stroke, intercerebral hemorrhage (ICH), and subarachnoid hemorrhage (SAH).

The WHO definition of stroke is a "rapidly developing clinical signs of focal (or global) disturbance of cerebral function, with symptoms lasting 24 hours or longer or leading to death, with no apparent cause other than of vascular origin" (Aho et al., 1980, p. 114). By comparing this definition to TIA, which is defined as lasting less than 24 hours, patients with stroke symptoms caused by subdural hemorrhage, tumors, poisoning, or trauma are excluded. This definition, first introduced in 1970, is still found in the WHO website.

■ UPDATED DEFINITION OF STROKE FOR THE 21ST CENTURY

"An Updated Definition of Stroke for the 21st Century: A Statement for Healthcare Professionals from the American Heart Association/American Stroke Association" (Sacco et al., 2013) incorporates 21st century science and knowledge amassed from research and technological advances in diagnostic imaging. The following is the 2013 definition of stroke from AHA/ASA (Sacco et al., 2013, p. 2066). The reader is directed to this 2013 document for more detailed information about the subtypes of stroke included in the new definition. The term *stroke* is broadly defined to include all of the following:

Definition of central nervous system (CNS) infarction: CNS infarction is brain, spinal cord, or retinal cell death attributable to ischemia based on the following:

1. Pathological, imaging, or other objective evidence of cerebral, spinal cord, or retinal focal ischemic injury in a defined vascular distribution; or
2. Clinical evidence of cerebral, spinal cord, or retinal focal ischemic injury based on symptoms persisting $\geq$24 hours or until death, and other etiologies excluded. (Note: CNS infarction includes hemorrhagic infarctions, types I and II.)

Definition of ischemic stroke: An episode of neurological dysfunction caused by focal cerebral, spinal, or retinal infarction. (Note: Evidence of CNS infarction is defined above.)

Definition of silent CNS infarction: Imaging or neuropathological evidence of CNS infarction, without a history of acute neurological dysfunction attributable to the lesion.

Definition of intracerebral hemorrhage: A focal collection of blood within the brain parenchyma or ventricular system that is not caused by trauma. (Note: Intracerebral hemorrhage includes parenchymal hemorrhages after CNS infarction, types I and II.)

Definition of stroke caused by intracerebral hemorrhage: Rapidly developing clinical signs of neurological dysfunction attributable to a focal collection of blood within the brain parenchyma or ventricular system that is not caused by trauma.

Definition of silent cerebral hemorrhage: A focal collection of chronic blood products within the brain parenchyma, subarachnoid space, or ventricular system on neuroimaging or neuropathological examination that is not caused by trauma and without a history of acute neurological dysfunction attributable to the lesion.

Definition of subarachnoid hemorrhage: Bleeding into the subarachnoid space (the space between the arachnoid membrane and the pia mater of the brain or spinal cord).

Definition of stroke caused by subarachnoid hemorrhage: Rapidly developing signs of neurological dysfunction and/or headache because of bleeding into the subarachnoid space (the space between the arachnoid membrane and the pia mater of the brain or spinal cord), which is not caused by trauma.

Definition of stroke caused by cerebral venous thrombosis: Infarction or hemorrhage in the brain, spinal cord, or retina because of thrombosis of a cerebral venous structure. Symptoms or signs caused by reversible edema without infarction or hemorrhage do not qualify as stroke.

Definition of stroke, not otherwise specified: An episode of acute neurological dysfunction presumed to be caused by ischemia or hemorrhage, persisting ≥24 hours or until death, but without sufficient evidence to be classified as one of the above.

▇▇ IMPLICATIONS OF THE UPDATED DEFINITIONS FOR STROKE

The updated definition of stroke is congruent with the science, technology, and knowledge of the 21st century as of 2013. As science, technology, and clinical knowledge continue to develop, there will no doubt be revisions to this definition in the future. But for now, the updated definitions have implications in the areas of clinical practice, education, research, and health policy.

Clinical Practice

In clinical practice, the focus for any type of acute stroke syndromes continues to be on rapid clinical and diagnostic assessment/evaluation and rapid treatment. Because stroke is a heterogeneous diagnosis, the clinician must rapidly sort through ischemic versus hemorrhagic etiology as well as the specific form of ischemic or hemorrhagic origin of the problem in order to select the appropriate treatment plan. Time is critical to preserve cerebral tissue as well as to reverse ischemia in potentially salvable tissue. Contemporary imaging techniques have provided a cadre of diagnostic tools that not only help to differentiate stroke mimics from stroke but also provide anatomic, temporal, and other characteristics about ischemia and pathophysiological responses to a stroke event. Computed tomography (CT) scans can quickly differentiate a hemorrhagic stroke from an ischemic stroke. A magnetic resonance imaging (MRI) scan is useful to differentiate stroke mimics such as migraines and brain tumors from ischemic and hemorrhagic stroke. Special techniques such as an MRI diffusion-weighted imaging (DWI) provide information about the timeline of the stroke which highlights tissue changes from minutes to days (Furlan, Marchal, Viader, Derlon, & Baron, 1996; Olivot & Albers, 2010). Multimagnetic resonance angiography, DWI, fluid attenuated inversion recovery (FLAIR), and perfusion-weighted MRI are useful diagnostics to detect "mismatch" areas which identify areas of potentially reversible ischemia known as the *penumbra*. Doppler imaging of the blood vessels in the neck and other vascular imaging procedures provide information about patency and structure of cerebral vessels (Chalela et al., 2007). A detailed discussion of diagnostics is found in Chapter 5, Diagnostic Testing in Stroke.

Diagnostics also create gray areas for clinicians to consider. For example, what should be done when small infarcts or microhemorrhagic areas are noted on a scan without the presence of clinical signs or symptoms in the patient? These areas are currently identified as *silent* areas but can also be considered markers of cerebrovascular disease, albeit noted in an asymptomatic patient. The current recommendation is that the patient should be followed, assessed, and managed for vascular risk factors as strategies for stroke prevention (Sacco et al., 2013).

The rapid development of science, technology, and clinical knowledge about stroke and research has provided the evidence from professional organizations such as AHA and ASA to develop clinical practice evidence-based guidelines to promulgate best practice for stroke patients. Clinical facilities have used the guidelines to develop their own algorithms and protocols to guide the care and management of the stroke patients that they serve. Clinicians must understand the methodological developmental process for guidelines in order to be informed consumers of guidelines. For example, questions to be answered include the following: "What is the strength of the evidence used to develop the guidelines?" "Are the guideline based on evidence or consensus?" and "How is bias addressed in the process of guidelines development?" There are models available to evaluate guidelines which should be used to determine the strength and quality of guidelines.

Education

The updated definition of stroke is a major change reflective of current science, technology, and knowledge with significant implications for practice, research, and health policy. How are all clinicians who care for stroke patients informed of changing best practices regardless if they practice in urban and rural settings or academic or non-academic centers? It is well known that change is a complex process that takes time. The usual routes for dissemination of professional information are publications, presentations, conferences, clinical practice guidelines, and other forms of educational methods such as webinars. However, to change practice in any setting, it takes change agents and champions to lead the change process. Leadership from professional organizations can help to promote dissemination of information and translation into practice to improve the outcomes for stroke patients through recommended effective strategies.

Research

Clear and consistent definitions of stroke, its subtypes, TIAs, and silent infarctions are critical for the interpretation of data from clinical trials, administrative stroke databases, and epidemiology in defining populations (Sacco et al., 2013). Operational definitions clarify variable attributes and suggest measurement criteria for variables and how the data can be recorded. The updates definition refocuses the former interest in time of development of symptoms to one of brain imaging tissue–based characteristics of ischemia and markers. The focus on brain imaging also influences the design of clinical investigations. For example, an appreciation of silent markers of asymptomatic cerebral infarction or microhemorrhagic areas noted on cerebral imaging broadens the scope of types of investigations to include prevention and longitudinal outcomes over multiple time points. Both documented strokes and asymptomatic silent markers provide opportunity for primary and secondary preventive strategies to be tested (Furie et al., 2011). The updated definitions of stroke have significant impact on stroke research for the future.

Health Policy

The change in the definition of stroke expands the scope of inclusion in the category of stroke. As a result, the disease prevalence will increase, but the mortality rate will most likely fall because milder forms of stroke will be included. When a definition of a disease is updated, the time of the definition change must be clearly noted for tracking of the disease over time for accurate interpretation of data and trends (Teutsch, 2010). With the updating of the definition of stroke, it will result in reclassification of stroke cases in incidence, prevalence, and mortality. In addition, the new definition has implications for public health, including surveillance and reporting, national and international statistics, disease classification coding systems, and existing health surveys (Sacco et al., 2013, p. 2081). Data collected through surveillance and registries will be different with the updated definition. This change will need to be taken in account when databases are mined for elucidating of trends and making projections for the future. This will also be an important consideration for researchers.

In summary, the updated definitions of stroke have a profound impact and ramifications for practice, education, research, and health policy especially how prevalence, incidence, and mortality are calculated and interpreted. It will be important to bear in mind when the redefinitions occurred and when it was incorporated into practice, education, research, and health policy arenas.

⬛ STROKE BURDEN AND SURVEILLANCE

Stroke Burden

The word *burden* means bearing of a heavy load. The concept of burden has been applied to multiple dimensions of health care at both the individual and population level such as treatment, family, disease, and economic burdens. Disease burden include incidence (yearly rate of onset, age of onset) and prevalence (the portion of the population found to have a condition). *Treatment burden* has been defined as "the self-care practices that patients with chronic illness must perform to respond to the requirements of their healthcare providers, as well as the impact that these practices have on patient functioning and well-being" (Gallacher et al., 2013, p. 1). As the level of treatment burden increases, patients may find it more difficult to adhere to the treatment plan, which can lead to poorer outcomes. The added "workload" of illness places demands on the patient's time and energy for activities such as medical appointments, diagnostic testing, and taking medications as well as self-care aspects of self-monitoring (e.g., blood pressure, blood glucose), dietary modifications, and exercise (Gallacher et al., 2013). Care is complex and multidimensional especially in chronic illness management, and burden is an integral part of the trajectory.

Almost half of stroke survivors have residual deficits including weakness or cognitive dysfunction 6 months after a stroke (Kelly-Hayes et al., 2003). The *impact* of the *workload* on the patient and family affects the patient's behavior and cognitive, physical, and psychological well-being (Eton et al., 2012; Shippee, Shah, May, Mair, & Mantori, 2009). Patients respond in different ways to what may appear as a similar burden to the outside observer so that a patient-centered approach is needed to appreciate the individual response, impact, and needs of each patient. With a chronic illness of a family member, the added burden on the family for caregiving, assistance with both activities of daily living (ADLs) as well as instrumental ADLs, redistribution of roles and responsibilities, and financial impact, the burden of a disease entity such as stroke is great. Treatment burden can also be viewed at the population level of the impact for needed health care and treatment on the health care resources at the local, national, or international level. The true impact of stroke must be viewed not only in terms of incidence and mortality rates but also from the lens of disability. Disability often persists for a long time and sometimes permanently after stroke (Norrving & Kissela, 2013).

Disease burden is the impact of a health problem and can be measured in terms of mortality, morbidity, treatment burden, economic burden, and other indicators. It is often quantified in terms of quality-adjusted life years (QALYs) or disability-adjusted life years (DALYs), both of which quantify the number of years lost due to disease. One DALY can be thought of as 1 year of healthy life lost, and the overall disease burden can be thought of as a measure of the gap between current health status and the ideal health status where the individual lives to old age and is free from disease and disability (Prüss-Üstün & Corvalán, 2006).

The *Global Burden of Diseases, Injuries, and Risk Factors Study* (GBD), published in 2010, reported that stroke was the second most common cause of death and the third most common cause of DALYs worldwide (Lozano et al., 2012). The study reported that although stroke mortality rates and mortality-to-incidence ratios have decreased in the past two decades, the global burden of stroke from a perspective of the absolute number of people affected every year, stroke survivors, related deaths, and DALYs lost are great and increasing, with most of the burden in low-income and middle-income countries. The investigators also reported that if these trends in stroke incidence, mortality, and DALYs continue, by 2030, there will be almost 12 million stroke deaths, 70 million stroke survivors, and more than 200 million DALYs lost globally as a result of stroke (Feigin et al., 2013). The human, health care resources, and economic burden of stroke is significant, but the projections for the future global burden are staggering and fall short of available health care resources.

Surveillance

From the perspective of public health, *surveillance* is the ongoing systematic collection, analysis, and interpretation of data, closely integrated with the timely dissemination of these data to those responsible for preventing and controlling disease and injury (Thacker & Berkelman, 1988). Public health surveillance is a tool to estimate the health status and behavior of the populations served by state agencies, federal health agencies, and ministries of health. Surveillance can directly measure actual activity in areas of interest within a population. It is, therefore, useful to measure both the need for interventions and the effects of interventions. The purpose of surveillance is to provide information to empower decision makers to make informed decisions. According to Mukherjee and Patil (2011), effective surveillance systems are most helpful when the health concern of interest is both a major public health problem and one that is thought to be preventable or modifiable.

At a basic level, all stroke surveillance systems should include data about incidence, case fatality, and mortality. More advanced systems include data on modalities of treatment, pre- and poststroke functional activity, categories of stroke, use of resources, access to care, and cost (Mukherjee & Patil, 2011). Unfortunately, even simple measures are not collected by many regions and countries, resulting in voids in data. In addition, storage of collected data may be an obstacle because of the lack of relational databases so that one database cannot be integrated with other databases. In creating stroke registries or other databases, it is important to have established common standards to address storage and integration of data for use at the population level. Need for surveillance and registries are critical for accurate data and data mining for research. Careful consideration of variables including how they are defined, operationalized, measured, and recorded is needed for standardization that will be useful for comparisons. Methods for extraction of clinical data from registries and combining those data with information-rich population data in a unified data stream are goals for the future. The AHA's *Get With The Guidelines* database is an ongoing, continuous quality improvement program that collects concurrent and retrospective patient-level adherence data within U.S. hospitals. The *Get With The Guidelines* database measures hospitals' adherence to secondary prevention guidelines (pharmacological and lifestyle interventions) for coronary artery disease, heart failure, and stroke (AHA, 2014). The contributions of data from facilities throughout the United States have made this a unique database for investigation of quality and quality improvement.

In summary, the burden of stroke can be considered at the individual and population level as well local, national, or global level. It is clear that stroke will continue to be a major health problem around the globe for the foreseeable future. Surveillance data are critical for monitoring population shifts and forecasting trends. As noted earlier, effective surveillance systems are most helpful when the health concern of interest is both a major public health problem and one that is thought to be preventable or modifiable. Stroke, in many cases, is preventable and modifiable. Efforts at prevention interventions to reduce the burden of stroke are being addressed.

PREVENTION OF STROKE

Prevention is classified into primary prevention and secondary prevention. Primary prevention of stroke and TIAs is directed at prevention of a first-time stroke. Secondary prevention of stroke and TIAs is directed at prevention of another stroke in persons who have had a stroke or who are experiencing TIAs. Both primary and secondary prevention will be addressed from the population and individual level and role of the interprofessional team.

From a global perspective, the INTERSTROKE study published in 2010 (O'Donnell et al., 2010) investigated risk factors for first-time acute stroke (e.g., all types of stroke) in 22 countries to set an agenda for targeted improvement. The five risk factors identified that contributed 80% to stroke risk were hypertension, smoking, waist-to-hip ratio, diet, and physical activity. Another 10% of stroke risk was due to diabetes mellitus, alcohol abuse, psychosocial factors (e.g., stress, depression), cardiac causes (i.e., atrial fibrillation, previous myocardial infarction, valvular heart disease), and ratio of apolipoprotein B to apolipoprotein A1 (O'Donnell et al., 2010). The response of the WHO was to propose five key components for stroke care that included the following: (1) primary care assessment and management of cardiovascular risk and TIA, (2) secondary prevention strategies, (3) education of the public and health care providers about stroke prevention and management, (4) access to stroke care and rehabilitation services, and (5) community and family support for patients with stroke and their caregivers (Mendis, 2010). In addition, the WHO has suggested a stepwise approach to stroke surveillance using standardized tools for data collection as a means to monitor progress (Norrving & Kissela, 2013). The INTERSTROKE study and the initiatives of the WHO applied to all forms of strokes.

Recent reports also indicate that in the last 40 years, there has been a shift in rates of stroke around the globe from the economically developed nations to the low- and middle-income countries. The rate of stroke has declined in the economically developed nations, whereas the rate has increased in the low- to middle-income countries.

In addition, the rates of disability and mortality are about 10 times greater in medically underserved regions compared to the most developed countries due to a lack of services and other resources to treat the continuum of stroke needs (Norrving & Kissela, 2013). Many organizations are developing public health approaches to address the maldistribution of stroke services directed at decreasing stroke rates and improving patient outcomes for stroke patients. A combination of preventive measures, access to care, and treatment resources are being addressed comprehensively.

Moving from a global focus to a U.S. focus for stroke prevention, AHA/ASA have taken the lead in the development of evidence-based clinical practice guidelines for stroke including the prevention of stroke. Because of the complexity of the processes of developing guidelines and the needed resources, some organizations such as AHA and ASA are collaborating to support the development of high-quality guidelines. In addition, other organizations provide endorsements of published guidelines, further adding to the credibility of the product.

In order to help health professionals and others to determine quality of guidelines, rating systems have been established to rate the strength and quality of the evidence used in writing guidelines. There are a number of tools available to rate the strength of evidence. For example, AHA/ASA uses a two-dimensional classification system, which includes an estimate of certainty of treatment effect and size of treatment effect (**Table 1-1**). This is the criteria that AHA/ASA expert panels employ in the evaluation of evidence when developing guidelines. Other organizations employ other grading systems. In most instances, a description of the scope and methodology used in the development of the guidelines is provided, which includes a description of the search

TABLE 1-1 Definition of Classes and Levels of Evidence Used in American Heart Association Stroke Council Recommendations

Class of Evidence for Treatment Effect

- **Class I**: Conditions for which there is evidence for and/or general agreement that the procedure or treatment is useful and effective
- **Class II**: Conditions for which there is conflicting evidence and/or a divergence of opinion about the usefulness/efficacy of a procedure or treatment
- **Class IIa**: The weight of evidence or opinion is in favor of the procedure or treatment.
- **Class IIb**: Usefulness/efficacy is less well established by evidence or opinion.
- **Class III**: Conditions for which there is evidence and/or general agreement that the procedure or treatment is not useful/effective and in some cases may be harmful

Therapeutic Recommendations

- **Level of Evidence A**: Data derived from multiple randomized clinical trials or meta-analyses
- **Level of Evidence B**: Data derived from a single randomized trial or nonrandomized studies
- **Level of Evidence C**: Consensus opinion of experts, case studies, or standard of care

Diagnostic Recommendations

- **Level of Evidence A**: Data derived from multiple prospective cohort studies using a reference standard applied by a masked evaluator
- **Level of Evidence B**: Data derived from a single grade A study, one case-control study, or studies using a reference standard applied by an unmasked evaluator
- **Level of Evidence C**: Consensus opinion of experts

strategy used for the literature review (e.g., inclusion/exclusion criteria, time period of literature included, types of studies included), internal peer review process, qualifications of the expert panel members, and any potential conflict of interest that would suggest bias of any panel member. The reader can then better judge the rigor of the process and credibility of the guidelines.

In reviewing guidelines, it is noted that often, a guideline is an update to a previously published guideline on the same topic, with recent guidelines reflective of new credible evidence and knowledge that is changing stroke care. In addition, a guideline introduction will report the inclusion dates of the literature reviewed and included in the development of the guidelines. For example, a guideline published in 2014 may include literature published only through 2012. The lag time is due to the process of reviewing, grading, and integrating evidence into the final guidelines and the rigorous internal peer review process of the final document before a guideline is approved and released for publication and circulation. In the current environment of continuous and rapid addition of new studies and knowledge being made available, keeping guidelines current for application to practice and care is an arduous responsibility for both sponsoring organizations that produce the guidelines as well as the individual practitioner who updates and sets standards for practice and care at the local level. Evidence-based national guidelines published by credible sources set a national standard for quality care. Monitoring achievement of nationally accepted, evidence-based guidelines on a population-based level is recommended as a basis for improving health promotion behaviors and reducing stroke health care disparities among high-risk groups (Kernan et al., 2014).

Primary Prevention

Primary prevention is addressed both at the population and individual level. At the population level, health policy drives strategies for prevention of stroke. Because stroke is ranked as the fourth major health problem in the United States, it receives attention at the national level. *Healthy People 2020* has set a national goal to "improve cardiovascular health and quality of life through prevention, detection, and treatment of risk factors for heart attack and stroke; early identification and treatment of heart attacks and strokes; and prevention of repeat cardiovascular events" (U.S. Department of Health and Human Services [USDHHS], 2010, para. 1). The monitoring of leading indicators related to this goal provides information of progress made. In addition to surveillance programs and registries that help to understand the problem at a population level, education of the general public about the nature of stroke, risk factors, warning signs and symptoms, and prevention is a major initiative. A variety of media are used to educate the general public about stroke and risk factors, including television, websites, billboards, health fairs, pamphlets, mass media exposures, and social media.

Primary prevention of stroke is also a major focus on the individual level as part of patient-centered primary care. The most recent evidence-based primary prevention guideline for stroke was published in 2014 by the AHA/ASA (Meschia et al., 2014). The previous guidelines published in 2006 and 2011 (Goldstein et al., 2006; Goldstein et al., 2011) focused on ischemic stroke (2006); and the 2011 guidelines added hemorrhagic stroke. The 2014 guidelines serve as a national standard for primary stroke prevention. In discussing these guidelines in this chapter, other pertinent evidence-based guidelines related to stroke prevention (James et al., 2014) are included. The aim of the 2014 guidelines is to provide comprehensive and timely evidence-based recommendations to prevent stroke in individuals who have not previously had a stroke or transient ischemic attack (Meschia et al., 2014). The updates include recommendations for the control of risk factors, interventional approaches to atherosclerotic disease of the cervicocephaic circulation, and prevention of thrombotic and thromboembolic stroke with the use of antithrombotic therapies. In addition, genetics and pharmacogenetic testing and the prevention of stroke in a variety of other specific conditions, including sickle cell disease and patent foramen ovale, are addressed (Meschia et al., 2014).

The 2011 guidelines approached risk of stroke from a classification of potential for modification of risk (i.e., nonmodifiable, modifiable, and potentially modifiable) (Goldstein et al., 2011). This classification of risk factors modification is discussed in the next section. The 2014 guidelines go a step further and recommend the use of a risk assessment tool such as the AHA/ACC CV Risk Calculator (http://my.americanheart.org/cvriskcalculator) to identify individuals who could benefit from therapeutic interventions and who may not be treated on the basis of any single risk factor (Meschia et al., 2014). This calculator is addressed below. Primary prevention is integral to the goals, focus, and responsibilities of all members of the interprofessional team through population health education about stroke including risk factors. Primary prevention strategies also included the application of interventions to address risk factors identified in individuals to prevent ischemic and hemorrhagic strokes and subarachnoid hemorrhage.

Risk Factor Modification

The various risk factors for stroke are included in **Table 1-2** according to nonmodifiable and modifiable risk factors with well-documented evidence and those that are potentially modifiable with less evidence to currently support its inclusion as a risk factor. The recommendations for addressing *modifiable risk factors* are found in **Table 1-3** and are based on the "Guidelines for the Primary Prevention of Stroke" (Meschia et al., 2014) and other related and pertinent evidence-based guidelines. Many of the recommendations are based on well-designed randomized controlled trials considered the gold standard for determination of efficacy and effectiveness of treatments. The sources of

---

TABLE 1-2 Risk Factors for Stroke Based on Modification and Strength of Evidence

Nonmodifiable Risk Factors	Modifiable Risk Factors, Well Documented	Potentially Modifiable
• Age	• Hypertension	• Metabolic syndrome
• Gender	• Exposure to cigarette smoke	• Excessive alcohol consumption
• Low birth weight	• Diabetes mellitus	• Drug abuse
• Race/ethnicity	• Atrial fibrillation and certain other cardiac conditions	• Oral contraceptives
• Genetic predisposition	• Dyslipidemia	• Sleep breathing disorders
	• Carotid artery stenosis	• Migraine headaches
	• Sickle cell disease	• Hyperhomocysteinemia
	• Postmenopausal hormone therapy	• Elevated lipoprotein(a)
	• Poor diet	• Hypercoagulability
	• Physical inactivity	• Inflammation
	• Obesity and body fat distribution	• Infection

Goldstein, L. B., Bushnell, C. D., Adams, R. J., Appel, L. J., Braun, L. T., Chaturvedi, S., . . . Pearson, T. A. (2011). Guidelines for the primary prevention of stroke: A guideline for healthcare professionals from the American Heart Association/American Stroke Association. *Stroke, 42*, 517–584.

TABLE 1-3 Modifiable Risk Factors with Recommendations for Both Primary and Secondary Prevention of Stroke in Patients with Stroke or Transient Ischemic Attacks

Modifiable Risk Factor	Recommendations for Primary Prevention of Stroke	Source of Recommendation (PP = Primary Prevention; SP = Secondary Prevention)	Recommendations for Secondary Prevention of Stroke in Patients with Stroke or Transient Ischemic Attacks (TIAs)
Hypertension	• In the general population, regular blood pressure (BP) screening and appropriate treatment of patients with hypertension, including lifestyle modification and pharmacological therapy are recommended. • Annual screening for high BP and health-promoting lifestyle modification are recommended for patients with pre-hypertesnsion (SBP of 120 to 139 mm Hg or DBP of 80 to 89 mm Hg). • Patients with hypertension should be treated with antihypertensive drugs to a target of BP of <140/90 mm Hg. • Reduction of BP is considered more important in reducing stroke risk than the choice of a specific agent, and treatment. And treatment should be individualized for the patient based on patient characteristics and medication tolerance. • Control of BP in accordance with an AHA/ACC/CDC Advisory to a target of <140/90 mm Hg is recommended in patients with type 1 or type 2 diabetes mellitus. • In the black hypertensive population, including those with diabetes, a calcium channel blocker or thiazide-type diuretic is recommended as initial therapy. • There is moderate evidence to support initial or add-on antihypertensive therapy with an angiotensin-converting enzyme inhibitor or angiotensin receptor blocker in persons with CKD to improve kidney outcomes (James et al., 2014).	**PP:** James et al., 2014; JNC 8 guidelines; Meschia et al., 2014 **SP:** Kernan et al., 2014	• BP reduction is recommended for previously untreated persons with an ischemic stroke or TIA who, after the first several days, have an established BP ≥140 mm Hg systolic or ≥90 mm Hg diastolic. • For previously treated persons with known hypertension, resumption of BP treatment for prevention of recurrent stroke and other vascular events in persons who have had an ischemic stroke or TIA and are beyond the first several days is recommended. • For patients with a recent lacunar stroke, it might be reasonable to target an SBP of <130 mm Hg. • An absolute target BP level and reduction is uncertain and should be individualized, but it is reasonable to use ≤140 mm Hg systolic and ≤90 mm Hg diastolic as targets (Kernan et al., 2014). • Lifestyle modifications have been associated with BP reduction. They include salt restriction; weight loss; consumption of a diet rich in fruits, vegetables, and low-fat dairy products; regular aerobic physical activity; and limited alcohol consumption. • The choice of specific drugs and targets should be individualized based on pharmacological properties and specific patient characteristics and comorbidities. • In diabetic patients, following existing guidelines for glycemic control and blood pressure targets in patients with diabetes is recommended.

Dyslipidemia

- In addition to theraputic lifestyle changes, treatment with HMG-coenzyme-A reductase inhibitors (statin) drugs is recommended for primary prevention of ischemic stroke in pateints estimated to have a high 10-year risk for cardiovascular events as recommended in the 2013 *ACC/AHA Guidelines for Treatment of Blood Cholesterol to Reduce Atherosclerotic Cardiovascular Risk in Adults* (Stone et al., 2013).
- Treatment of adults with diabetes mellitus with a statin, especially those with additional risk factors, is recommended to lower the risk of first stroke.

PP: Meschia et al., 2014; Stone et al., 2013
SP: Stone et al., 2013; Kernan et al., 2014

- The 2013 guidelines for the treatment of blood cholesterol (Stone et al., 2013) recommend statin therapy for people with a history of a cardiovascular event (heart attack, stroke, stable or unstable angina, peripheral artery disease, TIA, or coronary or other arterial revascularization).
- Statin therapy with intensive lipid-lowering effects is recommended to reduce risk of stroke and cardiovascular events among patients with ischemic stroke or TIA who have evidence of atherosclerosis, an LDL-C level ≥100 mg/dL, and who are with or without evidence of ASCVD (Kernan et al., 2014).
- Statin therapy with intensive lipid-lowering effects is recommended to reduce risk of stroke and cardiovascular events among patients with ischemic stroke or TIA presumed to be of atherosclerotic origin, LDL-C level <100 mg/dL, and no evidence for other clinical ASCVD.
- Patients with ischemic stroke or TIA with elevated cholesterol or comorbid coronary artery disease should be otherwise managed according to ACC/AHA 2013 guidelines, which include lifestyle modification, dietary recommendations, and medication recommendations (Grundy et al., 2004; Kernan et al., 2014).

Cigarette smoking

- Counseling, in combination with drug therapy using nicotine replacement, bupropion, or varenicline, is recommended for active smokers to assist in quitting smoking.
- Based on strong evidence of a relationship between smoking and ischemic stroke and SAH, abstention from cigarette smoking is recommended for patients who have never smoked.

PP: Meschia et al., 2014
SP: Furie et al., 2011

- A strong "stop smoking" message should be sent to any smoker.
- Counseling should be provided, as necessary.

(continued)

15

TABLE 1-3 Modifiable Risk Factors with Recommendations for Both Primary and Secondary Prevention of Stroke in Patients with Stroke or Transient Ischemic Attacks *(continued)*

Modifiable Risk Factor	Recommendations for Primary Prevention of Stroke	Source of Recommendation (PP = Primary Prevention; SP = Secondary Prevention)	Recommendations for Secondary Prevention of Stroke in Patients with Stroke or Transient Ischemic Attacks (TIAs)
Diabetes mellitus	• Control of BP in accordance with an AHA/ACC/CDC Advisory to a target of <140/90 mm Hg is recommended in patients with type 1 or type 2 diabetes mellitus. • For adults with diabetes mellitus, treatment with a statin, especially those with additional risk factors, is recommended to lower the risk of first stroke. • The usefulness of aspirin for primary stroke prevention for patients with diabetes mellitus but low 10-year risk of CVD is unclear.	**PP:** James et al., 2014; Meschia et al., 2014 **SP:** Kernan et al., 2014	• After a TIA or ischemic stroke, all patients should be screened for diabetes mellitus (HbA_{1c} is probably best choice). • Following existing guidelines for glycemic control in patients with diabetics who have had a stroke or TIAs is recommended. • BP targets for stroke or TIA patients with diabetes mellitus were not specifically addressed in 2014 guidelines. The American Diabetic Association recommends a goal of <140 mm Hg for SBP and <80 mm Hg for DBP but accepts that lower goals may be appropriate for selected individuals, such as young patients who tolerate the lower readings (Kernan et al., 2014).
Atrial fibrillation	• CHA_2DS_2-VASc score* is recommended to assess stroke risk (see below for description of score) and replaces the $CHADS_2$ score. • For patients with valvular AF at high risk for stroke, defined as a CHA_2DS_2-VASc score of ≥2 and acceptably low risk for hemorrhagic complications, long term oral anticoagulant therapy with warfarin at a target INR of 2.0 to 3.0 is recommended. • For patients with nonvalvular AF, a CHA_2DS_2-VASc score of ≥2, and acceptably low risk for hemorrhagic complications, oral anticoagulants are recommended with options which include warfarin (INR, 2.0 to 3.0), dabigatran, apixaban and rivaroxaban. • The selection of antithrombotic agent should be individualized on the basis of patient risk factors (particularly risk for intracranial hemorrhage), cost, tolerability, patient preference, potential or drug interactions, and other clinical characteristics, including the time that it takes for the INR to be in a therapeutic range for patients taking warfarin.	**PP:** January et al., 2014; Meschia et al., 2014 **SP:** Kernan et al., 2014; Culebras, Messe, Chaturvedi, Kase, & Gronseth, 2014	• For prevention of recurrent stroke in patients with nonvalvular AF, whether paroxysmal (intermittent) or permanent, anticoagulation with a vitamin K antagonist, apixaban, or dabigatran are recommended (Kernan et al., 2014). • For patients with ischemic stroke or TIA along with AF unable to take oral anticoagulants, aspirin alone is recommended. • The combination of clopidogrel plus aspirin therapy, compared to aspirin alone, might be reasonable. • For most patients with a stroke or TIA along with AF, the initiation or oral anticoagulation within 14 days after the onset of neurological symptoms is reasonable. • In patients at high risk for hemorrhagic conversion of an ischemic stroke, it is reasonable to delay initiation of oral anticoagulation beyond 24 days.

| Other cardiac conditions (MI and thrombus, cardiomyopathy, valvular heart disease, prosthetic heart valve) | • Statins are useful for primary and secondary prevention of ASCVD in higher risk patients.
• ACC/AHA practice guidelines providing strategies to reduce the risk of stroke in patients with a variety of cardiac conditions including valvular heart disease, unstable angina, chronic stable angina, and acute MI are endorsed. See guidelines.
• Anticoagulation is indicated in patients with mitral stenosis and a prior embolic event, even in sinus rhythm.
• Anticoagulation is indicated in patients with mitral stenosis and left atrial thrombus.
• Warfarin (INR target, 2.0–3.0) and low-dose aspirin are indicated after aortic valve replacement with bileaflet mechanical or current-generation, single-tilting-disk prostheses in patients with no risk factors; warfarin (INR target 2.5–3.5) and low-dose aspirin are indicated in patients with mechanical aortic valve replacement and risk factors; and warfarin (INR target 2.5–3.5) and low-dose aspirin are indicated after mitral valve replacement with any mechanical valve.
• Surgical excision is recommended for the treatment of atrial myxomas.
• Surgical intervention is recommended for symptomatic fibroelastomas and for fibroelastomas that are >1 cm or appear mobile, even if asymptomatic. | **PP and SP:** Antman et al., 2004; Fraker et al., 2007; Jneid et al., 2012; Nishimura et al. 2014
PP: Meschia et al., 2014
SP: Kernan et al., 2014 | • In patients with a stroke or TIAs *and* cardiac disease, treatment is more complex, and consideration of both problems must be factored into the treatment plan.
• Anticoagulants with a variety of drugs are recommended in some cases and not in others.
• Statins are useful for primary and secondary prevention of ASCVD in higher risk patients.
• Patients with stroke and cardiac disease should be managed by an interprofessional team with expertise in both areas of practice.
• ACC/AHA practice guidelines provide recommendations to reduce the risk of stroke in patients with a variety of cardiac conditions, including valvular heart disease, unstable angina, chronic stable angina, and acute MI. See specific guidelines. They also publish guidelines specific to the cardiac problem. |
| Asymptomatic carotid stenosis | • Patients with asymptomatic carotid artery stenosis should receive daily asprin and a statin.
• Recommendations for carotid endarterectomy in asymptomatic patients who have >70% stenosis of the internal carotid artery if the risk of perioperative stroke, myocardial infarction and death is low (<3%) may be considered although effectiveness compared to medical management is not clear.
• See Meschia et al. for further recommendations. | **PP:** Meschia et al., 2014
SP: Kernan et al., 2014 | • **Symptomatic extracranial carotid disease**
• Carotid angioplasty and stenting (CAS) is indicated as an alternative to CEA for symptomatic patients at average or low risk of complications associated with endovascular intervention when the diameter of the lumen of the internal carotid artery is reduced >70% as noted by noninvasive imaging, or >50% by catheter-based imaging, or noninvasive imaging with corroboration when the anticipated rate of periprocedural stroke or death is <6%. |

(continued)

TABLE 1-3 Modifiable Risk Factors with Recommendations for Both Primary and Secondary Prevention of Stroke in Patients with Stroke or Transient Ischemic Attacks *(continued)*

Modifiable Risk Factor	Recommendations for Primary Prevention of Stroke	Source of Recommendation (PP = Primary Prevention; SP = Secondary Prevention)	Recommendations for Secondary Prevention of Stroke in Patients with Stroke or Transient Ischemic Attacks (TIAs)
			• It is reasonable to consider patient's age in choosing between CAS and CEA. For older patients (i.e., older than ≈70 years of age), CEA may be associated with improved outcome compared with CAS, particularly when arterial anatomy is unfavorable for endovascular intervention. For younger patients, CAS is equivalent to CEA in terms of risk for periprocedural complication (i.e., stroke, MI, or death) and long-term risk for ipsilateral stroke. • See Kernan et al. (2014) for further specific recommendations.
Intracranial atherosclerosis	• Not specifically addressed.	**SP**: Kernan et al., 2014	• For patients with recent stroke or TIA (within 30 days) attributable to severe stenosis (70%–99%) of a major intracranial artery, the addition of clopidogrel 75 mg/day to aspirin for 90 days might be reasonable. • For patients with a stroke or TIA attributable to 50%–99% stenosis of a major intracranial artery, maintenance of SBP below 140 mm Hg and high-intensity statin therapy are recommended. • See Kernan et al. (2014) for further recommendations.
Postmenopausal hormone therapy	• The USPSTF recommends against the use of combined estrogen and progestin for the prevention of chronic conditions in postmenopausal women. • The USPSTF recommends against the use of estrogen for the prevention of chronic conditions in postmenopausal women who have had a hysterectomy.	**PP**: Bushnell et al., 2014; Goldstein et al., 2011; USPSTF, 2012 **SP**: Furie et al., 2011	• For women who have had an ischemic stroke or TIA, postmenopausal hormone therapy (with estrogen with or without a progestin) is not recommended.

Diet and nutrition	• Reduced intake of sodium and increased intake of potassium as indicated in the US Dietary Guidelines for Americans are recommended to lower BP.
	• A DASH-style diet, which emphasizes fruits, vegetables, and low-fat dairy products and reduced saturated fat, is recommended to lower BP.
	• A diet that is rich in fruits and vegetables and thereby high in potassium is beneficial and may lower the risk of stroke.
	• Reduce daily intake of sodium to <2,300 mg. In those 51 years of age and older and those of any age who are African American or who have hypertension, diabetes, or chronic kidney disease, reduced sodium intake to 1,500 mg/day is recommended to lower blood pressure.
	• Consume <10% of calories from saturated fatty acids and 300 mg/day of cholesterol.
	• If alcohol is consumed, up to one drink per day for women and two drinks per day for men is recommended.
		• Consume a dietary pattern that emphasizes intake of vegetables, fruits, and whole grains; includes low-fat dairy products, poultry, fish, legumes, no tropical vegetable oils and nuts; and limits intake of sweets, sugar-sweetened beverages, and red meats.
		  a. Adapt this dietary pattern to appropriate calorie requirements, personal and cultural food preferences, and nutrition therapy for other medical conditions (including diabetes).
		  b. Achieve this pattern by following plans such as the DASH dietary pattern, the USDA food pattern, or the AHA diet.
		• Aim for a dietary pattern that achieves 5%–6% of calories from saturated fat.
		• Reduce percent of calories from saturated fat.
		• Reduce percent of calories from *trans fats*.
		• In those 51 years of age and older and those of any age who are African American or who have hypertension, diabetes, or chronic kidney disease, reduced sodium intake to 1,500 mg/day is recommended to lower blood pressure.
		
		PP: Meschia et al., 2014; U.S. Department of Agriculture & U.S. Department of Health and Human Services (USDA & USDHHS), 2010
		SP: Eckel et al., 2014

Physical inactivity	• Healthy adults should perform at least moderate- to vigorous-intensity aerobic physical activity at least 40 min a day 3 to 4 d/wk.	• For patients with ischemic stroke or TIA who are capable of engaging in physical activity, at least 30 min of exercise, typically defined as vigorous activity sufficient to break a sweat or noticeably raise heart rate, 1–3 times a week (e.g., walking briskly, using an exercise bicycle) may be considered to reduce risk factors and comorbid conditions that increase the likelihood of recurrent stroke. • For persons with a disability following ischemic stroke, supervision by a health care professional, such as a physical therapist or cardiac rehabilitation professional, at least on initiation of an exercise regimen may be considered. **PP:** Meschia et al., 2014; USDA & HHS, 2010 **SP:** Furie et al., 2011

(continued)

19

TABLE 1-3 Modifiable Risk Factors with Recommendations for Both Primary and Secondary Prevention of Stroke in Patients with Stroke or Transient Ischemic Attacks (continued)

Modifiable Risk Factor	Recommendations for Primary Prevention of Stroke	Source of Recommendation (PP = Primary Prevention; SP = Secondary Prevention)	Recommendations for Secondary Prevention of Stroke in Patients with Stroke or Transient Ischemic Attacks (TIAs)

Obesity and body fat distribution	• Overweight and obesity have been defined.
	• Among overweight (BMI = 25 to 29 kg/m²) and obese (BMI >30 kg/m²) individuals, weight reduction is recommended for lowering BP.
	• Among overweight (BMI = 25 to 29 kg/m²) and obese (BMI >30 kg/m²) individuals, weight reduction is recommended for reducing the risk of stroke.
	• Advise overweight and obese adults that the greater the BMI, the greater the risk of CVD, type 2 diabetes, and all causes of mortality.
	• Counsel overweight and obese adults with cardiovascular risk factors that lifestyle changes that produce even modest, sustained weight loss of 3%–5% produce clinically meaningful health benefits, and greater weight losses produces greater benefits.
	• Prescribe a diet to achieve reduced calorie intake for obese or overweight individuals as part of a comprehensive lifestyle intervention. See specific recommendations based on patient characteristics and goals.
	• See specific recommendations for bariatric surgery and patient selection in secondary prevention column.
		PP: Jensen et al., 2013; Meschia et al., 2014
		
		SP: Jensen et al., 2013
			• Same information found in the primary prevention column applies to secondary prevention. In addition, there are recommendations for weight loss as listed below.
			• Prescribe a diet to achieve reduced calorie intake for obese or overweight individuals who would benefit from weight loss as part of a comprehensive lifestyle intervention. Any one of the following methods can be used to reduce food and calorie intake:
			  a. Prescribe 1,200–1,500 kcal/day for women and 1,500–1,800 kcal/day for men (kilocalorie levels are usually adjusted for the individual's body weight).
			  b. Prescribe a 500 kcal/day or 750 kcal/day energy deficit.
			  c. Prescribe one of the evidence-based diets that restricts certain food types (such as high-carbohydrate foods, low-fiber foods, or high-fat foods) in order to create an energy deficit by reduced food intake.
			• Prescribe a calorie-restricted diet, for obese and overweight individuals who would benefit from weight loss, based on the patient's preferences and health status and preferably refer to a nutritionist for counseling.
			• Advise overweight and obese individuals who would benefit from weight loss to participate for ≥6 months in a comprehensive lifestyle program that assists participants in adhering to a lower calorie diet and in increasing physical activity through the use of behavioral strategies.

- Prescribe on-site, high-intensity (i.e., ≥14 sessions in 6 months) comprehensive weight loss interventions provided in individual or group sessions by a trained interventionist.
- Advise adults with a BMI ≥40 kg/m^2 or BMI ≥35 kg/m^2 with obesity-related comorbid conditions who are motivated to lose weight and who have not responded to behavioral treatment with or without pharmacotherapy with sufficient weight loss to achieve targeted health outcome goals that bariatric surgery may be an appropriate option to improve health and offer referral to an experienced bariatric surgeon for consultation and evaluation.

*The **CHADS$_2$ score** is a clinical predictive rule for estimating the risk of a stroke in patients with nonrheumatic atrial fibrillation. The **CHA$_2$DS$_2$-VASc score** is a refinement of CHADS$_2$ score and extends the latter by including additional common stroke risk factors, as discussed below.

The maximum CHADS$_2$ score is 6, whereas the maximum CHA$_2$DS$_2$-VASc score is 9 (for age, either the patient is 75 years and older and gets 2 points, is between 65 and 74 years of age and gets 1 point, or is younger than 65 years of age and does not get points). Note that female gender only scores 1 point if the patient has at least one other risk factor and does not score any points in isolation.

CHA$_2$DS$_2$-VASc Score (Olesen et al., 2011)

	Description	Points
C	Congestive heart failure (or left ventricular systolic dysfunction)	1
T	Hypertension; blood pressure consistently above 140/90 mm Hg (or treated hypertension on medication)	1
A$_2$	Age 75 years and older	2
D	Diabetes mellitus	1
S$_2$	Prior stroke of TIA or thromboembolism	2
V	Vascular disease (e.g., peripheral artery disease, myocardial infarction, aortic plaque)	1
A	Age 65–74 years	1
Sc	Sex category (i.e., female sex)	1

Interpretation of Scores. A total score of 0, low risk; 1, moderate risk; and 2 or greater, high risk. Specific treatment recommendations are associated with each level of risk.

BF, blood pressure; SBP, systolic blood pressure; DBP, diastolic blood pressure; INR, international normalized ratio; MI, myocardial infarction; MRA, magnetic resonance angiography; USPSTF, U.S. Prevention and Services Task Force; DASH, dietary approaches to stop hypertension; BMI, body mass index; CVD, cardiovascular disease.

Note: This table focuses mostly on Class 1 and Levels of Evidence A and B recommendations from the AHA/ASA 2014 primary and secondary prevention guidelines; the reader is directed to these reports for a complete list of AHA/ASA recommendations. In addition, other pertinent prevention reports are cited in this table.

TABLE 1-4 Major Risk Factors for Intracerebral (Hemorrhagic) Stroke

Age and lifestyle	• Older age group especially with hypertension • Sedentary, overweight, smokers, and have diabetes mellitus • More common in men
Ethnicity	• All minorities including native Americans, Hispanics, and African Americans significantly higher risk • African Americans have twice the risk for first time ICH as Caucasians
Hypertension	• Major risk factor for ICH • Chronic hypertension is the most common cause of ICH.
Hyperlipidemia	• Vascular risk factor • Increases risk of atherosclerosis
Diabetes mellitus	• Vascular risk factor
Smoking	• Vascular risk factor • Smokers of a pack a day have 2.5 times greater risk of stroke than nonsmokers.
Medications	• Anticoagulants, antiplatelet agents, decongestants, antihypertensive medications, stimulants (including diet pills), and sympathomimetic drugs • Patient on warfarin must be carefully monitored for maintenance of therapeutic INR ranges.
Recent surgery	• Carotid endarterectomy or carotid stenting because of risk of hyperperfusion after such procedures
Dementia	• Associated with amyloid angiopathy
Alcohol or illicit drug use	• Excessive alcohol use • Cocaine, sympathomimetic drugs, and stimulants • Cocaine and methamphetamine are major factors for stroke in young people. • About 85%–90% of ICH in people in their 20s or 30s due to drug abuse
Coagulopathies	• Associated with liver disease, cancer • Hematological disorders including sickle cell anemia

INR, international normalized ratio.
Data from Morgenstern, L. B., Hemphill, J. C., III., Anderson, C., Becker, K., Broderick, J. P., Connolly, E. S., Jr., . . . Tamargo, R. J. (2010). Guidelines for the management of spontaneous intracerebral hemorrhage: A guideline for healthcare professionals from the American Heart Association/American Stroke Association. *Stroke, 41*, 2108–2129; Juvela, A., Hillbom, M., & Palomaki, H. (1995). Risk factors for spontaneous intracerebral hemorrhage. *Stroke, 26*, 1558–1564; National Stroke Association. (2009). *Hemorrhagic stroke fact sheet*. Retrieved from http://www.stroke.org

the recommendations are listed in the table. The reader can consult the references to determine the methodology followed to evaluate the strength of the evidence reviewed which formed the basis of the recommendations as well as review the full document and recommendations. In addition, **Table 1-4** lists the major risk factors for hemorrhagic stroke to further extract those risk factors most commonly associated with hemorrhagic stroke. SAH is most often related to the ruptured cerebral aneurysm. **Table 1-5** lists the SAH risk factors. Other causes are cerebral trauma and intracerebral hemorrhage stroke. SAH, including risk factors, is discussed in Chapter 8. Intracerebral hemorrhagic stroke is discussed in Chapter 7.

In addressing the *nonmodifiable risk factors*, a number of general recommendations are highlighted. They include the following:

● A three-generation family history to identify any risk factors should be included in a person's medical history.
● Referral for genetic testing counseling may be considered for patients with rare genetic causes of stroke for which the patient is at risk.
● Noninvasive screening for unruptured intracranial aneurysm in patient with two or more first-degree relatives with SAH might be considered.

TABLE 1-5 Major Risk Factors for Subarachnoid Hemorrhage

Presence of unruptured cerebral aneurysm	• The larger the aneurysm size, the more likely the aneurysm will rupture, resulting in SAH. • Aneurysms >7 mm are a significant risk factor for SAH. • Aneurysms <7 mm in size are a risk factor for SAH in patients with hypertension and/or smoking .
Age and lifestyle	• SAH incidence increases with age, with a majority of SAH cases occurring in adults over the age of 50 years. • Significant, stressful life events are associated with aneurysm rupture. • Use of sympathomimetic drugs is a risk factor for SAH. • High alcohol consumption is associated with SAH. • Consuming a diet rich in vegetables may lower the risk of SAH.
Gender	• SAH is more common in women than in men. • Incidence estimates 1.2 times higher in women than in men, although this number is declining from 1.6 times higher in women than in men between 1960 and 1994.
Ethnicity	• Higher incidence in African Americans and Hispanics compared to Caucasians
Hypertension	• Associated with aneurysm growth and SAH • Treatment of hypertension should be initiated to reduce the risk of SAH.
Smoking	• Smoking is associated with increased risk of SAH, regardless of age. • Risk of SAH will be equivalent of nonsmokers within 5 years of smoking cessation.

There are multiple *modifiable risk factors* supported by strong evidence for prevention and management. In **Table 1-3**, each modifiable risk factor is addressed, and the key recommendations related to stroke are briefly noted. The reader is referred to the "Guidelines for the Primary Prevention of Stroke" for the complete list of recommendations (Meschia et al., 2014).

There are also multiple *potentially modifiable risk factors* listed in **Table 1-2**. The reader is referred to "Guidelines for the Primary Prevention of Stroke" for a discussion of these factors (Meschia et al., 2014). The health provider must to be aware of these risk factors as applicable to a particular patient and consider these risk factors in the diagnostic workup and plan of care.

Cardiovascular Risk Calculation

The 2013 ACC/AHA Guideline on the Assessment of Cardiovascular Risk (Goff et al., 2014) is a new tool useful for estimating 10-year and lifetime risks for atherosclerotic cardiovascular disease (ASCVD), which is defined as coronary death or nonfatal myocardial infarction or fatal or nonfatal stroke. It is based on the Pooled Cohort Equations and the work of Lloyd-Jones et al. (2004, 2006). The information required to estimate ASCVD risk includes age, sex, race, total cholesterol, high-density lipoprotein cholesterol, systolic blood pressure, blood pressure–lowering medication use, diabetes status, and smoking status. A downloadable spreadsheet provides a means for the provider and patient to estimate 10-year and lifetime risk. The download is available as a companion to the "2013 ACC/AHA Guideline on the Assessment of Cardiovascular Risk" (Goff et al., 2014) at the AHA website.

The application of the estimates of 10-year risk for ASCVD to various race/ethnic groups is useful to take into account the nonmodifiable risk factor of race/ethnicity. The estimates are based on data from multiple community-based populations and are applicable to African American and non-Hispanic white men and women 40 through 79 years of age. For other ethnic groups, the recommendation is to use the equations for non-Hispanic whites, even though those estimates may underestimate the risk for persons from some race/ethnic groups, especially American Indians, some Asian Americans (e.g., south Asian ancestry), and some Hispanics (e.g., Puerto Ricans). The estimate may also overestimate the risk for other groups, including some Asian Americans (e.g., of East Asian ancestry) and some Hispanics (e.g., Mexican Americans). A calculation of risk higher than 7.5% is considered an elevated 10-year risk for ASCVD. Goff et al. (2014) noted that the use of the estimates of 10-year and lifetime risk is useful in primary care as a means of informing providers and patients of risk for ASCVD and for matching the intensity of preventive efforts with the individual's absolute risk. The 2013 guidelines for cholesterol (Stone et al., 2013) apply the ASCVD risk calculations model as a basis for their recommendations for management of cholesterol.

Gender-Specific Prevention Guidelines

According to the 2014 stroke statistics (Go et al., 2013), on a yearly basis, 55,000 more women than men have a stroke. Women have a higher lifetime risk of stroke than men. Among those 55 to 75 years of age, there is a one in five chance of stroke for women as compared to one in six for men. Part of the explanation for this difference is the fact that women live longer than men so that the lifetime risk of stroke in the 55- to 75-year age group is higher for women (20%) than for men (17%) (Seshadri et al., 2006). As a result, women are more likely to live alone as widows, more often institutionalized after stroke, and have a poorer recovery than men (Gall, Tran, Martin, Blizzard, & Srikanth, 2012; Gargano, Reeves, & Coverdell, 2007; Holroyd-Leduc, Kapral, Austin, & Tu, 2000; Kim, Lee, Roh, Ahn, & Hwang, 2010; Paolucci et al., 2006; Petrea et al., 2009; Roquer, Campello, & Gomis, 2003). These factors and others result in a greater burden from stroke for women as compared to men.

The "Guidelines for the Prevention of Stroke in Women" (Bushnell et al., 2014) is the first specific guideline ever published for primary prevention of stroke in women. The focus of this evidence-based guideline is stroke risk factors that are unique to women. This is important because of the differences in women that influence the impact of stroke such as genetic differences in immunity, coagulation factors, hormonal factors, reproductive factors (e.g., pregnancy, childbirth, menopause), and social factors (Bushnell et al., 2014). In addition, these guidelines provide more details specific to women than have been included in the current primary and secondary stroke prevention guidelines and cardiovascular prevention guidelines. However, the authors clearly note that other primary prevention guidelines should be consulted in conjunction with these guidelines in order to address both the gender-specific and general considerations that apply to all populations.

The major recommendations addressed in prevention of stroke in women (Bushnell et al., 2014) are listed in the following text. The reader is directed to the full guideline for further detailed information.

- Women with hypertension prepregnancy should be considered for low-dose aspirin and/or calcium supplement therapy to lower preeclampsia risks.
- Preeclampsia is a risk factor after pregnancy; other risk factors in these women such as smoking, high cholesterol, and obesity should be treated early.

- Depending on the level of high blood pressure in a pregnant woman, it is recommended that a blood pressure of 160/110 mm Hg or above should be treated. At 150 to 159 mm Hg/100 to 109 mm Hg, a decision to treat or not treat must be made.
- Before taking birth control pills, a woman should be screened for hypertension because of the increased risk with the combination of both risk factors.
- Women older than 75 years of age should be screened for atrial fibrillation (AF) because AF is a risk factor for stroke.

In summary, primary prevention is key to maintaining a healthy society. Authoritative guidelines help to promulgate the latest evidence from randomized controlled trials, meta-analysis, systematic reviews, and other forms of rigorous research for translation into evidence-based practice protocols. However, with the rapid development of new science and new knowledge, there is a constant need to update published guidelines. The rapid expansion of scientific knowledge related to stroke is changing how interprofessional team members practice and the treatment options available to patients. The overlap of risk factors for both cardiovascular disease and stroke is evident, so primary prevention strategies are not only beneficial for stroke but also for cardiovascular disease. For success with prevention on both fronts, the individual health care provider and patient must work together as partners. Healthy lifestyle changes and addressing of modifiable and potentially modifiable risk factors require a commitment from the patient and must be supported by the health care provider for ongoing success. Periodic screening and monitoring of progress is important in the primary care environment for prevention. Use of gender-specific guidelines, along with general primary prevention guidelines, offers a new dimension for special risk modification in women to prevent stroke.

Secondary Prevention

The secondary prevention of stroke in patients with stroke or TIAs is critical in the prevention of a recurrent stroke, which is often more severe, leaving the patient with more disabilities. Recommendations for secondary prevention in patients who had a stroke or TIAs are included in **Table 1-3**. The reader is directed to the cited references to review the recommendations in their entity. Originally, secondary prevention guidelines for stroke and TIAs were published in 2006 (Sacco et al., 2006), updated in 2011 (Furie et al., 2011), and more recently updated in 2014 (Kernan et al., 2014). With the rapid development of new knowledge, the 2014 guidelines can also be expected to be updated in the future. The reader is cautioned to review the most recent literature for updated guidelines.

In addition to practice-focused recommendations, Kernan et al. (2014) also addressed quality. Monitoring achievement of nationally accepted evidence-based guidelines on a population-based level is recommended as a basis for improving health promotion behaviors and reducing stroke health care disparities among high-risk groups. They recommend voluntary hospital-based programs for quality monitoring and improvement to improve adherence to nationally accepted evidence-based guidelines for secondary stroke prevention.

The role of the interprofessional team in secondary stroke and TIA prevention often begins in the acute care setting when a patient is admitted for treatment of a stroke. In addition to the diagnostic workup and acute care treatment, identification of risk factors is critical. This requires a detailed medical history to determine presence of previously identified risk factors including how they were being managed, goals of therapy, success in meeting target goals, and patient outcomes. Patients and their families may or may not be able to provide complete information regarding previous medical history.

The approach to patients must be patient centered to collect all relevant information to not only understand treatment but also to understand how the patient has responded and adhered to the treatment plan. In some instances, the hospitalization for an acute stroke precipitates the identification of new risk factors. In this case, a treatment plan is developed based on discussion with the patient and family about this new information. In other instances, the stroke and hospitalization may be the first encounter for the patient with health providers because the person has not had access to health care for a variety of reasons. Oftentimes, these patients have multiple comorbidities and require a comprehensive plan to address not only secondary stroke risk factors but also the coordination of other health care needs that extend well into the posthospitalization and recovery from stroke phase.

The members of the interprofessional team must work together to educate the patient and family about risk factors to prevent a secondary stroke. A well-designed plan with clear explanations to the patient/family is needed. All interprofessional team members must recognize their role to reinforce the information provided and help the patient to find ways to incorporate recommended strategies into his or her lifestyle. Other responsibilities of the interprofessional team are to coordinate care and transitions in care as the patient moves from acute care to rehabilitation, skilled nursing care facility, or home. It is at transition points that a coordinated plan of care often falls apart. The case manager or the transition coordinator member of the team is instrumental in making arrangements for a smooth transition. Follow-up appointments must be scheduled and the patient/family informed. Any appointment for physical therapy, occupational therapy, or other services including home health must be scheduled. If the patient is going to be managed by the primary care provider after acute hospitalization, a comprehensive transfer of critical information must be assured. Some patients will be seen in the stroke clinic for follow-up staffed by an interprofessional team with expertise in stroke care. Oftentimes, these are the same team members who cared for the patient in the acute care setting. These appointments serve two important purposes: (1) monitor of recovery from the stroke and (2) prevent a recurrent stroke. An interprofessional team with expertise in stroke care can improve patient outcomes and work effectively with the patient/family and primary care provider to prevent a second stroke.

SUMMARY

This chapter has set a framework for a discussion of stroke by addressing stroke statistics, the evolving changes in the definition of stroke and TIAs, the burden of stroke, stroke surveillance, risk factors, and primary and secondary prevention of stroke. The primary and secondary prevention of stroke and TIAs is based on the evidence-based guidelines available from several credible sources addressing general problems such as hypertension and cholesterol, known risk factors for stroke, as well as recommendations specific to stroke. The guidelines have been developed by interprofessional groups working collaboratively on panels to identify and translate the best evidence into evidence-based guidelines to guide practice and care. The refocusing of health care on prevention mobilize population and community-based strategies to keep people healthy. In addition, secondary prevention strategies, delivered by an interprofessional team, are directed at prevention of a recurrent stroke in those persons who have or have had a stroke or TIAs. Subsequent chapters will discuss the best practices for the care of patients with ischemic stroke, hemorrhagic stroke, and SAH.

REFERENCES

Ad Hoc Committee on Cerebrovascular Disease. (1975). A classification and outline of cerebrovascular diseases, II. *Stroke, 6*, 564–616.

Aho, K., Harmsen, P., Hatano, S., Marquardsen, J., Smirnov, V. E., & Strasser, T. (1980). Cerebrovascular disease in the community: Results of a WHO collaborative study. *Bulletin of World Health Organization, 58*, 113–130.

Albers, G. W., Caplan, L. R., Easton, J. D., Fayad, P. B., Mohr, J. P., Saver, J. L., & Sherman, D. G. (2002). TIA Working Group. Transient ischemic attack: Proposal for a new definition. *The New England Journal of Medicine, 347*, 1713–1716.

American Heart Association. (2014). *Get with the guidelines*. Retrieved from https://www.heart.org /HEARTORG/HealthcareResearch/GetWithTheGuidelinesHFStrokeResus/Get-With-The-Guidelines -Data-Request_UCM_319145_Article.jsp

Antman, E. M., Anbe, D. T., Armstrong, P. W., Bates, E. R., Green, L. A., Hand, M., . . . Ornato, J. P. (2004). ACC/AHA guidelines for the management of patients with ST-elevation myocardial infarction: A report of the American College of Cardiology/American Heart Association Task Force on Practice Guidelines (Committee to revise the 1999 guidelines for the management of patients with acute myocardial infarction). *Journal of the American College of Cardiology, 44*, E1–E211.

Bushnell, C., McCullough, L. D., Awad, I. A., Chireau, M. V., Fedder, W. N., Furie, K. L., . . . Walters, M. R. (2014). Guidelines for the prevention of stroke in women: A statement for healthcare professionals from the American Heart Association/American Stroke Association. *Stroke, 45*, 1–45. doi:10.1161/01 .str.0000442009.06663.48

Centers for Disease Control and Prevention. (2015). Classification of diseases, functioning, and disability. *International Classification of Diseases, Tenth Revision, Clinical Modification (ICD-10-CM)*. Retrieved from http://www.cdc.gov/nchs/data/icd/2015_icd10cm_preface.pdf

Centers for Disease Control and Prevention. (2014). *Deaths and mortality*. Retrieved from http://www.cdc .gov/nchs/fastats/deaths.htm

Chalela, J. A., Kidwell, C. S., Nentwich, L. M., Luby, M., Butman, J. A., Demchuk, A. M., . . . Warach, S. (2007). Magnetic resonance imaging and computed tomography in emergency assessment of patients with suspected acute stroke: A prospective comparison. *Lancet, 369*, 293–298.

Culebras, A., Messe, S. R., Chaturvedi, S., Kase, C. S., & Gronseth, G. (2014). Summary of evidence-based guideline update: Prevention of stroke in nonvalvular atrial fibrillation: Report of the Guideline Development Subcommittee of the American Academy of Neurology. *Neurology, 82*, 716–724.

Easton, J. D., Saver, J. L., Albers, G. W., Alberts, M. J., Chaturvedi, S., Feldmann, E., . . . Sacco, R. L. (2009). Definition and evaluation of transient ischemic attack: A scientific statement for healthcare professionals from the American Heart Association/American Stroke Association Stroke Council; Council on Cardiovascular Surgery and Anesthesia; Council on Cardiovascular Radiology and Intervention; Council on Cardiovascular Nursing; and the Interdisciplinary Council on Peripheral Vascular Disease. *Stroke, 40*, 2276–2293.

Eckel, R. H., Jakicic, J. M., Ard, J. D., de Jesus, J. M., Houston Miller, N., Hubbard, V. S., . . . Yanovski, S. Z. (2014). 2013 AHA/ACC guideline on lifestyle management to reduce cardiovascular risk. *Journal of the American College of Cardiology, 63*(25, Pt. B), 2960–2984. doi:10.1016/j.jacc.2013.11.003

Eton, D. T., Ramalho de Oliveira, D., Egginton, J. S., Ridgeway, J. L., Odell, L., May, C. R., & Montori, V. M. (2012). Building a measurement framework of burden of treatment in complex patients with chronic conditions: A qualitative study. *Patient Related Outcome Measures, 3*, 39–49.

Feigin, V. L., Forouzanfar, M. H., Krishnamurthi, R., Mensah, G. A., Connor, M., Bennett, D., . . . Murray, C. (2013). Global and regional burden of stroke during 1990–2010: Findings from the Global Burden of Disease Study 2010. *Lancet, 383*(9913), 245–254. doi:10.1016/S0140-6736(13)61953-4

Fisher, C. M. (1958). Intermittent cerebral ischemia. In I. S. Wright & C. H. Millikan (Eds.), *Cerebral vascular diseases* (pp. 81–97). New York, NY: Grune & Stratton.

Fraker, T. D., Jr, Fihn, S. D., Gibbons, R. J., Abrams, J., Chatterjee, K., Daley, J., . . . Yancy, C. W. (2007). 2007 chronic angina focused update of the ACC/AHA 2002 guidelines for the management of patients with chronic stable angina: A report of the American College of Cardiology/American Heart Association Task Force on Practice Guidelines Writing Group to develop the focused update of the 2002 guidelines for the management of patients with chronic stable angina. *Journal of the American College of Cardiology, 50*(23), 2264–2274.

Furie, K. L., Kasner, S. E., Adams, R. J., Albers, G. W., Bush, R. L., Fagan, S. C., . . . Wentworth, D. (2011). Guidelines for the prevention of stroke in patients with stroke or transient ischemic attack: A guideline for healthcare professionals from the American Heart Association/American Stroke Association. *Stroke, 42*, 227–276.

Furlan, M., Marchal, G., Viader, F., Derlon, J. M., & Baron, J. C. (1996). Spontaneous neurological recovery after stroke and the fate of the ischemic penumbra. *Annals of Neurology, 40*, 216–226.

Gall, S. L., Tran, P. L., Martin, K., Blizzard, L., & Srikanth, V. (2012). Sex differences in long-term outcomes after stroke: Functional outcomes, handicap, and quality of life. *Stroke, 43*, 1982–1987.

Gallacher, K., Jani, B., Morrison, D., Macdonald, S., Blane, D., Erwin, P., . . . Mair, F. S. (2013). Qualitative systematic reviews of treatment burden in stroke, heart failure and diabetes: Methodological challenges and solution. *BMC Medical Research Methodology, 13*, 10. doi:10.1186/1471-2288-13-10

Gargano, J. W., Reeves, M. J., & Coverdell, P. (2007). National Acute Stroke Registry Michigan Prototype Investigators. Sex differences in stroke recovery and stroke-specific quality of life: Results from a statewide stroke registry. *Stroke, 38*, 2541–2548.

Go, A. S., Mozaffarian, D., Roger, V. L., Benjamin, E. J., Berry, J. D., Borden, W. B., . . . Turner, M. B. (2013). Heart disease and stroke statistics—2013 update: A report from the American Heart Association. *Circulation, 127*, e6–e245.

Goff, D. C., Jr., Lloyd-Jones, D. M., Bennett, G., Coady, S., D'Agostino, R. B., Sr., Gibbons, R., . . . Wilson, P. W. (2014). 2013 ACC/AHA guideline on the assessment of cardiovascular risk. *Journal of the American College of Cardiology, 63*(25, Pt. B), 2935–2959. doi:10.1016/j.jacc.2013.11.005

Goldstein, L. B., Adams, R., Alberts, M. J., Appel, L. J., Brass, L. M., Bushnell, C. D., . . . Sacco, R. L. (2006). Primary prevention of ischemic stroke: A guideline from the American Heart Association/American Stroke Association Stroke Council: Cosponsored by the Atherosclerotic Peripheral Vascular Disease Interdisciplinary Working Group; Cardiovascular Nursing Council; Clinical Cardiology Council; Nutrition, Physical Activity, and Metabolism Council; and the Quality of Care and Outcomes Research Interdisciplinary Working Group. *Stroke, 37*, 1583–1633. doi:10.1161/01.STR.0000223048.70103.F1

Goldstein, L. B., Bushnell, C. D., Adams, R. J., Appel, L. J., Braun, L. T., Chaturvedi, S., . . . Pearson, T. A. (2011). Guidelines for the primary prevention of stroke: A guideline for healthcare professionals from the American Heart Association/American Stroke Association. *Stroke, 42*, 517–584.

Grundy S. M., Cleeman, J. I., Merz, C. N., Brewer, H. B., Jr., Clark, L. T., Hunninghake, D. B., . . . Stone, N. J. (2004). Implications of recent clinical trials for the National Cholesterol Education Program Adult Treatment Panel III guidelines. *Circulation, 110*, 227–239.

Holroyd-Leduc, J. M., Kapral, M. K., Austin, P. C., & Tu, J. V. (2000). Sex differences and similarities in the management and outcome of stroke patients. *Stroke, 31*, 1833–1837.

James, P. A., Oparil, S., Carter, B. L., Cushman, W. C., Dennison-Himmelfarb, C., Handler, J., . . . Ortiz, E. (2014). 2014 evidence-based guideline for the management of high blood pressure in adults: Report from the panel members appointed to the Eighth Joint National Committee (JNC 8). *Journal of the American Medical Association, 311*(5), 507–520. doi:10.1001/jama.2013.284427

January, C. T., Wann, L. S., Alpert, J. S., Calkins, H., Cigarroa, J. E., Cleveland, J. C., Jr., . . . Yancy, C. W. (2014). 2014 AHA/ACC/HRS guideline for the management of patients with atrial fibrillation: A report of the American College of Cardiology/American Heart Association Task Force on Practice Guidelines and the Heart Rhythm Society. *Circulation, 130*, e199–e267.

Jensen, M. D., Ryan, D. H., Apovian, C. M., Ard, J. D., Comuzzie, A. G., Donato, K. A., . . . Yanovski, S. Z. (2013). 2013 AHA/ACC/TOS guideline for the management of overweight and obesity in adults: A report of the American College of Cardiology/American Heart Association Task Force on Practice Guidelines and the Obesity Society. *Circulation, 129*, S102–S138.

Jneid, H., Anderson, J. L., Wright, R. S., Adams, C. D., Bridges, C. R., Casey, D. E., Jr., . . . Zidar, J. P. (2012). ACCF/AHA focused update of the guideline for the management of patients with unstable angina/non–ST-elevation myocardial infarction (updating the 2007 guideline and replacing the 2011 focused update): A report of the American College of Cardiology Foundation/American Heart Association Task Force on Practice Guidelines. *Circulation, 126*, 875–910.

Kelly-Hayes, M., Beiser, A., Kase, C. S., Scaramucci, A., D'Agostino, R. B., & Wolf, P. A. (2003). The influence of gender and age on disability following ischemic stroke: The Framingham study. *Journal of Stroke and Cerebrovascular Disease, 12*, 119–126.

Kernan, W. N., Ovbiagele, B., Black, H. R., Bravata, D. M., Chimowitz, M. I., Ezekowitz, M. D., . . . Wilson, J. A. (2014). Guidelines for the prevention of stroke in patients with stroke and transient ischemic attack: A guideline for healthcare professionals from the American Heart Association/American Stroke Association. *Stroke, 45*, 2160–2236.

Kim, J. S., Lee, K. B., Roh, H., Ahn, M. Y., & Hwang, H. W. (2010). Gender differences in the functional recovery after acute stroke. *Journal of Clinical Neurology, 6*, 183–188.

Lackland, D. T., Roccella, E. T., Deutsch, A. F., Fornage, M., George, M. G., Howard, G., . . . Towfighi, A. (2014). Factors influencing the decline in stroke mortality: A statement from the American Heart Association/American Stroke Association. *Stroke, 45*, 315–353. doi:10.1161/01.str.0000437068.30550.cf

Lloyd-Jones, D., Adams, R. J., Brown, T. M., Carnethon, M., Dai, S., DeSimone, G., . . . Wylie-Rosett, J. (2010). Heart disease and stroke statistics—2010 update: A report from the American Heart Association. *Circulation, 121*, e46–e215.

Lloyd-Jones, D. M., Leip, E. P., Larson, M. G., D'Agostino, R. B., Beiser, A., Wilson, P. W., . . . Levy, D. (2006). Prediction of lifetime risk for cardiovascular disease by risk factor burden at 50 years of age. *Circulation, 113*, 791–798.

Lloyd-Jones, D. M., Wilson, P. W., Larson, M. G., Beiser, A., Leip, E. P., D'Agostino, R. B., & Levy, D. (2004). Framingham risk score and prediction of lifetime risk for coronary heart disease. *The American Journal of Cardiology, 94*, 20–24.

Lozano, R., Naghavi, M., Foreman, K., Lim, S., Shibuya, K., Aboyans, V., . . . Memish, Z. A. (2012). Global and regional mortality from 235 causes of death for 20 age groups in 1990 and 2010: A systematic analysis for the Global Burden of Disease Study 2010. *Lancet, 380*, 2095–2128.

Mendis, S. (2010). Prevention and care of stroke in low- and middle-income countries: The need for a public health perspective. *International Journal of Stroke, 5*, 86–91.

Meschia, J. F., Bushnell, C., Boden-Albala, B., Braun, L. T., Bravata, D. M., Chaturvedi, S., . . . Wilson, J. A. (2014). Guidelines for the primary prevention of stroke: A statement for healthcare professionals from the American Heart Association/American Stroke Association. *Stroke, 45*, 3754–3832.

Mohr, J. P. (2004). Historical perspective. *Neurology, 62*(Suppl. 6), S3–S6.

Mukherjee, D., & Patil, C. G. (2011). Epidemiology and the global burden of stroke. *World Neurosurgery, 76*(65), s85–s90.

Nishimura, R. A., Otto, C. M., Bonow, R. O., Carabello, B. A., Erwin, J. P., III., Guyton, RA., . . . Thomas, J. D. (2014). 2014 AHA/ACC guideline for the management of patients with valvular heart disease: Executive summary: A report of the American College of Cardiology/American Heart Association Task Force on Practice Guidelines. *Circulation, 129*, 2440–2492.

Norrving, B., & Kissela, B. (2013). The global burden of stroke and need for a continuum of care. *Neurology, 80*(Suppl. 2), S1–S12.

O'Donnell, M. J., Xavier, D., Liu, L., Zhang, H., Chin, S. L., Rao-Melacini, P., . . . Yusuf, S. (2010). Risk factors for ischaemic and intracerebral haemorrhagic stroke in 22 countries (the INTERSTROKE study): A case-control study. *Lancet, 376*, 112–123. doi:10.1016/S0140-6736(10)60834-3

Olesen, J. B., Lip, G. Y., Hansen, M. L., Hansen, P. R., Tolstrup, J. S., Lindhardsen, J., . . . Torp-Pedersen, C. (2011). Validation of risk stratification schemes for predicting stroke and thromboembolism in patients with atrial fibrillation: Nationwide cohort study. *BMJ, 342*, d124. doi:10.1136/bmj.d124

Olivot, J. M., & Albers, G. W. (2010). Using advanced MRI techniques for patient selection before acute stroke therapy. *Current Treatment Options in Cardiovascular Medicine, 12*, 230–239.

Paolucci, S., Bragoni, M., Coiro, P., De Angelis, D., Fusco, F. R., Morelli, D., . . . Pratesi, L. (2006). Is sex a prognostic factor in stroke rehabilitation? A matched comparison. *Stroke, 37*, 2989–2994.

Petrea, R. E., Beiser, A. S., Seshadri, S., Kelly-Hayes, M., Kase, C. S., & Wolf, P. A. (2009). Gender differences in stroke incidence and poststroke disability in the Framingham Heart Study. *Stroke, 40*, 1032–1037.

Prüss-Üstün, A., & Corvalán, C. (2006). *Preventing disease through healthy environments: Towards an estimate of the environmental burden of disease.* Geneva, Switzerland: World Health Organization.

Rogers, V. L., Go, A. S., Lloyd-Jones, D. M., Benjamin, E. J., Berry, J. D., Borden, W. B., . . . Turner, M. B. (2012). Heart disease and stroke statistics 2012 update: A report from the American Heart Association. *Circulation, 125*(1), E2–E220.

Roquer, J., Campello, A. R., & Gomis, M. (2003). Sex differences in first-ever acute stroke. *Stroke, 34*, 1581–1585.

Sacco, R. L., Adams, R., Albers, G., Alberts, M. J., Benavente, O., Furie, K., . . . Tomsick, T. (2006). Guidelines for prevention of stroke in patients with ischemic stroke or transient ischemic attack: A statement for healthcare professionals from the American Heart Association/American Stroke Association Council on Stroke: Co-Sponsored by the Council on Cardiovascular Radiology and Intervention: The American Academy of Neurology affirms the value of this guideline. *Stroke, 37*, 577–617. doi:10.1161/01.STR.0000199147.30016.74

Sacco, R. L., Kasner S, E. Broderick, J. P., Caplan, L. R., Connors, J. J., Culebras, A., . . . Vinters, H. V. (2013). An updated definition of stroke for the 21st century: A statement for healthcare professionals from the American Heart Association/American Stroke Association. *Stroke, 44*, 2064–2089. doi:10.1161/STR.0b013e318296aeca

Seshadri, S., Beiser, A., Kelly-Hayes, M., Kase, C. S., Au, R., Kannel, W. B., & Wolf, P. A. (2006). The lifetime risk of stroke: Estimates from the Framingham Study. *Stroke, 37*, 345–350.

Shippee, N. D., Shah, N. D., May, C. R., Mair, F. S., & Mantori, V. M. (2009). Cumulative complexity: A functional, patient-centered model of patient complexity can improve research and practice. *Journal of Clinical Epidemiology, 65*, 1041–1051.

Stone, N. J., Robinson, J., Lichtenstein, A. H., Bairey Merz, C. N., Blum, C. B., Eckel, R. H., . . . Wilson, P. W. (2013). 2013 ACC/AHA guideline on the treatment of blood cholesterol to reduce atherosclerotic cardiovascular risk in adults. *Journal of the American College of Cardiology, 63*(25, Pt. B), 2889–2934. doi:10.1016/j.jacc.2013.11.002

Teutsch, S. M. (2010). Considerations in planning a surveillance system. In: L. Lee, S. Teutsch, S. Thacker, & M. St. Louis (Eds.), *Principles and practice of public health surveillance* (3rd ed., pp. 18–43). New York, NY: Oxford University Press.

Thacker, S. B., & Berkelman, R. L. (1988). Public health surveillance in the United States. *Epidemiologic Reviews, 10,* 164–90.

Towfighi, A., & Saver, J. L. (2011). Stroke declines from third to fourth leading cause of death in the United States. *Stroke, 42,* 2351–2355.

U.S. Prevention Services Task Force. (2012). Retrieved from http//:www.uspreventionservicestaskforce.org /uspstopics.htm.

U.S. Department of Agriculture & U.S. Department of Health and Human Services. (2010). *Dietary guidelines for Americans, 2010* (7th ed.). Washington, DC: U.S. Government Printing Office.

U.S. Department of Health and Human Services. (2010). *Heart disease and stroke.* Retrieved from https://www .healthypeople.gov/2020/topics-objectives/topic/heart-disease-and-stroke

World Heart Federation. (2014). *Stroke.* Retrieved from http://www.world-heart-federation.org/cardiovascular -health/stroke/

CHAPTER 2

Development of Stroke Systems of Care

Claranne Mathiesen and Sarah L. Livesay

Stroke is a significant cause of morbidity and mortality in the United States and worldwide (Jauch et al., 2013). Historically, stroke was a disease characterized by supportive care only. However, the last two decades has witnessed advances in treatment of the disease, necessitating the rapid identification and treatment of patients with stroke as well as an understanding that organized and interprofessional care improves outcomes for patients with ischemic stroke, intracerebral hemorrhage (ICH), and subarachnoid hemorrhage (SAH). These treatments and organization of care are predicated on the development of a stroke system of care that allows for early recognition of a stroke event and rapid transport to a hospital capable of providing organized stroke care. This chapter will review the development of a stroke system of care in the United States to date and highlight the role of coordination of emergency medical services (EMS), external program certification for hospitals with expertise in providing stroke care, and telemedicine in the development of a stroke system of care.

STROKE SYSTEM OF CARE DEFINED

A system of health care delivery represents the continuum of services offered to a patient or a population of patients (Institute for Healthcare Improvement [IHI], 2014). Within the United States, the development of systems of health care across geographical settings and for specific patient populations is currently conducted within the context of the IHI Triple Aim Initiative: Health care should be delivered in a system that improves the health of populations, improves the patient's experience of care, and reduces the per capita cost of health care (IHI, 2014). Prior to the discovery of intravenous (IV) thrombolysis as a treatment for ischemic stroke in the mid-1990s, there was no need to have an organized system of care to identify stroke patients and to facilitate care once identified. Care for patients with stroke was largely supportive and not time-sensitive. However, IV thrombolysis is now available for the treatment of acute ischemic stroke and must be administered within hours of the start of a stroke. Therefore, early recognition and transportation of a stroke patient to a hospital capable of providing thrombolysis became a paramount concern once this treatment was available. The American Heart Association/American Stroke Association (AHA/ASA) quickly began initiatives to develop such a system for the treatment of stroke. The AHA/ASA defines stroke system of care (SSC) as a coordinated continuum of care that addresses all aspects of care, from primary prevention to activation of EMS, acute care, secondary prevention, rehabilitation, and reentry into the community (Silva & Schwamm, 2013).

Several initiatives were underway between 1997 and 2005 to develop a system of care for stroke patients. However, the best conceptualization of an SSC was published in 2005, when the AHA/ASA introduced their Stroke System of Care Model (SSCM). The model proposed that all citizens should have access to organized and expert stroke care regardless of geographical location or other socioeconomic disparities. Significant progress has been made over the past decade toward the development of an SSC. Efforts to organize care resulted in increased use of IV tissue plasminogen activator (tPA), improved patient outcomes, and reduction in mortality (Silva & Schwamm, 2013). However, stroke continues to be a time-sensitive condition that has limited acute interventions, which require a systematic approach to patient triage, workup, and intervention. This is further challenged by a need for coordination of speedy access to multiple resources and specially trained teams to treat patients emergently. IV thrombolysis remains underused in the treatment of ischemic stroke (Alberts et al., 2005; Gorelick, 2013). Although great progress has been made, as of 2010, only a slight majority of patients in the United States had access to hospitals with stroke expertise through EMS routing protocols, suggesting much work remains to fully realize the AHA/ASA SSCM (Gorelick, 2013).

Early efforts to develop stroke programs have focused on identification of resources necessary to provide stroke care, development of care pathways, and cohorting of patients on stroke units. Formalized stroke certification by external organizations has continued to improve care by setting a minimum standard of program organization and evaluation, and rigorous evaluation process for any organization wishing to call themselves a stroke center. The definition of relationships between hospitals and the best organization of services in an SSC has evolved over years. However, the AHA/ASA, in conjunction with the Brain Attack Coalition and the National Stroke Association, have converged on a model with three distinct levels of stroke centers in the United States (Gorelick, 2013).

▌▊ DEVELOPING STROKE SYSTEMS OF CARE

After the approval of recombinant tissue plasminogen activator (rtPA) in 1996, there was an immediate need for integration of EMS as a key component of a successful SSC. The AHA/ASA and the National Stroke Association (NSA) have mobilized to develop and support efforts to improve symptom recognition, activation of 911 for EMS response, and the rapid treatment of stroke after hospital arrival (Gorelick, 2013). The NSA established in the mid-1990s the NSA Stroke Center Network program and developed foundational guidelines for the early recognition of stroke and delivery of EMS services to route patients to hospitals capable of providing emergent stroke care and thrombolysis. The Brain Attack Coalition formed shortly after and also worked to improve EMS services and the rapid detection and treatment of ischemic stroke.

The AHA/ASA, Brain Attack Coalition, and NSA continue to shape the delivery of organized stroke care through national advocacy efforts nearly a decade later. All three national societies support the concept of an SSC integrating care from prevention to acute treatment and rehabilitation. The attributes of an effective SSC include coordinated care, a customized system that fits local environment needs, use of available resources and programs with an emphasis on continual performance improvement, and quality assurance (Silva & Schwamm, 2013). The importance of coordination between the various components of a stroke system is essential and remains challenging because it spans usual lines of demarcation for medical care, reimbursement, and government jurisdiction as we now define it (Higashida et al., 2013). However, the development of a U.S. SSC to date attempts to coordinate care across care settings despite the barriers.

Brain Attack Coalition

The Brain Attack Coalition (BAC) provided foundational guidance for the development of an SSC and continues to guide the stroke field through recommendations on the development and organization of stroke care. The BAC is a multidisciplinary group composed of representatives from a number of major professional organizations involved in delivering stroke care. The BAC provided the initial framework for the formal development of a tiered stroke system in the United States through the publication of consensus papers with recommendations for organizing stroke care services (Alberts et al., 2000; Alberts et al., 2005). The BAC initially proposed the development of primary stroke centers (PSCs) as hospitals that offered organized stroke care 24 hours a day (Alberts et al., 2000). In this initial paper, the BAC surmised that organized stroke care in PSC hospitals would have a direct and measurable positive impact on the mortality and morbidity after stroke. A PSC would offer rapid assessment of a patient with stroke symptoms and access to stroke experts capable of providing thrombolysis to patients with ischemic stroke in a timely fashion. Beyond thrombolysis in the first few hours of ischemic stroke, the PSC would also coordinate early rehabilitation services and initiate secondary preventive measures according to the best evidence in managing patients with stroke (Alberts et al., 2000).

After the BAC's introduction of the PSC model, The Joint Commission (TJC), in collaboration with AHA/ASA, established minimum structural elements, standards of care, and performance measures to guide hospitals in developing a PSC program. In 2003, TJC began certifying PSCs, thus providing national recognition for centers demonstrating compliance with national standards, PSC recommendations, clinical practice guidelines, and ongoing performance improvement activities (Fonarow, Smith, Saver, Reeves, Bhatt, et al., 2011). Since the initial TJC certification in 2003, the PSC certification program has continued to grow, with approximately 1,600 centers currently certified as of 2014 (TJC, 2014a).

In 2005, the BAC published a second consensus paper calling for a second tier of stroke certification for centers that specialized in the surgical management of patients with ischemic stroke, ICH, and SAH. This new tier of stroke centers would be called *comprehensive stroke centers* (CSCs), and the recommendations outlined the interprofessional coordination of care necessary for the most acutely ill patients with stroke (Alberts et al., 2005). A CSC would incorporate neurosurgical services, endovascular services, and cardiovascular surgery services when appropriate with neurological services in the hospital. This additional tier of stroke certification recognized that not all PSC centers could offer neurosurgical, endovascular, and other advanced programs of care around the clock. A CSC represented concentrated and highly cost and time-intensive services. This model was similar to the trauma system in place in the United States and familiar to many

EMS providers and community leaders. In 2013, TJC finalized the standards and performance measures for CSCs and began certifying organizations. As of 2014, 73 centers in the United States had successfully completed initial CSC certification (TJC, 2014b).

In 2013, the BAC proposed a third tier of stroke centers to complete the model of the AHA/ASA SSCM. The third tier is the development of acute stroke–ready hospital (ASRH), where the most immediate and stabilizing stroke care could be provided and then patients would be mobilized to either a PSC or CSC as needed (Alberts et al., 2013). The development of a formal certification program by TJC or other external certifying bodies has yet to be developed.

Stroke program certification has played a key role in the development of an SSC in the United States by organizing care within a hospital. Beyond hospital certification, the development of regionalized models to dictate how EMS interacts with CSCs is also shaping the delivery of acute stroke care in the United States. This has included development of local and regional EMS regulations to route acute stroke patients to PSCs. By the end of 2010, it was estimated that 53% of U.S. population was covered by routing protocols (Song & Saver, 2012).

The evolution of organized stroke care has now spanned almost two decades with a stroke center model promoting use of structured care protocols and continuous performance improvement/quality assurance that spans the entire care continuum. Many parallels can be made to the currently developed trauma model of care delivery. Shared experiences can also be traced to the development of regionalized resources for heart attack and cardiac arrest centers. These multifaceted time-sensitive emergencies all share a similar need for coordination of care, public and EMS collaboratives, and ongoing care delivery system improvements. Data evaluating the impact of developing stroke programs in hospital suggest this model is improving stroke care. There are multiple studies that validate the efficacy of stroke units and stroke programs within hospitals in providing care to patients with acute stroke. In comparison to patients cared for in general medical units without a focus on stroke care, patient cared for in stroke units had up to a 28% reduction in mortality, a 7% increase in being able to return to home, and an 8% reduction in length of stay (Candelise et al., 2007; "Collaborative Systematic Review," 1997; Langhorne et al., 2013).

Although the tiered system of stroke care is the current model for delivering stroke care in the United States, the relationship between stroke centers has yet to be fully defined. The PSC level of care remains the most common stroke center certification in the nation and allows the most citizens access to general stroke care and thrombolysis when appropriate. Theoretically, all PSCs should then work with a CSC who would care for the most acutely ill stroke patients in need of the most intensive services. However, the types of patients who should receive care at a CSC versus a PSC and facilitating the timely transfer of patients remain undefined.

In addition to external certification, many states in the United States have developed policy and legislative initiatives guiding the regional routing of patients with stroke by EMS to only hospitals capable of providing care, such as a certified center (L. Schwamm et al., 2010). This is commonly referred to as *state designation of stroke centers and regional routing protocols*. The initiative to include state legislators in the development of regional stroke systems began in the early 2000s after the Stroke Treatment and Ongoing Prevention (STOP Stroke) Act failed to gain bipartisan support at a national level in 2003 (L. Schwamm et al., 2010). Regional AHA/ASA representative then began grassroots efforts at a regional and state level to influence the development of EMS routing protocols for stroke patients. As of 2013, over half the states in the United States have legislation guiding the designation of stroke hospitals and subsequent EMS routing of patients with stroke, with several additional states currently considering such legislation (Gorelick, 2013).

American Heart Association/American Stroke Association Establishment of Stroke System of Care Model

In 2005, the AHA/ASA conveyed a multidisciplinary group, the Task Force on the Development of Stroke Systems, to describe the state of stroke care fragmentation at the time and to define key components of a stroke system and recommend methods for implementation of a stroke system (L. H. Schwamm et al., 2005). This task force of experts in areas of stroke prevention, EMS, acute stroke treatment, stroke rehabilitation, and health policy development conducted an extensive review of stroke literature and developed the SSCM. Using a systems approach to stroke care, it was identified that the care delivery model in most areas of the United States failed to provide an integrated coordinated means of providing stroke prevention measures, acute treatment, and rehabilitation. The group identified key components of an SSC, including the development of stroke centers as already outlined earlier. However, the SSCM conceptualized care beyond a stroke center across the stroke continuum of care. Seven key components were identified as necessary to coordinate and promote patient access including the following:

- Primordial and primary prevention
- Community education
- Notification and response of EMS
- Acute stroke treatment, including hyperacute and emergency department processes
- Subacute stroke treatment and secondary prevention
- Rehabilitation
- Continuous quality improvement activities

Primordial prevention referred to interventions designed to decrease the development of disease risk factors and have broad impacts on health, whereas primary prevention referred to the strategies used to manage known disease risk factors. A well-organized SSC would include efforts to prevent stroke from ever occurring through such prevention strategies. Community education was also recognized as a critical element of an SSC, and the SSCM emphasized the need for increased awareness of stroke symptoms by the general community, timely presentation to a stroke center for treatment when a stroke occurred, and better adherence to risk reduction regimens.

The SSCM also recognized the key role of EMS in an organized SSC (L. H. Schwamm et al., 2005). Effective notification and response of EMS for stroke involves complex communication between the public, EMS programs, and hospital emergency departments. The field recognition of stroke symptoms, priority dispatch of EMS providers, triage, and transport to appropriate facilities require definition and coordination between the EMS services and the receiving hospital. ⊙ The model further recognized the importance of an interprofessional hospital-based acute stroke team (AST). The AST coordinates stroke care from arrival to discharge and requires ongoing training, supporting rapid identification, diagnosis, and initiation of acute stroke therapies to patients presenting to the hospital. The AST should operate using written protocols that outline evidence-based interventions, appropriate resources, and clearly delineate roles of hospitals and team members.

Finally, an SSC should include organized and standardized efforts to provide subacute care after hospitalization, with focus on risk factor reduction and prevention of poststroke complications. Stroke rehabilitation should be provided to optimize neu-rological recovery, including teaching compensatory strategies, relearning activities of daily living and skills required for community reintegration. Each phase of care in the SSCM should operate using a systems approach to stroke care and use continuous qual-ity improvement strategies to improve patient care processes and outcome. Process and outcome metrics should be identified through evidenced-based methods or driven by national consensus. Building stroke systems in the United States is the next step in im-provement of stroke outcomes in prevention, treatment, and rehabilitation of stroke (L. H. Schwamm et al., 2005).

The AHA/ASA Task Force on the Development of Stroke Systems made the follow-ing general recommendations:

- Stroke systems should ensure effective interaction and collaboration, promote orga-nized care, and identify performance measures to evaluation stroke systems.
- Care coordination requires development of tools to be used for stroke prevention, treatment, and rehabilitation.
- Decisions need to be based on what is in the best interest of the stroke patient and may require collaboration among entities transcending geopolitical or corporate affiliations.
- Stroke system should identify and address potential obstacles to implementation.
- The system should be customized for each state, region, and locality with recogni-tion of universal elements and should bridge disparities such as rural and neuro-logically underserved areas (L. H. Schwamm et al., 2005).

▊▊ COMPONENTS OF STROKE SYSTEMS OF CARE

Core Components of Certified Stroke Centers

All stroke centers, regardless of certification as a PSC or CSC, begin with some consis-tent structural elements that support the overall operations that are needed to provide stroke patient care. The initial coordination of services for a stroke program begins with the EMS team providing the first contact for medical care (The role of EMS in supporting stroke care is fully described in Chapter 4). A stroke program in a hospital must have a relationship with area EMS. This relationship includes the level of knowl-edge the EMS workers have related to stroke recognition and initial care, inbound communication, and handoff to the hospital team. Both the EMS and hospital stroke program must determine the necessary dedicated resources and administrative infra-structure needed between the EMS and the PSC or CSC (Alberts et al., 2000; Alberts et al., 2005).

The core recommendations for PSCs are organized around 11 aspects of stroke care and can be divided into direct patient care and support services (**Tables 2-1** and **2-2**) (Alberts et al., 2000). The core components listed for patient care have continued to offer an organizing framework and remains the building platform for both primary and comprehensive levels of care. The PSC continues to stabilize and provide emergency care to stroke patients 24 hours a day, 7 days a week. The CSC should offer the same services as a PSC as well as additional neurosurgical, endovascular, and critical care ser-vices for the most critical stroke patients that require advanced testing and intervention (Alberts et al., 2005). Development of effective notification of EMS and prehospital com-munication has been shown to increase the direction of patients to facilities equipped

TABLE 2-1 Major Elements of a Primary Stroke Center

ASTs
Written care protocols
EMS
Emergency department
Stroke unit
Neurosurgical services

Alberts, M. J., Hademenos, G., Latchaw, R. E., Jagoda, A., Marler, J. R., Mayberg, M. R., . . . Walker, M. D. (2000). Recommendations for the establishment of primary stroke centers. Brain Attack Coalition. *The Journal of the American Medical Association, 283*(23), 3102–3109.

with the right resources to manage stroke emergencies. Further development of regional partnerships and use of telemedicine continues to afford more patient-aggressive interventions and improved patient outcomes.

All stroke centers should coordinate EMS and emergency department interaction. This may be done through mutually agreed upon processes for patient identification and triage of stroke using validated scales, emphasizing gathering of key patient information on time of onset, medical history, and contact information. Additionally, the BAC and many states have developed emergent triage protocols routing stroke patients to only designated stroke centers to ensure appropriate care (Alberts et al., 2011). The benefits of having a dedicated inpatient stroke unit has been well supported with reductions in mortality, increased return to independence, and reduction in hospital length of stay (Alberts et al., 2011; Foley, Salter, & Teasell, 2007; Langhorne et al., 2013).

ASTs are a critical part of organizing and delivering emergent stroke care within stroke centers. There are several models of staffing and availability of AST staff, and the stroke program is at liberty to determine who staffs the AST and how communication occurs. At a minimum, the AST should include a physician or advanced practice provider and another health care provider, typically a nurse who is available 24 hours a day, 7 days a week, responding within 15 minutes of patient arrival (**Table 2-3**) (Alberts et al., 2011). Many centers staff the AST with a general neurologist or a neurologist with stroke expertise. However, in some centers, emergency department or internal medicine hospitalists provide these acute services. The AST should operate within predefined written care protocols to guide the roles of team members in the delivery of stroke care including stabilization, diagnostic workup, monitoring, and acute interventions (Alberts et al., 2011).

TABLE 2-2 Common Aspects of Stroke Certified Centers—Support Services

Support of medical organization
Stroke center director
Neuroimaging services
Laboratory services
Outcome and quality improvement
Continuing medical education

Stroke unit or designated stroke beds are required for those primary stroke centers that will provide ongoing inpatient care.
Alberts, M. J., Hademenos, G., Latchaw, R. E., Jagoda, A., Marler, J. R., Mayberg, M. R., . . . Walker, M. D. (2000). Recommendations for the establishment of primary stroke centers. Brain Attack Coalition. *The Journal of the American Medical Association, 283*(23), 3102–3109.

TABLE 2-3 Acute Stroke Team Timeliness of Care Benchmarks

National Institute of Neurological Disorders and Stroke Recommended Intervals for Care

Door-to-doctor first sees patient (10 min)
Door-to-CT completed (25 min)
Door-to-CT read (45 min)
Door-to-thrombolytic therapy starts (60 min)
Physician examination (15 min)
Neurosurgical expertise available* (2 hr)
Admitted to monitored bed (3 hr)

*On-site or by transfer to another facility.
Summers, D., Leonard, A., Wentworth, D., Saver, J. L., Simpson, J., Spilker, J. A., . . . Mitchell, P. H. (2009). Comprehensive overview of nursing and interdisciplinary care of the acute ischemic stroke patient: A scientific statement from the American Heart Association. *Stroke, 40*(8), 2911–2944. doi:10.1161/STROKEAHA.109.192362

All stroke centers regardless of PSC or CSC certification should meet minimum criteria for coordination of care between physician specialties, testing areas, and the provision of care as an interprofessional team. This may include access to neurological, neurosurgical, and neurocritical care expertise; cardiac monitoring; cerebral and cerebrovascular imaging; and laboratory services. The administrative support necessary to develop and sustain infrastructure and specialized personnel cannot be understated. Dedicated neurological expertise has been demonstrated in the literature to reduce morbidity and mortality in stroke centers. Advocacy efforts with local providers and policymakers at the local, state, and national levels can make a significant contribution to reducing poststroke disability by working to promote coordinated stroke network systems (Higashida et al., 2013). Emphasis on geographical appraisal of resources and potential benefit of strategic use of ground and aeromedical transportation should allow all citizens access to a stroke center within 60 minutes of symptoms onset.

All PSCs and CSCs centers should demonstrate the use of interprofessional care protocols. The use of written care protocols continues to gain popularity in many aspects of medical, surgical, and nursing care. Standardization of care by use of evidenced-based care protocols has been endorsed widely in the ongoing development of stroke centers and can be implemented across multihospital systems to reduce care variability (Alberts et al., 2011). Typical protocols detail care during the emergency care of ischemic and hemorrhagic stroke including stabilization of vital functions, diagnostic testing, and medications including IV tPA. Protocols should be reviewed by the interdisciplinary team annually and reflect published national guidelines. Compliance with protocols is often measured as part of the process and outcome metrics maintained by stroke centers.

■■ TIERED STROKE SYSTEM AND STROKE CENTER DIFFERENCES

SSCs include the development of various levels of stroke centers; the extended use of telemedicine technologies; advanced medical, endovascular, and neurosurgical interventions; and early rehabilitation strategies (Higashida et al., 2013). The impact of SSC in reduction of stroke-related deaths by just 2% to 3% annually would translate into 20,000 fewer deaths in the United States and 40,000 fewer deaths worldwide (Higashida et al., 2013). However, the ideal model for interaction between various tiers of stroke centers has yet to be identified. Theoretically, the fully operationalized SSC in the United States could include four different types of acute care facilities (CSC, PSC, ASRH, and non-stroke hospital), with formal relationships between stroke facilities and potentially would include establishing telemedicine relationships between facilities. Bridging the gaps in access to stroke experts across regions would allow communities access to experienced specialists that have ability to assist with acute stroke emergencies. A comparison of the characteristics of acute stroke inpatient facilities is summarized in **Table 2-4** (Higashida et al., 2013).

In 2011, the BAC published revised recommendations to PSC elements to further support best practices and evolving studies guiding the treatment of patients with stroke (Alberts et al., 2011). The importance of the AST in the initial care of the patient has been critical to accessing acute stroke therapies and should include at minimum a physician and one other health care provider available at bedside within 15 minutes. The emphasis on the presence and content in written care protocols was expanded. Written care protocols are thought to assist the interprofessional team in providing safe care and have been shown to be associated with decreased complications. The publication also emphasized that electronic order sets and documentation can reduce variations in care delivery. Additional emphasis was placed on the importance of activating 911, and use of validated EMS stroke scales can enhance effective and accurate communications to the receiving facilities. The guideline continued to support formal recommendations on transportation to stroke

TABLE 2-4 Some Characteristics of Typical Acute Inpatient Stroke Care Facilities

Characteristics	Non-Stroke Center	ASRH	PSC	CSC
Typical bed count	20–50	30–100	100–400	400–1500
Annual stroke admissions	10–50	25–50	50–300	>300
Rapid neuroimaging 24/7*	No	Performed and read within 45 min of order	Performed and read within 45 min of order	Performed and read within 45 min of order
IV tPA capability 24/7	No	60-min door-to-needle time	60-min door-to-needle time	60-min door-to-needle time
AST available	No	At bedside within 15 min	At bedside within 15 min	At bedside within 15 min
Stroke unit	No	No[†]	Yes	Yes
Neurocritical care unit	No	No	No	Yes[§]
Access to neurosurgical services	No	Yes, within 3 hr or by transfer[‡]	Yes, within 2 hr in house or by transfer	Yes, 24/7 coverage and call schedule

ASRH, acute stroke–ready hospital; PSC, primary stroke center; CSC, comprehensive stroke center; IV tPA, intravenous tissue plasminogen activator; AST, acute stroke team.
*24/7 Neurological expertise available through telemedicine, on site, or a combination.
[†]Some ASRHs may have the necessary resources on site or via telemedicine to support a stroke unit.
[‡]This may vary based on geographic and other considerations.
[§]Or a defined neurocritical care service operating within the context of a medical or surgical intensive care unit.
From Higashida, R., Alberts, M. J., Alexander, D. N., Crocco, T. J., Demaerschalk, B. M., Derdeyn, C. P., . . . Wood, J. P. (2013). Interactions within stroke systems of care: A policy statement from the American Heart Association/American Stroke Association. *Stroke, 44*(10), 2961–2984.

centers and routine use of telemedicine technologies continue to support hospital care. Stroke centers should continue to educate EMS and emergency department personnel and offer participation in educational activities related to the diagnosis and treatment at least two times per year. Finally, the guideline reiterated that neurosurgical coverage should be available and documented in a written plan that is approved by referring and receiving facilities. Diagnostic imaging with computed tomography (CT) or magnetic resonance imaging (MRI) needs to be available within 6 hours of order and results within 2 hours, and the early integration of rehabilitation should be part of all PSC care.

The 2011 BAC update for the establishment of PSCs also strengthened recommendations around the hospital's commitment and support of the program (Alberts et al., 2011). Hospital administration must demonstrate the availability and support of program infrastructure and funding. Additionally, physician leadership was seen as critical to program success, and the guideline noted that the designated physician director is necessary to provide administrative leadership and clinical guidance to the program. According to the guidelines, all PSCs should use a stroke registry, database, or similar monitoring program such as Get With The Guidelines-Stroke (GWTG-S) or the Paul Coverdell National Acute Stroke Registry for quality improvement purposes. The BAC strongly supported and endorsed certification programs as a means to validate components, protocols and level of care, and outcomes at a PSC (Alberts et al., 2011). The TJC standards for PSC were revised according to the most recent AHA/ASA and BAC guidelines.

Comprehensive Stroke Center

Adding to the already well-described PSC, the CSC provides additional care in the following four areas: (1) personnel with neurosurgical, neuroendovascular, and neurocritical care expertise; (2) specialized diagnostic and treatment; (3) facility infrastructure; and (4) programmatic areas to support complex patient needs (Alberts et al., 2005). Complex stroke patients requiring expertise of multispecialty services for large vessel ischemic stroke, ICH, and SAH are expected to benefit from the additional resources in the neurological intensive care at the CSC. To become certified as a CSC, the program must demonstrate adequate staffing, expertise with complex stroke patients, infrastructure to handle simultaneous stroke patients, and expanded programs to serve as a resource to PSCs in the region (Alberts et al., 2005).

A CSC functions as a resource center for other facilities in their area and often supports several PSCs. These areas are identified as eligibility requirements for CSCs and these include the following:

- Meet certification standards
- Maintain minimum volumes for coil embolization and surgical clipping of aneurysm, IV tPA, and other services
- Advanced imaging 24/7
- Post hospital care coordination
- Dedicated neurointensive care unit
- Peer review process for reviewing any patient care complications
- Participation in institutional review board (IRB)–approved stroke research
- Performance improvement beyond the PSC metrics

The diagnosis and treatment of some patients with complex types of stroke may require more resources and higher intensity of care than available at many hospitals and in most PSCs. A CSC has the specialized expertise, infrastructure, and programs necessary to meet the needs and to serve as a resource to PSCs in the region (**Table 2-5**) (Alberts et al., 2005).

TABLE 2-5 Components of a Comprehensive Stroke Center

Personnel with expertise in the following areas
Vascular neurology or neuroscience intensive care
Vascular neurosurgery or nursing director for stroke program
APN
Vascular surgery
Diagnostic radiology/neuroradiology
Interventional/endovascular physician(s)
Critical care medicine
Physical medicine and rehabilitation
Rehabilitation therapy (physical, occupational, speech therapy)
Staff stroke nurse(s)
RT
Swallowing assessment

Diagnostic techniques
MRI with diffusion (IA) or MR perfusion (IIB)
MRA/MRV (IA) or CT perfusion (IIIC)
CTA (IA) or Xenon CT (IIIC)
Digital cerebral angiography (IA) or SPECT (IIIC)
TCD (IA) or PET (IIB)
Carotid duplex U/S (IA)
Transesophageal echo (IA)

Surgical and interventional therapies
CEA (IA)
    Clipping of intracranial aneurysm (IA) or stenting/angioplasty of extracranial vessels (IIB)*
    Placement of ventriculostomy (IA) or stenting/angioplasty of intracranial vessels (IIIC)*
    Hematoma removal/draining (IIB–VC)
    Placement of intracranial pressure transducer (VC)
    Endovascular ablation of IAs/AVMs (IA)
    IA reperfusion therapy (IIB)
    Endovascular Rx of vasospasm (IIIC)

Infrastructure
Stroke unit[†] (IA)
ICU or stroke clinic
Operating room staffed 24/7 or air ambulance
Interventional services coverage 24/7 or neuroscience ICU
Stroke registry (IIIC)

Educational/research programs
Community education (IA) or clinical research
Community prevention (IA) or Laboratory research
Professional education or fellowship program
Patient education or presentations at national meetings

APN, advanced practice nurse; RT, respiratory therapist; MR, magnetic resonance; MRA, magnetic resonance angiography; MRV, magnetic resonance venography; CTA, computed tomography angiography; SPECT, single photon emission computed tomography; TCD, transcranial Doppler; PET, positron emission tomography; U/S, ultrasound; CEA, carotid endarterectomy; AVMs, arteriovenous malformations; Rx, prescription; ICU, intensive care unit.
*Although these therapies are currently not supported by grade IA evidence, they may be useful for selected patients in some clinical settings. Therefore, a CSC that does not offer these therapies should have an established referral mechanism and protocol to send appropriate patients to another facility that does offer these therapies.
[†]The stroke unit may be a part of an ICU.
From Alberts, M. J., Latchaw, R. E., Selman, W. R., Shephard, T., Hadley, M. N., Brass, L. M., . . . Walker, M. D. (2005). Recommendations for comprehensive stroke centers: A consensus statement from the Brain Attack Coalition. *Stroke, 36*(7), 1597–1616.

Acute Stroke–Ready Hospitals

Recent studies have shown that approximately 50% of U.S. population does not reside within 60 minutes of a PSC (Alberts et al., 2013). In 2013, Alberts et al. published a paper recommending from the BAC the formation and designation of ASRH to better cover the U.S. population. Formal development of resources that follow the same principles as PSC's in providing organized structured care protocols, resource allocation to support emergency care, and processes for access to expanded neurological expertise with telemedicine would further equip hospitals to offer rapid stroke intervention and coordinated interfacility transfer (Alberts et al., 2013). It is estimated that 1,000 or more hospitals would be eligible to become ASRHs and interact with nearby PSCs and CSCs and further increase the ability to treat stroke patients.

Several key components of a PSC should be provided at an ASRH as essential and core care for acute stroke patients presenting in any setting. This can be summarized as nine specific care areas and three ancillary or support areas. As mentioned earlier, the AST is a necessary component and provides necessary support to ensure ability to administer IV tPA. Staffing of the ASRH AST would include minimally a nurse and a physician with stroke training and available 24/7 within 15 minutes of patient arrival. In some facilities, this is accomplished by combining the roles of other emergency response team such as code team or rapid response team. Written stroke protocols ensure organized stroke care and include orders for laboratory, imaging, and IV tPA with performance parameters. The critical relationship between EMS and emergency department requires a plan to ensure appropriate communication to receiving facility and include transportation to a CSC when needed. The use of telemedicine and teleradiology provides support to ensure access to neurological expertise is available to support local AST in the diagnosis and treatment of acute stroke patients. The development of written treatment protocols provides opportunity for the ASRH to provide emergent therapies such as IV tPA or reversal of coagulopathy prior to transporting patients to a PSC or CSC.

A number of ASRH may not have dedicated stroke unit resources but at a minimum should include well-trained nursing staff, the capability to provide cardiac telemetry monitoring, care protocols to prevent complications, neurological assessment tools, and tracking of outcomes (Alberts et al., 2013). Given the remote and rural settings of most ASRH, a plan for transport for neurosurgical services within 3 hours of identified need should be available. Hospital administration should take an active role in ensuring key programmatic elements, providing resources to ensure successful program, and identifying a physician leader with cerebrovascular disease training. Additionally, transfer agreements with PSC or CSC should include detailed written plan that includes air and ground transfer options.

Outcome measures frequently used in PSC may be adapted to ASRHs (Alberts et al., 2013). Performance metrics such as hospital arrival to treatment time for IV tPA, initial imaging and physician assessment, as well as other standard metrics should be monitored to ensure ongoing adherence to guidelines. The appropriate threshold for compliance in an ASRH is still in development. Additional information monitored might include transfer and transportation protocols.

Presently, there are some states that are already incorporating the ASRH tier of hospital facilities into the overall systems of care. The BAC strongly supports the development of an ASRH certification program that would include certification to be performed by outside independent organization; onsite assessment of facility, protocols, and staff; and collection of at least four performance metrics. The BAC suggests ASRH certification should occur every 2 to 3 years (Alberts et al., 2013).

▮▮ BENEFITS OF A STROKE CENTER

The major benefits of stroke centers include improved organization of stroke care and improved patient outcomes after stroke (**Table 2-6**) (Alberts et al., 2000). Several studies demonstrate the impact of stroke centers in limiting poststroke disability and reducing health costs. Improving the timeliness of stroke care and number of patients receiving IV tPA are significant contributors to this decline in poststroke disability and health care cost. Research shows that receiving treatment with IV tPA earlier is associated with improved outcome. Quantitative estimates have cited that the typical patient loses 1.9 million neurons each minute in which a stroke is untreated (Saver, 2006). Studies demonstrate that with every 15-minute reduction in door-to-needle times, there was a 5% lower odds of risk-adjusted, in-hospital mortality (Fonarow, Smith, Saver, Reeves, Hernandez, et al., 2011). Results from clinical trials have encouraged multiple organizations to set targets for timely initiation of thrombolytic therapy after hospital arrival. Several recent studies demonstrate that stroke centers are more likely to administer IV tPA and to administer the medication faster than non-stroke centers (Gorelick, 2013).

The ASA GWTG-S database participation program provides a data solution that has been adopted by over 1,000 hospitals and has over 1 million patient records. This database serves as a national stroke registry and is believed to be representative of the national fee for service Medicare population (Gorelick, 2013). Hospitals can use this database to track key metrics, target areas for improvement, and benchmark against other groups. Centers for Medicare and Medicaid Services (CMS) has adopted stroke core measures, further supporting stroke performance improvement. A critical function of stroke systems approach to stroke care is the use of continuous quality improvement initiatives. Essential to quality efforts is data accessibility and transfer of data to providers and facilities. In 2005, the Task Force on Stroke Systems of Care endorsed the development of consensus performance measures and the evaluation of system components in collaboration with key stakeholders (L. H. Schwamm et al., 2005).

TABLE 2-6 Benefits of a Primary Stroke Center

Improved efficiency of patient care
Fewer peristroke complications
Increased use of acute stroke therapies
Reduced morbidity and mortality
Improved long-term outcomes
Reduced cost to health care systems
Increased patient satisfaction

Alberts, M. J., Hademenos, G., Latchaw, R. E., Jagoda, A., Marler, J. R., Mayberg, M. R., . . . Walker, M. D. (2000). Recommendations for the establishment of primary stroke centers. Brain Attack Coalition. *The Journal of the American Medical Association, 283*(23), 3102–3109.

The impact organized care at a stroke center can have at reducing mortality cannot be overemphasized. Patients treated at PSCs are more likely to be alive, independent, and living at home 1 year after stroke than those treated in general care hospitals (Silva & Schwamm, 2013). The organization of care provided on stroke units has been reported in multiple studies to reduce stroke-related morbidity, length of stay, and stroke-related mortality (Fuentes & Díez-Tejedor, 2009). Additionally, several meta-analyses confirm the number needed to treat with organized stroke care to prevent one death was 33, to prevent one patient being unable to live at home was 20, and to prevent one patient failing to regain independence was 20 ("Collaborative Systematic Review," 1997). Langhorne et al. (2013) completed a systematic review and meta-analysis confirming that patients with ICH benefit at least much as ischemic stroke patients from organized stroke care.

Development of a network of ASRHs, PSCs, and CSCs will increase the chances that patients will receive appropriate stroke treatment in a timely and effective manner, increasing the chance of better patient outcomes. The reality that only 5% to 7% of patients with ischemic stroke will receive treatment with IV tPA further supports a need to provide organized care. The regionalization of care will better coordinate resources such as EMS, telemedicine, and stroke centers, ensuring the most appropriate level of care (Higashida et al., 2013).

▌▌ RECOGNIZING STROKE CENTERS

Certification versus Designation as a Stroke Center

In health care, third-party certification has played an important role in the development of an SSC in the United States. However, hospital accreditation and certification are different processes often offered by the same external reviewers such as TJC. Hospital accreditation can be defined as an external peer assessment process used by accrediting bodies to evaluate whether a hospital satisfies established standards (Fonarow et al., 2010). Hospital accreditation is mandatory to receive federal dollars for health care reimbursement, whereas hospital certification programs are voluntary. To become certified, programs must meet structural, process, and performance standards for treating a specific disease population (Fonarow et al., 2010). Presently, hospitals can seek certification from a number of well-established programs. TJC accredits approximately 80% of U.S. hospitals and has partnered with the AHA, launching PSC certification in 2003. This certification is based on the recommendations from the BAC and the ASA/AHA. Certification is granted to a facility that demonstrates compliance with national standards and has developed care pathways based on clinical practice guidelines and performance measurement and improvement activities (Fonarow et al., 2010).

A large majority of stroke certified hospitals are certified by TJC. Additionally, Healthcare Facilities Accreditation Program (HFAP) and Det Norske Veritas (DNV) offer a similar certification process that involves on-site assessment of compliance with national standards, clinical practice guidelines, and performance measurement and improvement activities.

Several hospital recognition programs are available through participation with databases such as GWTG-S and Coverdell. Exemplary outcome reporting through GWTG-S may result in an award for performance such as the Silver Award, Gold Award, and Platinum Award for performance measures. These awards provide recognition to hospitals that achieve certain performance levels on standardized quality measures (Fonarow et al., 2010). However, they should not be confused with external certification programs.

Many states in the United States have also developed methods to recognize hospitals as stroke centers that are managed through direct reporting to state department of health. These programs are guided by state legislation, and requirements vary from state to state. The state designation process generally does not include on-site validation. Some states require attestation of program services and submission of performance data. The following websites will be helpful for certification criteria and details related to achieving certification:

- http://www.jointcommission.org/certification/primary_stroke_centers.aspx
- http://www.hfap.org/AccreditationPrograms/certificationProcess.aspx
- http://dnvglhealthcare.com/certifications/stroke-certifications

The SSCM recognizes the need for synergy between CSCs and noncertified hospitals in meeting the needs of patients residing in communities across the nation. All hospitals caring for stroke patients should have transfer protocols to ensure timely interfacility transport to meet patient needs. Careful consideration of patient transport and offering of tPA treatment will ensure that all patients are afforded full available treatments.

Role of Telemedicine

The SSCM recommends implementation of telemedicine and aeromedical transport to increase access to acute stroke care in underserved areas. Although a tiered system of stroke hospitals may cover a majority of counties nationally, not every county will have quick access to an ASRH or PSC staffed with stroke experts. Therefore, stroke telemedicine may bridge the geographical disparities and allow stroke victims' access to stroke experts through the use of technology. Telemedicine has been defined broadly as "the use of telecommunications technologies to provide medical information and services" (Perednia & Allen, 1995, p. 483). Telemedicine is integrated audio and visual remote assessment allowing two-way real-time conferencing between a patient and a caregiver. Telemedicine used for stroke care commonly includes patient access to stroke neurology and radiology services. Teleradiology supports stroke telemedicine by ability to obtain radiographic images at one location and transmit to another for diagnostic and consultative purposes (Jauch et al., 2013). The benefits of telestroke are several: increased use of IV tPA; decreased door-to-treatment times; has been proven to have similar safety as PSCs in symptomatic ICH 2% to 7%; and in-house mortality rate of 3.5% (Jauch et al., 2013).

Telestroke systems continue to supplement resources at participating sites in stroke systems promoting around the clock coverage for a health care facility and allow ongoing access to specialist that may not be on-site. The United States has approximately 4 neurologists per 100,000 persons, caring for more than 700,000 acute strokes per year (L. H. Schwamm et al., 2009). Remote services require contracts for services, credentialing and privileging, protocols for care, and ongoing performance improvement with both hub and spoke sites. Additionally, equipment maintenance and staff training are key areas that lend to successful use of this technology. Typical telestroke providers use two-way audiovisual communication through laptop computers, access to imaging archives, and communication systems that allow provider interaction with patient and family at remote sites of care (Higashida et al., 2013). Additionally, telemedicine can be used to provide ongoing care for subacute stroke, support intensive care surveillance and monitoring, and can improve transitions in care from acute to subacute levels.

Postacute Rehabilitation and Community Reintegration

The majority of patients after a stroke will require rehabilitation services, and a fully integrated SSC offers all stroke survivors access to rehabilitation services when needed. Rehabilitation should be started as early as possible in the hospital setting. Eligible patients should have access to acute rehabilitation professionals. Acute rehabilitation is best coordinated by an interprofessional team directed not only at restoration of function and compensation for lost function but also at preventing secondary complications (Rymer et al., 2014). Formal rehabilitative efforts may occur for months, whereas the adjustment and recovery process is lifelong. The current SSCM does not adequately address how to facilitate integrated rehabilitation services and community reintegration for all stroke patients. Further research and advocacy is needed to guide this end of the SCC continuum.

S U M M A R Y

Over the last two decades, the concept and definition of an integrated SSC has evolved. We now have established formal criteria for three levels of care, evidenced-based clinical practice guidelines to guide care in these centers, and performance improvement processes and outcome measures in stroke care. Additional efforts continue to define how centers within an SSC should interact to best provide timely access for emergency care and, offer specialty consultation using technology and advanced transport to support early and aggressive offering of treatment to reverse or limit disability from stroke. Building care teams that span the continuum is a priority to meet lifelong needs for enhanced care coordination post hospitalization.

R E F E R E N C E S

Alberts, M. J., Hademenos, G., Latchaw, R. E., Jagoda, A., Marler, J. R., Mayberg, M. R., . . . Walker, M. D. (2000). Recommendations for the establishment of primary stroke centers. Brain Attack Coalition. *The Journal of the American Medical Association*, *283*(23), 3102–3109.

Alberts, M. J., Latchaw, R. E., Jagoda, A., Wechsler, L. R., Crocco, T., George, M. G., . . . Walker, M. D. (2011). Revised and updated recommendations for the establishment of primary stroke centers: A summary statement from the brain attack coalition. *Stroke*, *42*(9), 2651–2665. doi:10.1161/STROKEAHA.111.615336

Alberts, M. J., Latchaw, R. E., Selman, W. R., Shephard, T., Hadley, M. N., Brass, L. M., . . . Walker, M. D. (2005). Recommendations for comprehensive stroke centers: A consensus statement from the Brain Attack Coalition. *Stroke*, *36*(7), 1597–1616. doi:10.1161/01.STR.0000170622.07210.b4

Alberts, M. J., Wechsler, L. R., Jensen, M. E., Latchaw, R. E., Crocco, T. J., George, M. G., . . . Walker, M. D. (2013). Formation and function of acute stroke-ready hospitals within a stroke system of care recommendations from the brain attack coalition. *Stroke*, *44*(12), 3382–3393. doi:10.1161/STROKEAHA.113.002285

Candelise, L., Gattinoni, M., Bersano, A., Micieli, G., Sterzi, R., & Morabito, A. (2007). Stroke-unit care for acute stroke patients: An observational follow-up study. *Lancet*, *369*(9558), 299–305. doi:10.1016/S0140-6736(07)60152-4

Collaborative systematic review of the randomised trials of organised inpatient (stroke unit) care after stroke. Stroke Unit Trialists' Collaboration. (1997). *British Medical Journal*, *314*(7088), 1151–1159.

Foley, N., Salter, K., & Teasell, R. (2007). Specialized stroke services: A meta-analysis comparing three models of care. *Cerebrovascular Diseases*, *23*(2–3), 194–202. doi:10.1159/000097641

Fonarow, G. C., Gregory, T., Driskill, M., Stewart, M. D., Beam, C., Butler, J., . . . Sacco, R. L. (2010). Hospital certification for optimizing cardiovascular disease and stroke quality of care and outcomes. *Circulation*, *122*(23), 2459–2469. doi:10.1161/CIR.0b013e3182011a81

Fonarow, G. C., Smith, E. E., Saver, J. L., Reeves, M. J., Bhatt, D. L., Grau-Sepulveda, M. V., . . . Schwamm, L. H. (2011). Timeliness of tissue-type plasminogen activator therapy in acute ischemic stroke: Patient characteristics, hospital factors, and outcomes associated with door-to-needle times within 60 minutes. *Circulation*, *123*(7), 750–758. doi:10.1161/CIRCULATIONAHA.110.974675

Fonarow, G. C., Smith, E. E., Saver, J. L., Reeves, M. J., Hernandez, A. F., Peterson, E. D., . . . Schwamm, L. H. (2011). Improving door-to-needle times in acute ischemic stroke: The design and rationale for the American Heart Association/American Stroke Association's Target: Stroke initiative. *Stroke, 42*(10), 2983–2989. doi:10.1161/STROKEAHA.111.621342

Fuentes, B., & Díez-Tejedor, E. (2009). Stroke units: Many questions, some answers. *International Journal of Stroke, 4*(1), 28–37. doi:10.1111/j.1747-4949.2009.00244.x

Gorelick, P. B. (2013). Primary and comprehensive stroke centers: History, value and certification criteria. *Journal of Stroke, 15*(2), 78–89. doi:10.5853/jos.2013.15.2.78

Higashida, R., Alberts, M. J., Alexander, D. N., Crocco, T. J., Demaerschalk, B. M., Derdeyn, C. P., . . . Wood, J. P. (2013). Interactions within stroke systems of care: A policy statement from the American Heart Association/American Stroke Association. *Stroke, 44*(10), 2961–2984. doi:10.1161/STR.0b013e3182a6d2b2

Jauch, E. C., Saver, J. L., Adams, H. P., Jr., Bruno, A., Connors, J. J., Demaerschalk, B. M., . . . Yonas, H. (2013). Guidelines for the early management of patients with acute ischemic stroke: A guideline for healthcare professionals from the American Heart Association/American Stroke Association. *Stroke, 44*(3), 870–947. doi:10.1161/STR.0b013e318284056a

Langhorne, P., Fearon, P., Ronning, O. M., Kaste, M., Palomaki, H., Vemmos, K., . . . Al-Shahi Salman, R. (2013). Stroke unit care benefits patients with intracerebral hemorrhage: Systematic review and meta-analysis. *Stroke, 44*(11), 3044–3049. doi:10.1161/STROKEAHA.113.001564

Perednia, D. A., & Allen, A. (1995). Telemedicine technology and clinical applications. *The Journal of the American Medical Association, 273*(6), 483–488.

Rymer, M. M., Anderson, C. S., Harada, M., Jarosz, J., Ma, N., Rowley, H. A., . . . Bornstein, N. M. (2014). Stroke service: How can we improve and measure outcomes? Consensus summary from a global stroke forum. *Acta Neurologica Scandinavica, 130*(2), 73–80. doi:10.1111/ane.12256

Saver, J. L. (2006). Time is brain—quantified. *Stroke, 37*(1), 263–266. doi:10.1161/01.STR.0000196957.55928.ab

Schwamm, L., Fayad, P., Acker, J. E., III., Duncan, P., Fonarow, G. C., Girgus, M., . . . Yancy, C. W. (2010). Translating evidence into practice: a decade of efforts by the American Heart Association/American Stroke Association to reduce death and disability due to stroke: A presidential advisory from the American Heart Association/American Stroke Association. *Stroke, 41*(5), 1051–1065. doi:10.1161/STR.0b013e3181d2da7d

Schwamm, L. H., Audebert, H. J., Amarenco, P., Chumbler, N. R., Frankel, M. R., George, M. G., . . . White, C. J. (2009). Recommendations for the implementation of telemedicine within stroke systems of care: A policy statement from the American Heart Association. *Stroke, 40*(7), 2635–2660. doi:10.1161/STROKEAHA.109.192361

Schwamm, L. H., Pancioli, A., Acker, J. E., III., Goldstein, L. B., Zorowitz, R. D., Shephard, T. J., . . . Adams, R. J. (2005). Recommendations for the establishment of stroke systems of care: Recommendations from the American Stroke Association's Task Force on the development of stroke systems. *Circulation, 111*(8), 1078–1091. doi:10.1161/01.CIR.0000154252.62394.1E

Silva, G. S., & Schwamm, L. H. (2013). Review of stroke center effectiveness and other get with the guidelines data. *Current Atherosclerosis Reports, 15*(9), 350. doi:10.1007/s11883-013-0350-8

Song, S., & Saver, J. (2012). Growth of regional acute stroke systems of care in the United States in the first decade of the 21st century. *Stroke, 43*(7), 1975–1978. doi:10.1161/STROKEAHA.112.657809

WEB REFERENCES

Institute for Healthcare Improvement. (2014). *Triple aim for populations.* Retrieved from http://www.ihi.org /Topics/TripleAim/Pages/default.aspx

The Joint Commission. (2014a). *Requirements for advanced primary stroke centers.* Retrieved from http://www .jointcommission.org/certification/primary_stroke_centers.aspx

The Joint Commission. (2014b). *Requirements for comprehensive stroke center advanced certification.* Retrieved from http://www.jointcommission.org/assets/1/6/CSC_DSC_March2014.pdf

CHAPTER 3

Interprofessional Teams in Stroke Care

Patricia A. Blissitt

As the fourth leading cause of death and the leading cause of disability, stroke necessitates care of the highest quality (Centers for Disease Control and Prevention, 2012; Miniño, Murphy, Xu, & Kochanek, 2011). Excellence in stroke care includes interprofessional teams who consistently demonstrate collaboration at the highest level. The stroke patient or the individual at risk for stroke may enter the health care system requiring different levels of care that change over time. In addition, multiple disciplines and subspecialties within each discipline have essential roles to fulfill, and within each discipline, the role of the health care professional may change depending on where the patient is in his or her disease trajectory and care setting.

Because of the many diverse and changing needs of the stroke patient, health care professionals who interface with stroke patients, both directly and indirectly, must include interprofessional collaboration as an essential competency in their practices. This chapter will (1) define interprofessional collaboration, (2) delineate the interprofessional practice model, (3) describe interprofessional stroke teams across the continuum, (4) identify team building competencies as well as barriers to interprofessional collaboration, (5) describe tools that may facilitate interprofessional collaboration, and (6)provide exemplars reflecting strong interprofessional collaboration.

INTERPROFESSIONAL COLLABORATION

Collaborative work between health care professionals has been assigned a number of terms as health care has evolved over the decades, including interdisciplinary, multi-disciplinary, interprofessional, multiprofessional, and transdisciplinary (Leathard, 2003; Mitchell, 2005; Nancarrow et al., 2013). All of these models of collaboration in health care are associated with teamwork. However, some distinctions have been made among the terms. The terms *interprofessional* and *multiprofessional* have a narrower focus than *interdisciplinary* and *multidisciplinary* (Atwal & Caldwell, 2002; McCallin, 2001). Interprofessional and multiprofessional are generally defined as consisting entirely of professionals from different disciplines, whereas interdisciplinary and multidisciplinary includes professional and nonprofessional staff (Nancarrow et al., 2013). Some authors go on to explain that interprofessional denotes collaboration, whereas multiprofessional and multidisciplinary do not (Goodman & Clemow, 2010). Transdisciplinary collaboration has been used to delineate the development of a new conceptual framework that diminishes the barriers to interprofessional work (Nowotney, 2005; Weaver, 2008). Transdisciplinary work diminishes traditional differences between disciplines and uses a holistic approach to collaborative work, with the result being more than the sum of the individual disciplines' contributions. New approaches, knowledge, products, or even new disciplines may result from transdisciplinary work (Weaver, 2008).

To further explain interprofessional practice, a number of related interprofessional operational definitions have been developed to provide the team members with a common language from which to develop a high-performing team. These terms include *interprofessionality, interprofessional education, interprofessional collaborative practice, interprofessional teamwork, interprofessional team-based care, professional competencies in health, interprofessional competencies in health care, interprofessional competencies,* and *interprofessional competency domain* (Interprofessional Education Collaborative Expert Panel, 2011) (**Table 3-1**). Interprofessionality is the fundamental concept used to explain the process that must occur for the patient's needs to be met. Characteristics of interprofessionality include continuous interaction, knowledge sharing to address

---

TABLE 3-1 Interprofessional Collaborative Practice Operational Definitions

Interprofessional education: "when students from two or more professions learn about, from and with each other to enable effective collaboration and improve health outcomes"*

Interprofessional collaborative practice: "when multiple health workers from different professional backgrounds work together with patients, families, carers [sic], and communities to deliver the highest quality of care"*

Interprofessional teamwork: the levels of cooperation, coordination, and collaboration characterizing the relationships between professions in delivering patient-centered care

Interprofessional team-based care: care delivered by intentionally created, usually relatively small workgroups in health care, who are recognized by others as well as by themselves as having a collective identity and shared responsibility for a patient or group of patients (e.g., rapid response team, palliative care team, primary care team, operating room team)

Professional competencies in health care: integrated enactment of knowledge, skills, and values/attitudes that define the domains of work of a particular health profession applied in specific care contexts

Interprofessional competencies in health care: integrated enactment of knowledge, skills, and values/attitudes that define working together across the professions, with other health care workers, and with patients, along with families and communities, as appropriate to improve health outcomes in specific care contexts

Interprofessional competency domain: a generally identified cluster of more specific interprofessional competencies that are conceptually linked and serve as theoretical constructs[†]

*ten Cate, O., & Scheele, F. (2007). Competency-based postgraduate training: Can we bridge the gap between theory and practice? *Academic Medicine, 82*(6), 542–547.

[†]World Health Organization. (2010). *Framework for action on interprofessional education and collaborative practice* (WHO Reference No. WHO/HRH/HPN/10.3). Geneva, Switzerland: Health Professions Network Nursing and Midwifery Office, Department of Human Resources for Health. Retrieved from http://www.who.int/hrh/resources/framework_action/en/

From Interprofessional Education Collaborative Expert Panel. (2011). *Core competencies for interprofessional collaborative practice: Report of an expert panel.* Washington, DC: Interprofessional Education Collaborative.

education and care issues, patient participation, an ethical code of conduct, and an integrated collaborative workflow (D'Amour & Oandasan, 2005).

INTERPROFESSIONAL PRACTICE MODELS

A number of interprofessional practice models have been developed. Although models may differ in their composition and roles, most interprofessional practice frameworks include a set of values and/or core competencies critical to their model. For example, an early model described by Ponte, Gross, Winer, Connaughton, and Hassinger (2007) consisted of only three team members: the nurse, physician, and hospital administrator. Yet, many of the concepts included in this model such as collaboration, decision making, patient- and family-centered care, patient safety, and priority setting are still considered essential to the effectiveness of the interprofessional practice model today (Ponte et al., 2007). In addition, earlier models of interprofessional teams embraced a style of interdisciplinary leadership that included empowerment of the individual in a nonhierarchical, nonthreatening environment and a partnership in which team members learn from each other and collectively become more effective than the individual contributions of each health care professional (Dietrich et al., 2010; Richardson & Storr, 2010). These principles are considered key to the work of interprofessional teamwork today as well.

In 2009, Hammick, Freeth, Copperman, and Goodsman stated that the core values of being interprofessional are respect, confidence, engagement with others, caring disposition, approachable attitude, and willingness to share. Competencies for being an interprofessional team member included (1) knowledge related to the work of others and teamwork; (2) collaborative and communicative skills and application of interprofessional education principles; and (3) appreciation and respect for others' collaboration, views, values, and ideas (Hammick et al., 2009). More recently, national and international interprofessional panels have developed formal frameworks calling for the urgent development of interprofessional collaborative practice and have detailed competency domains delineating specific attributes (Interprofessional Education Collaborative Expert Panel, 2011; World Health Organization [WHO], 2010). WHO (2010) defines the domains of interprofessional practice (and learning) as teamwork, roles and responsibilities, communication, learning and critical reflection, recognizing the needs of patients and developing a relationship with them, and ethical practice. Similarly in 2011, the Interprofessional Education Collaborative Expert Panel—composed of the American Association of Colleges of Nursing, American Association of Colleges of Osteopathic Medicine, American Association of Colleges of Pharmacy, American Dental Education Association, Association of American Medical Colleges, and the Association of Schools of Public Health—established competencies in four domains: values and ethics, roles and responsibilities, communication, and teams and teamwork.

More recently, Ash and Miller (2014) attributed successful interprofessional collaboration to many of the same characteristics described earlier, including shared purpose, shared decision making, reciprocal trust, team member recognition and value, high-level performance, role and responsibility clarity, collaborative work culture, strong leadership, effective communication, and conflict resolution. In addition, they added the concepts of emotional intelligence, transformational leadership, differentiation of leadership and management, and the role of change agent, continuous reflective learning, and the patient and family as members of the interprofessional team.

Emotional intelligence is one's awareness of the role emotion plays in relationships and how emotions can be used in a positive manner to facilitate communications and motivate others. Transformational leaders empower others to achieve shared goals using coaching and mentoring to inspire others toward a desired state (Institute of Medicine, 2011). The focus of leadership involves the development of relationships through modeling, inspiring, challenging, enabling others, and encouragement. In contrast, management concepts emphasize using resources to meet organizational goals rather than a concerted focus on the development of the team and its individual members to maximize outcomes. The interprofessional team must view themselves as change agents who continuously learn and reflect on that learning to adapt and change as needed to meet the team's goals. The team's inclusion of the patient and family as a member of the team, with full disclosure of the patient's condition, provision of meaningful and consistent patient and family education, and facilitation of an active patient and family voice in decision making, are conducive to patient- and family-centered care (Institute of Medicine, 2011). Patient- and family-centered care empowers the patient and family to maximally benefit from the work of the team with greater understanding of their disease and how they can make a difference in their recovery. Patient- and family-centered care also results in greater patient, family, and team satisfaction (Ash & Miller, 2014). The interprofessional practice models, described earlier and still evolving, are essential to ensure stroke care of the highest quality.

INTERPROFESSIONAL STROKE TEAMS ACROSS THE CONTINUUM OF CARE

The teamwork that occurs in stroke care depends on a number of factors, including the patient's clinical presentation, the type of stroke, treatment options, and the extent of disabilities. The roles of the interprofessional health team members may extend beyond a single acuity level and transition point. Stroke care often requires multiple interprofessional teams that provide a continuum of care within and across institutions without disruption to minimize risk of deterioration and poor outcomes. See **Table 10-2** for possible interprofessional team members and roles.

The levels of care for stroke patients include prehospital, telestroke, and emergency department (ED) care; acute care; critical care; electronic intensive care unit (ICU); progressive care; rehabilitation; skilled nursing facility care; long-term care; nursing home care; home care; secondary prevention; and palliative care. The goals of primary and secondary prevention include identification of risk factors and effective management of modifiable risk factors (see Chapter 1). Critical to effective management of modifiable risk factors is patient and family education and access to care to assist the patient with compliance (Goldstein et al., 2011).

Prehospital, telestroke, and ED personnel have shared roles, including identification of stroke, field response, transport, evaluation, emergent care, consultation, and referral for additional interventions and management (Audebert, 2006; Gorelick, Gorelick, & Sloan, 2008; Stradling, 2009). Depending on the emergency medical system within a geographic area, an emergency medical technician may be the first responder at the scene but may ask for additional support from paramedics with advanced life support training for the stroke patient with life-threatening cardiopulmonary disease. This will enable provision of airway protection and resuscitation including medication administration at the scene. After the initial workup and management at the first hospital, if the level of care needed by the patient is not available at the first hospital, the prehospital providers, including flight nurses and paramedics, may transport the patient from the original hospital without higher level stroke management expertise to a primary or comprehensive stroke center by ground or air.

EMERGENCY DEPARTMENT ADMISSION

In the ED, much of the interprofessional team work is performed by physicians, advanced practice nurses, physician assistants, nurses, and respiratory therapists. Medical specialties include emergency medicine, neurology, neurosurgery, neuro-radiology neurointerventionists, neurointensivists, hospitalists, physiatry, and other specialties that may be needed as consultants to make recommendations about the stroke patient's care. For example, risk factors that have contributed to the stroke may be problematic in managing the stroke, such as cardiac disease and diabetes mellitus. The stroke itself may have resulted in complications such as respiratory compromise, the inability to maintain a patent airway, ineffective breathing, aspiration, or a stunned myo-cardium in aneurysmal subarachnoid hemorrhage.

Once the patient has arrived in the ED, a stroke code may be called. However, the stroke neurologist or neurosurgeon may have already been informed about the in-coming patient and established a plan that includes continued stabilization and rapid neurological assessment including imaging, laboratory analysis, and determination of definitive treatment with attention to time-sensitive interventions. More than one facil-ity may be involved such as the receiving hospital with limited resources and a primary or comprehensive stroke center. The stroke neurologist at the primary or comprehensive stroke center may review imaging and clinical presentation with the physician at the receiving hospital. Inclusion and exclusion criteria for intravenous (IV) recombinant tissue plasminogen activator (rtPA) may be reviewed and a plan of care determined. For example, the IV rtPA may be started at the receiving hospital followed by a transfer to the primary or comprehensive stroke center. The pharmacist may be directly involved with rtPA dosing and blood pressure management strategies. Neurosurgery may be consulted for a hemorrhagic stroke or increased intracranial pressure from a large territory stroke. Interventional neuroradiology may also be consulted for endovascular therapies such as aneurysmal stenting and coiling (Summers et al., 2009).

ED nurses are responsible for assessing and monitoring the patient with attention to airway, breathing, and circulation; neurological status; responsiveness related to thera-pies; and blood pressure control. Neither physicians nor nurses can work in isolation to maximize the impact of their efforts without the involvement of other disciplines to accomplish mutual goals for the patient.

The respiratory therapist will assess the respiratory system, provide pulmonary hygiene, manage oxygen therapy, or collaborate with the team regarding intubation and mechanical ventilation management. If the patient is awake and stable, a nurse-directed swallow screen may be performed to screen for safety from aspiration. If it is determined that the patient is at low risk for aspiration, oral medications can be safely administered. In the acute phase of stroke, respiratory therapists work to reduce risk of hypoxia, aspiration, and ventilator-associated pneumonia post stroke.

Although patient and family education begins in the ED and can be undertaken by any team members, the education is very focused on the stroke and immediate treatment decisions. Palliative care may be consulted as needed for comfort or end-of-life consid-erations as the patient's condition warrants (Creutzfeldt, Holloway, & Walker, 2012).

ADMISSION TO THE ACUTE CARE FACILITY

Upon admission to the critical care, acute care, or stroke unit in an acute care hospital, more team members become involved in patient care. An additional diagnostic workup and consultation by neurosurgery, interventional neuroradiology, or interventional neuroradiology may be required. A decompressive craniectomy may be indicated in a large territory ischemic stroke or hemorrhagic stroke. Insertion of an external ventricular drainage device may be indicated for subarachnoid hemorrhage or intraparenchymal stroke and may be performed at the bedside in critical care or in the operating room (OR).

Depending on the severity of the stroke and the level of consciousness, an initial evaluation by rehabilitation therapies may occur early on admission or postponed until the patient's condition stabilizes. If the patient did not pass the nurse swallow screen, the speech therapist will evaluate swallowing and also assess the patient's communication and cognitive functions. Respiratory therapy will continue to assess and intervene for airway and breathing issues, both directly related to the acute stroke and any prestroke pulmonary issues such as obstructive sleep apnea, a risk factor for stroke, and chronic obstructive pulmonary disease. Physical and occupational therapy will evaluate extremity strength, tone, and coordination and provide recommendations and interventions around such rehabilitation strategies as protective positioning, range of motion, mobilization, and working with perceptual deficits. Once tone returns to the affected extremities, occupational and physical therapists will evaluate and assist in the management of spasticity as needed (Miller et al., 2010). The rehabilitation physician may be consulted to assess abilities and recommend management post stroke but prior to rehabilitation.

In critical care, the patient's medical management may be directed by a neurocritical care intensivist or a general critical care intensivist. Advanced practice nurses and physician's assistants may also direct the care of the stroke patient. The staff nurse assesses, plans, intervenes, and evaluates the patient holistically with attention to physiologic, cognitive, and psychosocial needs. Respiratory therapy may not only continue to provide the management initiated in the ED but also work toward discontinuation of mechanical ventilation and intubation as the patient's condition allows. The pharmacist will review the patient's prestroke medication profile and current pharmacological needs and reconcile those needs while assessing for drug interactions or adverse effects.

Early in critical care (or acute care), the dietitian will assess the patient's nutritional status and develop a plan for nutritional support, depending on the patient's ability for oral intake, or recommend enteral feedings. Parental nutrition is rarely required. Later in critical care or acute care phase, the dietitian may counsel patients about dietary risk reduction strategies for hyperlipidemia, diabetes mellitus, or other recommended dietary modifications. The rehabilitation therapists begin their work in the critical or acute care setting with an initial patient assessment followed by progressive activity as soon as the patient's condition has stabilized (Cell, Hassan, Marquardt, Breslow, & Rosenfeld, 2001; Connolly et al., 2012; Jauch et al., 2013; Morgenstern et al., 2010). Rehabilitation therapists include speech, occupational, physical, and recreational therapists. The focus of the speech therapist is swallowing, cognition (including attention and memory), and communication (including speech and language). Speech therapists, also referred to as *speech and language pathologists*, address perceptual disorders, such as apraxia, along with occupational and physical therapists (Miller et al., 2010). Occupational and physical therapists work with the patient to recover lost motor and sensory abilities especially in relationship to performing activities of daily living (ADLs). Compensatory measures are taught for residual deficits to optimize independence in ADLs.

Assistive devices may be incorporated into the patient's plan of care. Occupational therapists focus on ADLs, preventive/corrective splinting and positioning, and adaptation of the home and workplace environments to accommodate disabilities (Langhorne, Bernhardt, & Kwakkel, 2011; Milller et al., 2010; National Institutes of Health, National Institute of Neurological Disorders and Stroke, 2013; Pinter & Brainin, 2012).

Transitions between settings in the hospital are critical, as transitions are often associated with missed communication and errors. Attention to detail and effective handoffs between critical care and acute care teams are essential to prevent deterioration, new complications, and return to critical care. If the patient was originally admitted to critical care but has been advanced to acute care, increased mobilization such as up to chair and walking, depending on the patient's neurological status, now becomes an immediate focus of care. ⊙ Previous team members such as the physician, nurse, pharmacist, respiratory therapist, dietician, and speech, occupational, and physical therapists will continue to move the patient toward the highest level of functional recovery possible and minimize risk of complications related to impaired mobility and hospitalization including venous thromboembolism, bowel and bladder incontinence, skin breakdown, falls, and delirium. Patient and family education, particularly regarding risk factors and secondary prevention, will be emphasized, including comorbidities such as cardiovascular disease, pulmonary disease, and diabetes; medications for blood pressure and hyperlipidemia; and antiplatelet/anticoagulant medications. Education around other interventions may be taught to family members as well, including participation in therapies. A hospitalist or the stroke neurologist or neurosurgeon-led team may direct care in acute care (Summers et al., 2009).

If the patient is discharged from an acute care hospital and admitted to an in-hospital rehabilitation facility, the focus will, more than ever, be on the functional recovery and teaching both the patient and family what they need to know to achieve the highest functionality and quality of life possible. ⊙ The team approach is never more evident than in rehabilitation with the involvement of the physiatrist; rehabilitation nurse; speech, occupational, and physical therapists; recreational therapist; and neuropsychologist as needed, if not consulted, in critical or acute care. Recreational therapists may work with the stroke patient to incorporate diversional activities into their recovery program. Recreational therapists assist in the recovery of previously learned skills and the acquisition of new skills with a focus on community reintegration (Miller et al., 2010; Williams et al., 2007). See Chapter 10 for a discussion of rehabilitation.

⊙ Discharge planning will be coordinated by social services or another health care professional, such as a nurse in the role of a case manager or discharge facilitator. If not consulted previously, the neuropsychologist will assess for poststroke depression and coping skills.

▮▮ MATCHING THE NEXT LEVELS OF CARE WITH PATIENT NEEDS

Following acute stroke care, the next level of care will depend on the individual's functional recovery at the time of discharge. ⊙ The team will assess if the patient's current condition at discharge best enables him or her to meet the goals of care that are fostered in rehabilitation, skilled nursing, long-term health care facility, nursing home, or home with or without outpatient rehabilitation or home health visits (Langhorne et al., 2011). Failure of the interprofessional stroke care team(s) to recognize the best placement of the stroke patient at this time may result in physical, cognitive, and emotional deterioration; failure to facilitate recovery; and wasted resources. Regardless of the discharge disposition, the focus of continued care is secondary stroke prevention to minimize recurrent stroke.

In the event that the patient is unable to participate in at least 3 hours of therapy and requires more direct nursing care, the patient may be discharged to a skilled nursing facility, nursing home, long-term care facility, or, possibly, home. At a skilled nursing facility, the patient may receive additional rehabilitation therapies to improve his or her readiness for rehabilitation. Regardless, the goal, depending on the patient's condition, will be to maintain the highest quality of life possible and minimize complications.

⊙ Neuropsychologists can evaluate cognitive deficits and assist with the management of cognitive and neurobehavioral dysfunction, including providing counseling for the patient and family regarding poststroke depression (Miller et al., 2010). Social workers and rehabilitation counselors also support the patient's recovery from stroke by identifying resources, facilitating coping, and assisting the patient's return to a meaningful life. The vocational rehabilitation counselor's focus is vocational counseling and placement, whereas the social worker's goal is less focused on returning the patient to work but rather in supporting the patient with the ability to function at the highest level in society (Miller et al., 2010). ⊙ Social workers may initially assess the patient's living situation while the patient is in critical care or acute care. However, they often continue to educate, inform, and counsel patients and their family as well as advocate for them beyond the acute phase of their stroke in rehabilitation, nursing home, long-term and skilled nursing facilities, and the community settings.

Finally, palliative care may provide an environment to assist the patient and family with end-of-life decisions. Palliative care has a broader scope in symptom detection and management to improve quality of life (Creutzfeldt et al., 2012). ⊙ Palliative care specialists provide expert recommendations regarding symptom management and goal setting and may be consulted anywhere along the continuum of stroke care (Holloway et al., 2014). Specific examples of the palliative care specialist's role in the care of the stroke patient include the management of refractory pain, dyspnea, agitation, and emotional distress as well as assisting in decision making regarding long-term nutrition and mechanical ventilation (Holloway et al., 2014).

▣ STRATEGIES FOR BUILDING AND SUSTAINING INTERPROFESSIONAL TEAM

Successful interprofessional collaboration in stroke care depends on a number of team-building and team-sustaining strategies and may be facilitated by implementation of formal team-building initiatives and positively reinforced by current regulatory requirements in stroke care. A number of characteristics have been assigned to successful interprofessional teams, including effective communication; mutual respect and understanding; trust; an appropriate combination of expertise and experience; a mutual goal orientation toward quality outcomes; efficient and effective resources; individual and group flexibility; clear purpose, role, and vision; leadership; a team culture; education and training opportunities; a positive presence; individual strengths; and value of the group work for the individual as well as the group as a whole (Clark, 2009; Molyneux, 2001; Nancarrow et al., 2013; Weaver, 2008). Individually and collectively, these characteristics are in alignment with successful interprofessional collaboration in stroke care. Formal programs, also referred to as *tool kits*, may be implemented to facilitate development of these attributes within stroke teams.

One program that may enhance interprofessional collaboration of stroke teams is Team Strategies and Tools to Enhance Performance and Patient Safety (TeamSTEPPS) Program, an evidence-based program developed by the Agency for Healthcare Research and Quality (AHRQ) and the U.S. Department of Defense, to train teams in four major competencies including communication, leadership, situation or performance monitoring, and mutual support. Originally developed for use in aviation-related issues, this course includes both didactic and simulation work for the health care participants (AHRQ, 2014; Clancy, 2007; Clapper & Kong, 2012; Stead et al., 2009). TeamSTEPPS tools to support development of the competencies include resource management; delegation, briefs, debriefs, and small group huddles; situation awareness; cross monitoring of other's needs; and providing feedback to correct the situation.

The basic TeamSTEPPS framework and concepts are congruent with and complementary to the interprofessional model. Key elements of TeamSTEPPS include the knowledge, skills, and actions (KSA) associated with teamwork, leadership, situation monitoring, mutual support, and communication (AHRQ, 2014) (**Table 3-2**). Effective teams are defined as work units with shared roles and responsibilities, strong leadership, goals, plans, and priorities. High-performing teams are interactive, dynamic, interdependent, and adaptive. Leaders of teams keep the team focused yet allow the team members, individually and collectively, to flourish. Effective leaders facilitate

TABLE 3-2 TeamSTEPPS Patient Safety Tool

Teamwork Competencies through TeamSTEPPS	TeamSTEPPS Tools	Example
Leadership	Resource management Delegation Brief and debrief Group huddle	Facilitate problem solving. Clarify team goals and objectives. Clarify roles and expectations. Use, model, and encourage TeamSTEPPS competencies.
Situation monitoring	Situation awareness Cross monitoring	Anticipate and predict others' needs. Watch each other's back and provide corrective feedback.
Mutual support	Task assistance feedback Advocacy and assertion CUS (I'm **C**oncerned, I'm **U**ncomfortable, for safety's sake, I'm **S**topping the line) Collaboration Two-challenge rule (voicing your concerns at least two times to ensure it has been heard)	Team members and leader receive and deliver constructive feedback. Correct workload distribution. Shift responsibilities to underutilized team members and assist those who are overwhelmed.
Communication	SBAR (Situation—Background—Assessment—Recommendation) Checkback (for accuracy and clarification) Handoff Callout	Ensure that communication is understood. Use structured and standardized communication techniques such as SBAR during codes.

TeamSTEPPS, Team Strategies and Tools to Enhance Performance and Patient Safety.
From Clapper, T. C., & Kong, M. (2012). TeamSTEPPS®: The patient safety tool that needs to be implemented. *Clinical Simulation in Nursing, 8*(8), e367–e373. doi:10.1015/j.ecns.2011.03.002

team actions, model exemplary behavior, communicate effectively, monitor situations, delegate, resolve conflict, and manage resources. The TeamSTEPPS model includes the use of such tools as briefs for planning work, huddles for updating the team on emergent situations, and debriefs to analyze events, change plans, and promote learning (AHRQ, 2014).

Situation monitoring is the continuous process of quickly assessing behavior and actions to evaluate a situation or environment. The goal is to identify potential or actual issues before they worsen or are incapable of being reversed. Situation monitoring may be performed by the leader or other team members. Tools to facilitate situation monitoring include application of the Status of the patient, Team members, Environment, and Progress (STEP) mnemonic; the I'M SAFE checklist of self-mnemonic; cross monitoring of others; and a shared mental model. The "I'M SAFE" checklist is a quick look at one's self regarding factors that can impact performance of the leader and team members, including Illness, Medications, Stress, Alcohol/drug use, Fatigue, and to meet nutritional (Eat) and Elimination needs. Cross monitoring and assessing the situation as it relates to another team member fosters mutual respect and accountability of the team. Teamwork necessitates incorporation of a shared mental model of the situation with mutual understanding, effective communication, and actions to monitor adequately.

An extension of situation monitoring is the concept of mutual support. Mutual support is provided to fellow team members through feedback, advocacy, and assertion, including invoking the two-challenge rule; voicing concerns a minimum of two times to ensure effective communication; and expression of one's concern, uncomfortable state, and stopping the work being done (abbreviated as CUS for Concern, Uncomfortable [state], and Stopping [the work being done]). Another technique to facilitate mutual support is summarized as DESC, a mnemonic which includes Description of a particular situation, Expression of concern, Suggestion of other alternatives, and the potential Consequences of failure to respond to the situation.

TeamSTEPPS provides direction to maximize communication, including a discussion delineating effective technique. Structured communication during handoffs and emergent situations may be enhanced using the Situation, Background, Assessment, Recommendation (SBAR) technique (Clapper & Kong, 2012). Another TeamSTEPPS strategy to enhance information exchange at handoffs is "I PASS THE BATON," a mnemonic for Introduction, Patient, Assessment, Situation, Safety concerns, Background, Actions, Timing, Ownership, and Next (AHRQ, 2014). The use of callouts, directing critical information to a specific individual in an emergent situation; checkbacks, closing the communication loop to verify actions were taken; and handoffs, transferring essential information to another team member who will be responsible for future care are recommended to ensure effective communication. Exemplars will be provided later to demonstrate the applicability of TeamSTEPPS as a tool to support interprofessional stroke team care.

Another program, Six Sigma Lean, developed from concepts, methods, and tools used in the automobile industry, has also been used with success in the health care industry to improve quality, maximize efficiency, minimize waste, resolve clinical issues, and engage and empower team members. Brainstorming, process mapping, standardization, and mistake-proofing are some of the principles of Six Sigma Lean (Ahmed, Manaf, & Islam, 2013; Cima et al., 2011; Holden, 2011). Although little research has been conducted applying either TeamSTEPPS or Six Sigma Lean specific to stroke care, both have yielded improved outcomes in trauma care, EDs, ORs, critical care units, and laboratory and radiology department areas where efficiency, effectiveness, and safety are critical.

Mandates and incentives driven by regulatory agencies, professional organization, and quality measurement programs may also foster the development of interprofessional collaboration in stroke care. Achievement of benchmarks, such as the American Heart Association/American Stroke Association (AHA/ASA) *Getting with the Guidelines* stroke quality measures (AHA/ASA, 2014) and The Joint Commission (TJC) are conducive to team building. Primary and comprehensive stroke core measures may best be demonstrated by a cohesive group working in concert with each other, resulting in shorter inpatient stays, fewer complications, and optimal outcomes. Examples of such agencies and organizations include TJC for health care organizations, Det Norske Veritas (DNV), state departments of health, U.S. Centers for Medicare and Medicaid Services (CMS), other third-party payers, American Nurses Association Credentialing Corporation Magnet Program, National Database of Nursing Quality Indicators (NDNQI), and professional organizations with evidence-based guidelines such as the ASA.

INTERPROFESSIONAL EDUCATION AND RESEARCH

Interdisciplinary collaboration requires that the health care professional acquire a broad base of knowledge, skills, and practiced actions applicable to diverse setting and clinical situations often referred to as *competencies*. Until recently, intraprofessional education has not routinely included interdisciplinary courses in the curriculum to provide a group of students from different discipline opportunities to learn and practice collaboration in a safe, nonthreatening environment. As of 1995, in the United States, less than 15% of nursing and medical schools included interdisciplinary courses in their curriculum (Institute of Medicine, 2003) despite the fact that a number of organizations, including the Institute of Medicine, Robert Wood Johnson Foundation, American Nurses Association, TJC, American Association of Colleges of Nursing, and the Interdisciplinary and the Pharmacy Deans Task Force on Professionalism, have proclaimed the need for interprofessional collaboration (Ash & Miller, 2014; Institute of Medicine, 2003).

A number of barriers to interprofessional collaboration have been cited, including current generations of practicing clinicians who have not participated in interprofessional education and lack of strong evidence that interprofessional collaboration makes a difference in patient care, outcomes, and patient and clinician satisfaction. Lack of direct monetary rewards for interprofessional collaboration has been noted as well. More subtle obstacles have included societal barriers such as gender, power, education, educational and cultural disparities, lack of understanding of the other disciplines' scope of practice, and fear of role and expertise infringement by other disciplines (Ash & Miller, 2014; Institute of Medicine, 2011).

Research evaluating the value of interprofessional collaboration in stroke regarding improved patient outcomes and financial savings is lacking. Published research on interprofessional collaboration in stroke has been sparse; the literature has primarily been anecdotal. Most published studies focused on identification of successful teamwork, education, and the professional's experience as a member of a team rather than patient and financial benefits. Case studies, interpretative phenomenology, ethnography, and retrospective medical record reviews were among the methods used (Barreca & Wilkins, 2008; Burton, Fisher, & Green, 2009; Cheung et al., 2012; Fens et al., 2013; Momsen, Rasmussen, Nielsen, Iversen, & Lund, 2012; Pierce, 2005; Seneviratne, Mather, & Then, 2009; Vanderzalm, Hall, McFarlane, Rutherford, & Patterson, 2013). Although most conclude that interprofessional collaboration in stroke care is a positive experience that requires education and training that improves, Fens et al. (2013) concluded that interprofessional collaboration was not effective for patients being discharged home.

A recent meta-analysis on the effect of interprofessional education on professional practice and health care outcomes in general revealed 15 small studies, some of which demonstrated positive outcomes (Reeves, Perrier, Goldman, Freeth, & Zwarenstein, 2013). The only stroke publication included in the review was in regard to the use of the interprofessional clinical pathway in stroke rehabilitation (Falconer, Roth, Sutin, Strasser, & Chang, 1993). The information in the meta-analysis was not generalizable regarding specific elements that may contribute to the success of interprofessional model. Randomized controlled trials and investigations that focus on the benefit of interprofessional interventions rather than intraprofessional interventions are needed.

ADDITIONAL TOOLS FOR INTERPROFESSIONAL COLLABORATION

A number of stroke assessment scales (**Table 3-3**) commonly used in stroke care can serve as effective communication tools for interprofessional collaboration. Such tools include $ABCD^2$ for prediction of stroke after transient ischemic attack (TIA) and $CHADS_2$ for atrial fibrillation–related stroke prediction; National Institutes of Health Stroke Scale (NIHSS) for both ischemic and hemorrhagic stroke; Hunt-Hess scale, World Federation of Neurological Surgeons (WFNS) Grading System, and Fischer scale for aneurysmal subarachnoid hemorrhage; ICH Score for intracerebral hemorrhage; Spetzler-Martin AVM Grading System for arteriovenous malformation; and modified Rankin Scale (mRS), Barthel Index, and Functional Independence Measure (FIM) scale for functional recovery measurement (Ghandehari, 2013; Harrison, McArthur, & Quinn, 2013; Hwang et al., 2010; Rosen & Macdonald, 2005). Standardized order sets, protocols, and procedures can also facilitate interprofessional collaboration by encouraging consistency in care as appropriate. In addition to stroke order sets, blood glucose and temperature management protocols are also beneficial (Summers et al., 2009). Clinical pathways provide a standardized approach to patient care with goals indicated to occur within specific time limits. Although clinical pathways have lessened in popularity over the past decade,

TABLE 3-3 Frequently Used Stroke Assessment Scales

Name of Scale	Type of Stroke
$ABCD^2$	Prediction of ischemic stroke after TIAs
$CHADS_2$ (See Chapter 1 for discussion)	Cardioembolic stroke/atrial fibrillation
National Institute of Health Stroke Scale (NIHSS)	Ischemic or hemorrhagic stroke
Hunt-Hess scale	Aneurysmal subarachnoid hemorrhage
World Federation of Neurological Surgeons (WFNS) Grading System	Aneurysmal subarachnoid hemorrhage
Fischer scale	Aneurysmal subarachnoid hemorrhage
ICH Score	Intracerebral hemorrhage
Spetzler-Martin AVM Grading System	Arteriovenous malformation
Modified Rankin Scale (mRS)	Functional recovery
Barthel Index	Functional recovery
Functional Independence Measure (FIM)	Functional recovery

they have value in keeping the team aware of where the patient should be on the pathway even though patient or system variances may have impeded progress.

▣ EXEMPLARS

The following scenarios demonstrate interprofessional collaboration in stroke care, incorporating key elements of TeamSTEPPS such as teamwork, leadership, situation monitoring, mutual support and communication, and various techniques including callback, callout, briefs, debriefs, huddle, CUS, DESC, and SBAR in the clinical setting, education, research, and quality improvement.

Clinical Exemplar 1

A patient with a right frontoparietal lobe ischemic stroke is 5 days post stroke. He has left upper extremity weakness, left homonymous hemianopsia, and apraxia. He is impulsive and exhibits poor judgment. He was assessed by the care team and deemed not yet ready for inpatient rehabilitation. When the physician, acute care nurse, pharmacist, and dietitian conduct routine team rounding for the patient, the acute care nurse states that the patient continues to be lethargic with a low blood pressure when he is sitting up in bed. In addition, even though he passed his swallow evaluation by speech therapy and the nurse received an order for a regular diet, he is eating poorly. The nurse expresses concern, stating that she is uncomfortable getting him out of bed and will not be getting him out of bed to pivot to a chair until his condition improves. The nurse uses the CUS technique to communicate concern. The physiatrist states he is not yet ready for rehabilitation because he cannot participate in a minimum of 3 hours of rehabilitation daily. The physiatrist's participation in rounds and expression of care plan exhibits mutual support and leadership. The physical or occupational therapist sees the patient daily, for about 20 to 30 minutes per session.

On rounds, the interprofessional team develops a plan as follows: ask speech therapist to reevaluate the patient's swallow function, and if the swallow test result is acceptable, ask the dietitian to visit the patient to obtain a list of his food and drink preferences. The neurology resident states that the patient's laboratory test and intake/output reflect some slight dehydration, which may be contributing to his unexpected orthostatic hypotension and the difficulty in adjusting his antihypertensive, again exhibiting mutual support. The attending physician, resident neurologist, pharmacist, and nurse collaborate to give the patient 2 L of normal saline over the next 16 hours and then perform postural vital signs. If the patient maintains his blood pressure with the head of bed up, the nurse plans to ask physical or occupational therapy to reevaluate the patient regarding advancing activity. The physical or occupational therapists will show the nurse how to reinforce their work with the patient, so the nurse has a shared mental model when caring for the patient. The sharing of the care plan between the therapists and the nurse occurs during briefs. After receiving a progress report from the neurologist, the physiatrist revisits the patient 2 days later, using the technique of checkback; the patient is ready for rehabilitation because he has made steady progress, which includes up in the chair, eating adequately, and following simple one-step commands. His blood pressure is stable and he is less impulsive than 2 days prior. The patient is discharged from acute care and admitted to rehabilitation with a detailed discharge summary and verbal handoff reports from physician to physician, therapist to therapist, and nurse to nurse. Handoff between staff occurs using the SBAR and I PASS THE BATON formats.

Clinical Exemplar 2

A patient has returned to the stroke clinic about a month after discharge from rehabilitation. The patient has been experiencing syncopal episodes, and the attending physician is considering decreasing what he believes to be his current antihypertensive. The pharmacist in the stroke clinic places a call to the patient's internal medicine physician and learns that the internal medicine physician has continued the antihypertensive agent the patient was taking prior to the stroke, not realizing the patient was also placed on a different antihypertensive by his stroke physician. The stroke physician had instructed the patient to stop the previous antihypertensives. The team working together to collect information and develop a plan exhibits both collaboration and mutual support. The internal medicine physician never received the patient's medical record from his stroke hospitalization. The pharmacist reports this to the neurologist, and the neurologist instructs the patient to stop one of the medications. The spouse is told to record the blood pressure and report results into the clinic over the next week and to immediately report any syncopal episodes. The blood pressure is stable and no further syncopal episodes occur. The hypotension is resolved. The pharmacist and physicians later huddle with the medical records department to discuss an action plan to lessen the likelihood of failure to receive or send documentation of care to providers in the community.

■■ EDUCATION

The following clinical scenario demonstrates interprofessional collaboration in a simulated educational setting.

Education Exemplar 1

The staff in the ED is practicing stroke codes in the simulation laboratory. The ED physician, neurologist, pharmacist, respiratory therapist, and stroke center coordinator and advanced practice nurse are present. The staff nurse notes the time when she saw the patient normal compared to the new onset of slurred speech and facial drop. His blood pressure is 190/115 mm Hg. His SpO_2 is 88%, and the respiratory therapist assesses his lungs and places the patient on a binasal cannula at 3 L/min. They notify the ED physician who states, "I just saw him; he was fine 15 minutes ago." The nurse restates the clinical presentation and adds, "I am concerned and uncomfortable, and he needs to be seen by a physician now." The nurse is expressing concern using the CUS technique. The ED physician examines him quickly and tells the nurse to call a stroke code, exhibiting leadership and collaboration. He asks the nurse to administer labetalol (Trandate) 10 mg IV push for blood pressure. The nurse quickly administers the medication and then verbalizes the labetalol has been administered, demonstrating the checkback technique for effective team communication.

The neurologist comes to the bedside, performs the NIHSS (score is 12), and agrees the patient's presentation is congruent with a stroke, demonstrating mutual support. A fingerstick glucose, other basic chemistries, coagulation studies, and toxicology laboratory studies are obtained, and the patient is taken immediately to the computed tomography (CT) scan. A CT scan of the head is negative for hemorrhage; the patient's clinical presentation has not improved. The staff nurse continues to obtain neurological checks and vital signs every 15 minutes. The cerebrovascular fellow, advanced practice nurse, and ED pharmacist review the patient's history with the inclusion and exclusion criteria for IV rtPA. The patient is deemed eligible. The neurologist, stroke center coordinator, and pharmacist agree on the amount of rtPA ordered, demonstrating team collaboration. The pharmacist returns with the rtPA and checks it with the staff nurse. The pharmacist asks for the patient's current blood pressure. It is now 180/105 mm Hg, which is sufficiently low enough to administer the rtPA. The team follow-up on critical physiological values prior to thrombolytic administration demonstrates the checkback technique. The nurse reviews rtPA administration with the pharmacist for the first 10% bolus to be given in the first minute followed by the remaining 90% over an hour. The ED physician and cerebrovascular fellow continue to assess the patient and ask the nurse's opinion about the patient's neurological status over the hour and blood pressure. The team monitoring of each other and the patient during a critical time in the patient's care demonstrates situation monitoring. The cerebrovascular fellow places post-rtPA orders into the computer. A neuroscience ICU (NICU) bed becomes available as the last of rtPA is infused, the NICU nurse receives a telephone report, and she goes to the ED to receive a more detailed handoff and transports the patient to the NICU. The patient's neurological status has improved. Simulation experience ends and a debrief is conducted regarding items performed well, led by the stroke coordinator and advanced practice nurse, including areas for improvement with attention to the timeline of care.

Education Exemplar 2

During simulation, a patient is undergoing coil embolization of a cerebral aneurysm in the virtual interventional radiology suite. During the procedure, the parent artery of the aneurysm is dissected, resulting in additional subarachnoid hemorrhage. The anesthesiologist notes a rapid widening of pulse pressure and bradycardia. The anesthesiologist notes the pupils to be fixed and dilated and immediately alerts the interventionalist of increased intracranial pressure. The anesthesiologist demonstrates situation monitoring and communicates with the neurointerventionalist using the DESC technique. Neurosurgery is called emergently to the interventional suite and a ventriculostomy is performed. The OR suite is prepared for a craniotomy for evacuation of a hematoma. Anesthesiology assesses coagulation and electrolytes, maintains oxygenation, and orders blood for the OR. The team's rapid response to an unexpected complication demonstrates collaboration and mutual support.

▉ QUALITY IMPROVEMENT

The following demonstrates interprofessional collaboration regarding a performance standard.

Quality Improvement Exemplar 1

Documentation compliance after cerebral angiogram, including neurological status, vital signs, site assessment, and distal pulses, has decreased. The stroke center quality improvement analyst, stroke center nurse manager, neuroradiologists, and stroke center neurologists meet to determine the issues and recommend corrective action. After brainstorming, they realize that the neuroradiology residents and nurses have not adapted to the new electronic order set and decide formal education is needed. Demonstrating collaboration, they review the computerized physician order set among themselves and then meet later with the nurse managers for the radiology nurses and NICU to better understand the rationale for the changes. Revisions in the order sets are made; however, the order sets are still different than the original hard copy paper order sets. The advanced practice nurse demonstrates mutual support by developing a learning module, and it is published for the neuroscience nurses to complete. Situation monitoring and ongoing debriefs reveal that as patients continue to undergo cerebral angiography, despite the learning module and posttest, documentation compliance is still below expectations. The nurse managers talk to the individual nurses, and the attending neuroradiologists talk to the neuroradiology residents, showing them where their documentation is inadequate regarding specific patients. This is extremely time-consuming as the attending physicians and nurse managers must look through each patient's chart individually before talking to the nurse or resident. They meet with the stroke center quality improvement nurse. Together, they develop a database that will abstract data from the nurses' documentation to allow aggregation of the data and more efficient review of the data demonstrating team collaboration. Within 4 months, checkback and monitoring reveals the nurses' compliance around angiogram documentation is greater than 90%, which was the goal.

Quality Improvement Exemplar 2

The patient is 7 days post-intracerebral hemorrhage and remains intubated with failure to wean from mechanical ventilation. Within the program, routine range of motion is generally the only intervention offered to bedridden stroke patients. However, the physical and occupational therapists believe that getting the patient out of bed while mechanically ventilated would benefit the patient physically and emotionally and is consistent with current evidence-based practice. Over the course of several days, the patient is more awake but weaker and appears depressed. The occupational and speech therapists speak to the neuropsychologist who also collaborates with the respiratory therapist and physiatrist. Together, they decide to advance the patient's activity level to dangling and then up in a chair. The team working together exhibits both leadership and team collaboration. With the assistance of the staff nurse, the respiratory therapist increases the activity level with the physician constantly monitoring the activity and the patient's response to the activity. Over the next few days, the occupational and physical therapists advance the patient to walking in the unit with a walker and portable cardiac monitor and ventilator.

RESEARCH

The NICU nurses plan to conduct a study on early mobility after stroke. Their hypothesis is that earlier mobility will lessen days in the NICU and lessen complications. There is currently an early mobility protocol in place for medical ICU patients. Five of the NICU nurses meet with the doctorally prepared neuroscience clinical nurse specialist (CNS), the nurse manager, neurointensivists, a neurosurgeon, and a neurologist in addition to the respiratory, physical, and occupational therapists. The staff nurses have been given a number of research studies to read ahead of time. Once the meeting occurs, they draft revisions of the existing protocol, determine inclusion and exclusion criteria for stroke patients, develop a research proposal including data collection sheets, and complete the forms for submission to the Institutional Review Board of the Committee for the Protection of Human Subjects. It is at this meeting that the team determines the role of each person's authorship for any publications and presentations. Meanwhile, the group ask to be included on the agenda of the next nursing research committee. The nurses in the NICU collect the data and periodically reconvene the original workgroup to discuss any difficulty with the study or patients lost from the study. The staff nurses work with the neuroscience CNS and university affiliated biostatistician during data analysis. (This is collaboration.)

No adverse events occur during data collection. (This is situation monitoring.) The research team decides to continue the protocol for all eligible NICU patients. Data analysis is completed and the staff nurses who draft the paper ask the other team members for input. All involved are included in the authorship, with those who provided the most work being listed first. (This is mutual support.) The various disciplines involved in the study prepare posters or presentations to take their work as a poster or presentation to various spring conferences before submitting the manuscript for peer review and publication.

SUMMARY

Stroke is a life-threatening and life-altering disease. Interprofessional teams facilitate functional recovery and provide the patient with expert coordinated care from a number of needed disciplines. The principles of interprofessional collaboration and teamwork must be learned. A number of tools exist to assist the health care professional with interprofessional collaboration efforts. The improved outcomes and advantages to interprofessional teams are yet to be fully realized. Research directed toward examining outcomes from interprofessional teams must be undertaken.

REFERENCES

Agency for Healthcare Research and Quality. (2014). *TeamSTEPPS® Team, strategies and tools to enhance performance and patient safety: An instructor's guide* 0.61 (AHRQ Publication No. 06-0020). Rockville, MD: Agency for Healthcare Research and Quality. Retrieved from http://www.usuhs.mil/cerps/TeamSTEPPS.html

Ahmed, S., Manaf, N. H. A., & Islam, R. (2013). Effects of Lean Six Sigma application in healthcare services: A literature review. *Reviews on Environmental Health, 28*(4), 189–194.

American Heart Association/American Stroke Association. (2014). *Stroke fact sheet*. Retrieved from http://www.heart.org/idc/groups/heart-public/%40wcm/%40private/%40hcm/%40gwtg/documents/downloadable/ucm_310976.pdf

Ash, L., & Miller, C. (2014). Interprofessional collaboration for improving patient and population health. In M. E. Zaccagnini & K. W. White (Eds), *The doctor of nursing practice essentials* (2nd ed., pp. 217–256). Burlington, MA: Jones & Bartlett.

Atwal, A., & Caldwell, K. (2002). Do multidisciplinary integrated care pathways improve interprofessional collaboration? *Scandinavian Journal of Caring Science, 16*(4), 360–367.

Audebert, H. (2006). Telestroke: Effective networking. *The Lancet Neurology, 5*(3), 279–282.

Barreca, S., & Wilkins, S. (2008). Experiences of nurses working in a stroke rehabilitation unit. *Journal of Advanced Nursing, 63*(1), 36–44.

Burton, C. R., Fisher, A., & Green, T. L. (2009). The organisational context of nursing care in stroke unit: A case study approach. *International Journal of Nursing Studies, 46*(1), 86–95.

Cell, L. A., Hassan, E., Marquardt, C., Breslow, M., & Rosenfeld, B. (2001). The eICU: It's not just telemedicine. *Critical Care Medicine, 29*(8 Suppl.), N183–N189.

Centers for Disease Control and Prevention. (2012). Prevalence of stroke—United States, 2006-2010. *MMWR. Morbidity and Mortality Weekly Report, 61*(20), 379–382.

Cheung, D., McKellar, J., Parsons, J., Lowe, M., Willems, J., Heus, L., & Reeves, S. (2012). Community re-engagement and interprofessional education: The impact on health care providers and person living with stroke. *Topics in Stroke Rehabilitation, 19*(1), 63–74.

Cima, R. R., Brown, M. J., Hebl, J. R., Moore, R., Rogers, J. C., Kollengode, A. . . . Deschamps, C. (2011). Use of lean and six sigma methodology to improve operating room efficiency in a high-volume tertiary-care academic medical center. *Journal of the American College of Surgeons, 213*(1), 83–94.

Clancy, C. M. (2007). TeamSTEPPS: Optimizing teamwork in the perioperative setting. *AORN Journal, 86*(1), 18–22.

Clapper, T. C., & Kong, M. (2012). TeamSTEPPS®: The patient safety tool that needs to be implemented. *Clinical Simulation in Nursing, 8*(8), e367–e373. doi:10.1015/j.ecns.2011.03.002

Clark, P. R. (2009). Teamwork: Building healthier workplaces and providing safer patient care. *Critical Care Quarterly, 32*(3), 221–231.

Connolly, E. S., Jr., Rabinstein, A. A., Carhuapoma, J. R., Derdeyn, C. P., Dion, J., Higashida, R. T., . . . Vespa, P. (2012). Guidelines for the management of aneurysmal subarachnoid hemorrhage: A guideline for healthcare professionals from the American Heart Association/American Stroke Association. *Stroke, 43*(6), 1711–1737.

Creutzfeldt, C. J., Holloway, R. G., & Walker, M. (2012). Symptomatic and palliative care for stroke survivors. *Journal of Clinical Internal Medicine, 27*(7), 853–860.

D'Amour, D., & Oandasan, I. (2005). Interprofessionality as the field of interprofessional practice and interprofessional education: An emerging concept. *Journal of Interprofessional Care, 19*(Suppl. 1), 8–20.

Dietrich, S. L., Kornet, T. M., Lawson, D. R., Major, K., May, L., & Riley-Wasserman, E. (2010). Collaboration to partnerships. *Nursing Administration Quarterly, 34*(1), 49–55.

Falconer, J. A., Roth, E. J., Sutin, J. A., Strasser, D. C., & Chang, R. W. (1993). The critical path method in stroke rehabilitation: Lessons from an experiment in cost containment and outcome improvement. *QRB Quality Review Bulletin, 19*(1), 8–16.

Fens, M., Vluggen, T. P., van Haastreg, J. C., Verbunt, J. A., Beusmans, G. H., & van Heugten, C. M. (2013). Multidisciplinary care for stroke patients living in the community: A systematic review. *Journal of Rehabilitation Medicine, 45*, 321–330.

Ghandehari, K. (2013). Challenging comparison of stroke scales. *Journal of Research in Medical Science, 18*(1), 906–910.

Goldstein, L. B., Bushnell, C. D., Adams, R. J., Appel, L. J., Braun, L. T., Chaturvedi, S., . . . Pearson T. A. (2011). Guidelines for the primary prevention of stroke: A guideline for healthcare professionals from the American Heart Association/American Stroke Association. *Stroke, 42*(2), 517–584.

Goodman, B., & Clemow, R. (2010). Working with other people. In B. Goodman & R. Clemow (Eds.), *Nursing and collaborative practice: A guide to interprofessional learning and working* (2nd ed.). Exeter, United Kingdom: Learning Matters.

Gorelick, A. R., Gorelick, P. B., & Sloan, E. P. (2008). Emergency department evaluation and management of stroke: Acute assessment, stroke teams and care pathways. *Neurologic Clinics, 26*(4), 923–942.

Hammick, M., Freeth, D., Copperman, J., & Goodsman, D. (2009). Being interprofessional: Models and meaning. In M. Hammick, D. S. Freeth, D. Goodsman, & J. Copperman (Eds.), *Being interprofessional* (pp. 7–24). Cambridge, United Kingdom: Polity.

Harrison, J. K., McArthur, K. S., & Quinn, T. J. (2013). Assessment scales in stroke: Clinimetric and clinical considerations. *Clinical Interventions in Aging, 8*, 201–211.

Holden, R. J. (2011). Lean thinking in emergency departments: A critical review. *Annals of Emergency Medicine, 57*(3), 265–278.

Holloway, R. G., Arnold, R. M., Creutzfeldt, C. J., Lewis, E. F., Lutz, B. J., McCann, R. M., . . . Zorowitzh, R. D. (2014). Palliative and end-of-life care in stroke: A statement for health professionals from the American Heart Association/American Stroke Association. *Stroke, 45*, 1887–1916.

Hwang, B. Y., Appelboom, G., Kellner, C. P., Carpenter, A. M., Kellner, M. A., Gigante, P. R., & Sander Connolly, E. (2010). Clinical grading scales in intracerebral hemorrhage. *Neurocritical Care, 13*(1), 144–151.

Institute of Medicine. (2003). In A. C. Greiner & E. Knebel (Eds.), *Health professions education: A bridge to quality*. Washington, DC: National Academies Press. Retrieved from http://iom.edu/Reports/2003/Health-Professions-Education-A-Bridge-to-Quality.aspx

Institute of Medicine. (2011). *The future of nursing: Leading change, advancing health*. Washington, DC: National Academic Press. Retrieved from http://iom.edu/Reports/2010/The-Future-of-Nursing-Leading-Change-Advancing-Health.aspx

Interprofessional Education Collaborative Expert Panel. (2011). *Core competencies for interprofessional collaborative practice: Report of an expert panel*. Washington, DC: Interprofessional Education Collaborative.

Jauch, E. C., Saver, J. L., Adams, H. P., Jr., Bruno, A., Connors, J. J., Demaerschalk, B. M., . . . Yonas, H. (2013). Guidelines for the early management of patients with acute ischemic stroke: A guideline for healthcare professionals from the American Heart Association/American Stroke Association. *Stroke, 44*(3), 870–947.

Langhorne, P., Bernhardt, J., & Kwakkel, G. (2011). Stroke care 2: Stroke rehabilitation. *Lancet, 377*(9778), 1693–1702.

Leathard, A. (2003). *Interprofessional collaboration: From policy to practice in health and social care*. London, United Kingdom: Brunner-Routledge.

McCallin, A. (2001). Interdisciplinary practice—A matter of teamwork: An integrated literature review. *Journal of Clinical Nursing, 10*(4) 419–428.

Miller, E. L., Murray, L., Richards, L., Zorowitz, R. D., Bakas, T., Clark, P., & Billinger, S. A. (2010). Comprehensive overview of nursing and interdisciplinary rehabilitation care of the stroke patient: A scientific statement from the American Heart Association. *Stroke, 41*(10), 2402–2448.

Miniño, A. M., Murphy, S. L., Xu, J., & Kochanek, K. D. (2011). Deaths: Final data for 2008. *National Vital Statistics Report, 59*(10), 1–126.

Mitchell, P. H. (2005). What's in a name? Multidisciplinary, interdisciplinary, and transdisciplinary. *Journal of Professional Nursing, 21*(6), 332–334.

Molyneux, J. (2001). Interprofessional teamworking: What makes teams work well? *Journal of Interprofessional Care, 15*(1), 29–35.

Momsen, A. M., Rasmussen, J. O., Nielsen, C. V., Iversen, M. D., & Lund, H. (2012). Multidisciplinary team care in rehabilitation: An overview of reviews. *Journal of Rehabilitation Medicine, 44*(11), 901–912.

Morgenstern, L. B., Hemphill, J. C., III, Anderson, C., Becker, K., Broderick, J. P., & Connolly E. S., Jr. (2010). Guidelines for the management of spontaneous intracerebral hemorrhage: A guideline. *Stroke, 41*(9), 2108–2129.

Nancarrow, S. A., Booth, A., Ariss, S., Smith, T., Enderby, P., & Roots, A. (2013). Ten principles of good interdisciplinary work. *Human Resources for Health,* 11, 19. Retrieved from http://www.human-resources-health.com/content/11/1/19

National Institutes of Health, National Institute of Neurological Disorders and Stroke. (2013). *Post-stroke rehabilitation fact sheet.* Retrieved from http://www.ninds.nih.gov/disorders/stroke/poststrokerehab.htm?css=print

Nowotney, H. (2005). *Rethinking interdisciplinary.* Retrieved from http://www.interdisciplines.org/interdisciplinary/papers/5/24

Pierce, L. L. (2005). Rehabilitation nurses working as collaborative research teams. *Rehabilitation Nursing, 30*(4), 132–139.

Pinter, M. M., & Brainin, M. (2012). Rehabilitation after stroke in older people. *Maturitas, 71*(2), 104–108.

Ponte, P. R., Gross, A. H., Winer, E., Connaughton, M. J., & Hassinger, J. (2007). Implementing an interdisciplinary governance model in a comprehensive cancer center. *Oncology Nursing Forum, 34*(3), 611–616.

Reeves, S., Perrier, L., Goldman, J., Freeth, D., & Zwarenstein, M. (2013). Interprofessional education: Effects on professional practice and healthcare outcomes (update). *The Cochrane Database of Systematic Reviews,* 3, CD002213. doi:10.1002/14651858.CD002213.pub3

Richardson, A., & Storr, J. (2010). A literature (corrected) review on the impact of nursing empowerment, leadership and collaboration. *International Nursing Review, 57*(1), 12–21.

Rosen, D. S., & Macdonald, R. L. (2005). Subarachnoid hemorrhage grading scales. *Neurocritical Care, 2*(2), 110–118.

Seneviratne, C. C., Mather, C. M., & Then, K. L. (2009). Understanding nursing on an acute stroke unit: Perceptions of space, time and interprofessional practice. *Journal of Advanced Nursing, 65*(9), 1872–1881.

Stead, K., Kumar, S., Schultz, T. J., Tiver, S., Pirone, C. J., Adams, R. J., & Wareham, C. A. (2009). Teams communicating through STEPPS. *Medical Journal of Australia, 190*(11 Suppl.), S128–S132.

Stradling, D. A. (2009). Telestroke: State of the science and steps for implementation. *Critical Care Nursing Clinics of North America, 21*(4), 541–548.

Summers, D., Leonard, A., Wentworth, D., Saver, J. L., Simpson, J., Spilker, J. A., . . . Mitchell, P. H. (2009). Comprehensive overview of nursing and interdisciplinary care of the acute ischemic stroke patient: A scientific statement from the American Heart Association. *Stroke, 40*(8), 2911–2944.

ten Cate, O., & Scheele, F. (2007). Competency-based postgraduate training: Can we bridge the gap between theory and practice? *Academic Medicine, 82*(6), 542–547.

Vanderzalm, J., Hall, M. D., McFarlane, L. A., Rutherford, L., & Patterson, S. K. (2013). Fostering interprofessional learning in a rehabilitation setting: Development of an interprofessional clinical learning unit. *Rehabilitation Nursing, 38*(4), 178–185.

Weaver, T. E. (2008). Enhancing multiple disciplinary teamwork. *Nursing Outlook, 56*(3), 108–114.

Williams, R., Barrett, J., Bercoe, H., Maahs-Fladung, C., Skalko, T., & Skalko, T. (2007). Effects of recreational therapy on functional independence of people recovering from stroke. *Therapeutic Recreation Journal, 41*(4), 326.

World Health Organization. (2010). *Framework for action on interprofessional education and collaborative practice* (WHO Reference No. WHO/HRH/HPN/10.3). Geneva, Switzerland: Health Professions Network Nursing and Midwifery Office, Department of Human Resources for Health. Retrieved from http://www.who.int/hrh/resources/framework_action/en/

Stroke Care across the Continuum of Care

CHAPTER 4

Prehospital Care

Sarah L. Livesay

The prehospital recognition and treatment of patients with stroke is essential and represents a rapidly evolving science in the continuum of stroke care. As in-hospital stroke treatment has changed dramatically over the past two decades, the evolution necessitated a prehospital system of recognition, stabilization, and transport to hospitals capable of providing rapid stroke treatments (Acker et al., 2007). The development of prehospital systems of care is covered in detail in this chapter as well as the prehospital interprofessional care priorities for patients with ischemic stroke, intracerebral hemorrhage (ICH), and aneurysmal subarachnoid hemorrhage (aSAH).

■■ CHANGING PARADIGMS OF TREATMENT

Care of the patient with a diagnosis of acute stroke has changed substantially over the past two decades. Prior to the 1990s, stroke was not considered a treatable disease. The care of a patient with stroke used to be supportive in nature, aimed at minimizing complications. With the advent of intravenous (IV) fibrinolysis for the treatment of ischemic stroke, the nature of ischemic stroke treatment shifted dramatically (Jauch et al., 2013). Fibrinolysis offered the first treatment aimed at destroying the offending clot and improving function. However, the treatment was only safe and effective when offered in the first few hours of the ischemic stroke onset. Suddenly, the recognition and rapid transport of a patient with stroke signs and symptoms became paramount and directly linked to both treatment and functional outcome (Jauch et al., 2013).

Since the U.S Food Drug Administration (FDA) approval of IV tissue plasminogen activator (tPA) to treat ischemic stroke, the delivery of rapid stroke care has continued to evolve. The research guiding rescue therapies such as endovascular treatment of stroke is ongoing and may offer additional time-sensitive interventions to improve stroke outcomes. Endovascular treatment options include intra-arterial treatment of large vessel ischemic stroke with tPA administered directly into a clot using a catheter threaded through the femoral artery (Jauch et al., 2013). Using the intra-arterial approach, mechanical thrombectomy of a large vessel clot is also an option in some stroke centers. Although the science supporting these practices has yielded conflicting outcomes, both therapies are time-sensitive and require rapid recognition and transport to a recognized stroke facility where these treatment options are offered.

The science guiding treatment of ICH and subarachnoid hemorrhage (SAH) also continues to develop and necessitates early symptom recognition and access to treatment. Blood pressure–lowering therapies, reversal of procoagulant therapy, and management of elevated intracranial pressure (ICP) are associated with better outcomes in patients with ICH when instituted early and aggressively (Morgenstern et al., 2010). The paradigm of treatment for aSAH has also undergone a transformation, with coil embolization being an option to eliminate a cerebral aneurysm in addition to surgical clipping (Connolly et al., 2012). Most patients with SAH will require a transfer to a stroke center with capabilities to manage endovascular and surgical treatment of the aneurysm and the complex disease process following the hemorrhage. Therefore, the role of organized prehospital care in the chain of stroke survival is essential to both survival and improved outcomes in all types of stroke.

EMERGENCY MEDICAL SERVICE SYSTEMS

Organized and efficient prehospital health care is a relatively recent concept, developing rapidly after the World Wars and experiencing significant shifts in focus in the past several decades (Simpson, 2013). Organized prehospital care first developed in the 1960s, with improved understanding of the management of trauma associated with automobile accidents (Simpson, 2013). Prior to the 1960s, morticians largely provided transportation to or from the hospital. In 1966, morticians provided more than half of the recorded ambulance services to the hospital. The mortician service consisted solely of transport of injured person without the focus or responsibility to provide rescue medical care for stabilization (Simpson, 2013). The concepts of triage, medical stabilization, and transport of injured persons developed and were refined during the major wars of the 20th century (Goniewicz, 2013). The development of organized trauma care coupled with a national organization of services led to a significant shift in prehospital care. With the Emergency Medical Services Systems Act of 1973 developed by the National Academy of Sciences National Research Council, prehospital care shifted away from a voluntary transport service toward a regional trauma system planning and prehospital emergency care (Simpson, 2013). This shift necessitated an organized system, with a process to call for help and the expectation that the person responding to the call is a trained medical professional. Therefore, the concept of emergency medical staff organization, training, and competency are relatively new professional dimensions that continue to develop.

Emergency medical services (EMS) care and transportation are provided by a number of different staff members with different levels of training. EMS transport units consist mainly of ambulances, helicopter, and fixed-wing aircraft. The staff providing care on a ground or air transport may be composed of a mixture of technicians with various levels of expertise and competencies of the nursing staff and the physician staff. Generally, five levels of emergency medical technicians (EMT) are recognized (**Table 4-1**). The capabilities of an ambulance to care for varying levels of acuity depend on the EMT staffing and level of expertise (**Table 4-2**). The safe transport of stroke patients to the hospital or between hospitals necessitates that the caregivers in the region understand the distribution of EMT providers and work with the EMS organizations to ensure that proper level EMTs are available to transport patients.

TABLE 4-1 Emergency Medical Staff Training

Emergency Medical Technician Level	Educational Focus	Training and Certification
Emergency care attendant (ECA)	Basic emergency response, including cardiopulmonary resuscitation (CPR), splinting, managing hemorrhage	Minimum of 40 hr of training
EMT-basic	Basic life support, management of hemorrhage	Minimum of 140 hr of training, pass National Registry test prior to state certification
EMT-intermediate	Emergency stabilization prehospital and/or interfacility care; procedures including IV therapy, endotracheal intubation	Minimum of 160 hr of training, must pass National Registry test prior to state certification
EMT-paramedic	Emergency stabilization prehospital and/or interfacility care; procedures including IV therapy, endotracheal intubation, electrical cardiac defibrillation, cardioversion, and drug therapy	Minimum of 624 hr of training, must pass National Registry test prior to state certification
Licensed paramedic	Emergency stabilization prehospital and/or interfacility care; procedures including IV therapy, endotracheal intubation, electrical cardiac defibrillation, cardioversion, and drug therapy. Additionally, licensed paramedics hold an associate's or bachelor's degree from an accredited educational institution.	Minimum of 624 hr of training, associate's or bachelor's degree from accredited program, must pass National Registry test prior to state certification
First responder	Certified EMS personnel trained to respond to medical emergency situations who do not transport patients; generally work in tandem with transporting personnel	Varied

From Texas Department of State Health Services. (2014). *EMS-trauma systems.* Retrieved from http://www.dshs.state.tx.us/emstraumasystems/

TABLE 4-2 Emergency Medical Services Transport Staffing

Level of Care	Staffing
Basic life support (BLS)	Minimum of two ECAs
Advanced life support (ALS)	Minimum of one EMT-basic and one EMT-intermediate
Mobile intensive care unit (MICU)	Minimum one EMT-basic and one EMT-paramedic
BLS with ALS capability	Two ECAs, full ALS status active with the addition of an EMT-basic and EMT-intermediate
BLS with MICU capability	Two ECAs, full MICU status, staffed by at least one EMT-basic and a certified or licensed paramedic
ALS with MICU capability	One EMT-basic and 1 EMT-intermediate, full MICU status with addition of certified or licensed paramedic
Air transport	May be fixed-wing airplane or rotor wing helicopter depending on distance necessary to travel; generally staffed by a registered nurse with EMS certification and a licensed or certified paramedic

Texas Department of State Health Services. (2014). *EMS-trauma systems.* Retrieved from http://www.dshs.state.tx.us/emstraumasystems/

Regional EMS organizations operate within a larger emergency medical service system (EMSS), encompassing the entire spectrum of prehospital care, response to acute illness in the community, intrahospital transport, and coordination of multiple services within a region. As research into the treatment of stroke changed the paradigm of stroke care from support to acute and time-sensitive treatment, the EMSS had to adjust to serve the population. Stroke was no longer a disease for which only supportive care was available; stroke became an acutely treatable disease, highly dependent on early recognition and transport to a facility capable of stroke treatment. In 2004, a task force was convened by the American Heart Association (AHA) and American Stroke Association to determine the barriers to prehospital care of the stroke patient (Acker et al., 2007). In 2007, an expert panel proposed four critical components of an effective stroke system of care. These critical components are as follows:

- For activating and dispatching EMS response for stroke patients, stroke systems should require appropriate processes that ensure rapid access to EMS for acute stroke patients.
- EMSS should use protocols, tools, and training of EMS responders that meet current guidelines for stroke care.
- Prehospital providers, emergency physicians, and stroke experts should collaborate in the development of EMS training, assessment, treatment, and transportation protocols for stroke.
- Patients should be transported to the nearest stroke center for evaluation and care if a stroke center is located within a reasonable transport distance and time.

As the prehospital care of patients with stroke continues to develop, public policy and system planning efforts should focus efforts on improving the system of care in these four essential components of a stroke system of care.

The task force further outlined the scope of an EMSS focused on stroke treatment. A stroke-specific EMSS should include a full spectrum of services including community outreach aimed at educating the public, emergency medical personnel, engagement of public safety agencies including police and fire, emergency departments, as well as critical care units. This definition of EMSS aimed at the treatment of stroke patients fits well with the American Stroke Association's (ASA) Chain of Survival. The ASA Chain of Survival proposes that the critical steps of stroke care include the detection of symptoms; the dispatch of caregivers with knowledge in stroke detection and early management; the delivery of the patient to a facility with stroke treatment expertise; the experts meeting the stroke patient at the door of the facility; the communication of key patient data relevant to the treatment of stroke; the decision to provide early treatment including IV thrombolysis, if indicated; and the admission of the patient to the hospital or transfer to a higher level of care (**Table 4-3**). A breakdown in any link of the Chain of Survival could result in poor patient outcomes.

■ RECOGNITION OF STROKE

To facilitate timely transport of a stroke patient to the hospital, the recognition of stroke signs and symptoms is critical. The general public, as well as prehospital providers, must recognize the urgency of seeking treatment when stroke symptoms begin. Delayed time from symptom onset to seeking care is a major barrier to effective treatments in all stroke subtypes. A significant contributor delaying patients from seeking emergent care is the lack of symptom awareness (Crocco, 2007).

TABLE 4-3 Stroke Chain of Survival

Detection	Patient or bystander recognition of stroke signs and symptoms
Dispatch	Immediate activation of 911 and priority EMS dispatch
Delivery	Prompt triage and transport to most appropriate stroke hospital and prehospital notification
Door	Immediate ED triage to high-acuity area
Data	Prompt ED evaluation, stroke team activation, laboratory studies, and brain imaging
Decision	Diagnosis and datermination of most appropriate therapy; discussion with patient and family
Drug	Administration of appropriate drugs or other interventions
Disposition	Timely admission to stroke unit, intensive care unit, or transfer

From Jauch, E. C., Saver, J. L., Adams, H. P., Jr., Bruno, A., Connors, J. J., Demaerschalk, B. M., . . . Yonas, H. (2013). Guidelines for the early management of patients with acute ischemic stroke: A guideline for healthcare professionals from the American Heart Association/ American Stroke Association. *Stroke, 44*(3), 870–947.

A seminal study of stroke system awareness was conducted in 2003. A phone survey of over 61,000 adults spanning 17 states was conducted by the Behavioral Risk Factor Surveillance System (BRFSS) assessing knowledge of stroke signs and symptoms. Study findings indicated that less than 20% of respondents could identify all signs and symptoms of stroke and possessed the knowledge of when to call 911 (Greenlund et al., 2003). Additionally, few recognized that stroke symptoms indicated a medical emergency necessitating rapid transport to the hospital. Recognition of symptoms and necessary action was significantly less common in ethnic minorities, those of older and younger age, those reporting less education, and respondents who smoked. The findings have been replicated in multiple regional and national surveys with similar findings.

Patients who experience an acute stroke continue to struggle with stroke symptom awareness in the months and years after their stroke event. Despite experiencing a stroke, many stroke survivors continue to have difficulty articulating the signs and symptoms of stroke and the need to rapidly mobilize to the emergency department. Therefore, community education and awareness is a significant priority for hospitals with organized stroke programs. Educational initiatives aimed at the general public as well as patients who have survived a stroke and are at risk of another stroke event must focus on both the signs and symptoms associated with stroke as well as the urgency with which a victim should seek medical care (Crocco, 2007). Target audiences for stroke education and outreach include populations at risk for stroke, the general public, as well as large employers (Rymer, 2005).

The ideal vehicle for public education remains a matter of continued debate. Certified stroke centers are required to provide community outreach education to maintain certification. However, data are unclear regarding the efficacy of such education. Generally, large media outreach campaigns are thought to be superior in reaching the public. Yet, studies show that even large media campaigns are not always effective. A recent systematic review of 10 media outreach campaigns designed to educate the public on stroke revealed mixed results. Media campaigns to educate the public were found to increase public awareness of signs and symptoms of stroke, without impacting public awareness of the need for emergency response to the symptoms (Lecouturier et al., 2010). In studies that targeted both the public and the professionals caring for stroke patients, outreach seemed to impact the providers more than the public (Lecouturier et al., 2010). Additional research is needed to guide initiatives to increase general awareness of symptoms associated with stroke as well as mobilization for transport to the hospital.

■ EMERGENCY MEDICAL SERVICES NOTIFICATION AND DISPATCH

Once a person is identified as having new onset of symptoms consistent with a stroke, he or she should activate EMS by calling 911. Transport by ambulance to a hospital with identified capabilities to treat a patient with acute stroke has clearly shown to result in faster treatment times than a patient or family member driving the patient to the hospital. However, dispatch staff answering at the call center must be educated about stroke signs and symptoms. EMS dispatch workers staff the call center and are responsible for sending EMTs to the patient. Studies have shown that when dispatch staff members are educated in recognizing signs and symptoms of stroke, they mobilize EMT staff to the scene much faster. Therefore, EMS dispatch workers must be included in any education and program planners as key members of the prehospital team.

■ PREHOSPITAL STROKE CARE CLINICAL PRIORITIES

As with any other critical or emergent disease process, the first priority of care is to assess and manage the airway, breathing, and circulation (ABCs). Patients with larger ischemic stroke, ICH, or SAH may experience a rapid decline in their level of consciousness, necessitating an oral airway and mechanical ventilation. Any indication of altered circulation should be rectified according to the AHA advanced cardiac life support (ACLS) protocol (Jauch et al., 2013).

At the time of prehospital activation for a suspected stroke, treating staff will be unable to determine with certainty if the stroke is ischemic, ICH, or SAH in nature until a computed tomography (CT) image of the head is obtained (Jauch et al., 2013). The general approach to a patient with suspected stroke requires specific treatment goals. Patients with suspected stroke should receive supplemental oxygen therapy to maintain oxygen saturations greater than 94%. The routine administration of oxygen therapy to patients without demonstrated hypoxia is not recommended (Jauch et al., 2013).

Blood pressure should be assessed frequently and extreme hypertension or hypotension should be addressed. Should the patient present with hypotension, the head of bed should be maintained flat and isotonic fluid administered. If the patient with suspected stroke has an elevated blood pressure, hypertension should not be corrected unless the systolic blood pressure (SBP) is greater than 220 mm Hg (Jauch et al., 2013). If the patient is experiencing an ischemic stroke, the blood pressure is allowed to elevate to support collateral circulation and minimize further infarction. For patients with ICH stroke or SAH, a lower blood pressure is currently preferred to minimize hematoma expansion or rebleeding from the aneurysm in the first few days after the hemorrhage (Connolly et al., 2012). However, prehospital staff cannot differentiate between stroke subtypes without neuroimaging and therefore cannot identify the need to decrease blood pressure in the prehospital setting. Therefore, blood pressure is generally allowed to be elevated as long as it does not exceed SBP greater than 220 mm Hg until neuroimaging is obtained upon arrival to the hospital (Jauch et al., 2013).

All patients with signs and symptoms suggestive of stroke should undergo routine testing of blood glucose. Patients with hypoglycemia may experience unilateral weakness or decreased level of consciousness, presenting in a similar manner to a patient with stroke (Jauch et al., 2013). If the blood glucose is decreased below 60 mg/dL, dextrose should be administered to correct the low glucose level, and the patient should be reassessed. Otherwise, dextrose-containing fluid should not be routinely administered because hyperglycemia is associated with worse outcomes in patients with stroke, and dextrose-containing fluids may exacerbate cerebral edema and other complications. The prehospital team should establish IV access, placing two large-bore IVs, when possible, to facilitate rapid treatment once the patient arrives at the hospital. When possible, the prehospital team should draw blood for laboratory analysis for expedited testing upon arrival to stroke center (Jauch et al., 2013).

The prehospital team interview and assessment of the patient's surroundings is critical to expediting care upon arrival to the hospital. The team should obtain the history of symptom onset or the time that the patient was last known well. A focused health history and review of symptoms may assist in determining the presence of stroke risk factors and ischemic stroke treatment exclusion including hypertension, diabetes mellitus, hyperlipidemia, atrial fibrillation or other cardiac dysrhythmias, trauma at onset, seizure at onset, history of seizures, or hypoglycemia (Jauch et al., 2013). Emergent treatment for all stroke types is predicated on a reliable history and, at times, consent for treatment. Therefore, the prehospital team should collect contact information for families with knowledge of the patient's medical care or onset story, particularly if persons are not transported with EMS in the ambulance to the hospital.

Finally, the prehospital team should conduct a stroke-specific secondary survey, assessing the patient's head and neck for sign of trauma, auscultating heart and lungs for any abnormalities, and assessing limbs for trauma or ecchymosis (Jauch et al., 2013). A focused history and physical examination conducted by the EMT staff and reported to hospital providers upon arrival to the emergency department (ED) will help the stroke team caregivers identify stroke risk factors as well as potential stroke mimics and provide treatment accordingly.

Ideally, the time spent at the scene when treating and transporting a patient with suspected stroke should be minimal. The ASA guidelines for the early management of acute ischemic stroke indicate that on-scene time should not exceed 15 minutes (Jauch et al., 2013). On-scene time is measured as the time from ambulance arrival at the scene of a patient with stroke symptoms to the time the patient is loaded in the ambulance and en route to the nearest stroke center. This time is often nicknamed *out of the chute* by EMS providers (Jauch et al., 2013).

PREHOSPITAL NOTIFICATION AND STROKE CENTER REFERRAL

The prearrival notification of the ED and stroke team of a suspected stroke patient en route to the hospital is a best practice and is associated with decreased time to lifesaving treatment once the patient arrives to the hospital. Once the EMT staff has identified a suspected stroke patient and loaded the patient into the ambulance, a call is generally placed during transport to the stroke center ED and stroke team staff with key patient information and an expected time of arrival. The largest trial to date studying the association between prehospital notification and treatment upon arrival was a retrospective review of nearly 400,000 patient encounters entered into the ASA's Get With The Guidelines database spanning the 8 years between 2003 and 2011 (Lin et al., 2012a). Prehospital notification occurred in 67% for patients. When hospitals were notified of a suspected stroke patient en route, the patient was significantly more likely to receive IV tPA within 3 hours ($p = .0001$) and have a National Institutes of Health Stroke Scale documented ($p = .0001$). Multivariate analysis of patients receiving IV tPA demonstrated that when hospitals were prenotified, patients were more likely to receive IV tPA in less than 60 minutes from hospital door to bolus, less than 120 minutes from onset to tPA bolus, and CT imaging in less than 25 minutes from arrival at the hospital door (Lin et al., 2012a). Prehospital notification allows the hospital team to initiate the cascade of events to provide care for a patient with stroke prior to patient arrival.

A follow-up analysis of the same *Get With The Guidelines* data set revealed significant variation in the patterns of prehospital notification. Wide variations in notification trends were noted between hospital organization, by region, and by state (Lin et al., 2012b). Prehospital notification occurred in 90% to 100% of cases in California, Colorado, Arizona, and Illinois, whereas notification occurred in 0% to 59% of patient cases in a majority of the northeastern United States. Patient factors appeared to factor into prehospital notification decisions, with older age and African American patients less likely to be called with suspected stroke symptoms (Lin et al., 2012b). As attention to stroke systems of care grew over the past decade, a modest overall increase in prehospital notification was noted, with notification occurring in 58% of patient in 2003 to 67.3% in 2011 ($p < .0001$).

Prehospital notification should follow preestablished protocols and include notification of ED staff and the stroke team in the receiving hospital. This process should be identified and detailed in stroke planning meetings in collaboration including area EMS and hospital stroke caregivers. To facilitate consistency, regional plans may be developed including all hospitals in the area to allow for uniform processes from the perspective of EMS staff. Generally, the city or regional committees overseeing prehospital emergent care conduct planning for regional protocols. In addition to prehospital notification, processes and protocols should be in place to dictate destination protocols to bypass hospitals that are not certified stroke centers or designated as capable of providing acute care to stroke patients through some alternate means. Most states in the United States have destination protocols dictating the bypass of non-stroke-certified hospitals in favor of a hospital with stroke certification. However, the relationships between various levels of certified stroke centers are less clear. For example, The Joint Commission currently certifies two levels of stroke centers: primary stroke center (PSC) and comprehensive stroke center (CSC). The ideal process for bypass of a PSC in favor of a CSC is still debatable. Best practice protocols are still evolving, and research is needed to best identify which patients should be referred to PSCs versus CSCs.

Stroke care in urban centers is generally provided by ground transport agencies. In more rural areas, air medical transport plays a vital role in the treatment and transport of patients with stroke. The guidelines for the early management of ischemic stroke indicate that it is reasonable to engage air medical transport when ground transport to the nearest stroke hospital exceeds 1 hour (Jauch et al., 2013). Air medical transport may also be appropriate to transfer a patient to a higher level of care when time sensitive-interventions are necessary, including intra-arterial treatment of acute ischemic stroke, surgical decompression of a hemorrhage, or management of an aneurysm associated with SAH.

Air medical transport priorities for care should follow prehospital treatment guidelines for the management of acute ischemic stroke, ICH, or SAH (Jauch et al., 2013). Blood pressure should be managed according to guidelines, and care should be taken to monitor frequent neurological assessments in addition to routine vital signs monitoring. Patients transported via helicopter or fixed-wing flight often receive sedation to assist with agitation associated with pain and the motion of flight. Sedation and analgesia should be used judiciously and with care not to mask the neurological examination. When sedation or anxiolysis is necessary, short-acting agents are preferred over long-acting agents.

FRAGMENTATION IN PREHOSPITAL CARE OF STROKE

The 2007 ASA task force identified multiple areas of breakdowns in the care of patients with stroke in the prehospital setting and suggested multiple strategies for overcoming challenges and barriers. The collaboration, communication, and program organization and relationships between in-hospital and prehospital providers clearly decrease treatment times and improve outcomes for patients with stroke. The task force recommended all EMS agencies create and implement predefined processes and protocols to guide prehospital care and dispatch. This includes the education of staff and use of validated screening tools for any patient with signs and symptoms suggestive of stroke. All caregivers involved in the care of a stroke patient from the dispatcher to the EMT should be knowledgeable regarding the urgency of stroke and the appropriate ambulance and technician level of care that should be dispatched to the scene.

The task force also recommended all EMS agencies engage in quality monitoring and a quality improvement program related to stroke identification and response times. The 2013 updated AHA/ASA guidelines for the early treatment of ischemic stroke proposed the following prehospital timeline (Jauch et al., 2013): the time between receipt of the call and the dispatch of response team less than 90 seconds; EMS response time to the scene is less than 8 minutes from dispatch, with properly equipped and staffed ambulance; dispatch time is less than 1 minute; turnout time defined as the time from dispatch call to unit en route is less than 1 minute; on-scene time is less than 15 minutes barring extenuating circumstances; and travel time is equivalent to trauma or acute myocardial infarction calls. Data should be collected, collated into aggregate data, and reviewed for improvement opportunities using rapid quality improvement methodologies.

The AHA/ASA EMS task force developed a recommendation stating that prehospital stroke quality data should be recorded on 100% of prehospital calls for suspected stroke, and prehospital organizations should be compliant with prehospital stroke process measures at least 90% of the time (Acker et al., 2007). Suggested prehospital measures include stroke history obtained when indicated, stroke assessment performed using validated stroke tool when indicated, a stroke history checklist that documents eligibility for acute therapies completed when indicated, on-scene time less than 15 minutes, and hospital transport destination appropriate according to regional guidelines. When an EMSS organization is unable to meet the suggested prehospital quality measures, rapid quality improvement methodologies should be employed to fix processes and improve performance.

The AHA/ASA EMS task force recommendations for improvement in stroke systems of care also recommended standard education for all prehospital personnel, and the training of prehospital caregivers should be based on national clinical practice guidelines (Acker et al., 2007). The ASA recommends that 100% of EMS providers complete a minimum of 2 hours of stroke assessment and care as part of the required continuing medical education(CME) for certification and relicensure. Further, prehospital and hospital stroke experts should collaborate to develop training, assessment, treatment, and transport protocols for potential stroke patients. Once patients with suspected stroke are identified and en route to a stroke center, the region should use predefined prehospital diversion or hospital bypass protocols to deliver stroke patients to the nearest stroke center.

A significant source of fragmented prehospital care is caused by the lack of EMS infrastructure and 911 coverage. The task force to improve prehospital care of the stroke patient recommended that all people have landline and wireless 911 access (Acker et al., 2007). The task force supported the development of stroke system transport and nonstroke facility diversion protocols. These protocols should outline when nonstroke facilities should be bypassed to deliver a suspected stroke patient to a stroke facility.

Finally, further discussion and deliberation regarding the relationships between PSCs and CSCs is necessary. State legislation plays a key role in outlining destination and bypass protocols and should be present in all 50 states (Schwamm et al., 2010). Currently, only 19 states endorse legislation guiding stroke systems of care and prehospital bypass. In addition to prehospital protocols, regional and state providers should determine transfer guidelines for the rapid transfer of stroke patients to a higher level of care when indicated.

THE FUTURE OF PREHOSPITAL STROKE CARE

As indicated throughout this chapter, new treatments for acute ischemic stroke, ICH, and SAH have changed the prehospital stroke treatment paradigm and changed prehospital care over the past decade. Prehospital stroke care best practice continues to evolve. Current prehospital treatment of a patient with stroke is limited by the inability to conduct a CT scan of the brain to identify if the symptoms are caused by an ischemic or hemorrhagic stroke. Recent advances in technology has made the CT scanner smaller and portable, ultimately resulting in a scanner successfully being installed in a prehospital ambulance. The first randomized clinical trial evaluating the use of an ambulance outfitted with a CT scanner was recently completed in Berlin, Germany (Ebinger et al., 2014). In the trial, an ambulance with CT scan capabilities and point-of-care laboratory testing was dispatched for patients calling 911 with symptoms of a stroke within 4 hours of symptom onset. Call response and treatment by the CT ambulance were compared to control weeks where routine ambulance response was used. The trial included 3,215 patients treated in the CT ambulance compared to 2,969 patients treated during control weeks (Ebinger et al., 2014). Patients were randomized with 200 patients who received IV thrombolysis treatment and transportation in the CT ambulance compared with 220 patients who received routine transportation and IV thrombolysis. As expected, patients who received care via the CT ambulance received IV thrombolysis significantly faster than routine care. Time to IV thrombolysis treatment was reduced by 15 minutes in patients (95% confidence interval [CI], 11 to 19). The thrombolytic treatment rate was higher in patients treated and transported in the CT ambulance (32.6% vs. 29%, $p < .001$). There was no difference in adverse events including symptomatic ICH following thrombolysis or 7-day in-hospital mortality (Ebinger et al., 2014).

The German study is currently being replicated in the United States in centers in Houston, Texas and Cleveland, Ohio. In addition to evaluating the timeliness of treatment, the U.S. trials will also evaluate the role of early intervention for ICH and SAH as well as attempt to quantify the economic impact of such treatment. These studies potentially set a new standard for the prehospital treatment and transport of patients with suspected stroke. However, the feasibility of widespread implementation remains unknown.

SUMMARY

The prehospital management of patients with stroke signs and symptoms in a critical link in the stroke Chain of Survival and coordinated care improves outcomes for stroke patients. Coordination of care is key, but the current system remains fragmented. Stroke caregivers must work with prehospital personnel to define processes and educate caregivers on stroke recognition, treatment, and transport.

REFERENCES

Acker, J. E., III., Pancioli, A. M., Crocco, T. J., Eckstein, M. K., Jauch, E. C., Larrabee, H., . . . Stranne, S. K. (2007). Implementation strategies for emergency medical services within stroke systems of care: A policy statement from the American Heart Association/American Stroke Association Expert Panel on Emergency Medical Services Systems and the Stroke Council. *Stroke*, *38*(11), 3097–3115. doi:10.1161 /STROKEAHA.107.186094

Connolly, E. S., Jr., Rabinstein, A. A., Carhuapoma, J. R., Derdeyn, C. P., Dion, J., Higashida, R. T., . . . Vespa, P. (2012). Guidelines for the management of aneurysmal subarachnoid hemorrhage: A guideline for healthcare professionals from the American Heart Association/American Stroke Association. *Stroke*, *43*(6), 1711–1737. doi:10.1161/STR.0b013e3182587839

Crocco, T. J. (2007). Streamlining stroke care: From symptom onset to emergency department. *The Journal of Emergency Medicine*, *33*(3), 255–260. doi:10.1016/j.jemermed.2007.02.056

Ebinger, M., Winter, B., Wendt, M., Weber, J. E., Waldschmidt, C., Rozanski, M., . . . Audebert H. J. (2014). Effect of the use of ambulance-based thrombolysis on time to thrombolysis in acute ischemic stroke: A randomized clinical trial. *Journal of the American Medical Association*, *311*(16), 1622–1631. doi:10.1001 /jama.2014.2850

Goniewicz, M. (2013). Effect of military conflicts on the formation of emergency medical services systems worldwide. *Academic Emergency Medicine*, *20*(5), 507–513. doi:10.1111/acem.12129

Greenlund, K. J., Neff, L. J., Zheng, Z. J., Keenan, N. L., Giles, W. H., Ayala, C. A., . . . Mensah, G. A. (2003). Low public recognition of major stroke symptoms. *American Journal of Preventive Medicine*, *25*(4), 315–319.

Jauch, E. C., Saver, J. L., Adams, H. P., Jr., Bruno, A., Connors, J. J., Demaerschalk, B. M., . . . Yonas, H. (2013). Guidelines for the early management of patients with acute ischemic stroke: A guideline for healthcare professionals from the American Heart Association/American Stroke Association. *Stroke*, *44*(3), 870–947. doi:10.1161/STR.0b013e318284056a

Lecouturier, J., Rodgers, H., Murtagh, M. J., White, M., Ford, G. A., & Thomson, R. G. (2010). Systematic review of mass media interventions designed to improve public recognition of stroke symptoms, emergency response and early treatment. *BMC Public Health*, *10*, 784. doi:10.1186/1471-2458-10-784

Lin, C. B., Peterson, E. D., Smith, E. E., Saver, J. L., Liang, L., Xian, Y., . . . Fonarow, G. C. (2012a). Emergency medical service hospital prenotification is associated with improved evaluation and treatment of acute ischemic stroke. *Circulation. Cardiovascular Quality and Outcomes*, *5*(4) 514–522. doi:10.1161 /CIRCOUTCOMES.112.965210

Lin, C. B., Peterson, E. D., Smith, E. E., Saver, J. L., Liang, L., Xian, Y., . . . Fonarow, G. C. (2012b). Patterns, predictors, variations, and temporal trends in emergency medical service hospital prenotification for acute ischemic stroke. *Journal of the American Heart Association*, *1*(4), e002345. doi:10.1161/JAHA.112.002345

Morgenstern, L. B., Hemphill, J. C., III., Anderson, C., Becker, K., Broderick, J. P., Connolly, E. S., Jr., . . . Tamargo, R. J. (2010). Guidelines for the management of spontaneous intracerebral hemorrhage: A guideline for healthcare professionals from the American Heart Association/American Stroke Association. *Stroke*, *41*(9), 2108–2129. doi:10.1161/STR.0b013e3181ec611b

Rymer, M. M. (2005). Organizing stroke systems of care. *Stroke*, *36*(7), 1358–1359; author reply 1359.

Schwamm, L., Fayad, P., Acker, J. E., III., Duncan, P., Fonarow, G. C., Girgus, M., . . . Yancy, C. W. (2010). Translating evidence into practice: A decade of efforts by the American Heart Association/American Stroke Association to reduce death and disability due to stroke: A presidential advisory from the American Heart Association/American Stroke Association. *Stroke*, *41*(5), 1051–1065. doi:10.1161/STR.0b013e3181d2da7d

Simpson, A. T. (2013). Transporting Lazarus: Physicians, the state, and the creation of the modern paramedic and ambulance, 1955-73. *Journal of the History of Medicine and Allied Sciences*, *68*(2), 163–197. doi:10.1093/jhmas/jrr053

CHAPTER 5

Diagnostics for Stroke

Cynthia Bautista and Sarah L. Livesay

Diagnostic testing is necessary to deliver evidence-based diagnosis and management of stroke as it provides invaluable information about the disease process and pathophysiology that impacts disease treatment and prevention of future disease. The interprofessional team providing care to a stroke patient is greatly extended when undergoing diagnostic testing. Many professionals are necessary to provide safe and effective diagnostic testing for patients with stroke. This chapter will highlight the most common diagnostic tests in stroke, including indications, contraindications, and periprocedural considerations for the interprofessional team providing stroke care.

▌▋ GENERAL DIAGNOSTIC TESTING CONSIDERATIONS

Indications

Diagnostic testing is indicated when it contributes to the diagnosis or management of the patient. Specific to the management of stroke, diagnostics may assist the interprofessional team with determining the time of stroke onset, the stroke subtype, as well as the location and distribution of the stroke. Even the best clinicians cannot distinguish between an ischemic stroke and intracerebral hemorrhagic (ICH) stroke or subarachnoid hemorrhage (SAH) by physical assessment and patient history alone. Diagnostic imaging is necessary to verify the stroke pathology and determine the next steps in managing the patient (Jauch et al., 2013). Test results may also assist the caregivers in ruling out common mimics of a stroke and may provide and contribute valuable information about the underlying pathophysiology of the stroke. Diagnostic imaging studies can assess the status of intracranial vessels and may be useful when conducted at any time along the stroke care continuum by influencing decision making for primary or secondary prevention options as well as acute intervention treatment options (Jauch et al., 2013).

Advanced neuroimaging may also reveal the degree of reversibility of the stroke, thereby immediately impacting treatment decisions and directly impacting the course of care for the patient with stroke. Finally, diagnostic testing assists the interprofessional care team in the monitoring of stroke evolution and complications during the inpatient and posthospital care period.

Testing Considerations

The need for information to guide patient diagnosis and management and other advantages of testing must be weighed against the potential risks associated with testing (Dillon, 2012). All tests carry a degree of risk, and the risk should be weighted with the benefit in any clinical case. The clinician must consider all factors, including the patient's condition prior to performing a diagnostic test, how well the patient is expected to tolerate the diagnostic test, and the contribution of knowledge gained from the test results to the overall care of the patient. If the patient is not hemodynamically stable at the time of diagnostic testing, collaboration between the care team members should occur to evaluate the need and appropriate timing for the test.

General Interprofessional Team Testing Considerations

The patient's understanding of the need for the diagnostic test, risks or side effects associated with testing, and alternatives to testing are central to informed decision making and the responsibility of all team members. Patients with cognitive deficits as a result of their stroke may require surrogate decision makers and will need frequent reinforcement of information for continued comprehension. Some diagnostic tests contain procedural components and are invasive in nature, necessitating additional consent and more complex care during and after the procedure. Informed and written consent should be obtained when indicated. To address patient safety issues associated with invasive procedures, organizations have embraced a Universal Protocol (UP) or a bundle of patient safety interventions aimed to reduce the risk of harm associated with procedures. A time-out or pause before a procedure to verify patient identity, procedure to be conducted, and potential complications has become a critical component of UP and should be completed with any invasive diagnostic procedure according to organizational protocol.

When the administration of contrast medium is necessary to complete a diagnostic test, an allergy screen should be conducted, and the patient should be monitored for any signs of distress. Patients receiving iodine contrast and have history of iodine allergy may require a steroid prophylaxis preparation due to 5% incidence of allergic reaction to contrast (Hickey & Murphy, 2010). Preprocedure evaluation should include a baseline assessment of liver and kidney function because the liver metabolizes most contrast media and the kidneys secrete most contrast media. In patients with underlying liver or kidney disease, the benefit of information afforded by the test should be weighed against potential worsening of the liver or kidney disease. For patients with underlying renal insufficiency, periprocedural hydration should be administered when certain intravenous (IV) contrast media are administered. Although administration of Mucomyst or sodium bicarbonate to provide renal protection is a common practice, evidence does not show that this practice provides a benefit beyond additional hydration.

NONCONTRAST COMPUTED AXIAL TOMOGRAPHY OR COMPUTED TOMOGRAPHY SCAN

Technique

A computed tomography (CT) scan of the brain uses attenuated x-ray imaging of tissues in a 360-degree rotation. X-ray attenuation determines tissue density from many different angles and is processed by a computer to create cross-sectional slices of brain and spine. CT imaging is conducted in a helical sequence; modern CT devices are able to obtain helical slices at 0.5 to 1 mm thick. All tissues in the brain and spine have different densities and are represented on CT imaging according to their density and are quantified in Hounsfield units (Deshmukh & Yafai, 2008). Tissue density varies from hyperdense, or the most dense; isodense; to hypodense, or the least dense. The CT image represents different densities with gradations of white to black (Dillon, 2012). Hyperdensity appears white in color and may represent bone, calcium deposits, or fresh blood. Isodensity appears gray in color and may represent cerebral tissue or subacute blood, about 1 week after the initial bleeding. Hypodensity is dark gray in color and may represent cerebral edema, fat, or chronic blood older than 2 weeks. Black seen on CT scan indicates cerebrospinal fluid (CSF) or air. CT imaging of the brain may also be obtained with contrast, providing a pictorial representation of vessels in the brain, as well as perfusion imaging, providing a color map representing the perfusion of blood to and away from the tissue of the brain (Dillon, 2012). The sophistication of CT imaging devices as well as software for image processing has improved significantly in recent years, resulting in improved images and increased use in stroke diagnosis and management.

Indication

CT imaging of the brain is a fast and noninvasive test to examine brain and spine anatomic structures (Dillon, 2012). CT of the brain without contrast is the preferred test to provide quick anatomic imaging of the brain for any patient with suspected stroke (Jauch et al., 2013). Noncontrast CT of the brain is generally the first imaging test done on any patient with suspected stroke and may be repeated to monitor the progress or complications associated with the stroke event. Hemorrhage may be seen on CT imaging within moments of it occurring. Ischemia is not immediately apparent and may take 6 hours or longer to be visible on a noncontrast CT of the brain (Jauch et al., 2013). The addition of IV contrast allows superior imaging of blood flow within cerebral arteries as well as areas of increased blood flow or capillary leakage. Cerebral edema or brain tissue herniation may also be detected on CT imaging of the brain. Therefore, noncontrast CT of the brain is used to detect a hemorrhagic stroke or SAH regardless of onset, ischemic stroke that is older than at least 6 hours, as well as cerebral edema, hydrocephalus, shift in brain structures from edema or hemorrhage, and herniation associated with any type of stroke. CT of the brain is less reliable in posterior fossa injury due to skull bone artifact.

As indicated earlier, ischemic stroke may be detected on noncontrast CT of the brain, although the appearance will differ according to the age of the infarct (Dillon, 2012). Age of the infarct is classified as acute (<24 hours), subacute (24 hours up to 5 days), and chronic (weeks) ischemic. An acute ischemic stroke that is less than 24 hours may be visualized on CT imaging because of the loss of gray-white matter differentiation in the insular ribbon area caused by vasogenic edema. Effacement of sulci can also be an early sign of ischemia causing edema. A hyperdensity noted in a large vessel may indicate an acute clot and is most often seen in the M1 or M2 branches of the middle cerebral artery (MCA) and the basilar artery. A subacute ischemic stroke that is 1 to 5 days old will appear as a defined area of infarcted tissue and may continue to have edema apparent on imaging. After 5 to 7 days, a chronic ischemic stroke is visualized on CT imaging of the brain, with clear territory margins and associated loss of brain tissue.

Blood is immediately apparent on noncontrast CT of the brain and is seen as hyperdense or white on imaging (Jauch et al., 2013). Associated edema may be visualized on imaging, with shifting of brain structures from the hemorrhage, edema, or both. Hydrocephalus or enlarged ventricles may be seen with any type of stroke and is more common with ICH, SAH, and posterior fossa ischemic stroke. Several different cerebral herniation syndromes are possible depending on the type, size, and location of the stroke and will be apparent on CT imaging.

Testing Considerations

CT scan is a noninvasive diagnostic test with minimal discomfort. The test has a short imaging time and is sensitive to motion artifact. The biggest risk associated with CT imaging is exposure to radiation, and this is of particular concern with repeated exposure for younger patients (Dillon, 2012). The radiation dose is higher with extended tests, such as CT angiography and/or perfusion CT, and risk of renal injury is higher due to IV contrast administration. Due to the radiation, there is a potential risk to fetal development if imaging is conducted while pregnant. Some patients experience claustrophobia or may be agitated during testing due to their stroke. These patients may require a short-acting sedative during the testing period. CT technologists and radiologists are involved in the planning and execution of CT imaging and should be consulted with any concerns related to radiation, indications, or contraindications to testing ⊙.

An additional consideration with higher acuity stroke patients is the safety of transport to CT imaging. A transport team may be necessary to safely transport the patient. The patient will have his or her head flat for at least several minutes. This may be a concern in patients with elevated intracranial pressure (ICP) and should be discussed by the care team when considering the test. ⊙ If contrast medium is going to be administered, the patient should be assessed for allergies to iodine, shellfish, or contrast dyes. Liver and renal function should be assessed if contrast medium is administered, and the patient should be well hydrated before and immediately after the test.

Patient education prior to CT of the brain should include indication and testing procedure, including the need to remain still during the test to avoid motion artifact. During the test, the patient may hear clicking sounds. The test should be completed in anywhere from 5 to 30 minutes, depending on the number of images ordered. If the patient receives contrast medium, he or she may feel a warm or flushed feeling when it is administered.

There are no significant short-term concerns with CT imaging. Cumulative radiation doses may be a consideration with repeated CT imaging. If contrast medium is administered during the test, patients should be monitored for allergic reaction, and fluid intake should be increased for a period of 6 to 8 hours to reduce the toxic effects of contrast on the kidneys and liver (Hickey & Murphy, 2010).

◼ COMPUTED TOMOGRAPHY ANGIOGRAM

Technique

A CT angiogram (CTA) is a CT scan as discussed earlier, with the addition of IV contrast (Dillon, 2012). The test is a quick and noninvasive means to visualize the details of the cerebral vessels and assess for large vessel occlusions. CTA offers multiplanar views of the cerebral vessels, and digital software allows three-dimensional (3D) reconstruction of the vessels. Slow or turbulent flow in a cerebral aneurysm can be visualized using the CTA. Plaque buildup, incomplete or complete occlusion of large- and medium-sized cerebral arteries, may also be visualized on CTA.

Testing Considerations

Testing considerations for CT are discussed at length earlier and are similar for a CTA. CTA may be added to a noncontrast CT of the brain to detect an ischemic stroke, cerebral aneurysm, or other vascular abnormality or to determine the extent of intracranial atherosclerosis.

◼ COMPUTED TOMOGRAPHY PERFUSION

Technique

A CT perfusion (CTP) is a CT of the brain with administration of IV contrast and calculation of several values to create a color map representing tissue perfusion (Dillon, 2012). CTP is composed of several values, including cerebral blood flow, cerebral blood volume (CBV), mean transit time (MTT), and time to peak (TTP). The four values provide a picture of speed and extent of blood flow, providing a picture of decreased or absent blood flow representing an ischemic stroke or other vascular abnormality.

Testing Considerations

Testing considerations for CT are discussed at length earlier and similar for a CTP. CTP may be added to a noncontrast CT of the brain to detect an ischemic stroke. A CTP also allows for the quantification of the ischemic penumbra or damaged tissue that is not yet infarcted. Therefore, CTP may be helpful for patients when additional rescue therapies are under consideration, such as endovascular therapy. A low-flow or oliguric blood flow state, indicative of ischemic penumbra, will appear as blue in color on the color map. A high-flow state will appear as red color on the map.

◼ MAGNETIC RESONANCE IMAGING

Technique

Magnetic resonance imaging (MRI) uses radiofrequency waves and magnetic fields to determine the hydrogen protons in tissues to produce images of various tissue densities. A cylindrical magnet surrounds the patient, and the magnet detects protons in the patient's tissue. Radiofrequency waves are delivered and protons become charged. With charged protons, vibration begins and the radiofrequency waves are stopped. Protons will realign, and the degree of tissue proton vibration is then measured. Brain or spinal tissue that is damaged will take a longer time to realign (Hickey & Murphy, 2010). The use of a gadolinium contrast medium can enhance images by highlighting leakage of contrast medium where the blood–brain barrier is compromised. There is an increased visibility of pathological processes with the use of contrast medium. The contrast enhancement has a bright or white appearance. The MRI of the brain represents a series of tests that comprises multimodal MRI testing modalities (Hickey & Murphy, 2010). These tests include the following:

- T1 weighted—vascular structures appear bright, whereas CSF appears dark; this image allows for a nice contrast between gray and white matter.
- T2 weighted—shows pathology such as edema; CSF appears white, whereas gray matter is white; cerebral white matter appears dark, and vascular structures are darker.
- Diffusion-weighted imaging (DWI)—demonstrates the extent of infarction within 5 to 10 minutes of onset; this test modality is useful for early diagnosis of ischemic stroke (Hickey, 2014).
- Perfusion-weighted imaging (PWI)—identifies abnormal cerebral blood flow and oligemic areas of brain tissue without permanent damage, which is also known as the *ischemic penumbra* (Summer & Malloy, 2011)
- Apparent diffusion coefficient (ADC)—is useful in defining the stage or acuity of infarcted tissue in ischemic stroke
- Gradient recalled echo (GRE)—is useful for detection of hemorrhage, including previous hemorrhages
- Fluid attenuated inversion recovery (FLAIR)—is the best sequence for visualizing edema, which appears white on this testing modality
- Contrast enhanced (CE)—Gadolinium contrast is often used to detect malignancy and meningitis.
- MR angiography (MRA)—assesses patency, stenosis, or occlusion of the arterial system
- Time of flight (TOF)—an image obtained during MRA and is particularly useful in imaging the large arteries of the circle of Willis and branching vessels.
- MR venography (MRV)—assesses patency, stenosis, or occlusion of the venous system

Indication

MRI of the brain can diagnose structural abnormalities and detect oxygen-deprived tissue within moments of onset (Hickey & Murphy, 2010). Therefore, it is sensitive for identification of ischemia from time of onset. The MRI is also superior for detection of ischemia in the brainstem, cerebellum, and other small structures of the brain as well as small ischemic areas (Jauch et al., 2013). MRIs take anywhere from 60 to 120 minutes to complete. Therefore, MRI is generally not conducted in the acute stroke setting where noncontrast CT of the brain is superior due to the limited time of the test. Most patients with ischemic stroke will undergo an MRI during the acute hospitalization to further quantify the stroke and vascular territory involved. Additionally, an MRI may be helpful in determining the underlying vascular abnormalities causing ICH or SAH.

The major benefit of using an MRI is its early detection of ischemia and sensitivity to edema. Another major benefit is its ability to capture the brainstem and cerebellar regions because it has high resolution, which is unobstructed by bone. It is also beneficial for the detection of small ischemic areas and/or ischemia in certain brain structures. The major disadvantage of this diagnostic study is the inability to have any metal (i.e., pacemaker) present in the body due to the use of magnetic fields. There is a risk of allergic reaction if contrast medium is administered, although the contrast medium is less nephrotoxic than the contrast medium used for CTs. Additionally, an MRI during the first trimester of pregnancy is generally avoided (Hickey & Murphy, 2010).

Testing Considerations

Due to the high risk of injury if a patient with metal implants such as pacemaker enters the magnetic field, an extensive safety screen is conducted prior to an MRI (Hickey & Murphy, 2010). MRI technologists and radiologists have expertise in determining which metal implants are safe for MRI and which are prohibited. Therefore, MRI technologists and radiologists are an important part of the interprofessional team and should be included in the screening and testing of patients with stroke ⊙. The interprofessional team should work to educate the patient about the test and disclosure of any metal implants. Most standard MRI machines have weight limitations. The patient's weight and neck girth should be assessed prior to mobilization to the MRI scanner. The patient will need to lie still and flat for an extended period of time. Patients must wear a metal frame around their head, and some patients experience anxiety and/or claustrophobia. Patients with known anxiety or claustrophobia may benefit from short-acting sedation or anxiolytics.

As with CT imaging, the patient's hemodynamic stability should be assessed as patients must mobilize to a different unit for several hours (Hickey & Murphy, 2010). Although hemodynamic monitoring is available in the MRI scanner suite, the ability to closely monitor and intervene, if a patient becomes unstable, is limited due to the magnet. If the patient requires mechanical ventilation or continuous IV medications, the team must arrange for use of an MRI-compatible ventilator and IV pumps. If contrast medium administration is planned, renal and liver function should be assessed. MRI posttest care is similar to CT scan posttest care.

▐▌ MAGNETIC RESONANCE ANGIOGRAM AND VENOGRAM

Indication

MR angiogram is indicated to assess cerebral arterial flow and detect high-grade atherosclerotic lesions of cerebral vessels (Hickey & Murphy, 2010). It is also used to detect arterial dissection of the carotid or vertebral arteries. An MRA can also detect other abnormalities such as fibromuscular dysplasia or vasculitis. An MR venogram is indicated to assess cerebral venous flow and evaluate for evidence of venous thrombosis or vascular malformation. Benefits, risks, and testing consideration are the same as for an MRI.

▐▌ DIAGNOSTIC CEREBRAL ANGIOGRAPHY

Technique

A diagnostic cerebral angiography is an invasive procedure to assess the cerebral vasculature (Jauch et al., 2013). The test involves the placement of a fluoroscopic catheter into the femoral artery, and radiopaque contrast medium is injected into the large cerebral arteries. The femoral artery is the preferred site of vessel access, although the brachial artery may also be used if the femoral artery is not available. Images of cerebral vasculature are produced using sophisticated x-ray imaging and injection of contrast material.

Indication

Cerebral angiography, often called an *arteriogram*, is used to evaluate vascular pathology and anatomy (Dillon, 2012). The test is more invasive than a CTA or an MRA and is indicated when either of these tests do not reveal the necessary information for patient diagnosis or management. It is the standard test for the detection of cerebral aneurysm, arteriovenous malformation (AVM), fistula, cerebral vasospasm associated with SAH, and a large vessel occlusion from any cause (Connolly et al., 2012; Jauch et al., 2013). Cerebral angiography can also assess collateral circulation to an ischemic area. It can be used as a diagnostic or a therapeutic modality. Cerebral angiography is often used in conjunction with a therapeutic intervention such as endovascular treatment of ischemic stroke with intra-arterial thrombolysis or mechanical thrombectomy or to treat vasospasm associated with SAH with vasodilator drugs. Cerebral angiography can also detect space-occupying lesions as evidenced by the displacement of vessels seen on imaging.

Testing Considerations

Cerebral angiography is an invasive test and therefore associated with additional risk of complications (Dillon, 2012). The procedure may damage blood vessels through a clot formation at the puncture site, or a vessel perforation, potentially resulting in a clot embolism, limb ischemia, or retroperitoneal hemorrhage. Patients should be monitored for vascular complications after the procedure. Additionally, renal and liver function should be assessed prior to administration of IV contrast, and patients should be appropriately hydrated before and immediately after the test.

The interprofessional team caring for a patient during cerebral angiography generally includes an interventional or neurointerventional radiologist, radiology technologist, and radiology nurse. The team should collaborate to obtain informed consent and generally educate the patient on the procedure ⊙. Patients undergoing cerebral angiography will receive conscious sedation at a minimum, and some may receive anesthesia. Therefore, patients generally need to be placed on nothing by mouth (NPO) for 8 to 12 hours pre-procedure. The patient should be assessed throughout the procedure and in the hours following the procedure for the complications discussed earlier. After the procedure, the patient will need to remain flat with the extremity extended for 6 hours with a pressure dressing in place. If a vascular closure device was used at the puncture site, see the manufacturer's instructions for monitoring and mobilization instructions. The patient will require frequent neurological assessment after cerebral angiography for any changes due to procedure. Additionally, the patient will require vascular assessments, including assessing the catheter site for signs of swelling, bleeding, or hematoma. Neurovascular checks on the catheter insertion extremity include assessment of pedal pulses and sensation.

▇▇ LUMBAR PUNCTURE

Technique

A lumbar puncture involves the insertion of a hollow-bore needle into subarachnoid space at the level of lumbar vertebrae 3 to 4 or 4 to 5 (Hepburn, 2014). A monometer is applied to the needle and pressure readings are noted. At this time, CSF samples can be obtained after the monometer is removed. The needle is then withdrawn and a bandage applied. To best access the lumbar space, the patient is positioned on his or her side with the knees flexed to the chest and with chin touching knees. This position results in arching of the lumbar spine. A lumbar puncture is a sterile procedure, and aseptic technique is used at all times. CSF samples are sent to the laboratory for analysis.

Indications

In the setting of stroke, lumbar puncture is used to determine the presence of subarachnoid blood and can confirm the diagnosis of an SAH (Hepburn, 2014). This procedure is generally indicated in low-grade SAH where CT scan of the brain is inconclusive for an SAH diagnosis. If the patient is complaining of a severe headache and the CT scan is negative for SAH, a lumbar puncture can be performed to assess for xanthochromia, a yellow color of the CSF, indicative of blood product breakdown. Frank red blood may also be noted and is most diagnostic for SAH when blood persists in the last CSF sample. Blood that clears while sampling CSF may be more indicative of a traumatic lumbar puncture. Additionally, lumbar puncture may be useful to rule out infection in patients with suspected stroke or patients with an external ventricular drain device to manage the stroke.

Testing Considerations

Lumbar puncture is an invasive procedure and requires informed consent. Risks associated with lumbar puncture include infection and bleeding (Hepburn, 2014). Bleeding risk is increased if there is a low platelet count or coagulopathy. There is a risk of herniation in the setting of significantly elevated ICPs when the lumbar puncture is performed. The team should collaborate with the physician or the advanced practitioner performing the procedure to record the opening and closing CSF pressures ⊙. After lumbar puncture, the patient will need to lie flat for about 6 hours. Assess for postprocedure headache which can occur in 30% of patients and administer analgesic and additional fluid, if necessary (Hickey, 2014). For several hours postprocedure, the patient should be monitored for motor and sensory neurological deficits of the lower extremities that may indicate bleeding into the spinal canal at the site of puncture or a new intracerebral event.

▮▮ TRANSTHORACIC ECHOCARDIOGRAM

Technique

Transthoracic echocardiogram (TTE) is a noninvasive ultrasonography of the heart from multiple angles to visualize the atria, ventricles, valves, and other structures (Jauch et al., 2013). The specificity of examination is limited by obesity, chronic lung disease, and a supine position due to the presence of a ventilator.

Indications

A TTE is used in a patient with stroke to identify cardiac pathology that may have contributed to the stroke etiology such as a thrombus, myxoma, or vegetation on the heart valves that may be associated with embolic ischemic stroke or left ventricular hypertrophy associated with chronic hypertension often seen in patients with sponta-neous ICH (Jauch et al., 2013; Morgenstern et al., 2010). Common cardiac conditions associated with a stroke include mitral stenosis, dilated left ventricle, a patent foramen ovale (PFO), valve vegetation, atrial enlargement, and intracardiac thrombus.

Testing Considerations

The interprofessional team caring for a patient during a TTE is expanded to include an echo-cardiography sonographer and, generally, a cardiologist ⊙. The stroke patient must turn to the left side while the sonographer conducts the ultrasound. If an agitated bubble study is indicated to assess for PFO, a nurse, advanced practice provider, or physician will administer agitated saline. This entails agitating normal saline to create bubbles using two syringes and a stopcock and then rapidly infusing this solution into a peripheral IV line (Hepburn, 2014). A TTE is noninvasive and is generally well tolerated without complications.

🔲 TRANSESOPHAGEAL ECHOCARDIOGRAM

Technique

A transesophageal echocardiogram (TEE) is an invasive form of cardiac echocardiog-raphy in which a probe is placed into the patient's esophagus to obtain cardiac imag-ing. A TEE is superior for providing retrocardiac views of the heart (Jauch et al., 2013). Agitated saline administration can also be used during this procedure.

Indications

The indications for this procedure are the same as for the TTE, and this test is generally indicated if there are unclear findings or inconclusive findings on the TTE or if retrocar-diac ultrasound views are specifically indicated.

Testing Considerations

As with a TTE, collaboration with physicians and ultrasound technologist needs to occur to provide safe patient care during this procedure ⊙. Moderate sedation is required when performing this procedure and appropriate monitoring should occur during and after the procedure. On rare occasions, significant complications may occur, including damage to the vocal cords or esophagus.

🔲 ELECTROENCEPHALOGRAPHY

Technique

Electroencephalography (EEG) is a noninvasive procedure that uses anywhere from 20 to 32 scalp electrodes to record electrical activity of cerebral cortex and amplify impulses into a measureable graph (Hickey & Murphy, 2010). The results are digitally processed and displayed on a computer screen. The frequency, amplitude, and waveform characteristics are all recorded. An EEG may be used intermittently or continuously depending on the purpose of the test (Hickey, 2014). The results of the EEG are used in conjunction with other tests to determine the diagnosis of the patient.

Indication

An EEG is the best test to monitor for seizure in the setting of stroke. All types of seizure activity are captured with an EEG, including frank seizures, nonconvulsive seizures, and status epilepticus. The EEG is especially useful when the patient is at risk for seizures and is pharmacologically paralyzed such as during induced hypothermia or undergoing treatment for refractory intracranial hypertension. An EEG may also be helpful in detecting vasospasm and ischemia after SAH, although clear indications for ongoing monitoring and treatment thresholds for EEG in vasospasm have yet to be developed. An EEG may help determine any injury that may be causing a lateral deficit. Generalized encephalopathy can also be detected using an EEG. Continuous EEG monitoring is useful for stroke patients with depressed levels of consciousness who may be experiencing nonconvulsive seizures.

Testing Considerations

An EEG technologist, in conjunction with either a neurologist with EEG expertise or an epileptologist, generally facilitates EEG monitoring. There are very few risks associated with EEG. It is difficult to obtain a reliable test when the patient becomes agitated or has significant movement. Additionally, it is difficult to obtain a reliable EEG waveform reading when the patient is receiving a large amount of sedation. Therefore, EEG testing must be correlated clinically with the patient's physical condition as well as medication administered at the time of the test. When the patient is receiving intermittent EEG monitoring, it is important to keep patient quiet and motionless during this time. Most intermittent EEG testing is completed within 20 to 60 minutes.

For the patient receiving continuous EEG monitoring, several additional considerations must be addressed. The nurse and the physician team should collaborate at least daily with the EEG technician to provide electrode maintenance. Electrode maintenance includes checking the skin under the electrodes for breakdown, assuring contact between the electrode and scalp to ensure accurate waveforms, and minimizing artifacts. Any signs of artifact should be brought to the EEG technician's attention. The patient's scalp integrity needs to be assessed every shift for signs of abrasions. If a head dressing is used to hold scalp electrodes in place, be sure to assess that two fingers can fit underneath the head dressing so not to put pressure on the scalp or forehead. If a video recording of the patient is also being used to record the patient's movements, the camera should be pointed toward the patient at all times. The nursing staff will be able to mark the EEG record when there is patient activity suspicious for seizure or medications are administered that may interfere with EEG monitoring.

CAROTID DUPLEX OR DOPPLER ULTRASOUND

Technique

Carotid duplex ultrasound, also known as *carotid Doppler ultrasound*, is a noninvasive ultrasound imaging test to assess patency of the carotid arteries (Jauch et al., 2013). Electrical energy is converted into ultrasound waves which have various acoustic impedances. The handheld probe or transducer sends echo waves back to the artery and back to the transducer. The Doppler effect, or sound waves, are transmitted and reflected onto a picture at varying intensities, reflecting the varied densities.

Indications

The ultrasound can detect and estimate the degree of vessel stenosis often caused by arthrosclerosis or vessel wall dissection (Jauch et al., 2013). Carotid duplex can also evaluate the collateral capacity of the circle of Willis. This procedure is least invasive test to assess the patency of the carotid arteries and is often used as a screening tool for patients at high-risk for vessel stenosis. However, carotid duplex frequently overestimates the amount of carotid stenosis. When stenosis is detected, confirmatory tests such as CTA, MRA, or catheter angiography, with better sensitivity and specificity, may be ordered.

Testing Considerations

As with TTE and TEE, carotid duplex ultrasonography is generally performed by an ultrasound technologist in conjunction with a cardiologist with ultrasonography training. This test is generally well tolerated without significant risk or side effects.

▮▮ TRANSCRANIAL DOPPLER

Technique

Transcranial Doppler (TCD) is a safe, noninvasive ultrasound test used to detect the velocity of the flow in the cerebral arteries (Harris, 2014). To perform this test, a trained technologist places a handheld probe over the thin skull area of the temporal bone. The probe is used to send low-frequency pulsed sound waves. These sound waves reflect back the velocity of blood flow for any artery in its path. The velocity is converted into a waveform and sound recordings of the cerebral vessels.

Indications

TCD is best established in the monitoring of patients with SAH for the development of vasospasm. As vasospasm occurs, vessel velocity will increase as the blood flow becomes more turbulent through the narrowed blood vessel. Early detection of vasospasm and response to vasospasm treatment can be detected using the TCD, particularly when monitoring occurs over a period of time, allowing velocity trends to develop. TCD is also useful to detect severe intracranial stenosis in carotid and vertebrobasilar vessels. Less frequent indications for TCD monitoring include assessing patterns and extent of collateral circulation supporting an area of ischemic infarct, microemboli detection during cardiac or carotid surgery, and in assessing acute ischemic stroke revascularization after IV thrombolysis.

Testing Considerations

TCD is noninvasive, painless, and generally well tolerated. One criticism of this test is that test results are highly operator dependent (Harris, 2014). Therefore, technologist competency is paramount and should be frequently assessed. Additionally, TCD can only capture the velocity of flow in the large cerebral vessels. TCD is not a reliable test to establish the presence of microvascular vasospasm.

▉ ELECTROCARDIOGRAM

Technique

A 12-lead electrocardiogram (ECG) is completed by placing electrodes at specific places over the thorax and the limbs to detect microscopic electric activity associated with the depolarization and repolarization of the heart with each heartbeat. Electrodes detect the electric activity and amplify the activity into a graph. Electrodes are placed throughout the body to best capture the hearts depolarization and repolarization from a variety of different directions, allowing different areas of the heart to be depicted from different leads or views.

Indication

A 12-lead ECG is recommended immediately upon admission with a stroke because cardiac disease has a high incidence in patients with a stroke, and patients with acute stroke may be experiencing cardiac dysfunction such as a myocardial infarct or heart failure. Although conducting an ECG on admission is a high priority, obtaining the ECG should not delay the initiation of acute stroke treatment. ECG monitoring should be continued using cardiac telemetry monitoring for at least the first 24 hours after stroke to screen for transient atrial fibrillation or other arrhythmias associated with acute ischemic stroke (Jauch et al., 2013). ECG changes can occur due to complications of a hemorrhagic stroke. A patient with SAH or ICH may experience ECG changes (Hickey, 2014). The patient with SAH should be assessed for Q-T prolongation and T-wave inversion associated with the catecholamine release during the hemorrhagic event.

S U M M A R Y

Diagnostic testing is critical in the diagnosis and management of all patients with stroke, regardless of the etiology. By understanding the indications, benefits, and risks associated with each test, all members of the interprofessional team can work together to provide safe and evidence-based care for the patient with stroke. Additionally, the team providing care to a patient with stroke will generally expand to include technologists and practitioners from other specialties including radiology, neuroradiology, cardiology, and epileptology. The team must coordinate care during the testing period to usher the patient safely through the stroke continuum of care.

R E F E R E N C E S

Connolly, E. S., Jr., Rabinstein, A. A., Carhuapoma, J. R., Derdeyn, C. P., Dion, J., Higashida, R. T., . . . Vespa, P. (2012). Guidelines for the management of aneurysmal subarachnoid hemorrhage: A guideline for healthcare professionals from the American Heart Association/American Stroke Association. *Stroke, 43*(6), 1711–1737. doi:10.1161/STR.0b013e3182587839

Deshmukh, M., & Yafai, S. (2008). Interpreting noncontrast head CT. *Advanced Emergency Nursing Journal, 30*(4), 297–302.

Dillon, W. P. (2012). Neuroimaging in neurologic disorders. In A. S. Fauci, D. L. Kasper, D. L. Longo, E. Braunwald, S. L. Hauser, J. L. Jameson, & J. Loscalzo (Eds.), *Harrison's principles of internal medicine.* New York, NY: McGraw-Hill.

Harris, C. (2014). Neuromonitoring indications and utility in the intensive care unit. *Critical Care Nurse, 34*(3), 30–39.

Hepburn, M. (2014). Stroke diagnostics. In S. Livesay (Ed.), *AANN comprehensive review for stroke nursing* (pp. 83–100). Chicago, IL: American Association of Neuroscience Nurses.

Hickey, J. V. (2014). Diagnostics for patients with neurological disorders. In J. Hickey (Ed.), *The clinical practice of neurological and neurosurgical nursing* (7th ed., pp. 93–113). Philadelphia, PA: Wolters Kluwer/ Lippincott Williams & Wilkins.

Hickey, J., & Murphy, K. P. (2010). Neurodiagnostic tests. In M. K. Bader & L. Littlejohns (Eds.), *AANN core curriculum for neuroscience nursing* (pp. 159–184). Glenview, IL: American Association of Neuroscience Nurses.

Jauch, E. C., Saver, J. L., Adams, H. P., Jr., Bruno, A., Connors, J. J., Demaerschalk, B. M., . . . Yonas, H. (2013). Guidelines for the early management of patients with acute ischemic stroke: A guideline for healthcare professionals from the American Heart Association/American Stroke Association. *Stroke, 44*(3), 870–947. doi:10.1161/STR.0b013e318284056a

Morgenstern, L. B., Hemphill, J. C., III, Anderson, C., Becker, K., Broderick, J. P., Connolly, E. S., Jr., . . . Tamargo, R. J. (2010). Guidelines for the management of spontaneous intracerebral hemorrhage: A guideline for healthcare professionals from the American Heart Association/American Stroke Association. *Stroke, 41*(9), 2108–2129. doi:10.1161/STR.0b013e3181ec611b

Summer, D., & Malloy, R. (2011). CT and MR imaging in the acute ischemic stroke patient: A nursing perspective. *Journal of Radiology Nursing, 30*(3), 104–115.

CHAPTER 6

Ischemic Stroke

Karen B. Seagraves and Sarah L. Livesay

Care of the ischemic stroke patient has evolved from the days of supportive care with little hope of recovery to become a treatable disease. Early recognition, use of advanced imaging, administration of intravenous and intra-arterial thrombolytics, and endovascular reperfusion provide patients with improved prognoses and often the ability to return to productive and satisfying lives. ⊙ To facilitate improved outcomes, it is essential that members of the interprofessional team are aggressive with early mobility, interaction, and education for the patient with ischemic stroke. The interprofessional team caring for the patient with ischemic stroke is composed of health professionals representing medicine and surgery, nursing, physical medicine and rehabilitation, physical and occupational therapy, speech and language pathology, case management, social work, nutrition support, and pharmacy. Their understanding of the pathophysiology and etiology of ischemic stroke as well as patient risk factors and comorbidities is imperative to anticipating the course of treatment and plan of care. With the expansion of understanding of stroke pathology and treatment over the past three decades, there has never been more availability of evidence-based guidelines and education for physicians, nurses, and interprofessional team members specific to stroke care that is easily accessible. The challenge facing all stroke practitioners is consistently implementing evidence-based stroke care in an organized fashion for all stroke patients across the nation.

This chapter will review the epidemiology and pathophysiology of stroke, initial and ongoing patient management, and interprofessional care of the stroke patient. Additionally, the organization of stroke care including stroke quality measures and evidenced-based best practices for optimal outcomes and care coordination across the continuum of care are discussed. This chapter will also discuss clinical recommendations for stroke care that come from the most recent guidelines available in early 2014 published by the American Heart Association and recommendations of the Brain Attack Coalition (BAC).

Clinical Pearl: Stroke information is available at your fingertips. There are comprehensive applications (apps) for your smart phone or tablet that include scales for ischemic and hemorrhagic stroke.

⬛ BACKGROUND

Stroke is the fourth leading cause of death in the United States. In 2010, 1 of every 19 deaths in the United States was from stroke. Each year, 795,000 people have strokes at a cost of $36.5 billion (Go et al., 2013). Of these, 610,000 are first strokes and 180,000 are recurrent strokes. Ischemic stroke is the most common type of stroke in the United States, comprising 87% of all strokes. Intracerebral hemorrhage (ICH) accounts for 10% of all strokes in the United States, and 3% are caused by subarachnoid hemorrhage (Go et al., 2013). Stroke carries a significant burden and is a disease that disproportionately impacts minority populations. Approximately 25% of patients who are 65 years of age and older will die within 1 year after their first stroke, and over 50% of patients who are 65 years of age and older will be dead within 5 years of their first stroke. Of patients between the ages of 45 and 64 years at the time of their first stroke, 14% of Caucasian men and 18% of Caucasian women will be dead at 1 year. Of African American patients having a first stroke between the ages of 45 and 64 years, 18% of men and 19% of women will be dead at 1 year. The death rate at 5 years is significantly higher for African American patients than white patients, with 40% of African American women versus 29% of Caucasian women and 41% of African American men versus 26% of Caucasian men dead within 5 years of their first stroke (Go et al., 2013). People living in the southeastern United States in the area known as the stroke belt have a 20% higher stroke mortality than the rest of the country. The number of adults between the ages of 20 and 54 years having strokes has increased, whereas a decline in other age groups has been noted. As the baby boomer population ages, it is anticipated that by 2030, an additional 3.4 million people will have had a stroke (Go et al., 2013). For additional information on stroke epidemiology and risk, refer to Chapter 1 on Stroke Epidemiology, Definition, Burden, and Prevention.

⬛ PATHOPHYSIOLOGY

Ischemic stroke occurs through a number of mechanisms that all result in the blockage of an artery and subsequent cell death. Several common ischemic stroke subtypes are recognized, and the etiology of a patient's stroke will determine how care is customized for the patient (**Table 6-1**).

Regardless of the etiology, during an acute ischemic stroke, 2 million neurons die every minute (Hickey, 2013). Neuronal death from ischemia is rapid because the brain cannot store glucose and without oxygen does not have any mechanism to create its own energy supply. The degree and duration of limited blood flow impact the brain cells differently. Oligemia is a reduction in the volume of blood flowing to the brain. The progression to ischemia occurs when the reduction in blood flow causes insufficient volume to perfuse the tissue. This results in infarction. This continuum creates a phenomenon known as the *ischemic penumbra*. The core of the infarct is the area of little to no perfusion that progresses to neuronal death and is considered unsalvageable. The penumbra is the

TABLE 6-1 Stroke Etiology

Percentage	Etiology of Stroke
20%	Atherothrombotic cerebrovascular disease of the large vessels including extra- and intracranial stenosis, dissection, and vasculitis
25%	Lacunar or small vessel ischemic disease of the penetrating arteries
20%	Cardioembolic related to atrial fibrillation, dilated cardiomyopathy, patent foramen ovale (PFO), and endocarditis
30%	Cryptogenic or no identifiable cause
5%	Venous thrombosis, hypoperfusion from hypotension related to shock or myocardial infarction (MI), hypercoagulability, cocaine use

From Albers, G. W., Amarenco, P., Easton, J. D., Sacco, R. L., & Teal, P. (2001). Antithrombotic and thrombolytic therapy for ischemic stroke. *Chest, 119*(1)(Suppl.), 300S–320S.

area surrounding the core infarct that although is experiencing a limited supply of oxygen and glucose has several hours of potential viability should blood flow be restored.

A sudden onset of sustained ischemia is more detrimental to brain tissue than one either of short duration or one that progresses slowly. Initially, the brain attempts to compensate using cerebral autoregulatory mechanisms by vasodilating, expanding collateral vessels, and increasing the oxygen and glucose extraction from the blood. If compensatory mechanisms fail, and brain cells are without oxygenated blood flow, tissue becomes ischemic and will progress to cell death or infarct if uncorrected (Shah, 2002). The availability of collateral circulation greatly influences the individual response to ischemia. Collateral circulation refers to a network of small arterial vessels that develop to support the arterial perfusion of brain tissue (Liebeskind, 2003). Much remains unknown about collateral cerebral circulation. However, patients with chronic atherosclerosis and ischemia may have developed an extensive network of small artery growth that supports the blood perfusion to the chronically affected brain tissue. When an acute ischemic stroke occurs, recruitment of collateral circulation begins immediately (Liebeskind, 2003). However, the degree to which each individual develops a collateral network of circulation varies for reasons not well understood.

Ischemic stroke may occur in large or small cerebral arteries, although the mechanism of ischemic stroke is generally different in large versus small arteries. Large artery vessel disease impacts both the intra- and extracranial arteries through a process of atherosclerosis. Fatty streaks full of foam cells as well as circulating lipids turn to plaques in the artery walls. When plaque forms in the lining of the blood vessels, it causes narrowing of the lumen. Through an acute process often mediated by inflammation, the plaques may ulcerate and thrombose, developing an acute occlusion of the artery. Additionally, atherosclerotic plaque may calcify, increasing the risk for rupture. The plaque disrupts the smooth surface of the artery and can become sites for thrombus formation. The narrowing or even complete blockage of the artery lumen limits blood flow, resulting in ischemia in the brain tissue distal to the obstruction. In the smaller arterioles and capillaries, stroke is caused by tiny thrombi formed when there is a release of vasoactive enzymes from the endothelium, leukocytes, and platelets. The endothelial cells swell, reducing the patency of the vessel lumen. Therefore, larger artery strokes generally result from atherosclerotic processes, and small artery strokes generally result from chronic vessel disease resulting from hypertension and diabetes mellitus.

Emboli from plaque or vegetation in the heart or aorta may be the etiology of large vessel obstruction resulting in ischemic stroke. Embolic strokes most often affect the middle cerebral artery (MCA) because of its anatomic proximity to the carotid arteries. Eighty percent of the blood carried to the brain through the large arteries of the neck passes through the MCAs (**Fig. 6-1** shows a detailed view of cerebral arteries). Therefore, when obstruction is noted in the large vessels of the brain, particularly the MCA, but also the posterior circulation, a full cardiac workup is indicated to identify the potential source for an embolism (Ustrell & Pellisé, 2010).

Regardless of the mechanism, within minutes of ischemia, the leukocytes that migrate to the area activate oxygen-free radicals, cytokines, and nitric acid. These mediators result in cellular and vessel changes that result in the vessels becoming more permeable, resulting in cerebral edema. This occurs within 1 hour of ischemia and is the beginning of cellular apoptosis (Shah, 2002). When brain tissue becomes ischemic, cell death and subsequent intracellular edema occurs. The edema compromises capillaries, which even further deprive the brain of blood and much needed oxygenation. The

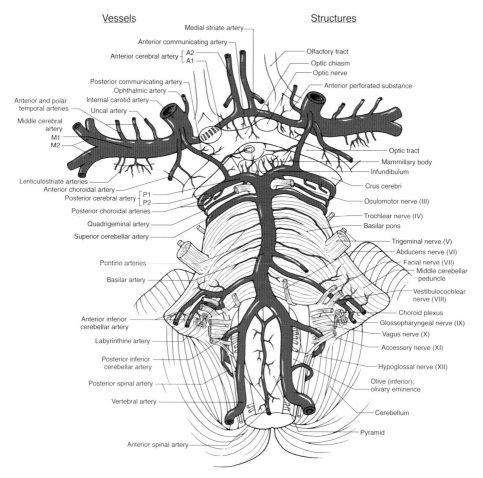

FIGURE 6-1 Cerebral arteries. The cerebral arteries covering the ventral surface of the brain, including the circle of Willis. *(From Haines, D. E. [2004]. Neuroanatomy: An atlas of structures, sections, and systems [6th ed.]. Baltimore, MD: Lippincott Williams & Wilkins.)*

larger the stroke size and territory of infarct, the more likely the development of cerebral edema. Cerebral edema generally peaks 72 hours after initial injury. Therefore, the patient may worsen clinically in days 1 to 3 following the initial event.

Additional neurological injury may occur after the initial stroke event, resulting from vasospasm triggered by the presence of emboli in a large vessel as well as hemorrhagic transformation of the ischemic stroke. Infarcted brain tissue is friable and sensitive to pressure changes associated with fluctuations in perfusion. Hemorrhagic transformation of an ischemic stroke results from abnormal bleeding into the brain tissue in the region of ischemia and infarct. If the thrombus or embolus causing the ischemia or infarct migrate or dissolve either spontaneously or as a result of thrombolytics, there can be resulting reperfusion to an area of cerebral tissue no longer able to support circulation (Shah, 2002). Hemorrhagic conversion of ischemic strokes is discussed in greater detail in Chapter 7.

In small vessel strokes, the smaller arteries are involved, and the changes to the blood vessel are typically the outcome of thickening of the vessel lining as a result of lipohyalinosis. These infarcts lead to the lacuna seen on imaging and reported as lacunar infarcts. These infarcts are typically found in the basal ganglia, thalamus, white matter of the internal capsule, and the pons (Hickey, 2013). Hypertension is the leading cause of small vessel ischemic strokes. Again, the impact of the stroke will depend on the size and territory of the infarct, which is based on where along the artery the occlusion occurs. In conclusion, the variables that impact the size of the infarct are collateral circulation available in the individual brain and the speed with which reperfusion of the penumbra is established.

Clinical Pearl: Only 50% of people have a complete circle of Willis joining the anterior and posterior circulation of the brain, which explains the variability of human response to strokes in similar territories due to availability of collateral circulation.

STROKE LOCATION

Localization of an ischemic stroke lesion involves recognizing syndromes or patterns of stroke based on location of affected arteries. This can help to predict or interpret the neurological deficits in acute stroke. The patient with stroke will experience symptoms based on which artery is occluded and how much brain tissue is without arterial circulation. Presenting symptoms can be used to predict complications, morbidity, and mortality in the stroke patient. In a left MCA stroke, the patient presents with aphasia, a left gaze preference, and right hemiplegia. In a right MCA stroke, the patient presents with a right gaze preference, left hemiplegia, and neglect. Neglect is the phenomenon that occurs when patients are unable to recognize, pay attention to, or acknowledge the existence of one side of the body. Anterior cerebral artery (ACA) strokes presents on the right side with apathy and left arm and leg weakness and on the left side with aphasia, apathy, and right arm and leg weakness. A patient presenting with a basilar artery stroke may exhibit quadriplegia or hemiplegia, locked-in syndrome, nystagmus, vertigo, diplopia, nausea and vomiting, or ataxia. The same symptoms without paralysis may indicate vertebral artery stroke (**Fig. 6-2** shows the motor cortex homunculus).

Clinical Pearl: Approach patients from the unaffected side when they have homonymous hemianopsia (loss of vision in half of each visual field) to avoid startling the patients.

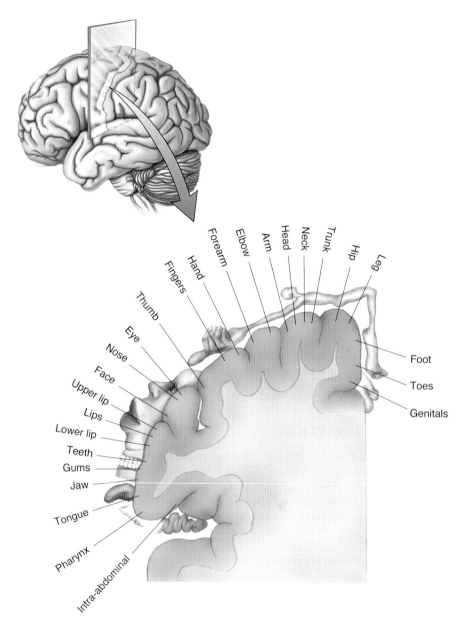

FIGURE 6-2 Motor cortex homunculus. The regions of the brain correlate with sensory receptors in specific areas of the body. The map of the cortex, commonly called the *homunculus*, illustrates the areas of the cortex commonly associated with sensory receptors on the skin. *(From Archer, P., & Nelson, L. A. [2013]. Applied anatomy & physiology for manual therapists. Philadelphia, PA: Lippincott Williams & Wilkins.)*

THE CONTINUUM OF STROKE CARE

The care of the patient with acute ischemic stroke is often categorized into three distinct phases based on the pathophysiology as discussed earlier and therapeutic goals of care (Summers et al., 2009). The hyperacute stroke period refers to the first several hours after an acute ischemic stroke. During the hyperacute phase of care, the interprofessional team is focused on efforts to treat the ischemic stroke and open the obstructed artery, when possible. The acute stroke phase generally begins 12 to 24 hours after the stroke begins and continues through the first several days after stroke. The goals of care during the acute phase of stroke include identifying the cause of the stroke, preventing and managing complications of the stroke, and initiating secondary prevention strategies to prevent another stroke event. The subacute phase of stroke care starts approximately 3 to 5 days after the stroke and continues for the first several weeks after the stroke. The goals of care during the subacute phase include the continued management of complications, continuation of secondary prevention measures to prevent another stroke event, aggressive rehabilitation to regain function, and reintegration of the stroke survivor back into the community (Summers et al., 2009).

STROKE PREVENTION: BEGINNING THE CONTINUUM

When a patient presents with acute ischemic stroke, clinicians employ a multitude of diagnostic tests to determine the source of the embolus or cause of the thrombus. Although viewed as comorbidities, these often preventable disease processes are the primary contributors to stroke. Up to 80% of strokes can be prevented (Go et al., 2013). Although age, sex, race, and family history cannot be changed, other risk factor modifications, with the guidance of a health care professional, can reduce stroke risk and increase awareness of signs and symptoms of acute stroke. High-impact risk factor modifications include controlling blood pressure, cholesterol, and blood glucose. Atrial fibrillation management, controlling diabetes, smoking cessation, maintenance of a healthy weight and body mass index, and eating a healthy diet can reduce risk of stroke. Stress, depression, oral contraceptive and hormone replacement therapy use, illegal drug use, and alcohol abuse can also contribute to stroke and are modifiable risk factors. Secondary prevention focuses on the management of modifiable risk factors through pharmaceutical measures, behavior modification, education, and community support and resources. See Chapter 1 for further discussion of preventive strategies.

TRANSIENT ISCHEMIC ATTACK

Patients may enter the hospital as direct admissions or through the emergency department after having had symptoms of stroke that subsequently resolved or are rapidly improving. A transient ischemic attack (TIA) occurs when blood flow to part of the brain is interrupted for a brief period of time (Easton et al., 2009). Since 2009, a tissue-based definition has been used for TIA pointing to transient deficit in neurological function caused by focal brain, spinal cord, or retinal ischemia without acute infarction. Prior to 2009, TIAs were thought to be defined by an absence of deficits or symptoms within 24 hours of onset. Newer imaging technology has demonstrated that one third of patients with traditionally resolving TIAs have actually had tissue infarction. Therefore, defining TIA based on time to tissue resolution alone results in an inadequate diagnosis (Easton et al., 2009).

A TIA is an indicator of significant risk for subsequent stroke. Ten percent to 15% of patients with TIA will go on to have a stroke within the following 90 days and half of those occur within 48 hours (Easton et al., 2009). Patients experiencing TIA are at high risk and need neurodiagnostic imaging, preferably diffusion magnetic resonance imaging (MRI), within 24 hours of symptom onset. Every effort should be made to determine the cause of ischemia and associated damage. Noninvasive imaging of the cervical vessels should be performed to assess for carotid stenosis and is typically done using magnetic resonance angiography (MRA) or carotid duplex. It is essential to uncover the mechanism that contributed to the event to determine the plan of care, the potential course of the disease process, and appropriate treatment. Blood work should mirror the workup including complete blood count, blood chemistry, prothrombin time (PT), partial thromboplastin time (PTT), and a fasting lipid profile. TIAs of unknown origin after diagnostic workup may need cardiac studies such as Holter monitoring, generally completed in the outpatient setting.

In the patient experiencing TIA, the ABCD^2 score can predict the likelihood of a subsequent stroke and may be used to tailor care (Johnston et al., 2007). The score is determined by assigning a value to risk factors such as age 60 years and older, blood pressure, type and duration of neurological symptoms, and presence of diabetes. The score does not include findings from imaging studies. Some stroke programs use the ABCD^2 score to determine the need for acute hospitalization versus follow-up in an outpatient setting within a few days of the TIA episode. Regardless of complete resolution of symptoms, if not admitted to the hospital, then patients should have diagnostic imaging scheduled as soon as possible after leaving the emergency department. Recently, a variety of TIA clinics have been designed for expeditious follow-up that allow for completion of MRI with diffusion-weighted imaging (DWI) and other neurodiagnostic studies including transcranial Doppler and carotid ultrasound. Clinic follow-up for TIA also allows an opportunity for risk factor review, planning, and teaching for medical management and consultation as needed for surgical treatment options.

HYPERACUTE STROKE CARE TREATMENT

The hyperacute phase of stroke care begins with stroke symptom recognition by the patient or witness and mobilization to the hospital for acute stroke care. Emergency department (ED) care occurs faster if the patient is brought to the hospital by local emergency medical services (EMS) (Jauch et al., 2013). Once the stroke patient has arrived at the ED, care should be provided according to the recommendation in the "Guidelines for the Early Management of Patients with Acute Ischemic Stroke" from the American Heart Association (Jauch et al., 2013). The guidelines reference National Institute of Neurological Disorders and Stroke (NINDS) recommendations from a 1996 symposium outlining specific time frames for the delivery of key elements of care.

Initial Emergency Department Response

Quick recognition of acute stroke symptoms and mobilization of the interprofessional team is paramount to the rapid treatment of the stroke event. Recommendations are for a patient to see a physician in 10 minutes or less from arrival and stroke team activation within 15 minutes. A computed tomography (CT) scan of the head should occur in 25 minutes or less, with results reported within 45 minutes or less from hospital ED arrival. In eligible patients, intravenous tissue plasminogen activator (tPA) should be administered within 60 minutes or less from arrival (**Table 6-2**) (Jauch et al., 2013). The same goal parameters for assessment and treatment apply to inpatients exhibiting signs and symptoms of acute stroke. One successful model to achieve time-based interventions includes prehospital notification of an inbound stroke patient from EMS and activation of the interprofessional team from the EMS phone call ⊙. The team converges on the patient location and provides rapid assessment, ordering of diagnostic studies, and acute interventions.

The urgent goal of ED treatment of a patient with new stroke symptoms is to identify the type of stroke (e.g., ischemic vs. hemorrhagic stroke) and evaluate the patient for urgent intervention, including intravenous fibrinolysis and endovascular procedures to open the occluded vessel. This process includes the rapid completion of neurological assessment, diagnostic imaging, and diagnostic testing including essential laboratory values. Within the aforementioned time frames, a thorough history and physical assessment should be conducted with a standardized neurological exam such as the National Institutes of Health Stroke Scale (NIHSS) (Meyer, Hemmen, Jackson, & Lyden, 2002).

TABLE 6-2 Intravenous Thrombolysis Exclusion Criteria

Contraindication	Warning (may increase the risk of unfavorable outcome but not an absolute contraindication)	Additional Contraindication in 3–4.5-Hr Window
SBP >185 or DBP >110 mm Hg	Advanced age	Age >80 years
CT finding suggests ICH, SAH, or well-established major ischemic stroke	Unable to determine eligibility	History of prior stroke and diabetes
Suspicion for SAH	Glucose <50 or >400 mg/dL	Any anticoagulant use prior to admission, even if INR <1.7
Seizure at onset unless diagnosis of vascular occlusion is established	Pregnancy	NIHSS >25
Recent intracranial or spinal surgery, head trauma, or stroke (<3 months)	Septic thrombophlebitis	CT finding demonstrates stroke involves more than one third of the MCA territory
Major surgery or trauma (within 3 months)	Acute pericarditis, bacterial endocarditis	
History of ICH, brain aneurysm, vascular malformation, or brain tumor		
Recent active internal bleeding including arterial puncture at a noncompressible site		
Platelets <100,000/mm³; heparin use within 48 hr with PTT >40 sec or exceeding upper range; INR >1.7		
Known bleeding diathesis or other major disorder associated with increased bleeding risk		

SBP, systolic blood pressure; DBP, diastolic blood pressure.
Adapted from Jauch, E. C., Saver, J. L., Adams, H. P., Jr., Bruno, A., Connors, J. J., Demaerschalk, B. M., . . . Yonas, H. (2013). Guidelines for the early management of patients with acute ischemic stroke: A guideline for healthcare professionals from the American Heart Association/American Stroke Association. *Stroke, 44*(3), 870–947.

The assessment helps to confirm suspicion for stroke and rule out any disease processes that present like stroke. These are often referred to as *stroke mimics*. Stroke mimics include hypoglycemia, seizures, migraine, tumors, drug intoxication, and psychogenic causes. All potential stroke patients should have a noncontract CT scan of the brain or brain MRI. The noncontrast CT of the brain is sensitive for detection of ICH and subarachnoid hemorrhage (SAH) and will help the clinician determine if hemorrhage is causing stroke symptoms or if ischemic stroke is the expected mechanism. Many stroke centers are including CT angiography and CT perfusion emergently with or immediately following the initial CT imaging.

Initial Diagnostics and Blood Pressure Control

The ED workup should include the assessment of blood glucose, oxygen saturation, and blood work including serum electrolytes, renal function tests, a complete blood count, platelet count, activated partial thromboplastin time (aPTT), and PT with international normalized ratio (INR). An electrocardiogram (ECG) and cardiac markers should also be completed as acute myocardial infarction may occur with ischemic stroke. Blood pressure management in the first hour of stroke treatment will depend on whether the patient receives treatment with intravenous recombinant tissue plasminogen activator (rtPA). Seventy-seven percent of patients experiencing a first stroke have blood pressure reading greater than 140/90 mm Hg (Go et al., 2013). For an ischemic stroke patient not receiving rtPA, current guidelines recommend that blood pressure not be lowered during the first 24 hours of stroke unless it is greater than 220/120 mm Hg. If the blood pressure requires reduction in the first 24 hours, it may be lowered by 15% of the presenting elevated pressure with concurrent monitoring for any sign or symptoms of neurological deterioration (Jauch et al., 2013). In order to administer intravenous rtPA, the blood pressure must be gently lowered to less than 185/110 mm Hg using agents such as labetalol or nicardipine. Once given, the blood pressure must be maintained below 180/105 mm Hg to minimize the risk of intracranial hemorrhage. Frequent monitoring is necessary to maintain the blood pressure within the safe range. Blood pressure should be monitored with neurological checks every 15 minutes for 2 hours, then every 30 minutes for the next 6 hours, and hourly for the remainder of the 24 hours from the administration of intravenous rtPA. This is a class I, level of evidence B recommendation in the most recent iteration of the American Heart Association "Guidelines for the Early Management of Patients with Acute Ischemic Stroke" (Hacke et al., 2008; Jauch et al., 2013). If elevated during the first 24 hours, blood glucose should be managed to a target range of between 140 and 180 mm Hg.

Initial Treatment

Fibrinolytic Therapy

Background

Intravenous (IV) fibrinolysis with tPA is the only approved treatment for ischemic stroke. Stroke treatment with IV tPA was approved by the U.S. Food and Drug Administration (FDA) after the 1996 NINDS Stroke Trial demonstrated that treatment with IV tPA within 3 hours of stroke symptom onset was associated with significantly improved outcome when measured at 90 days (The National Institute of Neurological Disorders and Stroke rt-PA Stroke Study Group, 1995). Patients who received IV tPA were more likely to have less global disability, improved measures of activities of daily living, and less neurological deficit 90 days after drug administration. Hemorrhage, particularly ICH, is the major complication associated with tPA treatment. ICH occurred in 6% of patients treated with tPA in the NINDS Stroke Trial compared to 0.6% who were not treated in the NINDS trial. There was no significant difference in mortality between the groups at 90 days or 1 year. The medication was approved for use by the FDA in 1996 and has become the standard of care for patients who are eligible for treatment (Jauch et al., 2013).

Since the approval of tPA for treatment of ischemic stroke, several trials and retrospective reviews have influenced fibrinolytic treatment. The European Cooperative Acute Stroke Study (ECASS III) trial demonstrated that tPA could be safely given to patients who present up to 4.5 hours after stroke symptom onset with a few additional exclusion parameters (Hacke et al., 2008). Patients receiving oral warfarin regardless of INR, patients with diabetes and a history of stroke, and patients older than age 80 years may be eligible for IV tPA if they present within 3 hours of stroke but should be excluded in the 3- to 4.5-hour time frame. The American Heart Association/American Stroke Association (AHA/ASA) endorsed the extended treatment window. However, the FDA has yet to approve the drug for usage in the extended window. Most organizations have embraced the extended time window and treat patients who present within 4.5 hours of stroke symptom onset.

Additionally, several retrospective case reviews have resulted in modifications to the original NINDS Stroke Trial inclusion and exclusion criteria for tPA treatment of patients who present within 3 hours of stroke treatment (**Table 6-2**). For example, the original trial excluded patients who had an NIHSS score higher than 4. However, experience with tPA treatment and stroke disease has revealed that patients with NIHSS less than 4 often experience debilitating strokes and often worsen after the first few hours of stroke. Therefore, most practitioners no longer consider this an absolute contraindication and treat patients with low NIHSS. As the inclusion and exclusion criteria continue to evolve, please refer to the most recent AHA/ASA clinical practice guideline for a detailed review of the literature.

Care during Fibrinolytic Administration

In the ED, the decision to administer IV rtPA must be made quickly because early and rapid treatment of ischemic stroke with IV tPA is associated with improved outcomes. Trials consistently demonstrate that IV tPA is most effective if given within the first 60 minutes of the acute stroke and has less benefit if treatment is delayed (Ahmed et al., 2010).

Clinical Pearl: The maximal success of IV tPA treatment cannot be determined in the acute phase but rather at 90 days post stroke.

IV rtPA administration should not be delayed by additional neuroimaging beyond a noncontrast CT of the brain. The radiologist and technician teams may be helpful in determining which patients may benefit from advanced imaging and facilitate completion of these imaging tests without delaying administration of IV tPA when indicated ⊙. Additionally, studies not essential to the decision to administer IV tPA, such as ECG and chest x-ray, should not delay administration of the medication. To facilitate rapid treatment when a patient is a candidate, essential laboratory and CT imaging results should be available within 45 minutes of patient arrival to the ED. However, delayed results from blood work should not prohibit administration of tPA unless there is suspicion of a bleeding disorder or a patient taking anticoagulants (Jauch et al., 2013).

To facilitate quick administration of fibrinolytics when indicated, the team should discuss treatment options with the patient and family early in the acute workup. The stroke team may mobilize all necessary equipment and information for tPA administration including the patient's weight, an IV pump and connecting tubing, normal saline, and two IV access sites, with one preferably with a 16- to 18-gauge needle in the antecubital vein. The correct dose of IV tPA must be calculated by the team, as it is a weight-based medication. Any additional tPA that will not be administered to the patient according to weight should be discarded. The medication is administered in two steps, with a bolus dose of 10% of the total dose administered over 1 minute and the remaining dose administered through the IV pump over 1 hour (Activase [Alteplase], 2014). The patient receiving IV tPA should not receive anything by mouth during administration and is monitored by the team at least every 15 minutes. Assessment priorities include monitoring for orolingual angioedema, bleeding, worsening of neurological symptoms, decrease in level of consciousness, onset of severe headache, nausea and vomiting, and a change in the NIHSS score. Blood pressure should be monitored and managed as discussed in the previous section. The patient is generally transferred to a neurocritical care unit or a stroke unit capable of post-thrombolytic monitoring for at least the first 24 hours post-IV rtPA. At that time if the patient is hemodynamically stable and does not require airway management, the patient should be transferred to the stroke unit for care.

Clinical Pearl: Because the 3- to 4.5-hour window is considered off-label use by the FDA, many organizations require written signed consent be obtained prior to administering the rtPA.

Endovascular Therapy

Patients who are outside the window for IV rtPA or ineligible for IV tPA for any reason may benefit from an endovascular intervention. Recanalization of a large vessel, restoring blood flow in select patients, has been shown to be effective for reperfusion and restoration of function in the large vessel ischemic stroke patient (Jauch et al., 2013). This involves an invasive procedure whereby a catheter is inserted into the femoral artery and threaded to the large vessel occlusion. Once the catheter is at the site of the occlusion, a number of therapeutic techniques are available. The clot may be mechanically disrupted using a variety of embolectomy products, including stent retrievers and suction devices. Using catheters to guide medication administration, tPA may also be delivered directly into the clot (Jauch et al., 2013). By inserting a catheter and mechanically disrupting and removing the clot, blood flow is reestablished. Devices for mechanical embolectomy include suction and entrapment devices similar to cardiac stents and are used to reach and remove clots without damaging the lumen of the vessel.

Recently, two trials evaluate the role of endovascular therapy and call into question the role of the endovascular thrombectomy in acute stroke treatment (Broderick, Tomsick, & Palesch, 2013; Ciccone & Valvassori, 2013). The Interventional Management of Stroke (IMS III) trial and the Systemic Thrombolysis for Acute Ischemic Stroke (SYNTHESIS) trial both evaluated the role of endovascular therapy compared to IV tPA treatment. The IMS III trial included patients treated within 3 hours of symptom onset, whereas the SYNTHESIS trial included patients treated with endovascular therapy within 6 hours of symptom onset. The IMS III trial was stopped early due to futility when interim analysis revealed no significant difference between the IV tPA and the endovascular treatment groups. The SYNTHESIS trial showed no difference in outcome between IV tPA alone and endovascular therapy at 90-day follow-up. Further review of both studies revealed methodological concerns that have caused some in the stroke field to question the results. Nevertheless, the studies have called endovascular treatment into question, and many programs have amended their treatment protocols accordingly.

Although the evidence to support mechanical endovascular revascularization is still being reviewed and debated, many programs continue to provide endovascular treatment to patients with large vessel ischemic stroke. Any organization providing endovascular therapy should monitor outcomes closely. Therefore, The Joint Commission (TJC) has incorporated quality measures to evaluate outcomes for the stroke patients who receive these treatments. TJC standards and the AHA/ASA guidelines suggest that all patients receiving endovascular treatment should be monitored to measure outcome as well as complications associated with the procedure (TJC, 2014). Further studies are underway with the goal of better defining the role of endovascular treatment in acute stroke management.

Antithrombotic Therapy

The majority of ischemic stroke patients will receive neither IV tPA nor endovascular treatment. For patients who are not eligible for thrombolytic or endovascular treatment, care is aimed at preventing complications and instituting secondary stroke prevention measures. Studies have shown that patients with ischemic stroke benefit from early antithrombotic administration (Jauch et al., 2013). Patients who received IV tPA or endovascular treatment should not receive additional antiplatelet medication until 24 to 48 hours after thrombolysis or endovascular treatment. However, patients who do not receive IV tPA or endovascular therapy should receive 325 mg of aspirin orally within 24 to 48 hours of stroke event. This is a class I, level of evidence A recommendation (see Chapter 1 for grading system). For the most current treatment recommendations, refer to the online version of the "Guidelines for the Early Management of Patients with Acute Ischemic Stroke" from the AHA.

ACUTE STROKE CARE

Once patients have passed the first several hours of their ischemic stroke, care priorities shift. The treatment priority shifts from acute treatment of vessel occlusion in the hopes of reestablishing arterial perfusion and move toward the monitoring and management of complications and initiation of secondary prevention strategies to prevent another stroke from occurring. Patients will generally be admitted to the neuroscience intensive care unit (ICU) or stroke unit according to their acuity and the organization's monitoring policies. Additionally, the interprofessional team works collaboratively to institute early rehabilitation and develops a plan for transitioning the patient back into the community as a stroke survivor.

ADDITIONAL DIAGNOSTIC WORKUP

Patients with ischemic stroke should undergo physiological monitoring including ECG monitoring for at least 24 hours after the stroke event to monitor for underlying cardiac dysfunction and dysthymia that may have caused the stroke event. A cardiac workup including echocardiogram is indicated for any patient with a suspected cardiac stroke etiology. The patient should be placed on telemetry monitoring at minimum for the initial 24 hours to assess for dysrhythmias often associated with stroke such as atrial fibrillation. A 12-lead ECG should be obtained if not already completed in the emergency setting. In atypical stroke presentations, such as stroke in a patient younger than the age of 50 years, a hypercoagulable workup and atypical stroke etiology workup may be indicated. Therefore, much of the stroke team's efforts in the days following the stroke onset are aimed at determining the underlying cause of the stroke event. The diagnostic workup should incorporate tests to determine the cause of stroke as well as rule out stroke mimics (Jauch et al., 2013).

SUPPORTIVE CARE

To facilitate medication safety, the team should obtain a list of medications the patient was taking at home and any currently prescribed medications along with the administration time. Standard fall and aspiration precautions should be initiated to minimize risk of these complications. ASA stroke guidelines indicate supplemental oxygen only if the patient's oxygen level is below 94% on room air. Implement routine skin assessments using a standardized tool such as the Braden Scale, as stroke patients are at risk for the development of pressure ulcers as a result of loss of sensation and mobility (Bergstrom, Braden, Laguzza, & Holman, 1987). Temperature management including surface cooling and antipyretic medications may be indicated for fever. Blood glucose management is essential as diabetes is a risk fact for stroke, and elevated glucose may impact patient outcomes. Apply intermittent external compression devices if ordered for patients who cannot receive anticoagulants.

Patients with large vessel ischemic stroke must be monitored for the development of cerebral edema and potential herniation that may contribute to neurological decline in the days following the stroke (Jauch et al., 2013). Large territory MCA and basilar artery strokes are vascular territories with known risk for the development of cerebral edema, although edema may complicate the recovery of any stroke of significant size regardless of location. Patients younger than the age of 80 years with large stroke infarct volume and minimal cerebral atrophy are at higher risk for the development of cerebral edema after an ischemic stroke.

SECONDARY PREVENTION

In addition to stroke diagnostic workup, multiple secondary prevention strategies are initiated during the acute stroke hospitalization. Blood pressure is commonly elevated during acute ischemic stroke and continues to be a concern beyond the initial management in the ED. Treatment is recommended for blood pressures greater than or equal to 220/120 mm Hg. IV medication is typically used because of the rapid ability to decrease the blood pressure and because often swallowing is impaired in the acute stroke patient. Patients receiving thrombolytic therapy may be treated with IV labetalol 10 to 20 mg infused over 1 to 2 minutes and may be repeated. For hypertension refractory to labetalol, nicardipine is the recommended agent. For mild to moderately elevated pressures, after 24 to 48 hours of permissive hypertension, blood pressure is gently lowered with oral antihypertensive drugs to the normotensive range. After beginning to drop the blood pressure back to the normotensive range, monitor the patient for worsening neurological symptoms with lower blood pressures and titrate accordingly (Jauch et al., 2013).

There is little research to guide which oral antihypertensive medication to initiate after a stroke, and often, the cardiac guidelines are used to guide this decision. The Joint National Committee (JNC) guideline can be used to help guide the appropriate choice for oral antihypertensives (James et al., 2014). It is important to take into consideration any antihypertensives that the patient may have been taking at home.

Hyperlipidemia should be treated using a variety of approaches and may include treatment with a statin medication. Statins have been shown to decrease low-density lipoprotein (LDL) in patients with elevated levels, a known ischemic stroke risk factor. However, treatment of a stroke survivor with a statin medication, regardless of LDL level, has been shown to decrease subsequent stroke risk, and statin treatment should be considered in patients with ischemic stroke. Antithrombotic, anticoagulant, or antiplatelet medications should be initiated as appropriate for the patient's care. Aspirin (ASA) 325 mg is recommended as the initial agent for all patients with ischemic stroke. A patient who failed ASA therapy may be placed on clopidogrel 75 mg or dipyridamole. For patients with atrial fibrillation, enoxaparin followed by warfarin is appropriate, as are newer medications such as thrombin inhibitors (dabigatran 150 mg twice a day or 75 mg twice a day for the renally impaired patient). Acute or subacute anticoagulation may be indicated in patients with an active cardiac thrombus, end-stage heart disease, or other cardiac etiologies and should be done in accordance with AHA/ASA treatment guidelines (Jauch et al., 2013).

Patients with ischemic stroke are often dehydrated upon admission to the hospital and should be hydrated using IV fluid with a goal of achieving euvolemia. Hypotonic fluids may exacerbate the development of cerebral edema, and dextrose-containing fluids may contribute to poststroke hyperglycemia. Any hypotonic IV fluid such as 1/2 or 1/4 normal saline and fluid containing glucose should be avoided during acute stroke management (Jauch et al., 2013). Fluid resuscitation should be accomplished using normotonic fluids.

Surgical Treatment

Patients with ischemic stroke may require neurosurgical intervention for the placement of an external ventricular drain (EVD), intracranial pressure (ICP) monitor, or surgical decompression of the skull known as *craniectomy* to relieve elevated ICP and impending herniation syndromes (Jauch et al., 2013). A subset of patients with ischemic stroke may require placement of an EVD to monitor and manage ICP or to relieve obstructive hydrocephalus associated with edema or mass effect from an infarct. Patients with an EVD are generally managed in the ICU, with consultation from the neurosurgical team ⊙. Additionally, a fraction of patients with acute ischemic stroke may be considered for carotid revascularization surgery (Jauch et al., 2013). The role of carotid endarterectomy and carotid stenting in the acute setting remains unclear and controversial. However, emergent or urgent carotid surgery may be considered in special clinical situations and requires coordination and consultation with the cardiovascular surgery team ⊙.

When cerebral edema is present after an ischemic stroke and contributing to neurological decline, management should follow the stepwise approach to managing elevated ICP, including elevating the head of bed, pharmacological interventions including osmotic diuretic and hypertonic saline, and placement of EVD to provide cerebrospinal fluid (CSF) drainage (Jauch et al., 2013). For a detailed review of the management of ce-rebral edema, please refer to Chapter 9. Surgical decompression has been studied in the management of malignant cerebral edema associated with MCA territory infarcts as well as posterior circulation infarcts. The interprofessional team should identify patients at high risk for neurological deterioration from cerebral edema, and a neurosurgical team should be available and involved in the patient's care prior to deterioration ☉. The team should work together to identify the best timing for surgical intervention, if indicated.

Prevention of Complications

Patients with ischemic stroke are at high risk for complications, including the develop-ment of venous thrombosis, fever, aspiration and resulting pneumonia, hyperglycemia, and other infections that result from invasive procedures and monitoring (Jauch et al., 2013). Patients with ischemic stroke are also at risk for the development of poststroke depression. A quarter of patients admitted to the hospital for acute stroke will worsen due to myriad of complications during their hospital stay. For a detailed review of com-mon complications seen after stroke, as well as management strategies, please refer to Chapter 9.

Stroke Education

Standardized stroke education developed for stroke patients and their family members should be provided upon admission and throughout the duration of the patients' stay. Educational priorities include the pathophysiology of stroke with basic illustrations, in-formation about diagnostic testing and all consulting practitioners, medications, and risk factors. Prior to discharge, the interprofessional team educates the patient and fam-ily on the signs and symptoms of stroke, when and how to activate emergency systems such as calling 911, community resources, and follow-up information. Education is cus-tomized to the individual patient including the etiology of his or her stroke, risk factors, goals, and resources. The patient must understand both the modifiable and nonmodifi-able risk factors that contributed to his or her stroke (TJC, 2013).

In-Hospital Care Organization

Patient handoff between caregivers is a prime time for breakdown in communications that can hinder patient safety and delivery of care. Several best practices for handoff of a stroke patient are available for use by interprofessional stroke team members, includ-ing verbal and written communication, as well as including a neurological exam at the time of handoff. Upon arrival to the stroke unit, handoff communication take place at the bedside between the ED nurse and the inpatient unit nurse. A comprehensive report includes information about the last known well time and any details about the symptoms at onset. Communications include documentation of a neurological assessment such as the NIHSS or similar examination completed by both nurses along with verification of any changes in neurological deficits since the initial presentation. The physical examina-tion includes assessment of level of consciousness, cognition, motor and sensory func-tion, as well as speech and language ability. If the family is not present, communicate family contact information or the status of efforts to contact the family.

Vital signs including blood pressure, heart rate and rhythm, pulse oxygenation, respiratory rate, and temperature are assessed at the time of handoff and compared to the same physiological parameters collected during the ED stay. Care priorities for the team include the completion of a full review of systems and a swallowing assessment or sip test if not already completed prior to admission to the unit (Donovan et al., 2013). Should the stroke patient arrive as a direct admission from an outpatient setting, the team attempts to collect similar information from the transporting EMS providers and via telephone with the referring physician's office.

For the post-IV rtPA or endovascular patient who no longer needs to be cared for in the critical care environment, the handoff may vary slightly. The interprofessional team members involved in care include the patient's course of treatment and NIHSS score before and after rtPA treatment as well as the ongoing neurological status in the handoff communication. The interprofessional model of care should follow the patient throughout the hospital stay regardless of the geographical unit. The team works collaboratively to move the patient along the continuum of care. These interprofessional team members generally include physical, occupational, or speech therapists; nutritional support; respiratory therapy; case management; social work; psychology; diabetes education; pharmacist; stroke navigators; and others, as needed ⊙. Pharmacists may be routinely consulted to review anticoagulant and antithrombotic orders for patients with stroke and can provide important collaboration with the members of the interprofessional team regarding medication management. The team should review the education provided to patients and families daily and provide ongoing reinforcement of teaching. Finally, the interprofessional team should have a daily plan for discharge and work together to achieve the discharge plan.

Admission orders and order sets used throughout the hospital stay should be stroke-specific, based on national clinical practice guidelines, and have standardized elements to meet all evidence-based needs of the acute or subacute stroke period. The AHA guidelines endorse the use of stroke order sets as a class I, level of evidence B recommendation (Jauch et al., 2013). Orders should support the clinical pathway or stroke protocols and include activities of the interprofessional stroke team. In addition, all care must be patient- and family-centered throughout the multiple decision-making points in the stroke continuum of care.

INTERPROFESSIONAL CARE OF THE ISCHEMIC STROKE PATIENT

The care of the patient with ischemic stroke throughout the continuum of care should be executed using an interprofessional team approach. The members of the interprofessional team may vary according to the phase of care. In addition to the diagnostic workup for stroke, acute treatment, and management of complications, the interprofessional team should address the need for rehabilitation and discharge planning soon after admission and throughout the acute hospital stay. Team members with expertise in rehabilitation and discharge planning include physiatrists, physical and occupational therapists, speech and language pathology, case management, and social work ⊙. Other team members who may contribute to the care of patients with stroke include neuropsychology, practitioners with expertise in diabetes education, pharmacists for warfarin (Coumadin) or enoxaparin (Lovenox) education, chaplain, respiratory therapy for smoking cessation, or other physician specialties including cardiology, vascular surgery, endovascular neurology, or physical and rehabilitative medicine. Traditionally, rehabilitation was thought to be helpful in the days and weeks following the stroke event and generally seen as a distinctly different phase of care following the acute hospitalization. However, instituting early rehabilitation early in the acute hospitalization in the form of mobilization and ambulation has proved to improve outcomes. The A Very Early Rehabilitation Trial (AVERT phase II) study demonstrated that it is safe to begin mobilization of the stroke patient within the first 24 hours of the event. Early mobilization can prevent complications, improve long-term functionality, and improve the discharge disposition of stroke patients (Cumming et al., 2011).

An interprofessional team approach to stroke patient care should be used for every patient admitted with a diagnosis of stroke (Summers et al., 2009). Communication between physicians, physical therapy, occupational therapy, speech and language pathology, case management, social work, and nursing should be ongoing in both structured and informal processes, with documentation of the shared information in the medial record visible to all disciplines participating in the patients' care ⊙. Due to the complex nature of stroke care and the many members of the interprofessional team contributing to care, communication between team members can be challenging. Interprofessional communication may occur through interprofessional patient rounds, direct communication between staff, as well as written communication in the medical record. The interprofessional approach to care and prioritization of communication ensures that no elements of care necessary for recovery, treatment of comorbidities, and secondary stroke prevention are overlooked.

The interprofessional plan of care should be accessible to all caregivers across all departments, disciplines, and services following the stroke patient. The many specialties guiding medical care for the patient, including neurology, vascular surgery, neurointerventional and neurocritical care physicians, neurosurgery, as well as clinical nurse specialists, nurse practitioners, and physician's assistants should have ongoing and open communication with each other as well as with the rest of the interprofessional team. Some of the best practices surrounding documentation of the interprofessional plan of care include the use of electronic health records to create comprehensive interdisciplinary note templates, separate tabs for rounding logs, or notes in the electronic medical record. Advanced options such as importing data from different fields into a collaborative note, smart phrases, or linking the notes from different providers into a centralized tab or page vary by electronic medical record capabilities. Regardless of the mechanisms used to share information, the objective should be that all members of the interprofessional team are informed, collaborative, and able to facilitate a smooth and seamless transition of care to the community and home environment for the stroke patient.

▓ COORDINATION ACROSS THE CONTINUUM OF CARE

The patients' discharge disposition will vary depending on their ability to provide self-care, family resources, economic status, ongoing medical and nursing care needs, and patient preference. Qualification for an acute rehabilitation facility (ARF) requires the patient to be able to participate in 3 hours of rehabilitation therapy daily including physical, occupational, and speech. Although some patients may qualify for ARF, restrictions by facilities related to ability to pay and Medicare or Medicaid status may require the patient to receive care at a skilled nursing facility (SNF) instead. Case managers and social workers should begin assessing needs and resources upon admission in order to optimize placement for long-term recovery. Other potential levels of postdischarge care include long-term acute care (LTAC), hospice, or home with outpatient rehabilitation or visiting nurses. Please refer to Chapter 10 for a detailed review of stroke rehabilitation and Chapter 11 for discussion regarding reintegration of the stroke survivor into the community.

Postdischarge follow-up is essential to support the education, lifestyle changes, and medical management prescribed after acute ischemic stroke. Discharge phone calls are a best practice that can impact the long-term success of recovery from acute stroke. Assessment by a nurse through a series of questions can inform the stroke team if appropriate and sufficient information and teaching was provided to the patient and family prior to discharge. Discharge phone calls are an opportunity to evaluate understanding of medications, follow-up care, recognition of symptoms of recurrent stroke, as well as personal risk factors. It is imperative that the discharge phone calls are made by a health care professional who has knowledge of appropriate resources such as case management, social work, and prescription assistance. The nurse should also have the ability to access the discharged patients' medical record for reinforcement and clarification of discharge instructions. Additionally, reassessment or screening for development of signs of depression may be appropriate at this time (Moulds & Epstein, 2008).

The interprofessional team should ensure that appointments are scheduled for timely follow-up after hospital discharge. New postdischarge models are emerging, such as bridge clinics, advanced practice nursing clinics, continuity or transitions clinics, and early neurology outpatient clinic appointments. Surgery scheduling and presurgery assessment information may be necessary for patients who will return for carotid endarterectomy or carotid artery stenting, which is usually scheduled within 2 weeks of the initial event. Pharmacy, nursing, case management, or social workers may see the patient in postdischarge follow-up in addition to the physician or advanced practice nurse. Upon returning home, patients and families often identify cognitive deficits and physical limitations that were not evident during the acute hospital stay and need further interaction with the health care team to successfully reintegrate into the community setting. Patients may also have adaptive equipment needs or require caregiver support services. Priorities for such postdischarge clinic visits include a detailed review of symptoms, medication compliance, and understanding of discharge education. The team may also review compliance with prescribed therapies and potential barriers and offer financial resources such as discount prescriptions or alternative therapies. Assessment for side effects from new medications such as muscle pain with a statin or excessive bruising with anticoagulants should be made and addressed. Encourage patients and their families to attend hospital-, rehabilitation-, or community-based stroke support groups.

ISCHEMIC STROKE QUALITY CARE

TJC has established sets of measures for primary and comprehensive stroke centers that when implemented consistently result in improved patient outcomes (see Chapter 12 for further information on outcome measures). These measures are also used by the Centers for Medicare & Medicaid Services (CMS) for mandatory reporting on stroke. A hospital may choose stroke as an accountability or core measure when submitting data for CMS reporting and TJC accreditation. Recommendations for standards that would constitute exceptional care delivered at stroke centers were developed from recommendations provided by the BAC (Alberts et al., 2005). Elements of care that support the measures are incorporated into standardized order sets. Additional measures included in the *Get With The Guidelines* (GWTG) database are also tracked because of their positive impact on outcomes when represented through direct patient care (AHA & ASA, 2014). Several individual states have developed stroke standards that enable individual hospitals to be deemed stroke centers for critical access as acute stroke ready, primary, or comprehensive levels of care (Higashida et al., 2013). The designations reflect the initial ability of a hospital to provide consistent and evidence-based care to stroke patients emergently. Additional levels of certification or state designation are achieved through demonstrated level of care progressing from primary through comprehensive care of complex stroke patients.

TJC-certified stroke centers undergo on-site reviews to assess compliance with consensus-based national standards, which cover program management, clinical information management, delivering or facilitating care, supporting self-management, and measuring and improving performance. They are also reviewed for effective use of evidence-based clinical practice guidelines to manage and optimize care and must have an organized approach to performance measurement and quality improvement (TJC, 2014). Please refer to Chapter 12 for a detailed discussion of stroke program quality indicators, patient outcomes, and program evaluation.

Although Primary Stroke Center (PSC) certification has been available through TJC since 2002, Comprehensive Stroke Center (CSC) certification only became available in 2012. TJC collaborates with the AHA who incorporates recommendations from the BAC. Other organizations offer versions of stroke center certification as well, including individual state-run programs, Det Norske Veritas (DNV), and the Healthcare Facilities Accreditation Program (HFAP). Benefits of comprehensive certification include recognition of administrative commitment to additional significant resources, staff, and training that are necessary to care for complex stroke patients. CSCs function in a collaborative and interprofessional manner to provide the specialized care necessary for better patient outcomes. The CSCs s should provide regional guidance and advanced treatment for complex stroke patients in addition to initiating and participating in groundbreaking research to improve care and outcomes of the stroke patient.

Clinical Pearl: Computer-based learning modules are convenient and comprehensive ways to educate interprofessional staff throughout the hospital to recognize the signs and symptoms of acute stroke and how to respond when they are identified.

FUTURE TRENDS IN PRACTICE

There is an abundance of information surrounding secondary prevention, emerging risk factors, and lifestyle changes for stroke survivors. The amount of information regarding resources, access to equipment, community services, respite care, and follow-up therapy can be overwhelming for both patients and their families. Perhaps even more challenging is the ability for hospital staff providing the information to deliver comprehensive, written, clear, and concise instruction in a limited amount of time. Inpatient stays are increasingly brief. The time allotted to discharge teaching is often abbreviated in order to reduce length of stay and turn over rooms for incoming patients. The recognition of a need for human resources to enable a strong transition back to the community has led to new roles for individuals dedicated to teaching, facilitating resources, and following up with patients after discharge. Stroke navigators, care coordinators, and stroke liaisons have joined ranks with bedside nurses, case managers, and social workers. Constructing a strong discharge plan with access to immediate responses to clinical, financial, and emotional needs is essential for a successful transition of care. This helps reduce the need for readmission to the hospital or even recurrent stroke. Trends in follow-up care in addition to poststroke neurology consultation include nurse practitioner– or clinical nurse specialist–run clinics. Review of education and medications, pharmacy support, rehabilitative therapies, and assessment for depression are incorporated into the poststroke outpatient visits.

Research studies are examining the role of external and intravascular cooling of patients immediately after the acute ischemic event. There is an ongoing search for neuroprotective agents, pharmaceutical thrombolytics, and novel ways to dissolve clots or improve perfusion including sonothrombolysis, transcranial near-infrared laser therapy, and flow diversion devices. Trials to clearly determine the benefits of thrombectomy for recanalization of arteries and very early carotid endarterectomy also hope to expand the capability of endovascular and surgical options to lessen the burden of stroke (Brethour et al., 2012; Horn et al., 2014; Nahab et al., 2013). Population studies continue to determine the discrepancies in the incidence of stroke that are linked to geography, race, genetics, and economic status (White et al., 2005). Studies are also investigating early detection and diagnosis with imaging reconstruction software, transcranial Doppler ultrasound for emboli detection, rapid transfer protocols, and improved provider education (Anderson, Smith, Ido, & Frankel, 2013; Sun et al., 2013). Physical medicine and rehabilitation experts are examining the benefits of very early mobilization devices that perform movement to restore limb function, pharmaceutical antispasmodics, and longer poststroke rehabilitation periods.

SUMMARY

Stroke is a global public health concern that impacts millions of people worldwide. In the United States, the aging population lives longer and subsequently has an increased likelihood of experiencing an ischemic stroke. Primary prevention and controlling modifiable risk factors are the keys to minimizing long-term disability associated with this disease. Early recognition of signs and symptoms of stroke and activation of stroke systems of care including EMS and acute stroke response teams increases the likelihood of good outcomes when stroke occurs. Hospitals should be prepared to rapidly obtain blood work, diagnostic imaging, and a comprehensive neurological examination by an interprofessional team with stroke expertise. IV rtPA should be readily available with monitoring by nurses trained in the NIHSS and blood pressure management. When available, early intervention for large vessel strokes including endovascular therapy cooling, blood glucose control, and reversal of hypercoagulability should be considered. Patients who experience stroke require care in areas or units that specialize in stroke care, early mobilization, and prevention of complications such as deep vein thromboses (DVTs), hospital-acquired pressure ulcers (HAPUs), and aspiration pneumonia. Attention to TJC quality measures and a strong focus on education and transitions of care are of the utmost importance for the long-term success of the stroke survivor.

REFERENCES

Activase (Alteplase). (2014). Retrieved from http://www.gene.com/download/pdf/activase_prescribing.pdf

Ahmed, N., Wahlgren, N., Grond, M., Hennerici, M., Lees, K. R., Mikulik, R., . . . Ringleb, P. (2010). Implementation and outcome of thrombolysis with alteplase 3-4.5 h after an acute stroke: An updated analysis from SITS-ISTR. *The Lancet Neurology, 9*(9), 866–874.

Alberts, M. J., Latchaw R. E., Selman, W. R., Shephard, T., Hadley, M. N., Brass, L. M., . . . Walker, M. D. (2005). Recommendations for comprehensive stroke centers: A consensus statement from the Brain Attack Coalition. *Stroke, 36*(7), 1597–1616. doi:10.1161/01.STR.0000170622.07210.b4

American Heart Association & American Stroke Association. (2014). *Frequently asked questions for Get With The Guidelines-stroke and ASTP.* Retrieved from http://www.strokeassociation.org/STROKEORG /Professionals/Frequently-Asked-Questions-for-Get-With-The-Guidelines-Stroke-and-ASTP _UCM_315318_Article.jsp

Anderson, E. R., Smith, B., Ido, M., & Frankel, M. (2013). Remote assessment of stroke using the iPhone 4. *Journal of Stroke and Cerebrovascular Diseases, 22*(4), 340–344. doi:10.1016/j.jstrokecerebrovasdis.2011.09.013

Bergstrom, N., Braden, B. J., Laguzza, A., & Holman, V. (1987). The Braden Scale for predicting pressure sore risk. *Nursing Research, 36*(4), 205–210.

Brethour, M. K., Nyström, K. V., Broughton, S., Kiernan, T. E., Perez, A., Handler, D., . . . Alexandrov, A. W. (2012). Controversies in acute stroke treatment. *AACN Advanced Critical Care, 23*(2), 158–172. doi:110.1097/NCI.0b013e31824fe1b6.

Broderick, J. P., Tomsick, T. A., & Palesch, Y. Y. (2013). Endovascular treatment for acute ischemic stroke. *The New England Journal of Medicine, 368*(25), 2432–2433. doi:10.1056/NEJMc1304759

Ciccone, A., & Valvassori, L. (2013). Endovascular treatment for acute ischemic stroke. *The New England Journal of Medicine, 368*(25), 2433–2434.

Cumming, T. B., Thrift, A. G., Collier, J. M., Churilov, L., Dewey, H. M., Donnan, G. A., & Bernhardt, J. (2011). Very early mobilization after stroke fast-tracks return to walking: Further results from the Phase II AVERT randomized controlled trial. *Stroke, 42*(1), 153–158.

Donovan, N. J., Daniels, S. K., Edmiaston, J., Weinhardt, J., Summers, D., & Mitchell, P. H. (2013). Dysphagia screening: State of the art: Invitational conference proceeding from the State-of-the-Art Nursing Symposium, International Stroke Conference 2012. *Stroke, 44*(4), e24–e31. doi:10.1161/STR.0b013e3182877f57

Easton, J. D., Saver, J. L., Albers, G. W., Alberts, M. J., Chaturvedi, S., Feldmann, E., . . . Sacco, R. L. (2009). Definition and evaluation of transient ischemic attack: A scientific statement for healthcare professionals from the American Heart Association/American Stroke Association Stroke Council; Council on Cardiovascular Surgery and Anesthesia; Council on Cardiovascular Radiology and Intervention; Council on Cardiovascular Nursing; and the Interdisciplinary Council on Peripheral Vascular Disease: The American Academy of Neurology affirms the value of this statement as an educational tool for neurologists. *Stroke, 40*(6), 2276–2293.

Go, A. S., Mozaffarian, D., Roger, V. L., Benjamin, E. J., Berry, J. D., Blaha, M. J., . . . Turner, M. B. (2013). Heart disease and stroke statistics—2014 update: A report from the American Heart Association. *Circulation, 129*(3), e28–e292. doi:10.1161/01.cir.0000441139.02102.80

Hacke, W., Kaste, M., Bluhmki, E., Brozman, M., Davalos, A., Guidetti, D., . . . Toni, D. (2008). Thrombolysis with alteplase 3 to 4.5 hours after acute ischemic stroke. *The New England Journal of Medicine, 359*(13), 1317–1329. doi:10.1056/NEJMoa0804656

Hickey, J. (2013). *Clinical practice of neurological & neurosurgical nursing* (7th ed.). Philadelphia, PA: Lippincott Williams & Wilkins.

Higashida, R., Alberts, M. J., Alexander, D. N., Crocco, T. J., Demaerschalk, B. M., Derdeyn, C. P., . . . Wood, J. P. (2013). Interactions within stroke systems of care: A policy statement from the American Heart Association/American Stroke Association. *Stroke, 44*(10), 2961–2984. doi:10.1161/STR.0b013e3182a6d2b2

Horn, C. M., Sun, C. H., Nogueira, R. G., Patel, V. N., Krishnan, A., Glenn, B. A., . . . Gupta, R. (2014). Endovascular reperfusion and cooling in cerebral acute ischemia (ReCCLAIM I). *Journal of Neurointerventional Surgery, 6*(2), 91–95. doi:10.1136/neurintsurg-2013-010656

James, P. A., Oparil, S., Carter, B. L., Cushman, W. C., Dennison-Himmelfarb, C., Handler, J., . . . Ortiz, E. (2014). 2014 evidence-based guideline for the management of high blood pressure in adults: Report from the panel members appointed to the Eighth Joint National Committee (JNC 8). *The Journal of the American Medical Association, 311*(5), 507–520. doi:10.1001/jama.2013.284427

Jauch, E. C., Saver, J. L., Adams, H. P., Jr., Bruno, A., Connors, J. J., Demaerschalk, B. M., . . . Yonas, H. (2013). Guidelines for the early management of patients with acute ischemic stroke: A guideline for healthcare professionals from the American Heart Association/American Stroke Association. *Stroke, 44*(3), 870–947. doi:10.1161/STR.0b013e318284056a

Johnston, S. C., Rothwell, P. M., Nguyen-Huynh, M. N., Giles, M. F., Elkins, J. S., Bernstein, A. L., & Sidney, S. (2007). Validation and refinement of scores to predict very early stroke risk after transient ischaemic attack. *Lancet, 369*, 283–292.

Liebeskind, D. S. (2003). Collateral circulation. *Stroke, 34*(9), 2279–2284. doi:10.1161/01.STR.0000086465.41263.06

Meyer, B. C., Hemmen, T. M., Jackson, C. M., & Lyden, P. D. (2002). Modified National Institutes of Health Stroke Scale for use in stroke clinical trials: Prospective reliability and validity. *Stroke, 33*(5), 1261–1266. doi:10.1161/01.str.0000015625.87603.a7

Moulds, K., & Epstein, K. (2008, August). Do post-discharge telephone calls to patients reduce the rate of complications? *The Hospitalist.* Retrieved from http://www.the-hospitalist.org/details/article/186124/Do_post -discharge_telephone_calls_to_patients_reduce_the_rate_of_complications.html

Nahab, F., Kingston, C., Frankel, M. R., Dion, J. E., Cawley, C. M., Mitchell, B., . . . Tong, F. C. (2013). Early aggressive medical management for patients with symptomatic intracranial stenosis. *Journal of Stroke and Cerebrovascular Diseases, 22*(1), 87–91. doi:10.1016/j.jstrokecerebrovasdis.2011.06.012

Shah, S. (2002). *Pathophysiology of stroke*. Retrieved from http://www.ferne.org/Lectures/pathophysiology%20 intro%200501.htm

Summers, D., Leonard, A., Wentworth, D., Saver, J. L., Simpson, J., Spilker, J. A., . . . Mitchell, P. H. (2009). Comprehensive overview of nursing and interdisciplinary care of the acute ischemic stroke patient: A scientific statement from the American Heart Association. *Stroke, 40*(8), 2911–2944. doi:10.1161 /STROKEAHA.109.192362

Sun, C. H., Nogueira, R. G., Glenn, B. A., Connelly, K., Zimmermann, S., Anda, K., . . . Gupta, R. (2013). "Picture to puncture": A novel time metric to enhance outcomes in patients transferred for endovascular reperfusion in acute ischemic stroke. *Circulation, 127*(10), 1139–1148. doi:10.1161/CIRCULA-TIONAHA.112.000506

The Joint Commission. (2013). *Facts about primary stroke center certification*. Retrieved from http://www .jointcommission.org/facts_about_primary_stroke_center_certification/

The Joint Commission. (2014). *Facts about advanced certification for comprehensive stroke centers*. Retrieved from http://www.jointcommission.org/certification/advanced_certification_comprehensive_stroke_centers.aspx

The National Institute of Neurological Disorders and Stroke rt-PA Stroke Study Group. (1995). Tissue plasminogen activator for acute ischemic stroke. *The New England Journal of Medicine, 333*(24), 1581–1587. doi:10.1056/NEJM199512143332401

Ustrell, X., & Pellisé, A. (2010). Cardiac workup of ischemic stroke. *Current Cardiology Reviews, 6*(3), 175–183. doi:10.2174/157340310791658721

White, H., Boden-Albala, B., Wang, C., Elkind, M. S., Rundek, T., Wright, C. B., & Sacco, R. L. (2005). Ischemic stroke subtype incidence among whites, blacks, and Hispanics: The Northern Manhattan Study. *Circulation, 111*(10), 1327–1331. doi:10.1161/01.CIR.0000157736.19739.D0

CHAPTER 7

Intracerebral Hemorrhagic Stroke

Christy L. Casper and Alexandra M. Graves

Stroke patients often have just hours to receive lifesaving treatment. Whether the stroke is ischemic or hemorrhagic, time to clinical expertise and treatment is crucial. Intracerebral hemorrhagic stroke or intracerebral hemorrhage (ICH) accounts for 1 out of 10 strokes and occur as a result of bleeding into brain tissue. Of all the stroke types, ICH carries the poorest prognosis for survival and functional recovery (Broderick, Brott, Tomsick, Miller & Huster, 1993). Stroke patients will present to hospitals of all sizes with varying levels of expertise and specialists available. The ability of health care providers to recognize focal neurological deficits, quickly obtain diagnostic imaging studies, initiate treatment, and, in some cases, transfer the patient to a higher level of care can make the difference in patient outcomes. Established pathways for treatment of ischemic stroke are in place at many hospitals. Conversely, many hospitals do not have clear guidelines for the acute management of ICH. Similar to prompt treatment of ischemic stroke, academic and experiential preparation of providers, definition of individual roles, and response time is critical to providing best practices and standardized care to ICH patients (Cooper, Jauch, & Flaherty, 2007). Emergency departments should be prepared to promptly treat or rapidly transfer these patients to a tertiary care facility, unless there is a do not resuscitate (DNR) order in place and the family wishes to move to comfort care.

Evidence suggests that "early, aggressive medical and surgical care" including admission to a structured neurocritical care unit with a full-time intensivist and dedicated nursing staff with specialty stroke training has a direct impact on ICH morbidity and mortality (Diringer & Edwards, 2001; Morgenstern et al., 2010). To date, no individual surgical or medical treatment for ICH has been proven effective for all ICH patients. ⊙ Despite this, providing coordinated care by a knowledgeable interprofessional team of physicians, nurses, nurse practitioners, physician assistants, pharmacists, rehabilitation therapists, radiology technicians, dietitians, respiratory therapists, case managers, social workers, and others can make the difference in the functional outcome of the individual patient with ICH.

The intent of this chapter is to provide an overview of the incidence and prevalence of spontaneous ICH, differentiate commonly used terms associated with this disease, list primary and secondary causes, discuss early diagnosis and diagnostic tools, review the continuum of care, summarize available medical and surgical treatments, examine predictors for prognosis, and outline posthospital care coordination. ⊙ Unlike other chapters written on ICH, the goals are also to highlight implications for the interprofessional team, include practical tips for caring for this patient population, and provide tools that can be implemented in practice. The interprofessional team collaborates closely with each discipline, bringing their expertise to the group to provide comprehensive care to the patient with an ICH.

▉ BACKGROUND

Spontaneous nontraumatic ICH is a major public health problem that affects over 2 million people worldwide each year. Although there are variations related to geography and race, ICH is believed to account for 10% of all strokes each year (Go et al., 2013). Asians are two times more likely than other ethnic groups to suffer from an ICH. Patients of African, Hispanic, and Native American decent have higher rates of ICH than Caucasian Americans (Mohr et al., 2011). Medically indigent people without easy access to medical care and blood pressure control are at higher risk (Daroff, Fenichel, Jankovic, & Mazziotta, 2012). ICH admissions to the acute hospital have increased due to factors such as the advancing age of the U.S. population, uncontrolled hypertension, and the increased use of anticoagulants and antiplatelet agents (Qureshi, Mendelow, & Hanley, 2009).

▉ INTRACEREBRAL HEMORRHAGE QUALITY OF CARE

In 2002, about 77% of U.S. counties lacked hospitals with neurological services (Go et al., 2013). To address the need for a more organized approach, primary and comprehensive stroke centers have emerged. Primary stroke centers (PSCs) provide acute care to most stroke patients, whereas some patients need specialized care not available at PSCs. Comprehensive stroke centers (CSCs) are tasked with providing specialized care to the more complex patients. CSCs tend to have a higher percentage of hemorrhagic strokes because of transfers from outside facilities. A University of Texas study found that the majority of the patients transferred to the CSC were ICH cases (Albright et al., 2013). CSCs are required to have neurocritical care units, an intensivist available 24/7, protocols, policies, order sets, and acute stroke teams that respond promptly to manage acute stroke patients.

▉ TERMS AND DEFINITIONS

It is important to differentiate the types of hemorrhage within the cranium because each type has different causes and management (shown in **Figs.** 7-1 and 7-2 and listed in **Table** 7-1).

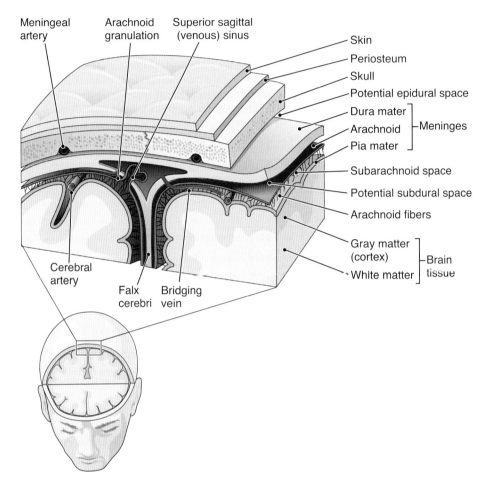

FIGURE 7-1 A cross-section of the skull, meninges, and cerebrum demonstrate the multiple layers covering the cortex. *(From McConnell T. H. [2013]. The nature of disease: Pathology for the health professions [2nd ed.]. Baltimore, MD: Lippincott Williams & Wilkins.)*

■■ CAUSES OF SPONTANEOUS NONTRAUMATIC INTRACEREBRAL HEMORRHAGE

Depending on the underlying cause of the hemorrhage, ICH is classified as primary or secondary. *Primary ICH* originates from the spontaneous rupture of small arterioles damaged by chronic hypertension and cerebral amyloid angiopathy. Additionally, modifiable risk factors including diabetes mellitus, cigarette smoking, heavy alcohol use, and illicit drug use can also lead to blood vessel damage and rupture. *Secondary ICH* is associated with vascular malformations, abnormal coagulopathies, bleeding into a tumor or ischemic stroke, cerebral venous sinus thrombosis, vasculitis, or moyamoya disease. **Figure 7-3** shows the typical hemorrhage location based on etiology and **Table 7-2** provides a summary of primary and secondary causes of ICH.

The Tentorium Cerebelli

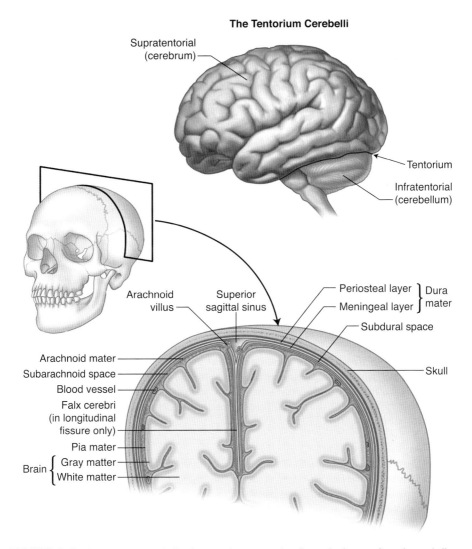

FIGURE 7-2   The tentorium cerebelli. The tentorium, separating the cerebral cortex from the cerebellum.

Primary Causes

Hypertension

ICH is tragic and costly and, in many cases, preventable. Despite the availability of potent antihypertensive medications, many of which are on the "4-dollar list" at local pharmacies, hypertension is the leading cause of ICH (Qureshi & Palesch, 2011; Qureshi et al., 1997). Chronic hypertensive "wear and tear" of vessel degeneration at arterial bifurcations is by far the leading cause of primary ICH, especially in patients between the ages of 40 and 70 years. The vessel wall weakens and ruptures, and

TABLE 7-1 Terms and Definitions

Terms	Definition
Intracranial hemorrhage	Any bleeding within the confines of the skull
Intracerebral hemorrhage (ICH) or intraparenchymal hemorrhage (IPH)	Bleeding into the brain parenchyma (distinctive tissue of an organ)
Intraventricular hemorrhage (IVH)	Bleeding in the ventricles of the brain. This is either a primary hemorrhage where bleeding starts in the ventricles or secondary hemorrhage due to invasion of blood into the ventricles from a nearby hematoma.
Extra-axial hemorrhage	Bleeding outside of the brain tissue
Intra-axial hemorrhage	Bleeding within the brain tissue. This includes ICH and IVH.
Epidural hemorrhage	Bleeding on top of the dura mater, under the skull
Subdural hemorrhage	Bleeding under the dura, on top of the brain
Subarachnoid hemorrhage	Bleeding under the arachnoid layer, on top of the pia mater and brain tissue
Supratentorial hemorrhages	Hemorrhages that occur within the cerebrum and above the dural layer that separates the occipital lobes from the cerebellum. This tough leather-like membrane is called the tentorium.
Infratentorial hemorrhage	Hemorrhage below the tentorium, primarily in the cerebellum

blood leaks into the surrounding tissue, causing a mass effect and toxic effects of blood products on the surrounding tissue. Elevated arterial pressure damages the intimal and subependymal layer of the arteriole, and the vessel becomes diseased and degenerates (Aguilar & Brott, 2011). Tiny end-vessel arteries, called penetrating arteries, which bifurcate from the larger more muscular vessels, are less equipped to handle the persistent abuse of high blood pressure. Charcot-Bouchard aneurysms (also known as *microaneurysms*) were described in neuropathological studies of brain specimens in 1868 in patients with ICH (Mohr et al., 2011). Hypertensive hemorrhages tend to result in a smaller volume of hematoma (≤30 cc) (Lang et al., 2001).

Common arterial locations for vascular disease are the lenticulostriate arteries and the pontine arteries. The lenticulostriate arteries come off the first branch of the middle cerebral artery and perfuse the deep structures of the brain including the basal ganglia, internal capsule, and thalamus. The lenticulostriate arteries are nicknamed "the arteries of stroke" because they can thrombose and cause an ischemic lacunar infarct or they may rupture under pressure and cause a classic deep hypertensive hemorrhage. The pontine perforators arise from the basilar artery and dive deep into the belly of the pons. Pontine hemorrhage is very often fatal.

Deep hemorrhages in the basal ganglia, the internal capsule, and the pons account for about two thirds of spontaneous ICH cases and occur in the classic locations for hypertensive hemorrhages. Lobar hemorrhages at the junction of white and gray matter account for the remaining one third (Flaherty et al., 2005; Grysiewicz, Thomas, & Pandey, 2008). Although hypertension is exclusively associated with deep hemorrhages, there is evidence that lobar hemorrhages can also be attributed to hypertension (Broderick, Brott, Tomsick, & Leach, 1993). **Table 7-3** lists a summary of typical locations of hypertensive hemorrhages.

Cerebral Amyloid Angiopathy

Cerebral amyloid angiopathy (CAA) is a disease process that primarily affects the elderly, and it is the second leading cause of ICH. In patients older than 65 years of

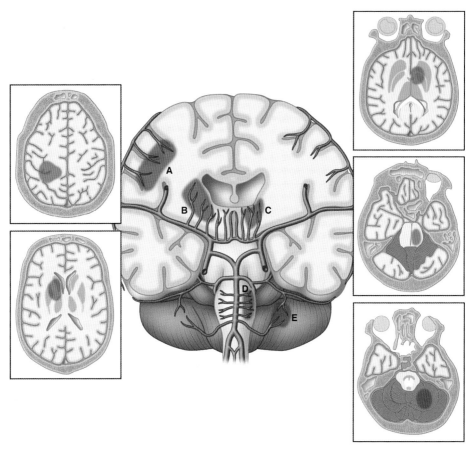

FIGURE 7-3 Hemorrhagic location based on etiology. Hemorrhages are often classified by location. In this figure, hemorrhages in locations B to E are often due to hypertension, whereas A is most often caused by CAA. Hemorrhage due to tumor, AVM, and other etiologies can occur anywhere. *(From Hemphill, J. C., Bonovich, D. C., Besmertis, L., Manley, G. T., & Johnston, S. C. [2001]. The ICH score: A simple, reliable grading scale for intracerebral hemorrhage. Stroke, 32[4], 891–897.)*

TABLE 7-2 Primary and Secondary Causes of Intracerebral Hemorrhage

Primary	Secondary
Hypertension	Vascular malformations: AVM, aneurysm, cavernous angioma
CAA	Hemorrhage into ischemic infarct
Sympathomimetic drugs, cigarette smoking, moderate to heavy alcohol use	Hemorrhage into a tumor
	Coagulopathy
	Cerebral venous sinus thrombosis
	Vasculitis
	Moyamoya disease

TABLE 7-3 Typical Locations of Hypertensive Hemorrhages

Sites	Percentage	Commonly Affected Arteries
Basal ganglia/putamen/ caudate head	50%	Originating from the ascending lenticulostriate branches of the MCA
Thalamus	10%–15%	Originating from the ascending thalamogeniculate branches of the PCA
Lobar	25%	Penetrating cortical branches of the ACA, MCA, or PCA
Cerebellum	5%–10%	Originating from the penetrating branches of the AICA, PICA, and SCA
Pons	5%	Originating from the paramedian branches of the basilar artery

PCA, posterior cerebral artery; ACA, anterior cerebral artery; AICA, anterior inferior cerebellar artery; PICA, posterior inferior cerebellar artery; SCA, superior cerebellar artery.
From Kase, C. S. (2012). Vascular diseases of the nervous system: Intracerebral hemorrhage. In R. B. Daroff, G. M. Fenichel, J. Jankovic, & J. C. Mazziotta (Eds.), *Bradley's neurology in clinical practice* (6th ed., pp. 1003–1106). Philadelphia, PA: Saunders Elsevier.

age, CAA may exceed hypertension as the cause of ICH. CAA is caused by deposits of beta-amyloid peptides on the media and adventitial layers of the small- and medium-sized arteries in the brain and the leptomeninges (the pia and arachnoid layers of the meninges). The protein deposits adhere to the intimal wall of the blood vessel, causing degeneration of the vessel. In severe cases of CAA, the vessels may weaken to the point of rupture. Hemorrhages related to CAA tend to be larger, and the volume is often greater than 30 cc (Lang et al., 2001). These hemorrhages occur at irregular and unpredictable intervals, are predominantly lobar, and occur in different vascular territories. The gradient echo sequence of a magnetic resonance imaging (MRI) scan may show remnants of blood by-products of various ages in multiple vascular distributions. This picture is highly suggestive of CAA. However, CAA is a diagnosis of exclusion and can only be confirmed with a brain biopsy or during autopsy.

CAA is also thought to be associated with the genetic risk factor apolipoprotein E (ApoE). Other risk factors include leukoaraiosis (white matter disease), a family history of ICH, a previous ischemic stroke, and frequent alcohol use. CAA also has similar histopathological features of Alzheimer disease (Mohr et al., 2011). White matter disease is commonly seen in elderly patients and in patients with hypertension, and a correlation was found between white matter disease and amyloid-positive vessels (Gatchev et al., 1993). White matter disease is also associated with larger hematoma volume and the risk of expansion (Lou, Al-Hazzani, Goddeau, Novak, & Selim, 2010). A familial association has been recognized in young patients and is thought to be related to a mutant protein deposit that is unrelated to beta-amyloid but which promotes vascular dysfunction in a similar fashion (Levy, Lopez-Otin, Ghiso, Geltner, & Frangione, 1989).

Other Primary Causes

In addition to hypertension and CAA, other diseases such as diabetes mellitus and personal habits such as cigarette smoking affect the cerebral vasculature. Patients with diabetes are at a three- to fourfold increased risk for ICH due to macrovascular and microvascular complications of the disease (Kissela et al., 2005). Cigarette smoking is a well-established risk factor for both ischemic and hemorrhagic stroke. Heavy alcohol use, another risk factor, is thought to inhibit platelet function, disturb coagulation pathways, and raise blood pressure in a linear dose-response fashion (Juvela, Hillbom, & Palomäki, 1995). Illicit drug use, with stimulants such as methamphetamines and cocaine, are associated with ICH. The cause may be abrupt spikes in blood pressure and cardiac arrhythmias. Interestingly, former cocaine users are more likely to have large vessel atherosclerosis, but current illicit drug users are more likely to suffer from an ICH stroke (Toossi, Hess, Hills, & Josephson, 2010). The positive relationship to hypercholesterolemia is less clear in ICH than in ischemic stroke. Contrary to ischemic stroke risk, high cholesterol actually seems to decrease the risk of ICH. This may indicate that atherosclerosis is not the predominant cause of ICH; rather, fragility of the vessels is the underlying reason for the rupture of the vessel (Ariesen, Claus, Rinkel, & Algra, 2003).

Secondary Causes

Vascular Anomalies

Rupture of vascular anomalies such as arteriovenous malformations (AVMs), cerebral aneurysms, or cavernous angiomas can lead to ICH. Hemorrhages of vascular anomalies occur more frequently in the younger, predominately female population and tend to follow a distinctive pattern of blood product markings on scans. Other distinctive characteristics include associated subarachnoid hemorrhage or intraventricular hemorrhage (IVH), prominent vascular structures, calcifications, and atypical locations for hypertensive ICH (Daroff et al., 2012). Cerebral angiography and/or MRI/magnetic resonance angiography (MRA) should be performed to definitively identify an underlying lesion.

Oral Anticoagulation

Cerebral hemorrhage is a major concern for patients receiving oral anticoagulation therapy (OAT). There are multiple validated indications for prescribing OAT; the number of patients receiving full-dose anticoagulation has increased. Fully anticoagulated patients have an 8- to 11-fold increase in the incidence of ICH, with the occurrence of death or severe disability about 65% (Daroff et al., 2012). Combining anticoagulants such as warfarin or the new oral anticoagulants such as dabigatran, rivaroxaban, or apixaban with aspirin increases the risk of ICH twofold.

Mortality is substantially higher in warfarin-induced ICH in an associated dose-dependent correlation. Careful control of the international normalized ratio (INR) can limit the risk and the severity of ICH. The onset of stroke-like symptoms in elderly patients receiving OAT warrants urgent evaluation (Rosand, Eckman, Knudsen, Singer, & Greenberg, 2004). The risk of ischemic and ICH strokes should be weighed prior to the initiation of full anticoagulation therapy. Patient and family education regarding dietary restrictions, underscoring the importance of INR monitoring, and recognizing signs and symptoms of ICH is critical. Provider documentation should clearly reflect initial education and ongoing reinforcement for all patients. A clear plan for follow-up laboratory surveillance and provider oversight should be arranged prior to discharge.

Hemorrhage into a Tumor

Intracranial tumors can be highly vascular and can lead to hemorrhage. The most common bleeding metastatic intracranial tumor is a metastatic melanoma. MRI scans are helpful when trying to identify a lesion under the hematoma (Daroff et al., 2012). For patients with either papilledema noted at the presentation of an acute ICH, an atypical location of ICH, or a ring-like high-density hemorrhage enhancement on the scant, an underlying tumor should be suspected.

Hemorrhage into an Ischemic Infarct

Hemorrhagic transformation of an ischemic stroke can occur spontaneously or after administration of tissue plasminogen activator (tPA) for acute ischemic stroke symptoms. Approximately 10% of patients with an ischemic stroke will have some hemorrhage within the stroke bed. The hemorrhage can range from a petechial hemorrhage to a parenchymal space-occupying hemorrhage with a large volume of blood. Prior to giving intravenous (IV) tPA, the risk for intracranial hemorrhage should be discussed with the patient and family. For patients who present within 3 hours of symptom onset, approximately 6% will have a symptomatic ICH compared to a rate of 0.6% of symptomatic ICH in the control group. These hemorrhages are classified as either symptomatic or asymptomatic based on clinical deterioration (Paciaroni, Bogousslavsky, & Levine, 2013). A *symptomatic hemorrhage* is defined as intracerebral blood along with a 4-point worsening in the National Institutes of Health Stroke Scale (NIHSS). Symptomatic ICHs are more commonly associated with higher NIHSS scores, cerebral edema, or mass effect on the baseline head computed tomography (CT) scan. An NIHSS score higher than 20 has a 17% change of hemorrhage (The NINDS t-PA Stroke Study Group, 1997). The European Cooperative Acute Stroke Study (ECASS III) clinical trial conducted in Europe showed that IV tPA was safe to be given up to 4.5 hours from onset of symptoms (Hacke et al., 2008). The risk of symptomatic hemorrhage in this expanded time window is 8%. Hospitals of every size and location can safely treat stroke victims with IV tPA if they have access to consultation and transfer agreements with experienced stroke centers.

Other Secondary Causes

Other less common secondary causes of ICH include a venous hemorrhage related to cerebral venous sinus thrombosis (CVST), vasculitis, and moyamoya disease. ICH occurs in the setting of CVST due to the blockage of the normal outflow of the venous blood via the venous sinuses. This buildup of pressure in the venous system can lead to rupture of the nearby veins and formation of a hematoma. The treatment for CVST is full anticoagulation, which is difficult when there is intracranial bleeding already present.

Another secondary cause, vasculitis, is characterized by inflammation and necrosis of the cerebral vessels and is mainly associated with autoimmune disorders such as giant cell arteritis and classic polyarteritis nodosa. These inflamed and necrotic vessels become damaged and can hemorrhage. The laboratory workup for inflammation includes an increased sedimentation rate and C-reactive protein (CRP) levels. Conventional angiography may show signs of large vessel angiitis. MRI, including apparent diffusion coefficient (ADC) maps, diffusion/perfusion measurements, and gradient echo sequence, can show evidence of both ischemic and hemorrhagic lesions of varying ages. Lumbar puncture and analysis of cerebrospinal fluid (CSF) may be performed if vasculitis is suspected and if the laboratory findings are inconclusive (Berlit, 2010).

Moyamoya disease is a chronic and progressive vasculopathy that presents with intracranial hemorrhagic or ischemic stroke. The term *moyamoya*, the Japanese word for "puff of smoke," describes the angiographic appearance of fragile collateral vessels that develop adjacent to severely stenotic cerebral arteries. The intima has duplicate or even triplicate layers of elastic lamina, which may be related to proliferation of smooth muscle cells in the vessel. These thin and dilated collaterals may develop vessel wall necrosis and microaneurysms and are the likely etiology of hemorrhages. Morbidity and mortality for patients with moyamoya disease with ICH is substantial (Zipfel, Fox, & Rivet, 2005).

◼ DIAGNOSIS WITH COMPUTED TOMOGRAPHY AND MAGNETIC RESONANCE IMAGING

Imaging with CT or MRI is the only definitive way to differentiate ischemic stroke from hemorrhagic stroke because symptoms can be similar. A CT scan without contrast medium is the imaging modality of choice in the diagnosis of acute ICH. CT scans without contrast media are highly sensitive and specific for the detection of acute blood products in the brain and can typically be done very quickly. CT is less sensitive in detecting subacute and old ICHs (Mohr et al., 2011). Most hospitals, even critical access hospitals with less than 25 beds, will have a CT scanner readily available 24/7. When viewing a noncontrast CT, the hyperdense appearance of fresh blood is easy to detect. If available, obtaining a CT angiogram (CTA) is helpful for detecting an underlying aneurysm, AVM, or venous thrombosis. Cerebral angiography should be obtained if clinical suspicion of a vascular anomaly is high or if there is an unusual appearance of the hemorrhage (Morgenstern et al., 2010). In addition, a CTA can help predict hematoma growth early in the course of illness. By using the CTA source images, a "spot sign" or contrast leaking in the vessel that appears hyperdense compared to the surrounding hematoma may be detected (Mohr et al., 2011).

The MRI is also recognized for its accuracy in detection of blood products as well as identification of underlying lesions such as intracranial tumors, cerebral vein thrombosis, cavernous angiomas, and other vascular malformations. The appearance of blood on an MRI depends on the evolution of the blood breakdown products. Several studies have demonstrated that an MRI is as reliable as noncontrast CT in the detection of acute blood. However, patients must be able to tolerate lying still for a longer period of time and screened for any contraindications for the MRI. In patients without a clear underlying etiology or in hemorrhages occurring in unusual locations, an MRI with contrast is indicated.

Clinical Pearl: Radiology

- An MRI checklist must be completed to check for any contraindications for the study. Obtain information about contraindications for an MRI from the family, when they are available, in order to avoid having to track them down if an MRI is ordered.
- Safely transporting critically ill patients requires coordination by multiple team members. The central coordinator of this activity is the primary nurse who will need to alert the charge nurse, call the radiology technicians, arrange transportation help, and notify respiratory therapy who will need to bring a portable ventilator for transport.
- Ordering serial CT scans in the first 24 hours is a common practice. Anticipate that the patient will need to be transported several times during the first few days of hospitalization.
- "Three B's"—*Blood, bone, and bling* appear white on CT images.

▊▊ THE CONTINUUM OF INTRACEREBRAL HEMORRHAGE STROKE CARE

Stroke Prevention: Beginning the Continuum

Hypertension is one of the most preventable contributors of ICH. Rigorous review of randomized controlled trials is summarized, and recommendations are provided in the Eighth Joint National Committee (James et al., 2014) on the management of hypertension. ⊙ These recommendations are designed to provide clear guidance especially for the primary care clinician who is the gatekeeper for treatment of hypertension. The JNC 8 recommendations include a stepwise progression of drug classes based on individual demographics and response to treatment (James et al., 2014). Close monitoring of anticoagulant doses with appropriate titration by a skilled provider also reduce the risk of ICH. Anticoagulation clinics have been shown to reduce the number of bleeding events and the number of thromboembolic events as well as decrease cost by reducing the number of hospitalizations and emergency department visits (Chiquette, Amato, & Bussey, 1998). Patients with known CAA should not be placed on any antithrombotic therapy if possible, and caution should be used in initiating antithrombotic therapy in patients with large ischemic strokes. Lifestyle modifications including avoidance of sympathomimetic drugs and cigarette smoking as well as controlling blood glucose can decrease the chance of an ICH.

The Stroke Care Continuum: Prehospital to the Emergency Department

Early identification of stroke symptoms and mobilization of emergency medical services (EMS) are critical in order to avoid delays in care. Large public campaigns (e.g., the 5 suddens, F-A-S-T) were launched in order to increase public knowledge about stroke symptoms and to call 911 for urgent transport. Dispatch of EMS and rapid transportation to the closest appropriate hospital should be tracked as performance measures. Prehospital stroke assessment scales such as the *Cincinnati Prehospital Stroke Scale* and the *Los Angeles Prehospital Stroke Scale* are widely used to educate EMS providers. See Chapter 4 for further discussion of prehospital care.

Hippocrates, the father of medicine, first recognized the symptoms of stroke and called it *apoplexy*, which is translated as "struck down by violence." The onset of focal neurological deficits with clinical signs of increased intracranial pressure (ICP) including severe headache, vomiting, loss of consciousness/coma, and systolic blood pressure greater than 220 mm Hg are strongly suggestive of ICH (Aguilar & Brott, 2011). Unlike ischemic stroke or subarachnoid hemorrhage, neurological symptoms related to ICH may not be at their maximum at onset. The hematoma can grow over minutes to hours, and symptoms progress and worsen depending on a mass effect on surrounding structures as different vascular territories become affected. Early hematoma growth and subsequent perihematomal edema contribute to increased ICP and deterioration in the neurological examination. Patients with hemorrhage below the tentorium may have signs of brainstem dysfunction, gaze abnormalities, cranial nerve deficits, and contralateral motor deficits. Ataxia, nystagmus, and dysmetria are common with cerebellar hemorrhages (Qureshi et al., 2001).

⊙ All members of the interprofessional team should be diligent during this time to conduct frequent neurological assessments and monitor vital signs closely to assess for signs of increasing ICP due to hematoma expansion, mass effect, and/or development of hydrocephalus. Understanding the typical timeline for the development of complications will help the whole team in planning the course of treatment. Realizing that hydrocephalus and hematoma expansion frequently occurs in the first hours, but that cerebral edema does not peak until around day 5, helps the team members to focus on the probable causes of neurological changes.

Nurses are present at the bedside 24/7 during the hospitalization of a patient. One topic of debate is the neurological assessment tool and the frequency of the examination. Nurses should conduct a detailed neurological examination at the beginning of their shift and during handoff to an oncoming nurse. Best practice is to conduct a bedside assessment with both nurses present. Once the baseline examination is established and the deficits are identified, conducting a focused examination throughout the shift allows the nurse to quickly identify deterioration in the exam. Changes in the focused bedside examination should lead to repeating the detailed neurological examination (**Table 7-4**). Knowing what is normal and anticipating deficits based on knowledge of the location of the ICH will help the nurse complete both the focused and the detailed neurological examination. Although the NIHSS is most commonly used in the ischemic stroke population, it is also used to assess patients with intracranial hemorrhage (Hinkle, 2014).

TABLE 7-4 Neurological Examination of the Unconscious Patient

Nursing Implications: Neurological Exam of the Unconscious Patient

- **Level of consciousness**
  - What was the stimulus? What was the response to escalating stimuli?
    - Presence in the room
    - Verbal stimuli: say name, loud clapping over head
    - Tactile: light touch
    - Central pain: trapezius squeeze, sternal rub, nasal tickle, supraorbital pressure. Uncover patient and watch for all responses.
    - Peripheral pain: may elicit a spinal reflex like triple flexion
- **Cranial nerves**
  - Pupils (CN II, III)
    - Size: pinpoint—pontine hemorrhage, opiate overdose
    - Shape: oval usually indicates increased ICP
    - Reaction to light: sluggish represents pressure on the oculomotor nerve (CN III)
  - Vision (CN II): blink to threat
  - Extraocular movements and vestibulo-ocular reflex (CN III, IV, VI, VIII)
  - Open eyelids to inspect position and movement of eyes. Oculocephalic reflex (doll's eyes): Rotate head side to side (if no contraindication). If eyes are fixed, brainstem is not working—"negative doll's eyes."
  - Corneal reflex, facial symmetry, grimace response (CN V, VII)
    - Observe facial movement with central pain, nasal tickle (insert a cotton swab into nostril and observe facial contraction)
  - Gag reflex (CN IX, X)
- **Motor response**
  - Purposeful versus nonpurposeful versus unresponsive
  - Localize, withdraw, stereotyped posturing (decorticate, decerebrate)
- **Muscle tone**
  - Spasticity: increased resistance to passive movement more pronounced in the extremes of range and followed by gradual release of resistance; reflects injury to corticospinal tract
  - Rigidity: state of increased resistance
  - Flaccidity: Muscle is weak, soft, and flabby.
- **Reflexes**
  - Deep tendon reflexes
  - Plantar response (Babinski)
  - Triple flexion (spinal reflex only)

The earliest neurological change is often a decrease in level of consciousness. If the patient is intubated and sedated, sedatives should be lightened/interrupted hourly to assess the response to stimulation. The ICP should be monitored carefully if there is an ICP monitor in place because the ICP will likely rise while off sedation. There are many choices of sedative agents and quickly reversible drugs that are often used in the neurological population due to the need for frequent neurological examination. Sedatives such as propofol (Diprivan) or dexmedetomidine (Precedex) provide the opportunity to provide the patient with a "sedation vacation." However, avoid sudden discontinuation of these drugs; the patient may awaken abruptly and become agitated due to pain and fear. Instead, decrease the dose by 50% every 5 to 10 minutes to allow the patient to awaken smoothly. Once the neurological examination has been completed, the drug can be restarted and titrated as needed. The sedation vacation is an opportunity to assess the patient's tolerance of both sedatives and narcotics. Just because the patient was on a high dose of sedation does not mean he or she will continue to require the same dose. Persistent deep sedation can lead to delirium and persistent cognitive impairment and is known to increase ventilator days, prolong intensive care unit (ICU) days, and increase complications and cost of care (Girard, Pandharipande, & Ely, 2008; Kress, Pohlman, O'Connor, & Hall, 2000).

The neurological examination is conducted in some capacity during any interaction with the patient by members of the interprofessional team. All observations of the neurological function can give the team a more complete understanding of the patient's condition. However, standardization of documentation requirements should be in place. The standard of care for assessments of a patient with an acute ICH includes neurological assessments and vital signs upon admission and then every 15 minutes for 1 hour then hourly once stable. Once admitted to the ICU, the standard is hourly for 24 hours then every 2 hours once stable. With any neurological change, the cycles should begin again (Hickey, 2011).

⊙ It is beneficial for all interprofessional team members to understand the neurological status of the patient and a collaborative team approach is essential when caring for the ICH patient. This knowledge will not only guide the medical and surgical decisions but will also help shape the team's conversations with the family (and patient as able) regarding morbidity and mortality, functional deficits, and future care needs. The case manager and the social worker are essential members of the care team and help the family navigate the mass of medical lingo and cope with the emotional stress of critical illness. Rehabilitation therapists including physical therapy (PT), occupational therapy (OT), and speech therapy (ST) are integral to the assessment of functional deficits and make recommendations about appropriate level of care and supervision needed after the acute hospitalization. Therapists should be consulted after elevated ICP has subsided, and the patient can start to be mobilized. Therapists work with the patient and family to set realistic goals for functional recovery including cognition and the eventual return to the prior level of independence, if possible. If independence is not possible, the interprofessional team members work with the family to plan for the next step in the continuum of care, whether that is placement in a facility or home with 24-hour supervision.

◼ TREATMENT

Surgical Treatment

Surgical decompression of ICH remains controversial except in cases of large (>3 cm) cerebellar hematomas. Multiple randomized controlled trials show that surgical evacuation of large cerebellar hematomas is superior to medical treatment. CSF diversion with an external ventricular drainage alone, in lieu of immediate surgical evacuation of a cerebellar hematoma, is not recommended (Morgenstern et al., 2010). There is no clear evidence for surgical evacuation of supratentorial ICH. The STICH trial (Surgical Trial in IntraCerebral Hemorrhage) was a European study that compared surgery within 72 hours versus initial nonsurgical management of patients with supratentorial ICH (Vespa, Martin, Zuccarello, Awad, & Hanley, 2013). The overall trial results showed that surgery, for the entire study population, did not provide benefit or cause harm. There were trends in two subgroups toward better outcome for patients with hemorrhage which extended to 1 cm of the cortical surface and were taken for evacuation within a median time of 30 hours and patients with a Glasgow Coma Scale (GCS) between 9 and 12. However, surgical evacuation did not reach statistical significance for either of these subgroups, and the debate continued. A follow-up study, STICH II, looked at evacuating superficial 10- to 100-mL hemorrhages in conscious patients who had no IVH. Similar to the predecessor trial, results were equivocal, with a small trend toward survival for patients undergoing surgery (Gaberel, Gakuba, Emery, & Touze, 2013).

Neurosurgeons are generally more inclined to perform a craniotomy to evacuate the hematoma if the ICH is in the nondominant hemisphere, the hematoma is large, the location is lobar and near the surface of the brain, or if the patient is clinically deteriorating (Mohr et al., 2011). If the decision for surgery is made, the surgeon may choose to leave the bone flap off (decompressive hemicraniectomy) in order to allow brain swelling outside of the skull rather than risk a herniation syndrome and potential death. The majority of studies on decompressive hemicraniectomy have been conducted on the malignant middle cerebral artery (MCA) ischemic stroke population, but one study on ICH patients showed that the procedure might be safe and effective for patients with a large hematoma and severe neurological impairment (Takeuchi, Wada, Nagatani, Otani, & Mori, 2013). Decompressive hemicraniectomy is controversial because patients are often very sick and tend to have many complications. The procedure may decrease overall mortality but leave the patient with overwhelming neurological impairment (Mayer, 2007). Patient selection is important, and none of the randomized trials included patients older than 60 years of age (Staykov & Gupta, 2011).

Other less invasive techniques for reducing the volume of the hematoma have been studied and other trials are ongoing. The MISTIE (Minimally Invasive Surgery plus rt-PA for ICH Evacuation) trial studied the use of stereotactic catheter placement directly into a deep hemorrhage, instilling a dose of tPA every 8 hours over 2 to 3 days and aspirating the hemolyzed clot. MISTIE reported improved long-term functional outcomes with decreased length of stay and decreased cost. The ICES (Intraoperative CT-Guided Endoscopic Surgery for ICH) trial is investigating the use of an endoscope to remove deep hemorrhage, and the SLEUTH trial (Safety of Lysis with EKOS Ultrasound in the Treatment of Intracerebral and Intraventricular Hemorrhage) used the EKOS endoscopic catheter to deliver ultrasonic waves along with tPA to break down the hematoma (Newell et al., 2011). The CLEAR IVH (Clot Lysis: Evaluating Accelerated Resolution of Intraventricular Hemorrhage) phase II trial showed improved outcomes for patients who received placement of external ventricular devices coupled with instillation of tPA into the ventricular system to break down IVH (Naff et al., 2011). The CLEAR III trial is currently enrolling patients. Even as studies show decreased overall mortality, no minimally invasive trials have consistently demonstrated improved functional outcomes.

Acute hydrocephalus (HCP) is a common complication of ICH. With an incidence of 40% to 50%, acute HCP is an independent predictor of poor outcome. Acute HCP generally occurs in the face of intraventricular extension of a basal ganglia hematoma, primary IVH, or mass effect which leads to obstruction of CSF drainage and reabsorption (Qureshi et al., 2009). Patients with small hemorrhages without IVH are less likely to need CSF diversion with an external ventricular device (EVD). Obstructive HCP is particularly relevant in patients with hemorrhages in the posterior fossa, which create mass effect and obstruction of the fourth ventricle. CSF diversion with an EVD should be considered early in the treatment course for patients with decreased level of consciousness, posterior fossa hemorrhage, and any signs of early HCP. ⊙ Physician providers of the interprofessional team will often order serial CT scans 6 hours apart to monitor for hematoma expansion and developing HCP. Late HCP may also develop over days and weeks, and caregivers should be mindful of this possibility especially if the patient has had intraventricular blood. Patients should be monitored for persistent decline in their neurological examination that is not related to sedating medications, infection, or other factors. Providers should have a low threshold of tolerance to look for late HCP by ordering a surveillance CT scan, especially in patients with any intraventricular blood.

For patients with ICH, the decision to take a patient for surgical evacuation or to place an EVD at the bedside may be made emergently such as in the case of evidence of a large cerebellar hemorrhage, acute HCP, or clinical deterioration of the patient. ⊙ The interprofessional team needs to anticipate these decisions and plan accordingly by ensuring that equipment is readily available, staff can be quickly mobilized, and necessary paperwork (preoperative check list, consent forms) is completed.

Medical Treatment

⊙ Early assessment and management of the airway, blood pressure, and circulation followed by measures to treat ICP and limit hematoma expansion including blood pressure control and prompt reversal of anticoagulants are pivotal in the first 24 hours after the ICH. Frequently, patients will be somnolent or will have significant bulbar dysfunction requiring intubation for airway protection. Patients may vomit and aspirate acidic gastric content, which can lead to pneumonia. In general, patients will need airway protection when the GCS is less than or equal to 8.

Hematoma Expansion

In addition to the ICH score, expansion of the hematoma is an independent predictor of mortality and disability (Davis et al., 2006). Studies have shown that 26% of patients will experience hematoma expansion within the first hour after the initial hemorrhage. Overall, 72% of patients have some degree of hematoma expansion during the first 24 hours, and 38% of patients will expand the hematoma by about one third of the total initial volume (Brott et al., 1997; Davis et al., 2006). Noncoagulopathic hematomas tend to expand early in the course, whereas coagulopathic hemorrhages can expand up to 24 hours or longer after initial hemorrhage (Aguilar et al., 2007).

Treatment targets to prevent hematoma expansion include the following: determining goals for blood pressure, defining how quickly the blood pressure can be reduced without risking cerebral ischemia, choosing appropriate antihypertensives to reach target blood pressures quickly, reversing coagulopathy, predicting who will have hematoma expansion, and identifying hemostatic agents to prevent hematoma expansion.

The FAST trial (Factor Seven for Acute Hemorrhagic Stroke) was the largest ICH medical trial ever conducted (Mayer et al., 2008). The study used recombinant factor

VIIa, which activates the extrinsic pathway of the coagulation cascade. Recombinant factor VIIa is U.S. Food and Drug Administration–approved for use in hemophilia to initiate hemostasis, and there was great hope that, if given no later than 4 hours after onset of symptoms, it would limit hematoma growth and improve clinical outcomes in non-OAT-related hemorrhages. Patients with a history of vasoocclusive disease, but without symptoms for the 3 months prior to ICH, were eligible for enrollment. The FAST trial compared placebo ($n = 268$) versus 20 mcg/kg ($n = 276$) versus 80 mcg/kg ($n = 297$) of recombinant factor VII. The 80-mcg/kg dose led to significant reduction in hematoma expansion at 24 hours, but unfortunately, there was no difference in the functional outcome at 3 months. The higher dose also correlated with significantly higher rates of arterial thrombotic events (Mayer et al., 2008). One hypothesis for the failure to show significant difference was that the trial included patients with known predictors of poor outcome including patients older than 80 years of age and patients with very large hematoma volumes of greater than 60 mL. The investigators also noted that the treatment arm had a greater number of patients with IVH. The American Heart Association/American Stroke Association (AHA/ASA) ICH guidelines published in 2010 suggest that further research is needed to identify a particular subgroup of patients who would benefit from this therapy (Morgenstern et al., 2010).

Blood Pressure Management

Blood pressure management in ICH is a topic of much debate by experts in the field. It remains unclear if elevated blood pressure contributes to hematoma expansion, and there is concern that aggressively lowering the blood pressure and the cerebral perfusion pressure (CPP) leads to further injury of surrounding tissue which is ischemic but not yet infarcted. Current guidelines recommend keeping systolic blood pressure (SBP) less than 180 mm Hg in patients without clinical signs of increased ICP. In patients with signs of elevated ICP, it is recommended to place an external ventricular drain and reduce the blood pressure while maintaining a CPP greater than 60 mm Hg. If the SBP is greater than 200 mm Hg, the recommendations are to monitor blood pressure every 5 minutes while aggressively titrating a continuous IV infusion (Morgenstern et al., 2010).

Two trials (ATACH [Antihypertensive Treatment of Acute Cerebral Hemorrhage] and INTERACT [Intensive Blood Pressure Reduction in Acute Cerebral Hemorrhage Trial]) investigated aggressive reduction of SBP to less than 140 mm Hg compared to the SBP goal of less than 180 mm Hg in order to reduce the likelihood of mortality and disability at 3 months (Anderson et al., 2008; Qureshi, 2007). Both studies showed that lowering SBP to less than 140 mm Hg was feasible. Unfortunately, a follow-up study (INTERACT II) failed to showed reduction of the primary outcome of death or severe disability (Anderson et al., 2008). ATACH-II was designed to address the efficacy of early and aggressive treatment with IV nicardipine for an SBP goal of less than 140 mm Hg. ATACH–II is currently recruiting participants and is estimated complete in July 2015 (http://www.clinicaltrials.gov). The ASA 2010 ICH guidelines state "acute lowering of systolic BP to 140 mm Hg is probably safe" (Morgenstern et al., 2010, p. 2115).

Interprofessional team members work closely together to determine and achieve targeted blood pressure goals. Caution should be used not to drop blood pressure precipitously, and the team should have a low threshold to start a continuous infusion of vasoactive medications because a bolus of an antihypertensive drug can lead to wide swings in the blood pressure. Continuous infusion of nicardipine resulted in less blood pressure variability, fewer dose adjustments, and required fewer additional agents in order to meet targets (Liu-Deryke et al., 2008). The medical staff will also consider placing an arterial line for close monitoring of the blood pressure. Of note, it is not a requirement for a patient on nicardipine to have an arterial line, but the need for line placement is evaluated on a case-by-case basis. ⊙ Additionally, close communication with the ICU pharmacist prevents delays in medication availability, especially medications that require mixing. The pharmacist also plays a key role in determining when to begin oral agents in order to initiate downward titration of continuous IV antihypertensive drips.

⊙ When PT and OT become involved and begin to mobilize the patient, problems with blood pressure control often become more exaggerated. The interprofessional team will need to work together to determine the best time to begin out of the bed orders as well as implement appropriate timing for medications in order to balance arousability with pain and anxiety.

Reversal of Anticoagulation

Unlike blood pressure management, experts are very clear about the need for prompt reversal of anticoagulation. Patients on full-dose anticoagulation are at higher risk for hematoma expansion. Any ICH patient on warfarin with an INR of 1.4 or higher is considered to have a life-threatening condition and should receive emergent reversal of anticoagulation. For patients on oral anticoagulants, fresh frozen plasma and vitamin K have been staples of treatment. In recent years, prothrombin complex concentrates (PCCs) have been increasingly recommended. PCCs are plasma-derived factors; have a high concentration of coagulation factors II, VII, IX, and X; and have been shown to quickly normalize the INR (Morgenstern et al., 2010). Anticoagulation with dabigatran (a direct thrombin inhibitor) in patients with atrial fibrillation and well-controlled hypertension was shown to have fewer fatal ICHs and fewer traumatic hemorrhages. Patients with subdural hemorrhage were included in this study (Hart et al., 2012). Concomitant aspirin use with warfarin independently predicted spontaneous ICH (Hart et al., 2012). ⊙ The ICU pharmacist collaborates closely with the team during rounds and throughout the day in order to address the appropriate antithrombotic choice for the patient.

Perihematomal Edema

Perihematomal edema typically peaks within 3 to 5 days but can persist for weeks after the initial hemorrhage (Aguilar & Brott, 2011). Both vasogenic and cytotoxic edema lead to disruption of the blood–brain barrier and possible cell death. Studies show that regular use of IV mannitol does not change mortality or functional outcome in ICH patients (Morgenstern et al., 2010). Steroids have no role in the management of cerebral edema or treating increased ICP and should be avoided unless there are other clinical indications (Poungvarin et al., 1987).

Other interventions that can decrease edema and elevated ICP include the following:

- Positioning
    - Elevate head of the bed to 30 degrees.
    - Keep head midline.
    - Avoid tight tape around neck that can occlude drainage of the jugular veins (i.e., taping to secure endotracheal tube).
    - Avoid severe hip flexion.

- Sedation and pain management
  - Limit stimulation and try to group interventions together.
  - Premedicate prior to interventions.
  - Monitor for signs and symptoms of pain.
- If a ventriculostomy or fiberoptic ICP monitor is in place, monitor and treat per physician orders.

Although lobar hemorrhages are more likely to invoke seizure activity, deep hemorrhages are also associated with seizure activity. Vespa et al. (2003) applied continuous electroencephalographic (EEG) monitoring to 63 ICH patients. Of the group, 28% of the patients showed signs of nonconvulsive status epilepticus within the first 72 hours of the hemorrhage. However, not all seizure activity has clinical signs. Patients who have significant neurological injury with midline shifting of normal structures are more likely to suffer nonconvulsive status epilepticus, which has few, if any, physical signs. Nonconvulsive status should also be considered for patients who have poor neurological function or who appear worse neurologically than the stroke would predict (Vespa et al., 2013). Unfortunately, it is unclear whether early identification and treatment of nonconvulsive status epilepticus and other electrographic abnormalities improves overall outcome. Despite the lack of evidence, the current recommendations for continuous EEG monitoring in the ICU state that continuous EEG monitoring is preferred over intermittent EEG in patients in status epilepticus to rule out nonconvulsive status in patients who are either at risk for nonconvulsive status or in patients with unexplained and persistent altered consciousness (Claassen et al., 2013). Prophylactic antiepileptics are often used, but there is little evidence to support this practice. Additionally, there is growing evidence that prescribing antiepileptics (especially phenytoin) to patient without evidence of seizures is linked to an increase in morbidity and mortality (Messé et al., 2009).

Clinical Pearl: Medication orders are often written without an end date. All health care providers should review the medication list and consider discontinuation of antiepileptics when they are no longer indicated.

Glucose Control

Elevated blood glucose upon admission is linked to expansion of the hematoma and increased overall morbidity and mortality for ICH patients. Response to these data led the medical community to focus on tight blood glucose control and aim for a range of 80 to 100 mg/dL. Unfortunately, episodes of systemic and cerebral hypoglycemia related to targeted therapy may lead to increased mortality (Morgenstern et al., 2010). Normoglycemia is recommended, but a specific target goal has yet to be identified.

Venous Thromboembolism Prophylaxis

The question of when it is "safe" to start pharmaceutical anticoagulation is a difficult one. All patients should have intermittent compression stockings in addition to elastic stockings to prevent venous clotting in the legs. Pharmaceutical prophylaxis may be considered in 1 to 4 days once the hematoma has stabilized and there are no signs of active bleeding (Morgenstern et al., 2010).

Clinical Pearl:

- Sequential compression devices are a must even when the patient complains.
- Monitor extremities for swelling and evidence of deep vein thrombosis.
- Peripherally inserted central catheter (PICC) care is extremely important because occlusion can lead to bloodstream infections and other complications. Be sure to check for blood return and actively flush each port with pulsatile flushing, even ones with continuous infusions running.

METRICS AND DATA

Along with the programmatic requirements, additional metrics were proposed for CSCs by Leifer et al. (2011). The Joint Commission adopted eight of the measures in March of 2014. Metrics specific to treat ICH are as follows:

- Modified Rankin Score (mRS) at 90 days
- Severity measurement performed for subarachnoid hemorrhage and ICH patients (overall rate). The ASA currently recommends the use of the ICH score (**Table 7-5**).
- Procoagulant reversal agent initiation for ICH

PROGNOSIS

ICH carries the poorest prognosis of all stroke types for survival and functional outcome. The overall mortality rate for ICH is 40% at 30 days, with over half of the deaths in the first 48 to 72 hours from neurological complications and withdrawal of care (Aguilar & Brott, 2011). For the survivors of the initial hemorrhage, only 12% to 39% were able to function independently at 1 year (Ikram, Wieberdink, & Koudstaal, 2012). Grading scales can be useful to improve communication and consistency between health care

TABLE 7-5 Intracerebral Hemorrhage (ICH) Score

Components		ICH Score Points
GCS score	3–4	2
	5–12	1
	13–15	0
ICH volume (mL)	≥30	1
	<30	0
IVH	Yes	1
	No	0
Infratentorial origin	Yes	1
	No	0
Age	≥80	1
	<80	0
Total ICH score		0–6

Data from Hemphill, J. C., Bonovich, D. C., Besmertis, L., Manley, G. T., & Johnston, S. C. (2001). The ICH score: A simple, reliable grading scale for intracerebral hemorrhage. *Stroke, 32*(4), 891–897.

TABLE 7-6 Calculating Intracerebral Hemorrhage Volume

Here is how to calculate the ICH volume:

$$\frac{A \times B \times C}{2}$$

Select the CT slice with the largest ICH
A = longest axis (cm)
B = longest axis perpendicular to A (cm)
C = number of slices × slice thickness (cm)

Data from Hemphill, J. C., Bonovich, D. C., Besmertis, L., Manley, G. T., & Johnston, S. C. (2001). The ICH score: A simple, reliable grading scale for intracerebral hemorrhage. *Stroke, 32*(4), 891–897.

providers, promote standardization of clinical treatment and research protocols, and aid providers in predicting prognosis. The ICH score was designed so that providers, who were not stroke neurologists or neurosurgeons, could easily and accurately make outcome predictions at the time of initial presentation.

The strongest predictors of outcome for ICH were identified and used as variables in the development of the ICH score (**Table 7-5**). Weighted values were assigned based on the strength of the association (Hemphill, Bonovich, Besmertis, Manley, & Johnston, 2001). The presenting GCS, age, presence of infratentorial hemorrhage (**Fig. 7-3**), calculated volume of the hematoma (**Table 7-6**), and the existence of IVH make up the components of the ICH score. The GCS has the strongest association with outcome and was, therefore, given the most weight. **Figure 7-4** demonstrates that a higher ICH score

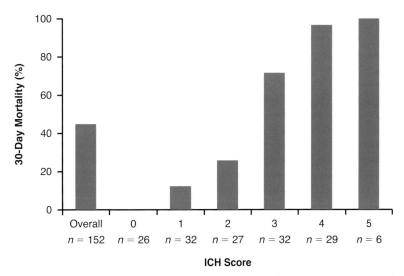

FIGURE 7-4 Mortality and ICH score at 30 days. Thirty-day mortality increases as ICH score increases. No patient with an ICH score of 0 died. All patients with an ICH score of 5 died. No patient in the University of California, San Francisco ICH cohort had an ICH score of 6, although this would be expected to be associated with mortality. *(From Hemphill, J. C., Bonovich, D. C., Besmertis, L., Manley, G. T., & Johnston, S. C. [2001]. The ICH score: A simple, reliable grading scale for intracerebral hemorrhage. Stroke, 32[4], 891–897.)*

is associated with a higher 30-day mortality. An ICH score of 5 or 6 equates with 100% mortality and a score of 0 equates with 0% mortality.

Precise prediction of functional outcome in patients with severe neurological insults, such as ICH, is difficult. Most deaths from ICH occur during the acute hospitalization, and these patients are more likely to have DNR orders in place. There is concern that overly pessimistic prognostication leads to self-fulfilling prophecy when care limitations and withdraw of care are ordered early in the course of the illness (Hemphill et al., 2001). Experts recommend "great caution" when instituting DNR orders in the first 24 hours after ICH (Morgenstern et al., 2010). The 2010 ASA guidelines recommend aggressive full care and postponement of DNR orders until at least the second hospital day. Patients who present to the hospital with DNR orders in place should not be included in this population, and their expressed wishes should be respected (Morgenstern et al., 2010).

POSTHOSPITAL CARE COORDINATION FOR THE INTRACEREBRAL HEMORRHAGE PATIENT

Patients with ICH have about a 20% chance of regaining their prior level of functioning. Planning for posthospital care and providing education for the patient and family is, therefore, extremely important and comes with challenges. Hospitals must have a coordinated interprofessional care process to provide a plan for posthospital care for these complicated patients. Thorough and well-coordinated discharge planning can be challenging and requires thoughtful planning. Advanced practice nurses (APNs) and/or physician assistants (PAs) are an integral part of the delivery of comprehensive stroke care and active participants in performance improvement processes. APNs and PAs collaborate closely with social workers, case managers, physical therapists, occupational therapists, and speech therapists along with pharmacists with neurological expertise in order to devise a plan for an appropriate and safe discharge.

A discharge planning team can help the patient, the family, or caregivers identify available medical and community resources. Patient and family/caregiver goals of care and discharge goals also need to be a part of the discharge plan. For patients going home who are not self-sufficient, their family's or caregiver's resources, knowledge, and commitment to providing ongoing safe care must be assessed. PT and OT provide an assessment of functional deficits and make recommendations regarding the level of supervision, ongoing needed therapy, and discharge disposition. If necessary, ongoing ST, swallowing evaluation, and special diet or feeding needs are provided including education and training of the patient and the families/caregivers. Because stroke patients frequently suffer from depression and cognitive decline, changes in mood and cognition is assessed. An individualized discharge plan of care should be documented in the patient's chart and patient-specific risk factors and treatment should be easily identified.

ICH patients will often need placement in skilled care facilities (e.g., acute inpatient rehabilitation, long-term acute care, or skilled nursing facilities), and the interprofessional team should identify high-risk patients early in the hospitalization. High-risk patients are not only those who have ICH with severe deficits but also those patients who are uninsured or underinsured, undocumented, homeless, or without family support. The social worker, case manager, and financial counselor are in communication with the interprofessional health team early in the hospitalization to work closely together around the anticipated discharge plan and the available options. This may help decrease length of stay and assist in providing a safe discharge plan.

Interprofessional discharge planning should be documented in the record. Hospitals can consider a somewhat scripted approach to use everyone's time and for documentation purposes. **Table 7-7** shows an interprofessional discharge template.

TABLE 7-7 Interprofessional Discharge Template

General statistics	1. Brief patient story 2. Anticipated plan of care with anticipated length of stay
Therapies assessment	1. Evaluations by PT/OT/SLP completed? 2. What are the final disposition recommendations? 3. Are there new cognitive deficits? Has a cognitive evaluation been done? 4. If acute rehab is recommended, has the physiatrist been consulted? 5. Do they need outpatient therapy, including physical therapy, occupational therapy, and speech therapy? 6. If going home, does family need training? Is this scheduled?
Case management assessment	1. Does the patient have insurance? 2. If no insurance, status of applications for aid (Medicaid, SSI, etc.) 3. What are the financial resources? 4. Can they afford their medications? 5. If LTAC, SNF, or home health is recommended, do they have benefits that will cover?

Social work assessment	1. Where is the patient from?
	2. Is family willing and able to provide care if needed?
	3. If patient is going directly home, does the family have the knowledge and resources necessary to care for the patient? Provide problem-solving strategies.
	4. Does the patient need public/community resources to facilitate integration into the community?
	   a. Support groups
	   b. Social services
	   c. Vocational rehabilitation
	   d. Behavioral health services
	   e. Family therapy services
	   f. Respite care services
	   g. American Heart Association and American Stroke Association

Nursing assessment	1. Are there signs that the patient is depressed? If so, what is the treatment plan? 2. Is pain control an issue? 3. DVT prophylaxis addressed? 4. Dysphagia screen performed? 5. Initial and ongoing stroke education performed and documented? 6. Other issues?

Dietary assessment	1. Is the patient undernourished or malnourished?
	   a. Calorie count needed?
	   b. Supplements needed?
	2. Tube feeding?
	3. Does the patient need warfarin teaching?

Follow-up	1. Does the patient have a PCP? 2. Will they be discharged on warfarin and need close monitoring of the INR? 3. Do they need a follow-up appointment made?
All	1. Goals of posthospital care

SLP, speech and language pathologist; SSI, Social Security Income; LTAC, long-term acute care; SNF, skilled nursing facility; DVT, deep vein thrombosis; PCP, primary care physician.

SUMMARY

The best treatment for stroke is to prevent a recurrent stroke from happening. Hypertension is the single highest cause of ICH. In order to prevent ICH stroke, which has the highest morbidity and mortality of all strokes, treatment of high blood pressure is paramount. The treatment and research described in this chapter focuses on the posthemorrhagic stroke management. Yet, a definitive evidence-based treatment has not been identified. Removing of blood products, controlling blood pressure, and giving homeostatic medications are interventions that have not consistently shown improvement in the functional outcome for ICH patients. ⊙ What has been shown to improve recovery is early aggressive care provided by an interprofessional team of physicians, nurses, pharmacists, social workers, case managers, therapists, and others with special training and expertise in the treatment of stroke. Coordination of acute interventions, provision of meticulous ICU care, and organization of a collaborative interprofessional team approach to caring for the ICH patient across the continuum of care are current best practices. These are the elements that make a difference in the functional outcome of the patient and the experience of the family who support them.

REFERENCES

Aguilar, M. I., & Brott, T. G. (2011). Update in intracerebral hemorrhage. *The Neurohospitalist*, 1(3), 148–159.

Aguilar, M. I., Hart, R. G., Kase, C. S., Freeman, W. D., Hoeben, B. J., García, R. C., . . . Yasaka, M. (2007). Treatment of warfarin-associated intracerebral hemorrhage: Literature review and expert opinion. *Mayo Clinic Proceedings*, 82(1), 82–92.

Albright, K. C., Boehme, A. K., Mullen, M. T., Seals, S., Grotta, J. C., & Savitz, S. I. (2013). Changing demographics at a comprehensive stroke center amidst the rise in primary stroke centers. *Stroke*, 44(4), 1117–1123.

Anderson, C. S., Huang, Y., Wang, J. G., Arima, H., Neal, B., Peng, B., . . . Chalmers, J. (2008). Intensive blood pressure reduction in acute cerebral haemorrhage trial (INTERACT): A randomised pilot trial. *The Lancet Neurology*, 7(5), 391–399.

Ariesen, M. J., Claus, S. P., Rinkel, G. J. E., & Algra, A. (2003). Risk factors for intracerebral hemorrhage in the general population a systematic review. *Stroke*, 34(8), 2060–2065.

Berlit, P. (2010). Diagnosis and treatment of cerebral vasculitis. *Therapeutic Advances in Neurological Disorders*, 3(1), 29–42.

Broderick, J., Brott, T., Tomsick, T., & Leach, A. (1993). Lobar hemorrhage in the elderly. The undiminishing importance of hypertension. *Stroke*, 24(1), 49–51.

Broderick, J. P., Brott, T., Tomsick, T., Miller, R., & Huster, G. (1993). Intracerebral hemorrhage more than twice as common as subarachnoid hemorrhage. *Journal of Neurosurgery*, 78(2), 188–191.

Brott, T., Broderick, J., Kothari, R., Barsan, W., Tomsick, T., Sauerbeck, L., . . . Khoury, J. (1997). Early hemorrhage growth in patients with intracerebral hemorrhage. *Stroke*, 28(1), 1–5.

Chiquette, E., Amato, M. G., & Bussey, H. I. (1998). Comparison of an anticoagulation clinic with usual medical care: Anticoagulation control, patient outcomes, and health care costs. *Archives of Internal Medicine*, 158(15), 1641–1647.

Claassen, J., Taccone, F. S., Horn, P., Holtkamp, M., Stocchetti, N., & Oddo, M. (2013). Recommendations on the use of EEG monitoring in critically ill patients: Consensus statement from the neurointensive care section of the ESICM. *Intensive Care Medicine*, 39(8), 1337–1351.

Cooper, D., Jauch, E., & Flaherty, M. L. (2007). Critical pathways for the management of stroke and intracerebral hemorrhage: A survey of US hospitals. *Critical Pathways in Cardiology*, 6(1), 18–23.

Daroff, R. B., Fenichel, G. M., Jankovic, J., & Mazziotta, J. C., Eds. (2012). *Bradley's neurology in clinical practice* (6th ed.). Philadelphia, PA: Saunders Elsevier.

Davis, S. M., Broderick, J., Hennerici, M., Brun, N. C., Diringer, M. N., Mayer, S. A., . . . Steiner, T. (2006). Hematoma growth is a determinant of mortality and poor outcome after intracerebral hemorrhage. *Neurology*, 66(8), 1175–1181.

Diringer, M. N., & Edwards, D. F. (2001). Admission to a neurologic/neurosurgical intensive care unit is associated with reduced mortality rate after intracerebral hemorrhage. *Critical Care Medicine*, 29(3), 635–640.

Flaherty, M. L., Woo, D., Haverbusch, M., Sekar, P., Khoury, J., Sauerbeck, L., . . . Broderick, J. P. (2005). Racial variations in location and risk of intracerebral hemorrhage. *Stroke, 36*(5), 934–937.

Gaberel, T., Gakuba, C., Emery, E., & Touze, E. (2013). Surgery for cerebral haemorrhage—STICH II trial. *The Lancet, 382*(9902), 1400–1401.

Gatchev, O., Råstam, L., Lindberg, G., Gullberg, B., Eklund, G. A., & Isacsson, S. O. (1993). Subarachnoid hemorrhage, cerebral hemorrhage, and serum cholesterol concentration in men and women. *Annals of epidemiology, 3*(4), 403–409.

Girard, T. D., Pandharipande, P. P., & Ely, E. W. (2008). Delirium in the intensive care unit. *Critical Care, 12*(Suppl. 3), S3.

Go, A. S., Mozaffarian, D., Roger, V. L., Benjamin, E. J., Berry, J. D., Borden, W. B., . . . Turner, M. B. (2013). Heart disease and stroke statistics—2013 update: A report from the American Heart Association. *Circulation, 127*(1), e6.

Grysiewicz, R. A., Thomas, K., & Pandey, D. K. (2008). Epidemiology of ischemic and hemorrhagic stroke: Incidence, prevalence, mortality, and risk factors. *Neurologic Clinics, 26*(4), 871–895.

Hacke, W., Kaste, M., Bluhmki, E., Brozman, M., Dávalos, A., Guidetti, D., . . . Toni, D. (2008). Thrombolysis with alteplase 3 to 4.5 hours after acute ischemic stroke. *The New England Journal of Medicine, 359*(13), 1317–1329.

Hart, R. G., Diener, H. C., Yang, S., Connolly, S. J., Wallentin, L., Reilly, P. A., . . . Yusuf, S. (2012). Intracranial hemorrhage in atrial fibrillation patients during anticoagulation with warfarin or dabigatran: The RE-LY trial. *Stroke, 43*(6), 1511–1517.

Hemphill, J. C., Bonovich, D. C., Besmertis, L., Manley, G. T., & Johnston, S. C. (2001). The ICH score: A simple, reliable grading scale for intracerebral hemorrhage. *Stroke, 32*(4), 891–897.

Hickey, J. V. (2011). Neurological assessment. In J. Hickey (Ed.), *Clinical practice of neurological and neurosurgical nursing* (pp. 154). Philadelphia, PA: Lippincott Williams & Wilkins.

Hinkle, J. L. (2014). Reliability and validity of the National Institutes of Health Stroke Scale for neuroscience nurses. *Stroke, 45*(3), e32–e34.

Ikram, M. A., Wieberdink, R. G., & Koudstaal, P. J. (2012). International epidemiology of intracerebral hemorrhage. *Current Atherosclerosis Reports, 14*(4), 300–306.

James, P. A., Oparil, S., Carter, B. L., Cushman, W. C., Dennison-Himmelfarb, C., Handler, J., . . . Ortiz, E. (2014). 2014 evidence-based guideline for the management of high blood pressure in adults: Report from the panel members appointed to the Eighth Joint National Committee (JNC 8). *The Journal of the American Medical Association, 311*(5), 507–520.

Juvela, S., Hillbom, M., & Palomäki, H. (1995). Risk factors for spontaneous intracerebral hemorrhage. *Stroke, 26*(9), 1558–1564.

Kissela, B. M., Khoury, J., Kleindorfer, D., Woo, D., Schneider, A., Alwell, K., . . . Broderick, J. P. (2005). Epidemiology of ischemic stroke in patients with diabetes: The Greater Cincinnati/Northern Kentucky Stroke Study. *Diabetes Care, 28*(2), 355–359.

Kress, J. P., Pohlman, A. S., O'Connor, M. F., & Hall, J. B. (2000). Daily interruption of sedative infusions in critically ill patients undergoing mechanical ventilation. *The New England Journal of Medicine, 342*(20), 1471–1477.

Lang, E. W., Ren Ya, Z., Preul, C., Hugo, H. H., Hempelmann, R. G., Buhl, R., . . . Mehdorn, H. M. (2001). Stroke pattern interpretation: The variability of hypertensive versus amyloid angiopathy hemorrhage. *Cerebrovascular Diseases, 12*(2), 121–130.

Leifer, D., Bravata, D. M., Hinchey, J. A., Jauch, E. C., Johnston, S. C., Latchaw, R., . . . Zorowitz, R. (2011). Metrics for measuring quality of care in comprehensive stroke centers: Detailed follow-up to brain attack coalition comprehensive stroke center recommendations a statement for healthcare professionals from the American Heart Association/American Stroke Association. *Stroke, 42*(3), 849–877.

Levy, E., Lopez-Otin, C., Ghiso, J., Geltner, D., & Frangione, B. (1989). Stroke in Icelandic patients with hereditary amyloid angiopathy is related to a mutation in the cystatin C gene, an inhibitor of cysteine proteases. *The Journal of Experimental Medicine, 169*(5), 1771–1778.

Liu-DeRyke, X., Janisse, J., Coplin, W. M., Parker, D., Jr., Norris, G., & Rhoney, D. H. (2008). A comparison of nicardipine and labetalol for acute hypertension management following stroke. *Neurocritical Care, 9*(2), 167–176.

Lou, M., Al-Hazzani, A., Goddeau, R. P., Novak, V., & Selim, M. (2010). Relationship between white-matter hyperintensities and hematoma volume and growth in patients with intracerebral hemorrhage. *Stroke, 41*(1), 34–40.

Mayer, S. A. (2007). Hemicraniectomy: A second chance on life for patients with space-occupying MCA infarction. *Stroke, 38*(9), 2410–2412.

Mayer, S. A., Brun, N. C., Begtrup, K., Broderick, J., Davis, S., Diringer, M. N., . . . Steiner, T. (2008). Efficacy and safety of recombinant activated factor VII for acute intracerebral hemorrhage. *The New England Journal of Medicine, 358*(20), 2127–2137.

Messé, S. R., Sansing, L. H., Cucchiara, B. L., Herman, S. T., Lyden, P. D., & Kasner, S. E. (2009). Prophylactic antiepileptic drug use is associated with poor outcome following ICH. *Neurocritical Care, 11*(1), 38–44.

Mohr, J. P., Grotta, J. C., Wolf, P. A., Moskowitz, M. A., Mayberg, M. R., & Von Kummer, R. (2011). *Stroke: Pathophysiology, diagnosis, and management (expert consult-online).* Philadelphia, PA: Elsevier Health Sciences.

Morgenstern, L. B., Hemphill, J. C., Anderson, C., Becker, K., Broderick, J. P., Connolly, E. S., . . . Tamargo, R. J. (2010). Guidelines for the management of spontaneous intracerebral hemorrhage: A guideline for healthcare professionals from the American Heart Association/American Stroke Association. *Stroke, 41*(9), 2108–2129.

Naff, N., Williams, M. A., Keyl, P. M., Tuhrim, S., Bullock, M. R., Mayer, S. A., . . . Hanley, D. F. (2011). Low-dose recombinant tissue-type plasminogen activator enhances clot resolution in brain hemorrhage: The intraventricular hemorrhage thrombolysis trial. *Stroke, 42*(11), 3009–3016.

Newell, D. W., Shah, M. M., Wilcox, R., Hansmann, D. R., Melnychuk, E., Muschelli, J., & Hanley, D. F. (2011). Minimally invasive evacuation of spontaneous intracerebral hemorrhage using sonothrombolysis. *Journal of Neurosurgery, 115*(3), 592.

Paciaroni, M., Bogousslavsky, J., & Levine, S. R. (2013). Hemorrhagic transformation of ischemic stroke. *Neurology Medlink Clinical Summary.* Retrieved from http://www.medlink.com/medlinkcontent.asp

Poungvarin, N., Bhoopat, W., Viriyavejakul, A., Rodprasert, P., Buranasiri, P., Sukondhabhant, S., . . . Strom, B. L. (1987). Effects of dexamethasone in primary supratentorial intracerebral hemorrhage. *The New England Journal of Medicine, 316*(20), 1229–1233.

Qureshi, A. I. (2007). Antihypertensive treatment of acute cerebral hemorrhage (ATACH). *Neurocritical Care, 6*(1), 56–66.

Qureshi, A. I., Mendelow, A. D., & Hanley, D. F. (2009). Intracerebral haemorrhage. *The Lancet, 373*(9675), 1632–1644.

Qureshi, A. I., & Palesch, Y. Y. (2011). Antihypertensive Treatment of Acute Cerebral Hemorrhage (ATACH) II: Design, methods, and rationale. *Neurocritical Care, 15*(3), 559–576.

Qureshi, A. I., Suri, M. A., Safdar, K., Ottenlips, J. R., Janssen, R. S., & Frankel, M. R. (1997). Intracerebral hemorrhage in blacks. Risk factors, subtypes, and outcome. *Stroke, 28*(5), 961–964.

Qureshi, A. I., Tuhrim, S., Broderick, J. P., Batjer, H. H., Hondo, H., & Hanley, D. F. (2001). Spontaneous intracerebral hemorrhage. *New England Journal of Medicine, 344*(19), 1450–1460.

Rosand, J., Eckman, M. H., Knudsen, K. A., Singer, D. E., & Greenberg, S. M. (2004). The effect of warfarin and intensity of anticoagulation on outcome of intracerebral hemorrhage. *Archives of Internal Medicine, 164*(8), 880–884.

Staykov, D., & Gupta, R. (2011). Hemicraniectomy in malignant middle cerebral artery infarction. *Stroke, 42*(2), 513–516.

Takeuchi, S., Wada, K., Nagatani, K., Otani, N., & Mori, K. (2013). Decompressive hemicraniectomy for spontaneous intracerebral hemorrhage. *Neurosurgical Focus, 34*(5), E5.

The NINDS t-PA Stroke Study Group. (1997). Intracerebral hemorrhage after intravenous t-PA therapy for ischemic stroke. *Stroke, 28*(11), 2109–2118.

Toossi, S., Hess, C. P., Hills, N. K., & Josephson, S. A. (2010). Neurovascular complications of cocaine use at a tertiary stroke center. *Journal of Stroke and Cerebrovascular Diseases, 19*(4), 273–278.

Vespa, P. M., Martin, N., Zuccarello, M., Awad, I., & Hanley, D. F. (2013). Surgical trials in intracerebral hemorrhage. *Stroke, 44*(6 Suppl. 1.), S79–S82.

Vespa, P. M., O'Phelan, K., Shah, M., Mirabelli, J., Starkman, S., Kidwell, C., . . . Martin, N. A. (2003). Acute seizures after intracerebral hemorrhage: A factor in progressive midline shift and outcome. *Neurology, 60*(9), 1441–1446.

Zipfel, G. J., Fox, D. J., Jr., & Rivet, D. J. (2005). Moyamoya disease in adults: The role of cerebral revascularization. *Skull Base, 15*(1), 27.

CHAPTER 8

Subarachnoid Hemorrhage

Mary L. King

Subarachnoid hemorrhage (SAH) is most commonly the result of cerebral trauma; however, most people are familiar with SAH as a description of a ruptured intracranial vessel due to an aneurysm or an arteriovenous malformation (AVM). Traumatic subarachnoid hemorrhage (tSAH) occurs in up to 55% of patients with moderate to severe cerebral injury and is a strong predictor of patient mortality and adverse outcomes (Wong et al., 2012). The second most common cause of SAH is the rupture of cerebral aneurysm, occurring in 30,000 to 35,000 cases per year. A precise incidence of aneurysmal subarachnoid hemorrhage (aSAH) is difficult to monitor due to the number of people who die from the rupture prior to hospital arrival. Therefore, most annual incidence statistics are underestimated. aSAH comprises 5% to 10% of all strokes in the United States. Additionally, cerebral hemorrhage is often the clinical presentation of a patient with an AVM. SAH due to AVMs is estimated at 2% to 4% per year. Once a person experiences an AMV-related hemorrhage, the annual risk of rehemorrhage increases to 6% to 18% per year (Crowley, Ducruet, McDougall, & Albuquerque, 2014). There are no known risk factors for AVM because this entity is thought to be congenital in origin and affects about 10 per 10,000 adults. The annual incidence is about 2% of all hemorrhagic strokes (Ferrara, 2011).

SAH carries a significant mortality and morbidity burden, far exceeding ischemic stroke and intracerebral hemorrhage (ICH). The mortality rate for aSAH within the first 24 hours of the initial hemorrhage is 25% (Le Roux & Wallace, 2009). In the past, the mortality rates during the first month were around 50%. Recent studies have indicated a decline in mortality to around 33% to 45%. Reasons for the decreased mortality rate are unclear but may be related to improvements in blood pressure control, a decline in cigarette smoking, and better primary health care. Of those who survive aSAH, nearly 30% of morbidity and mortality is related to secondary complications related to delayed cerebral ischemia, also known as *vasospasm*, and more than half have experienced a significant decline in their quality of life and remain dependent on others for care (Le Roux & Wallace, 2009).

According to recent studies, the prevalence of intracranial aneurysm (IA) in the general population ranges from 1% to 3%; however, a meta-analysis found that the prevalence was approximately 3.2% of a population with an average age of 50 years (Washington, Vellimana, Zipfel, & Dacey, 2011). In the United States, approximately 25,000 to 35,000 people are affected by aSAH annually, with an estimated incidence of 8 to 10 per 100,000 (Bautista, 2012). The National Hospital Discharge Survey (NHDS) has collected data since 1965. The NHDS used hospital discharge records based on the *International Classification of Diseases*, 9th Revision, Clinical Modification (*ICD-9-CM*) code 430 from hospitals in all 50 states and the District of Columbia (not including Veterans Administration [VA] hospitals and federal and military hospitals). This study reviewed data from a 30-year time frame (1979 to 2008) that represents about 1% of all hospitalizations, or 350,000 discharges per year. The findings, although observational, demonstrated that the rate of admission for patients with a primary diagnosis of SAH (612,500 patients) has remained stable over the 30-year time frame with a significant decrease in in-hospital mortality and total deaths after SAH (Rincon, Rossenwasser, & Dumont, 2013).

SAH may be further defined as subarachnoid blood on computed tomography (CT) scan, blood or xanthochromic cerebrospinal fluid (CSF), or red blood cells in the final tube of CSF sample and positive angiography findings (Perry et al., 2013). Prehospital care is critical and includes basic care for airway, breathing, and circulation (ABCs) and triage to deliver the patient to the nearest medical center with neurological/neurosurgical services including CT scan, angiography, neurosurgical consultation, and comprehensive care from emergency department (ED) through rehabilitation. Large, tertiary medical centers are often regional treatment centers and have the specialized interprofessional health care teams to accept aSAH patients as the need arises (Zebian, Kulkami, & Kazzi, 2013).

RISK FACTORS

The incidence of aSAH increases with age, and females are affected more than males particularly in the 45- to 55-year age group when the risk is nearly doubled (Ganti et al., 2013). Studies have demonstrated a regional variance with aSAH, with an increased incidence among the Japanese and Finnish compared to more southern regions closer to the equator. The incidence is doubled in African Americans compared to Caucasians. In addition to age and ethnic background, risk factors for aSAH include smoking, cocaine abuse, excessive alcohol consumption, and hypertension (Bautista, 2012). Other risk factors for aSAH include family history, genetics, or congenital conditions. Marfan syndrome, Ehlers-Danlos disease, neurofibromatosis type I, and autosomal dominant polycystic kidney disease are among the collagen vascular diseases that may predispose a person to aneurysm formation (Patel & Samuels, 2012).

Although the population is aging, the elderly are in better health and have longer life expectancies, thus the number of elderly patients with aSAH is increasing. A recent review found that the annual incidence of aSAH in people older than 70 years of age has exceeded a rate of 25 per 100,000 people. Despite the age and regional variations, aSAH is a neurosurgical emergency that carries high morbidity and mortality. Research indicates a mortality rate of approximately 50% within a month of the event, with the remaining 50% suffering from disabling functional and cognitive deficits (Washington et al., 2011).

Older age (>60 years), cigarette smoking, female gender, posterior circulation location, atherosclerosis, hypertension, and larger IA size (>5 mm) are contributing factors for an IA to rupture. A family history of IA or SAH, previous history of SAH, or the presence of autosomal dominant polycystic kidney disease increases the risk of IA rupture (Washington et al., 2011). However, studies in animal models and preclinical subjects have demonstrated that inflammation and the complement system activation may have a role in IA formation and rupture (Abate & Citerio, 2014).

PATHOPHYSIOLOGY

IAs are generally found at vessel bifurcations within the circle of Willis. The most common locations are at the bifurcation of the basilar artery, at the junction of the ipsilateral posterior inferior cerebellar artery (PICA) and vertebral artery (VA), or on the anterior communicating artery. The hemodynamic changes caused by increased blood pressure and other risk factors promote changes in the vessels and contribute to the formation and rupture of an IA (Penn, Komotar, & Connolly, 2011). In addition, endothelial dysfunction is thought to be the result of hemodynamic stress that leads to the inflammatory response in the arterial walls. This endothelial dysfunction ultimately results in vascular remodeling and cell death. Macrophages and apoptosis of smooth muscle cells in conjunction with further degradation of the extracellular matrix contribute to the progressive weakening of the arterial wall (Chalouhi, Hoh, & Hasan, 2013). Heavy alcohol use with its effects on blood pressure and hemodynamic factors is considered an independent risk factor for aSAH. Cocaine and similar drug abuse increases the risk of aSAH due to the strong vasoconstrictor effects and the resulting extreme hypertension (Diringer, 2009) (**Fig. 8-1**).

GRADING SCALES

A number of grading scales are used in practice to standardize the clinical classification of patients with SAH and to monitor progression and change in condition. These scales are based on the initial clinical neurological examination and the appearance of blood on the initial head CT. These scales include the Glasgow Coma Scale, the Hunt and Hess grading scale, the WFNS scale, the Fisher grading scale, and the modified Fisher grading scale. The *Glasgow Coma Scale* (GCS), introduced in 1974, was designed as a reliable and objective scale of neurological function in three subscales of level of consciousness, eye opening, and motor function (Teasdale & Jennett, 1974; Teasdale, Murray, Parker, & Jennett, 1979) (**Table 8-1**). The patient is assessed against the criteria of each scale, and the resulting points are added together to give a patient score between 3 and 15. In interpreting the score, the higher score correlates to a better patient's condition. The GCS is used for initial and ongoing assessment of a patient with possible or confirmed cerebral trauma to determine neurological deficits and any changes in neurological condition over time.

The World Federation of Neurosurgical Societies (WFNS) developed the WFNS grading scale, which describes the clinical presentation of SAH patients. The scale combines consciousness and motor deficit in its scoring system. The WFNS grading system uses a combination of consciousness and motor deficits from the GCS and presence of focal neurological deficits to grade the severity of SAH (Teasdale et al., 1988) (**Table 8-2**). The scale is useful for predicting recovery and response to treatment. For example,

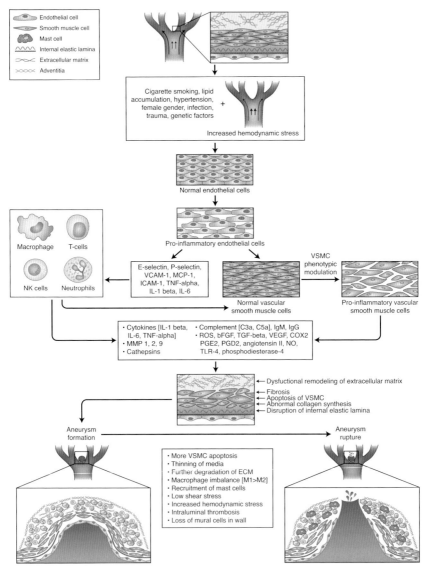

FIGURE 8-1 Cerebral aneurysm (CA) formation and rupture. Aneurysm formation is initiated by hemodynamically triggered endothelial dysfunction. An inflammatory response implicating several cytokines and inflammatory mediators as well as macrophages, T cells, and mast cells ensues. Concurrently, smooth muscle cells (SMCs) undergo phenotypic modulation to a proinflammatory phenotype. The inflammatory response in vessel wall leads to disruption of internal elastic lamina, extracellular matrix digestion, and aneurysm formation. Loss of mural cells and further inflammation and vessel wall degeneration ultimately lead to CA rupture. *bFGF*, basic fibroblast growth factor; *COX2*, cyclooxygenase-2; *ECM*, extracellular matrix; *ICAM*, intercellular adhesion molecule; *IL*, interleukin; *MCP*, monocyte chemoattractant protein; *MMP*, matrix metalloproteinase; *NK*, natural killer; *NO*, nitric oxide; *PGD*, prostaglandin D; *PGE*, prostaglandin E; *ROS*, reactive oxygen species; *TGF*, transforming growth factor; *TLR*, toll-like receptor; *TNF*, tumor necrosis factor; *VCAM*, vascular cell adhesion molecule; *VEGF*, vascular endothelial growth factor; *VSMC*, vascular smooth muscle cell. *(From Chalouhi, N., Hoh, B. L., & Hasan, D. [2013]. Review of cerebral aneurysm formation, growth, and rupture. Stroke, 44, 3613–3622.)*

TABLE 8-1 Glasgow Coma Scale

The GCS is the most common scoring system used to describe the level of consciousness following a brain injury. It is used to help gauge the severity of an acute brain injury. The scale is a simple, reliable, and objective way of recording initial and subsequent neurological function and correlates well with outcome following severe brain injury. The GCS has three subscales that measure the following functions:

Eye opening (E)
- 4 = spontaneous
- 3 = to voice
- 2 = to pain
- 1 = none

Verbal response (V)
- 5 = normal conversation
- 4 = disoriented conversation
- 3 = words, but not coherent
- 2 = no words, only sounds
- 1 = none

Motor response (M)
- 6 = normal
- 5 = localized to pain
- 4 = withdraws to pain
- 3 = decorticate posture (an abnormal posture that can include rigidity, clenched fists, legs held straight out, and arms bent inward toward the body with the wrists and fingers bend and held on the chest)
- 2 = decerebrate (an abnormal posture that can include rigidity, arms and legs held straight out, toes pointed downward, head and neck arched backward)
- 1 = none

Clinicians use this scale to rate the best eye opening response, the best verbal response, and the best motor response an individual makes. The final GCS score or grade is the sum of these numbers.

Adapted from Teasdale, G., & Jennett, B. (1974). Assessment of coma and impaired consciousness: A practical scale. *The Lancet, 2*(7872), 81–84; Teasdale, G., Murray, G., Parker, L., & Jennett, B. (1979). Adding up the Glasgow Coma Score. *Acta Neuroschirurgica. Supplementum, 28*(1), 13–16.

elderly patients who have a WFNS score of I to III have the best clinical recovery and seemed to benefit from aggressive treatment when compared to patients younger than age 70 years with a WFNS score of IV or V (Schöller et al., 2013).

The *Hunt and Hess grading scale*, introduced in 1968, helps to classify the severity of an SAH based on the patient's clinical condition. It is used as a predictor of a patient's prognosis/outcome; higher score (grade) correlates to a lower survival rate (Hunt & Hess, 1968) (**Table 8-3**).

TABLE 8-2 World Federation of Neurosurgical Societies Grading Scale

Grade	Glasgow Coma Scale	Motor Deficit
I	15	Absent
II	14–13	Absent
III	14–13	Present
IV	12–7	Present or absent
IV	6–3	Present or absent

From Teasdale, G. M., Drake, C. G., Hunt, W., Kassell, N., Sano, K., Pertuiset, B., & De Villiers, J. C. (1988). A universal subarachnoid hemorrhage scale: Report of a committee of the World Federation of Neurosurgical Societies. *Journal of Neurology, Neurosurgery, and Psychiatry, 51*(11), 1457.

TABLE 8-3 Hunt and Hess Grading Scale for Subarachnoid Hemorrhage

Grade	Hunt and Hess Scale
I	Asymptomatic or mild headache
II	Moderate to severe headache, nuchal rigidity, with or without cranial nerve deficits
III	Confusion, lethargy, or mild focal symptoms
IV	Stupor and/or hemiparesis
V	Comatose and/or decerebrate posturing

From Hunt, W. E., & Hess, R. M. (1968). Surgical risk as related to time of intervention in the repair of intracranial aneurysms. *Journal of Neurosurgery, 28*(1), 14–20.

SIGNS AND SYMPTOMS

aSAH usually occurs without warning as a sudden cataclysmic event that changes the lives of the patient and the family. This hemorrhagic stroke is a neurosurgical emergency and often described as devastating, catastrophic, and often fatal. Clinical signs and symptoms may range from a slight headache and nuchal rigidity to coma and death. Patients presenting with IA rupture often complain of the "worst headache of my life" or a thunderclap headache and may have associated nausea and vomiting (often projectile), photophobia, and nuchal rigidity. Depending on the size of the rupture, neurological deficits may be present and range in severity from a focal deficit to coma. The presence of an unruptured IA or increased intracranial pressure (ICP) postrupture may cause cranial nerve palsies from compression on the third and/or sixth cranial nerve (CN III, CN VI). Some patients experience seizures with IA rupture (Diringer, 2009).

aSAH may be classified using scales including the GCS, the WFNS scale, and Hunt and Hess grading scale, which reflect the clinical condition of the patient. The *Hunt and Hess grading scale* and the *WFNS* scale are predictors of outcomes, with the higher the score, the poorer the prognosis (Green, Burns, & DeFusco, 2013). The Hunt and Hess grading scale is often shown in conjunction with the WFNS scale because they correlate SAH grades with the GCS. **Table 8-4** provides a comparison of these scales with patient survival (Rosen & Macdonald, 2005). However, the *Fisher grading scale* is a numerical scale from 0 to 4 that provides insight to the amount of subarachnoid blood on CT scan (**Table 8-5**). These grading scales demonstrate a direct link to the severity of the hemorrhage, the clinical grade of the IA, and incidence of vasospasm after the SAH. In comparison, the modified *Fisher grading scale* provides more specific descriptions of the amount and location of blood seen on CT scan. **Table 8-6** shows a comparison of the Fisher and modified Fisher grading scales (Claassen et al., 2001). The percentages associated with each grade on the modified scale are slightly higher for symptomatic vasospasm.

Clinical Pearl: All patients having signs and symptoms of stroke should be transported to the nearest primary stroke center or hospital with a similar designation for the available acute therapeutic interventions (American Heart Association/American Stroke Association). Patients with SAH may require transport to the nearest comprehensive stroke center to receive specialized care from vascular neurologists and neurosurgical and neurocritical care teams.

TABLE 8-4 Comparison of World Federation of Neurosurgical Societies Grading Scale, Hunt and Hess Grading Scale, and Glasgow Coma Scale with Survival

World Federation of Neurosurgical Societies Grading Scale	Grade	Hunt and Hess	Glasgow Coma Scale	Survival
No motor deficit	I	Asymptomatic or minimal headache and slight nuchal rigidity	15	70%
No motor deficit	II	Moderate to severe headache, nuchal rigidity, no neurological deficit other than cranial nerve palsy	13–14	60%
Motor deficit	III	Drowsiness, confusion, or mild focal deficit	13–14	50%
With or without motor deficit	IV	Stupor, moderate to severe hemiparesis, possibly early decerebrate posturing	7–12	20%
With or without motor deficit	V	Deep coma, decerebrate posturing, moribund appearance	3–6	10%

From Patel, V. N., & Samuels, O. B. (2012). The critical care management of aneurysmal subarachnoid hemorrhage. In Y. Murai (Ed.), *Aneurysm*. InTech. doi:10.5772/48474

▌▌ DIAGNOSTICS

Some patients may have a "warning" or sentinel headache that occurs hours to weeks before the SAH. Accurate diagnosis and early identification of a sentinel headache decreases morbidity and mortality related to SAH (Zebian et al., 2013). Approximately 2% of all ED admissions are for complaint of headache. Making the diagnosis of SAH in a patient with headache and a new neurological deficit is a straightforward process, but the diagnostic algorithm for headache alone without a neurological deficit becomes more challenging because the provider must decide which alert, neurologically intact patient needs further investigation. Half of all SAH patients present in this manner. Basic CT scan (without contrast) of the brain is performed, followed by a lumbar puncture (LP) if the CT scan is negative and SAH is suspected. The side

TABLE 8-5 Fisher Grading Scale

Grade	Fisher Scale*
1	Focal thin layer of blood
2	Diffuse thin SAH
3	Thick SAH
4	Focal or diffuse, thin SAH with extensive intracerebral or intraventricular hemorrhage

*The Fisher grading scale classifies the appearance of SAH on CT scan. This scale has been modified by Claassen and coworkers (2001), reflecting the additive risk from SAH size and accompanying intraventricular hemorrhage (0, none; 1, minimal SAH without IVH; 2, minimal SAH with IVH; 3, thick SAH without IVH; 4, thick SAH with IVH).
From Fisher, C., Kistler, J., & Davis, J. (1980). Relation of cerebral vasospasm to subarachnoid hemorrhage visualized by computerized tomographic scanning. *Neurosurgery*, *6*(1), 1–9; Patel, V. N., & Samuels, O. B. (2012). The critical care management of aneurysmal subarachnoid hemorrhage. In Y. Murai (Ed.), *Aneurysm*. InTech. doi:10.5772/48474.

TABLE 8-6 Fisher and Modified Fisher Grading Scale

Grade	Fisher Scale	% with Symptomatic Vasospasm	Modified Fisher Scale	% with Symptomatic Vasospasm
1	Focal thin	21%	Focal or diffuse thin SAH, no IVH	24%
2	Diffuse thin SAH	25%	Focal or diffuse thin SAH, with IVH	33%
3	Thick SAH present	37%	Thick SAH present, no IVH	33%
4	Focal or diffuse thin SAH with significant ICH or IVH	31%	Thick SAH present, with IVH	40%

From Claassen, J., Bernardini, G. L., Kreiter, K., Bates, J., Du, Y. E., Copeland, D., . . . Mayer, S. A. (2001). Effect of cisternal and ventricular blood on risk of delayed cerebral ischemia after subarachnoid hemorrhage: The Fisher Scale revisited. *Stroke, 32,* 2012–2020.

effect of an LP may result in a headache that is worse than the original headache (Perry et al., 2013). Digital subtraction angiography (DSA) has been considered the preferred method for diagnosing intracranial IAs for many years. Improvements in CT technology, that is, computed tomography angiography (CTA), have been integrated into the diagnosis and treatment algorithms for patients with SAH in many neurological centers in Europe and the United States as the CT technology has improved dramatically (Abate & Citerio, 2014). Magnetic resonance imaging (MRI) may be used for diagnosis but is not considered a first-line option because the length of time to complete the examination is much longer that CT or CTA. Patient limitations such as cardiac pacemakers or other metallic-based implants may preclude the use of MRI (Patel & Samuels, 2012).

When a patient is being considered for either an endovascular or surgical approach for the treatment of an IA, a number of diagnostics are ordered to assist with identification of treatment options and decision making about the best approach for the particular needs of the patient. An angiogram is performed prior to surgical clipping to determine the location and size of the IA. Additional imaging studies may be conducted to more fully appreciate the characteristics of the IA. CT scan (with and without contrast), CTA, and DSA may be ordered preoperatively (**Fig. 8-2**). MRI is usually not one of the first-line examinations due to availability, cost, and the inability to distinguish hemorrhage. MRI may be useful for patients who are several days postbleed or to identify small infarcts (American Association of Neuroscience Nurses [AANN], 2009). However, one small study compared susceptibility-weighted imaging (SWI) with standard CT techniques and fluid attenuated inversion recovery (FLAIR) to indicate SAH. The researchers found that by using a combination of SWI and FLAIR, MRI was able to detect SAH at higher rates than with CT alone (Verma et al., 2013). The neurosurgeon determines the surgical approach based on the location of the IA, with the main treatment options including clipping of an aneurysm or endovascular obliteration of the aneurysm. Clipping an IA is a major neurosurgical procedure that requires a craniotomy and generally lasts several hours. Research has shown that when a patient is anesthetized for long periods of time, there is an increased risk of complications due to physiological compromise and suppression of the immune system (Fox & Choi, 2009).

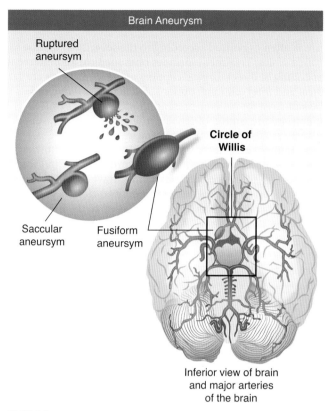

FIGURE 8-2 Aneurysms located on arteries of the circle of Willis. *(From Hickey, J. V. [2014]. The clinical practice of neurological and neurosurgical nursing [7th ed.]. Philadelphia, PA: Lippincott Williams & Wilkins.)*

Positioning the patient for the procedure requires meticulous attention to detail by the surgical staff. Neurosurgical procedures can last several hours, and improper positioning or inadequate padding of bony prominences can result in significant patient injury and complications. For example, peripheral nerve injury such as brachial plexus or ulnar nerve compression can result in permanent damage that causes numbness, tingling, or intractable pain (Gerken, 2013). Insufficient or improperly placed padding may result in a hospital-acquired pressure ulcer (HAPU). HAPUs are considered one of the Centers for Medicare and Medicaid Services (CMS) "never events," and the organization will not be reimbursed for any care or treatments to heal a HAPU (McKeon & Cardell, 2011). More importantly, the patient would be subjected to additional pain, the possibility of additional surgical procedures to debride or graft a severe HAPU, and a possible increased length of stay. See Chapter 5 on diagnostics.

Clinical Pearl: When educating the patient, family, or significant other, use the term *stroke* in addition to the term *subarachnoid hemorrhage* to help them understand that aSAH is a type of stroke.

▗▖ TREATMENT OVERVIEW

SAH patient care is often organized according to the severity of disease as measured on the aforementioned scales. Treatment includes both medical and interventional options of endovascular coiling or direct surgical clipping of the IA. Patients are generally treated with both medical and interventional options. More conservative or less invasive interventions may be sufficient for patients presenting with a grade I or II SAH. The key goals for all SAH patients are prevention of rehemorrhage (rebleeding), supportive care, pain management, and accurate diagnosis and treatment.

Although the immediate care is aimed at preventing rehemorrhage and securing the aneurysm, other common problems include hydrocephalus and vasospasm. Hydrocephalus is present in up to 30% of patients with intraventricular hemorrhage. In patients with a significant SAH and a higher (more severe) clinical grade, the incidence of rebleeding is higher and may be evident upon admission to the ED or intensive care unit (ICU). Hydrocephalus often occurs within the first 3 days post hemorrhage. Placement of an intraventricular external drainage device is required with the majority of patients showing signs of clinical improvement (Diringer, 2009). Approximately 60% of patients with aSAH have radiographic vasospasm defined as vasoconstriction and narrowing of the cerebral arteries evident with cerebral angiography with or without clinical signs or symptoms. About 39% of patients will have clinical manifestations of vasospasm.

Osmotic or loop diuretics and antihypertensive medications for blood pressure control may be sufficient to stabilize the patient until surgical or endovascular interventions can be initiated to secure the IA (Becske et al., 2013). Grades III, IV, or V require more aggressive and extensive care that may include intubation and mechanical ventilation to protect the airway and support respiratory effort in patients with decreased level of consciousness. Rapid-sequence intubation (RSI) is recommended for patients with SAH, including sedation and short-acting neuromuscular blockade and other agents that lessen the possibility of an increase in ICP. Intravenous access is necessary, and arterial blood pressure monitoring is preferred; central line access should be accomplished as soon as safely possible. Cardiac monitoring, pulse oximetry, and end-tidal carbon dioxide measurements provide additional data to the health care team to direct care. Other interventions may include an indwelling urinary catheter, seizure prophylaxis, and calcium channel blockers (Becske et al., 2013).

Medical Management

The major concerns after an aSAH are rebleeding, hydrocephalus, and vasospasm. The most immediate concern is rebleeding. The greatest risk of rebleeding and mortality is within the first 8 hours of the initial hemorrhage. About 9% to 17% of patients are at risk of rebleeding in the first 72 hours. Rehemorrhage carries a mortality rate up to 50% (Patel & Samuels, 2012). Nearly 15% of patients rebleed in the first few hours after the initial hemorrhage; however, the risk of rebleeding once the IA is obliterated is about 1% (Washington et al., 2011). Blood pressure control is a major component of prevention of rebleeding and is one of the major categories of drug therapy for management of aSAH. The following section discussed drug therapy used for aSAH, including blood pressure control, vasospasm, and anticoagulants.

Drug Therapy

Historically, large hospitals and academic medical centers have had specialized neuroscience units and staff. In recent years, smaller community hospitals who previously cared for neuroscience patients in general medical or surgical ICUs are progressively becoming more specialized and the number of neuroscience/neurological ICUs and specialty medical-surgical units are increasing. ⊙ The role for neuroscience-specialized pharmacists is growing, providing an additional level of expertise to understand the effects of neurological illness or injury, drug interactions, and the effects on the patient (Rhoney, 2010). The pharmacist is vital in managing dosing of drugs such as antiepileptics, anticoagulants, antibiotics, pain control, and medications that require pharmacy-dosing services. Patients in the ICU often have multiple continuous intravenous infusions for blood pressure control and sedation and pain medication in addition to scheduled medications for the prevention of seizures, treatment of hyponatremia, or other complications of aSAH. Neuroscience ICUs have evidence-based, drug-specific protocols to reduce medication errors and decrease the variability between providers. Optimizing drug protocols has the potential to increase patient safety and improve outcomes, and collaboration with the pharmacy team is essential (Rhoney, 2010).

Blood Pressure Control

Blood pressure control is critical to reduce the risk of rebleeding until the IA is secured and during the first 24 to 48 hours postoperative period (Becske et al., 2013). The sudden surge in central sympathetic stimulation associated with aSAH results in hypertension, and the generally accepted goal is to maintain the systolic blood pressure less than 160 mm Hg. The risk of rebleeding is highest in the first 24 hours of the initial hemorrhage and carries a mortality rate up to 78%. Opioid pain medications may help to decrease the blood pressure and promote patient comfort; however, administering rapid-acting intravenous (IV) antihypertensive medications given as needed or via continuous infusion work to maintain the blood pressure within ordered parameters (Becske et al., 2013). Nitrates and nitroprusside have fallen out of favor as first-line agents for blood pressure control due to the potential for increased ICP and toxic side effects, particularly with prolonged nitroprusside infusions (Abate & Citerio, 2014).

Labetalol (Normodyne) and hydralazine (Apresoline) are often the favored intermittent dosing medications, whereas nicardipine (Cardene) and clevidipine (Cleviprex) are continuous infusions used for blood pressure control (Diringer, 2009). Labetalol is a beta-blocker that may be administered over 2 minutes in doses ranging from 5 to 20 mg IV every 15 minutes (Labetalol, 2014). Nursing considerations for this medication include a maximum dose of 300 mg in 24 hours and a contraindication for patients with bradycardia. Beta-blocker antihypertensives should be held for heart rate of less than 60 beats per minute. Labetalol is contraindicated in patients with a history of asthma, obstructive airway disease, or cardiac conditions that are associated with bradycardia or heart block (Physician's Desk Reference [PDR], 2014). Hydralazine may be given in incremental IV doses of 20 to 40 mg every 30 to 60 minutes. The mechanism of action of hydralazine is also vasodilation, but with a direct effect on arterioles to decrease systemic resistance and reduce blood pressure. The duration of action is longer than labetalol and lasts 1 to 4 hours with a half-life of 2 to 8 hours. Contraindications include patients with coronary artery disease (CAD); it should be used with caution in patients with severe kidney impairment, hypovolemia, or stroke. The precaution for stroke patients is to avoid a sudden drop in blood pressure related to antihypertensive medications, particularly in ischemic stroke that may result in a hypoperfusion injury to the brain (PDR, 2014).

Nicardipine (Cardene) is given via continuous IV infusion in titrated doses from 5 to 15 mg/hr to maintain systolic blood pressure of maximum 150 to 160 mm Hg to prevent rebleeding. Some clinicians prefer to maintain the blood pressure less than 140 mm Hg to prevent rehemorrhage (Green et al., 2013). Nicardipine is a calcium channel blocker that inhibits transmembrane influx of extracellular calcium ions across vascular smooth muscle and cardiac cells without effect on serum calcium levels. Side effects may include symptomatic hypotension or tachycardia and should be used with caution in patients with congestive heart failure (CHF) or left ventricular dysfunction. Nicardipine has a rapid-acting onset of action and has been shown to be effective to reduce blood pressure in a controlled manner. The half-life of this medication is about 2 to 4 hours. It is recommended to change the peripheral infusing sites every 12 hours (PDR, 2014).

Clevidipine (Cleviprex) is also a calcium channel blocker with a similar mechanism of action as nicardipine. The onset of action is about 2 to 4 minutes, with a half-life of about 15 minutes. Dosing and titration begin at 1 to 2 mg/hr and may be doubled every 90 seconds. When the blood pressure is near the targeted goal, dosing is less than doubled and titration times are increased from the rapid titration interval to every 5 to 10 minutes. Clevidipine is in a lipid base without preservatives. Patients should be screened for allergy or hypersensitivity to soy or egg products prior to administration. This medication is contraindicated in patients with CHF (PDR, 2014).

Vasospasm Prevention and Treatment

The drug categories associated with the prevention and treatment of vasospasm include calcium channel blockers, magnesium, endothelin antagonists, and statins. These categories are reviewed in the following sections to describe their current use, if any, in vasospasm management.

Calcium Channel Blockers

Calcium channel blockers (CCBs) have been used for their effect to reduce contraction of cardiac and smooth muscle without an effect on skeletal muscle. The effectiveness of this classification of drugs has been a source of many studies over the years, but it is theorized that the abnormal vasoconstriction of cerebral vascular smooth muscle is mitigated by CCBs (Greenburg, 2010). Nimodipine (Nimotop) is a cost-effective agent as well as the drug of choice for use in patients with aSAH. A side effect of nimodipine is hypotension, especially if the patient is not well hydrated. Titration of vasoactive infusions may be necessary to augment blood pressure post dosing. Patients may be sensitive to blood pressure fluctuations. As a result, focal deficits and a decrease in blood pressure can occur after CCBs are administered to patients with vasospasm. The neuroscience nurse must be aware of this side effect and closely monitor the patient's vital signs and neurological assessment when this medication is given. Nimodipine is generally administered orally (PO) and recently became available in IV form. However, oral administration is generally preferred. Nimodipine is given in doses of 60 mg every 4 hours or 30 mg every 2 hours for 21 days. If hypotension is a recurring problem after dose is given, the recommendation is to administer smaller, more frequent dosing (Diringer, 2009).

Clinical Pearl: Sudden and severe decreases in blood pressure with associated focal neurological deficits have been reported anecdotally by neuroscience nurses when nimodipine has been given via a duodenal feeding tube. Start nimodipine at the lowest ordered dose to assess the patient's response to the medication.

Magnesium

Magnesium has been studied and found to have mixed results on neuroprotective and vasodilatation properties. Vasodilation results from an inhibition of calcium channel–mediated smooth muscle contractions. Various spasmogenic agents such as endothelin-1, norepinephrine, angiotensin II, and serotonin are counteracted by magnesium. Magnesium is thought to have some degree of neuroprotective effects because hypomagnesemia is associated with a worse outcome (PDR, 2014). Reportedly, more than one third of patients admitted with aSAH have hypomagnesemia that is related to the size of the hemorrhage. Studies with magnesium administration protocols in SAH have not determined dosing or optimal magnesium levels (Patel & Samuels, 2012). One consideration when infusing magnesium is the effect on the heart and arrhythmias, specifically the risk for torsades de pointes. Protocols for magnesium infusions for SAH generally include cardiac considerations and parameters for QT and QTc. The QT interval is the time between the start of the Q wave and the end of the T wave in the cardiac electrical cycle. This measurement provides information on how quickly the ventricles are repolarized and ready for a new cardiac cycle. The QTc is the measurement of time between the onset of ventricular depolarization and the completion of ventricular repolarization. Magnesium infusion should be limited in patients with a QTc less than 440 or 445 to avoid prolongation of the QT interval and the potential for lethal dysrhythmia (Frangiskakis et al., 2009).

The Magnesium for Aneurysmal Subarachnoid Hemorrhage (MASH-2) trial was a phase 3, randomized, placebo-controlled trial conducted in eight centers in Europe and South America. A total of 1,204 patients were enrolled. An updated Cochrane meta-analysis of seven prior randomized trials from MASH-2 and those randomized trials that were eligible for inclusion since the MASH-2 trial involved 2,047 patients and demonstrated that magnesium was not superior to a placebo in reducing poor outcomes after aSAH. Therefore, magnesium could not be recommended for routine administration in aSAH (Dorhout et al., 2012). Another prospective, randomized, placebo-controlled study found that the incidence of delayed ischemic neurological deficit was significantly lower in patients treated with magnesium infusion. Transcranial Doppler (TCD) and angiographically identified vasospasm was significantly reduced in the group receiving magnesium. However, it is of note that the outcome scores were measured by *Glasgow Outcome Scale* (GOS), and patients considered a "good outcome" was scored as a 4 or 5 on a scale of 1 to 5 after 6 months (Westermaier et al., 2010).

Endothelin Antagonists

Endothelin antagonists (ET-A) are another potential treatment under investigation. ET-A receptors mediate vasoconstriction in arterial smooth muscle. Clazosentan is a selective ET-A receptor antagonist that demonstrated a decrease and a reversal in vasospasm after SAH. One study, CONSCIOUS-1 (Clazosentan to Overcome Neurological Ischemia and Infarct Occurring after Subarachnoid Hemorrhage), found a significant dose-dependent effect on vasospasm when evaluated with angiography. The 413 patients in this study were randomized and given placebo or clazosentan within 56 hours and continued on their assigned protocol for up to 14 days (Rhoney, McAllen, & Liu-DeRyke, 2010). Subsequent studies with clazosentan have reported no benefit with this drug.

Statins

Research with statin drugs have also demonstrated a lack of efficacy and have shown no benefit in the treatment of vasospasm; however, studies are ongoing. To date, the recommendations have been to continue the statin medication if the patient had been taking it prior to the onset of the SAH (Abate & Citerio, 2014).

Anticoagulants

Patients presenting with SAH and who were on anticoagulant therapy for cardiovascular conditions have a worse prognosis and outcomes. Anticoagulants tend to increase the amount of bleeding at the time of rupture, thereby increasing the overall amount of blood in the subarachnoid space, basal cisterns, and the parenchyma (Rinkel, Prins, & Algra, 1997). On the other hand, thrombotic complications related to venous thromboembolism (VTE) may be equally as lethal in patients with stroke. Most of the literature regarding stroke and VTE does not differentiate between hemorrhagic and ischemic strokes. Members of the interprofessional team are charged with implementing preventive strategies upon admission that include mechanical (i.e., sequential compression devices) and pharmacological interventions (Field & Hill, 2011).

aSAH induces a prothrombotic state, thereby increasing the risk of VTE, a medical condition that includes deep vein thrombosis (DVT) and pulmonary embolism (PE). Over the past 10 years, the CMS in collaboration with The Joint Commission have focused on hospital-acquired conditions (HACs). HACs have since been tied to hospital reimbursements whereby the hospital is responsible for the costs associated with the care and treatment of the patient who develops one or more of the nine designated HACs. HACs may have additional implications for health care organizations by way of legal action, that is, malpractice lawsuits, and results that are publicly reported on websites such as Medicare Hospital Compare Quality of Care (http://www.hospitalcompare.hhs.gov) (Hight, 2010). Prevention of VTE is one of several quality measures set forth by government agencies to improve care and prevent HAC.

Interprofessional team members must understand the risks of prescribing anticoagulants for patients with SAH whether the IA is secured or unsecured. Accepted clinical practice is to initiate *pharmacological prophylaxis* therapy 24 to 48 hours after surgery with unfractionated or a low-molecular-weight heparin (Bautista, 2012). However, nonpharmacological interventions are recommended and should be implemented upon admission. VTE prevention measures are often supported by nurse-driven protocols to apply intermittent pneumatic compression (IPC) devices upon admission to the nursing unit. VTE prophylaxis may also include graded elastic compression stockings known in the United States as "TED stockings" and antiplatelet therapy. Additional measures may include early mobilization and prevention of dehydration. Stroke units that promote early mobilization have demonstrated lower rates of DVT. Patients with stroke are at high risk for dehydration due to dysphagia and inadequate oral intake or decreased level of consciousness (Field & Hill, 2011).

Pain Control

Pain management is an important aspect of patient care. Given the "worst headache of my life" complaint, the interprofessional health care team needs to provide interventions to make the patient as comfortable as possible. Nonopioid medications such as acetaminophen (650 mg PO or 1,000 mg IV) can be administered every 4 to 6 hours; however, consideration must be given to contraindications, that is, liver disease. Accurate monitoring by the pharmacist and nurse to ensure that the patient does not receive more than the maximum allowable dose of 3 g in a 24-hour time period is essential. Opioid medications such as fentanyl (12.5 to 25 mg IV every hour as needed), Dilaudid (0.2 to 4 mg IV every 3 to 4 hours as needed), and morphine sulfate (2 to 4 mg IV every 1 to 2 hours as needed) may provide pain relief as well as a degree of sedation and serve to decrease anxiety. Patient effect must be monitored closely to avoid oversedation and an inability to accurately assess the patients' neurological status. Pain management is essential but with caution so that worsening in neurological status is not masked (Green et al., 2013).

HYDROCEPHALUS

Hydrocephalus is a concern with low-grade aSAH and may impact the ability to effectively control blood pressure. Hydrocephalus is the result of the influx of blood into the ventricles and ventricular system in the brain that disrupts the absorption of CSF by the arachnoid villi. Clipping or coiling the IA does not influence development of hydrocephalus. Approximately 30% of patients with SAH have impaired reabsorption of CSF that requires urgent placement of an external ventricular drain (EVD). An EVD provides a means to manage hydrocephalus and monitor ICP. The intraventricular catheter attached to the external drainage system is placed by a physician or, in some institutions, a specially trained advanced practice nurse. The majority of patients demonstrate clinical improvement after EVD (Diringer, 2009). Hydrocephalus may persist past the acute phase and require placement of a permanent shunt. Interventions with fibrinolytics such as intraventricular recombinant tissue plasminogen activator (rtPA) have been used to facilitate faster clearance of bloody CSF (Diringer, 2009).

The interprofessional team, and especially nursing, must keep in mind multiple considerations for patients with EVDs, including accurate monitoring of ICP and cerebral perfusion pressure (CPP), assessment of the ICP waveform, and correlating the neurological examination findings with ICP changes or changes in level of consciousness when the level of the EVD is raised or the drainage system is closed in the presence of hydrocephalus. Prompt notification to the physician by the nurse is critical to prevent further deterioration. The nurse may anticipate orders for a CT scan to assess ventricle size and the reopening or lowering of the level of the drainage system to assist in draining the CSF. Protocols for EVD site care vary widely across the United States; variations include sterile, occlusive dressings to an open-to-air insertion site, with site care at specified intervals. The nurse should follow the institutional protocols for monitoring parameters and care of the drainage system.

Case Study: Mr. W., a 68-year-old patient with a ruptured anterior communicating artery IA, is postbleed day 12 and postendovascular coiling of aneurysm day 11. He is able to follow simple commands with all extremities, but his legs are weaker than his arms. His EVD is open to drain at 10 cm H_2O and draining approximately 10 to 15 mL/hr. The CSF color remains bloody but has progressed to a light pink color. The neurosurgeon ordered the EVD level to be raised to 15 cm H_2O yesterday; today he orders the level increased to 20 cm H_2O. After about 6 hours, the nurse notes Mr. W. to be more lethargic, slower to follow commands, and requires frequent stimuli (verbal and tactile) during the assessment. His ICPs had increased from an average of 8 to 10 mm Hg to 15 to 18 mm Hg. The neurosurgeon was notified immediately of the decline in neurological status, and a CT scan was ordered and completed "STAT." The CT scan demonstrated enlarged ventricles when compared to the last CT scan done 3 days prior. The surgeon ordered the level of the EVD to be decreased back to 10 cm H_2O. Within another 6 hours, Mr. W. was becoming more responsive and less lethargic, and the ICPs have returned to baseline of 8 to 10 mm Hg. Mr. W. required placement of a ventriculoperitoneal shunt prior to his transfer from the ICU for a permanent, internal means to control hydrocephalus (**Fig. 8-3**). ■

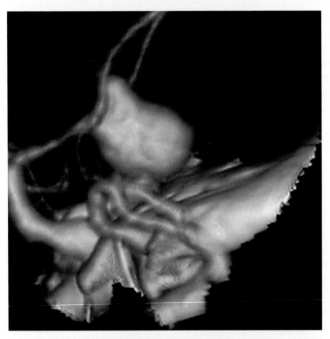

FIGURE 8-3 Computed tomography angiogram demonstrating 11-mm anterior communicating artery aneurysm. *(Courtesy: Christopher S. Ogilvy, MD, Massachusetts General Hospital, Boston, MA. From Hickey, J. V. [2014]. The clinical practice of neurological and neurosurgical nursing [7th ed.]. Philadelphia, PA: Lippincott Williams & Wilkins.)*

▊▊ VASOSPASM

As previously mentioned, approximately 60% of patients with aSAH will develop radiographic vasospasm defined as vasoconstriction and narrowing of the cerebral arteries evident with cerebral angiography with or without clinical signs or symptoms. About 30% of aSAH patients will have clinical vasospasm, which is also referred to as *delayed ischemic neurological deficit* (DIND). DIND or delayed cerebral ischemia (DCI) is gaining favor to describe the effects of vasospasm, which is described as worsening or new focal neurological deficits or obvious sites of ischemic damage on CT scan (Abate & Citerio, 2014). These patients will be symptomatic, with changes that are characterized by a decreased level of consciousness or confusion or focal neurological deficits (Greenburg, 2010). Patients with vasospasm and DCI have longer lengths of stay in the ICU and may have new onset of neurological deficits and an overall poorer prognosis and recovery. Vasospasm is the result of cerebral arterial narrowing that is thought to be triggered by the breakdown of hemoglobin in the subarachnoid space, which creates an inflammatory response, impairs autoregulation, and results in ischemia and infarction (Abate & Citerio, 2014; Bautista, 2012). The CT scan provides a means to measure the size of the subarachnoid blood and visualize blood in the cisterns or the ventricles. The *Fisher grading scale* and *modified Fisher grading scale* are helpful in predicting the risk of vasospasm (see Table 8-6).

Vasospasm begins at about postbleed day 3 and may last 21 days. The most severe vasospasm is seen between postbleed days 7 and 10. The neurological status of the patient may "wax and wane" throughout the period of vasospasm, testing the assessment skills of the neuroscience nurse and the expertise of the interdisciplinary team. Invasive monitoring devices to measure brain tissue oxygenation, cerebral microdialysis, thermal diffusion flow measurement, and near-infrared spectroscopy may be helpful in the management of patients with vasospasm but are not available in all neurological centers.

Noninvasive monitoring devices such as TCD measure blood flow velocities, thereby approximating the degree of narrowing in the anterior and posterior cerebral circulation. Determination of vasospasm via TCD relies on a ratio of flow velocities between the middle cerebral artery (MCA) and internal carotid artery (ICA). When the flow velocities are greater than 200 cm/sec and the MCA-to-ICA ratio is greater than 6, vasospasm is present. Vasospasm is a severe complication of aSAH that will result in death in about 25% of patients and leave another 50% with severe disabilities (Abate & Citerio, 2014).

In the past, the so-called triple H therapy was the mainstay of treatments for vasospasm. The use of triple H therapy employed a combination of hypertension, hypervolemia, and hemodilution aimed at "thinning" the blood (IV infusions of saline and/or albumin) with a goal of decreasing the hematocrit. The rationale for hemodilution is to decrease blood viscosity, thus increasing cerebral blood flow. However, multiple studies have demonstrated that hemodilution reduces the oxygen-carrying capacity of the red blood cells, resulting in a diminished cerebral oxygen delivery. Several adverse effects have been associated with hypervolemia; it has not shown efficacy over maintaining euvolemia (Abate & Citerio, 2014). As a result of the research, practitioners are changing the treatment to include hypertension but promote an overall state of euvolemia (Diringer, 2009).

As practitioners move to euvolemia, 24 to 48 hours after the aneurysm is secured, permissive hypertension is becoming part of the treatment; that is, the patient's blood pressure is naturally allowed to trend upward. When signs and symptoms of vasospasm occur, an IV infusion with vasoactive drugs can be initiated to further increase the blood pressure and, consequently, cerebral blood flow and perfusion. Hypertension is accomplished with IV fluids and the addition of vasoactive infusions such as phenylephrine (Neo-Synephrine) or norepinephrine (Levophed) to maintain the systolic blood pressure (SBP) to a level dependent on the patient's condition and provider practice preferences. Studies have shown that increasing the blood pressure to an individual goal or to a percent of the baseline blood pressure based on the presence or absence of the patient's clinical symptoms is the most effective means to manage the patient (Diringer, 2009). Additional vasoactive drugs may be needed to maintain SBP and cardiac output (e.g., dopamine, dobutamine, milrinone) depending on the patient's past medical history and the presence of preexisting or new-onset cardiac dysfunction.

Hypovolemia is a complication of the initial IA rupture. Management of fluids to avoid vasospasm is a balancing act to provide an adequate fluid volume status (i.e., at least maintaining a euvolemic state) and avoid hypervolemia that may induce cerebral edema, pulmonary edema, cardiac arrhythmias, CHF, or sepsis. Research has compared hypervolemia with euvolemia and found no significant differences in the clinical setting. Use of normal saline (0.9%) works well to maintain volume status; however, hypertonic saline (1.5%, 3%, or 7.5% concentrations) may be used for patients with hyponatremia (Green et al., 2013).

Recommendations for care of the patient with vasospasm include intravascular fluid monitoring with the use of invasive and/or noninvasive devices. Examples of invasive devices are central lines or pulmonary artery (PA) catheters. Central venous pressure can be measured with a central line or PA catheter, and caution should be used with central venous pressure values because use of these values has not been shown to be a reliable indicator of volume or of the cardiac response (Bautista, 2012). PA catheters are not recommended due to the high risk of complications with the catheter and the lack of evidence that its use have a positive impact on the patient's overall care. Noninvasive monitoring devices such as an arterial pressure–based monitor (Flo-Trac, Edwards Lifesciences, Irvine, CA) are available. It should be noted that the limitations with an arterial pressure–based monitoring device require a patient to be intubated and control-ventilated with an arterial line that has an accurate, consistent waveform.

Considerations for critical care nurses are blood pressure monitoring and maintaining blood pressure within the ordered parameters to optimize cerebral perfusion. Hypotension can be treated with bolus infusions of IV fluids and use of vasoactive infusions if hypotension persists. Obviously, hypertension should be avoided to prevent rebleeding if the IA has not been secured, and antihypertensive medications are indicated to maintain SBP less than 160 mm Hg.

Case Study: Mrs. T., a 56-year-old female with a left MCA stroke caused by aneurysmal SAH, is postbleed day 9. She was a Hunt and Hess grade III upon admission, with right-sided weakness, right upper extremity (UE) drift, and mild aphasia. Her SBP parameter has been increased and maintained above 160 mm Hg based on her TCD results that show mild to moderate vasospasm; she is on a low-dose phenylephrine. Since admission, her deficits had slowly resolved, but with onset of vasospasm and SBP less than 160 mm Hg, weakness is evident as is the UE drift. The ICU nurse administers the 10 a.m. dose of nimodipine 60 mg PO. The patient was educated about the name, purpose, and at least two side effects of the medication with the first dose; reinforcement of this education is provided again using "teach-back" techniques to ensure patient understanding. At 11:00 a.m., the nurse enters the room and Mrs. T. is unable to respond to the nurse's greeting despite attempts to speak; her SBP is 115 mm Hg. The nurse titrates the phenylephrine up according to the physician orders and remains with the patient to monitor the effect. The nurse explains that the lower blood pressure in vasospasm can result in lower blood flow to the affected area and weakness and speech difficulties reoccurred. By increasing the vasoactive infusion rate, the nurse anticipates the deficits will resolve as cerebral perfusion improves. As the SBP increases within minutes of the titration, the patient begins to regain strength, movement, and speech. The nurse notifies the physician of the side effect of the nimodipine 60 mg PO on the blood pressure and the neurological assessment. Orders are received for nimodipine 30 mg PO every 2 hours. The goal is to deliver the doses more frequently, in smaller doses, and reduce the risk of the significant SBP decrease. In addition to the dosage change, the nurse encourages the patient to move slowly, especially when getting out of bed to a chair or in working with the therapists. Moving and standing slowly will help to prevent orthostatic hypotension that can be caused by standing up too quickly and avoid a potential and significant drop in SBP and the risk for ischemia to the brain. ■

OTHER COMMON PROBLEMS

There are a number of other common problems encountered with aSAH that the interprofessional team must address. They include cardiac dysfunction, seizures, hyponatremia, fever, Terson syndrome, delirium, infections, and prevention of complications and patient safety. See also Chapter 9 for complications of stroke.

Cardiac Dysfunction

Cardiac abnormalities related to SAH have been well documented, but research continues on the frequency of different cardiac abnormalities and how these influence patient outcomes. Studies are underway to examine RNA molecular markers to determine if there is a genetic predisposition to cardiac side effects or vasospasm in patients with SAH. Cardiac changes may range from a mild alteration in the electrocardiogram (ECG) to a reversible left ventricular dysfunction (e.g., Takotsubo cardiomyopathy), non-ST-segment elevation myocardial infarction (NSTEMI), ST-segment elevation myocardial infarction (STEMI), or cardiac arrest. The severity of SAH is associated with the likelihood of cardiac changes and poor neurological outcomes. In 50% to 100% of patients with aSAH, T-wave inversion and QT interval prolongation is seen with elevation in troponin levels in 20% to 40% of cases. Further abnormalities of cardiac wall motion and decreased ejection fraction (EF) are noted in 10% of patients with aSAH. Cardiac dysfunction may lead to sudden death or require mechanical interventions to support heart function such as an intra-aortic balloon pump (IABP).

Neurogenic "stunned myocardium" or "neurogenic stress cardiomyopathy" or Takotsubo-like cardiomyopathy describes a reversible, acute cardiac condition that is found mainly in postmenopausal women with aSAH. *Takotsubo* or *Tako-tsubo* is a Japanese term that refers to a fishing pot used to catch octopus. *Tako* (octopus) *tsubo* (pot) is the shape of the fishing pot and the shape of the left ventricle during Takotsubo cardiomyopathy: The left ventricle resembles the neck of the pot (narrow), and the posterior or apical section of the ventricle dilates outward (like a balloon) to give the appearance of the base of the pot (Griffin & Logue, 2009).

Transient ST elevation or deep T-wave inversions are seen on the ECG, and echocardiography denotes an apical left ventricular ballooning that is difficult to distinguish from cardiac changes caused by myocardial ischemia in the absence of CAD. This phenomenon is thought to be caused by a catecholamine-mediated surge that accompanies SAH. The associated SAH-related damage to the cerebral cortex, hypothalamus, and brainstem stimulates disequilibrium within the neuroendocrine and autonomic nervous systems that results in dysfunction of the heart and other organs. The severity of the SAH is thought to be the main predictor of cardiac dysfunction in that the worse the hemorrhage, the higher the risk of cardiac dysfunction (Ando, Trio, & De Gregorio, 2010; Diringer, 2009). ECG changes do not correlate with a myocardial infarction (MI) or demonstrate a worse outcome; however, the presence of MI and elevated troponin level higher than 1.0 mcg/L is associated with poorer outcomes and increased mortality (Ahmadian et al., 2013).

⊙ Patients with neurogenic cardiac dysfunction present a unique challenge to the neuroscience nurse. Blood pressure is generally elevated with an SAH event, but with cardiac dysfunction, the management of the patient is comparable to that for pump failure, and the patient may be hypotensive and require the use of inotropic agents, fluid management, diuretics, and higher oxygen concentrations. The nurse should anticipate a cardiac consultation and possible cardiac catheterization for differential diagnosis to determine the presence or absence of coronary artery stenosis or obstructions.

⊙ An IABP may be used as an adjunctive therapy to support the patient's heart in light of wall motion abnormalities and low EF. Because these patients generally have suffered a more severe or higher grade SAH, the incidence of vasospasm is high. The challenges faced by the interprofessional team with the onset of vasospasm become more critical as the need to balance cardiac function while protecting the brain from DCI increases. Nurses who are specially trained in the care of the patient with IABP are used in some ICUs in collaboration with the neuroscience nurse to manage the IABP.

Clinical Pearl: In some cases, registered nurses (RNs) who are specially trained in the care of cardiac patients and IABPs help in caring for a patient with SAH and an IABP. The neuroscience nurse should be the lead in how vasoactive or inotropic medications are administered and titrated to prevent DCI. The purpose of vasoactive infusions is aimed at support of CPP and preservation of brain function through maximal blood pressure support as able with the infusions and IABP assist.

Seizures

Seizures may occur when an IA ruptures or after the bleeding occurs. Several factors increase the risk of seizure including older age (>65 years), the presence of a thick clot (with or without hematoma), rupture of an MCA, intraparenchymal hemorrhage, postoperative DCI due to vasospasm, and surgical clipping. The incidence of seizures with ruptured IA is estimated to be between 8% and 30%. In patients with high-grade SAH, nonconvulsive seizures are more prevalent (estimated at 10% to 20%) when continuous electroencephalographic (EEG) monitoring was used (Patel & Samuels, 2012).

In years past, prophylactic treatment of seizures was common, and phenytoin was the drug of choice. More recent studies have examined the risks and benefits of antiepileptic drugs (AEDs). Investigations of phenytoin have shown worse outcomes, and AEDs do not seem to prevent seizures after SAH. Seizures can cause increases in blood pressure, cerebral blood flow, and ICP which can increase the risk of rebleeding and further patient deterioration. Status epilepticus related to nonconvulsive seizures increases morbidity and mortality if not quickly identified and treated (Raper, Starke, Komotar, Allen, & Connolly, 2012).

The role and responsibilities of the neuroscience nurse is critical in conducting diligent assessments and recognizing subtle changes in the patient's condition. Patients with SAH may wax and wane in their day-to-day or even hour-to-hour neurological assessments. The nurse should be aware that a subtle change in level of consciousness, new-onset or increased confusion, or a focal deficit may herald the presence of subclinical or nonconvulsive seizure activity. Prompt notification of findings to the physician or other appropriate health care provider can result in initiation of prompt treatment or consultations, (i.e., neurology/epileptologist), EEG trend monitoring, and administration of AEDs and benzodiazepines such as lorazepam to assist in seizure identification and treatments. Some AEDs such as phenytoin require regular monitoring of blood levels for therapeutic effect.

Hyponatremia

Abnormalities in serum sodium levels are a common complication in SAH. Cerebral salt wasting (CSW) and syndrome of inappropriate secretion of antidiuretic hormone (SIADH) may occur in patients with SAH. Many studies have attributed hyponatremia to elevated levels of brain natriuretic peptides (BNPs) during the acute phase, specifically when ICP is elevated and vasospasm is present, but without an increase in antidiuretic hormone (ADH) secretion. The patient experiences a high urine output with high levels of sodium in the urine; therefore, close monitoring of serum sodium levels is critical in patients with SAH and vasospasm. If sodium is not corrected, the degree of hyponatremia worsens, and cerebral edema and the risk of seizures increase (Abate & Citerio, 2014). Euvolemia is the goal of therapy. Fluid restriction is not recommended to treat hyponatremia; however, mild hypertonic saline solutions can be used to correct sodium levels.

Determining the cause of hyponatremia is essential because the management of CSW and SIADH differs. CSW occurs with natriuresis, a loss of sodium that results in a loss of free water that leads to hyponatremia and is considered a hypovolemic hyponatremia state. Conversely, SIADH results when ADH is inappropriately secreted, resulting in a euvolemic hyponatremia and a decreased urinary output. Urine osmolality is usually normal to low in CSW but high in SIADH. Urine sodium levels are elevated in both syndromes. Overall fluid volume status is the best indicator for diagnosing CSW versus SIADH (Patel & Samuels, 2012) (**Table 8-7**).

TABLE 8-7   Cerebral Salt Wasting versus Syndrome of Inappropriate Secretion of Antidiuretic Hormone

	Cerebral Salt Wasting	Syndrome of Inappropriate Secretion of Antidiuretic Hormone
Urine osmolality	↑	↑
Urine sodium concentration	↑	↑
Extracellular fluid volume	↓	↑
Fluid balance	Negative	Neutral to slightly +
Sodium balance	Negative	Neutral to slightly +

From Yee, A. H., Burns, J. D., & Wijdicks, E. F. (2010). Cerebral salt wasting: Pathophysiology, diagnosis, and treatment. *Neurosurgical Clinics of North America, 21,* 339–352.

All interprofessional team members must understand the cause and treatments for hyponatremia. Close monitoring of serum sodium levels is an essential component of care for patients with SAH and vasospasm. The nurse should anticipate orders for sodium supplementation with mildly hypertonic saline solutions (i.e., 3% sodium chloride) and/or with oral salt tablets in addition to IV fluids to restore euvolemia. Additional supplementation with mineralocorticoids such as fludrocortisone may be used to increase volume levels and maintain serum sodium levels higher than 135 mEq/L (Patel & Samuels, 2012).

Patients with hyponatremia can suffer permanent neurological injury or death if this condition is missed or incorrectly diagnosed. Recognition of sodium dysfunction and the ability to distinguish between various treatments in the neuroscience patient population is crucial. Pharmacists are essential in the interprofessional approach to managing hyponatremia and ensuring safe and appropriate patient care (Murphy-Human & Diringer, 2010).

Fever

Fever is defined as a body temperature higher than 38.3°C or 100.9°F. Nearly 75% of patients with SAH will have a fever at some point following SAH. Fever occurs more frequently in patients with high-grade, poor prognosis SAH and nearly half have a fever unrelated to any type of infection. The risks of fever are related to the effects on cerebral metabolism from the increased temperature, which results in increased metabolic needs of the brain and exacerbation of cerebral ischemia. Fever control with medications (i.e., acetaminophen or low-dose nonsteroidal anti-inflammatory drugs [NSAIDS]), cooling blankets, or other types of noninvasive cooling devices are employed to bring the patient's temperature into a normothermic range. Intravascular cooling devices require special equipment to circulate cool/cold saline via the catheter, and the catheter itself is different from the commonly used central venous catheter. The equipment is expensive, and not all hospitals may have access to these devices.

Invasive cooling devices such as the intravascular catheter may be used; however, cooling interventions should not be delayed while waiting for the equipment or for the provider to insert the catheter. Several surface cooling machines are available such as cooling blankets or cooling wraps that adhere to the skin with a nonadhesive material or with hook-and-loop fasteners that hold the wrap device around the arms, legs, or torso. These devices are easy to use and generally readily available as a nursing intervention for fever control. Use of ice bags, cool baths, and fans in the room is another nursing intervention that generally can be implemented without a specific provider order. The nurse should follow organizational policies and procedures for fever management and device usage. Consideration must be given to patient shivering during any type of fever control interventions and may be mitigated by the use of neuromuscular blocking medications (intubated/mechanically ventilated patients only!), placement of warm blankets on arms and legs, and administration of meperidine in low doses.

Terson Syndrome

Terson syndrome is a complication of aSAH that causes vision loss that is potentially reversible. The incidence of Terson syndrome in patients with SAH is estimated to be 8% to 15%. After aSAH, there is a vitreous hemorrhage caused by a disruption in the retinal capillaries. The exact mechanisms are unknown but thought to be related to the rapid increase in ICP often associated with aSAH that may force CSF or blood to effuse through the optic nerve sheath. The result may be a dilation of the retrobulbar portion of the eye with compression and obstruction of the central retinal vein. The result is venous congestion, hypertension, and the rupture of the retinal vein and capillaries. Patients with more severe aSAH (GCS <8, Fisher grade >3, and Hunt and Hess grade >III) are most frequently associated with Terson syndrome. SAH in the anterior circulation is also a common cause of Terson syndrome and affects both eyes in up to 60% of patients.

Diagnosis can be made as soon as an hour after the initial SAH by funduscopic examination; these findings may be evident for months after the SAH. Orbital CT findings (e.g., retinal nodularity and crescentic hyperdensities) illustrate Terson syndrome; however, these findings may be subtle and overlooked. Visual evoked potential (VEP) may not be helpful for diagnosis (Middleton, Esselman, & Lim, 2012).

As the patient recovers from the SAH, gradual resolution of the hemorrhage and improvement in visual acuity occurs over months to years. One study noted improvement in 86% of the patients in 6 months; after a year, 45% had hemorrhage resolution, and by 2 years, the remaining patients had full visual acuity and resolution of the hemorrhage. Complications associated with conservative management may include retinal detachment, cataracts, and retinopathy. Surgical intervention with pars plana vitrectomy (PPV) may help to speed visual recovery and the overall rehabilitative course.

◉ Members of the interprofessional team should be aware of this condition in order to coordinate the care and rehabilitation of patients who develop vision loss and initiate a consult with an ophthalmologist for operative or nonoperative interventions. Physiatrists or occupational therapists may be the first to identify the visual loss and have the expertise to manage the deficit and assist the patient with compensatory strategies. Rehabilitation strategies for visual therapy focus mainly on treatments of central vision loss (e.g., visual field deficits or oculomotor impairment). Compensation strategies (e.g., learned techniques that use spared functions) and substitutive strategies (e.g., magnification, adaptive devices) are methods used to assist the patient in recovery. A systematic review of the rehabilitative methods found the most effective, cost-effective, and user-friendly therapy to be compensatory scanning therapy (Middleton et al., 2012).

Delirium

Delirium is defined as an acute confusional state characterized by fluctuating symptoms such as inattention, disturbances of consciousness, or disorganized thinking (Oh, Kim, Chun, & Yi, 2008, p. 143). Delirium is an acute change in one's mentation and is considered a problem of inattention and confusion that prevents the person from thinking clearly and making sense of what is going on around him or her. Other key features of delirium may include hallucinations, altered psychomotor activities, disorientation, memory impairment, and disturbances in the sleep–wake cycle. Delirium increases the costs of care by increased lengths of stay and increases the risk of falls.

Postoperative delirium (POD) is associated with longer lengths of stay and increased costs and is an unexpected and confounding complication, especially in the elderly. POD contributes to more frequent discharges to long-term care facilities. The interprofessional team should have an understanding of the differences between delirium and dementia for early recognition and intervention. Delirium has an acute onset, and symptoms fluctuate over the course of hours or days. Dementia has a slow, insidious onset and the patient progressively declines. The presence of delirium or dementia preoperatively predisposes the patient to POD, and the patient's ability to recover from POD is unlikely regardless of treatments provided (Oh et al., 2008).

The pathophysiology of POD is thought to be due to reversible neuronal dysfunction after metabolic or toxic alterations, activation and degranulation of vasoactive substances, and the development of perivascular edema resulting from an interaction between leukocytes and endothelial cells. Acetylcholine is a critical piece in the development of POD because of the role in the regulation of cerebral functions, that is, motor activity, rapid eye movement (REM) sleep, mood, attention, and memory. The decline in acetylcholine transmission is a physiological process that is age-dependent. In addition, any depletion in "cholinergic reserve" may play a role in the significantly higher incidence of delirium in the elderly (Oh et al., 2008).

In the neuroscience patient, delirium may be difficult to distinguish from a neurological change. In a patient with aSAH with vasospasm, it is not uncommon to have acute changes in neurological assessments or a pattern of wax and wane over the course of hours or days. The use of tools such as the *Confusion Assessment Method for the ICU* (CAM-ICU) may be used to identify delirium. The challenge with delirium assessment tools in neurological patients is the ability of the patient to communicate either verbally, by hand squeeze to prompts, or nodding/shaking the head to indicate "yes"/"no." Of note, patients who are aphasic due to stroke or suffering from confusion/disorientation related to traumatic brain injury may not be appropriate candidates for the delirium assessment tools based on their underlying disease process or injury. ⊙ The interprofessional team should consider the neurological disease process along with other factors that can contribute to delirium such as sleep deprivation, loss of day/night orientation, sedation, opioids, noise, and unfamiliar surroundings.

Approximately 80% of ICU patients will suffer delirium at some point in their stay. *ICU psychosis* is a term that has been used in reference to patients who have acute mentation changes due to medications, sleep deprivation, and noise levels generated by an ICU stay. Proactive interventions to prevent delirium are being incorporated into ICU routines as the education and research is more widely known. Among the research findings on delirium and the after-effects of critical illness and an ICU stay, it is known that:

- About 80% of survivors of critical illness will have residual effects on memory and judgment months or years later.
- Up to 50% of patients suffer from depression after an ICU stay.
- Critical illness polyneuropathy/muscle weakness occurs in about one third of patients who are mechanically ventilated, in about half of all patients with sepsis, and about half of the patients who have an ICU stay of 1 week.

Patients suffering from aSAH generally have lengthy ICU stays related to complications such as hydrocephalus and the need for an EVD, mechanical ventilation and ongoing sedation, or vasospasm. These patients are high risk for developing delirium, and prevention strategies are critical for the neuroscience nurse. Delirium is often misunderstood and thought to be interchangeable or the same as dementia. The differences are significant and key to understanding this potentially devastating side effect (ICU Delirium and Cognitive Impairment Study Group, 2014). Continued cognitive impairment may persist up to 1 year posthospitalization.

The Modifying the Impact of ICU-Associated Neurological Dysfunction-USA (MIND-USA) Study investigated the role of antipsychotics in critically ill patients with the hypothesis that the administration of medications such as haloperidol or ziprasidone to critically ill patients with delirium will improve their short- and long-term clinical outcomes, including days alive without brain dysfunction (Balas et al., 2014). Psychotropic drugs, neuroleptic medications (e.g., haloperidol, droperidol), may be administered when nonpharmacological interventions are not successful. Physostigmine and metrifonate are more recent medication interventions that are thought to decrease behavioral problems by improving cholinesterase activity (Oh et al., 2008).

Infections

Patients with aSAH must be monitored for infections related to indwelling medical devices. The most common forms of associated infections are central line–associated blood stream infections (CLABSIs) and catheter-associated urinary tract infections (CAUTIs).

CLABSI is a complication related to the presence of a centrally inserted, large-bore IV catheter and carries a mortality rate of 12% to 25%. Hospitals have adopted standards set forth by the Centers for Disease Control and Prevention (CDC) and The Joint Commission that focus not only on ICU concerns and insertion techniques but also on the maintenance of the lines and the care of the catheter. CLABSI is one of several never events identified by CMS that affects hospital reimbursements. As a result, the costs of the care of the patient with a central line infection (e.g., antibiotics, increased length of stay) are borne by the health care organization. These costs are estimated to be about $26,000. Between 2001 and 2009, the incidence of CLABSI was reduced by approximately 58%, a number that continues to decline. CLABSI incidence is publicly reported on the CMS Hospital Compare website.

Emphasis is now on the use of evidence-based bundles to ensure adherence of all components involved in line care (O'Grady et al., 2011). The components of the CLABSI bundle include (1) hand hygiene, (2) use of maximal sterile barriers during insertion, (3) chlorhexidine gluconate (CHG) site preparation, (4) daily documentation of line necessity, and (5) avoidance of femoral insertion site. Maximal sterile barriers include gowns, gloves, masks, and cap for the provider inserting the line as well as any other staff assisting (Dumont & Nesselrodt, 2012). Additional devices available to prevent infection are impregnated discs that are placed over the line insertion site and alcohol-saturated caps to cover IV access ports (used instead of "scrubbing the hub" for 15 seconds prior to each access). Central line kits contain all of the sterile items needed for site care and dressing changes accompanied by standardized organizational protocols. All interprofessional team members are educated about the CLABSI bundle, and often, central line dressing changes are included in annual skills or simulation labs to ensure that consistent and safe practices are maintained.

CAUTI is defined as a symptomatic urinary tract infection (UTI) or an asymptomatic bacteriuria and considered a never event by CMS. CAUTI may be underestimated by the interprofessional team because a UTI may be thought to be a "minor" in the scheme of possible problems as well as a minor compared to CLABSI, which carries a higher morbidity and mortality rate. The significance of a UTI is evident when the UTI or CAUTI converts to sepsis. Each year in the United States, there are over 1.7 million hospital-associated infections (HAIs), and of this number, over 99,000 resulted in death. Until recently, urinary catheters were not monitored. The majority of hospitals did not track the use or duration of urinary catheters. That has changed especially with the consequence of not being reimbursed for CLABSIs.

The CDC/Healthcare Infection Control Practices Advisory Committee (HICPAC) developed a *Guideline for Prevention of Catheter-associated Urinary Tract Infections* that has provided explanations on surveillance requirements and definitions of CAUTI. The National Healthcare Safety Network (NHSN) is the agency to which the UTI rates are reported. Specific indications are required as part of the provider order to account for the necessity of the indwelling catheter (**Table 8-8**). The expectation is that when the patient

TABLE 8-8 Indications for an Indwelling Urinary Catheter

Acute urinary retention: due to medication (anesthesia, opioids, paralytics) or nerve injury

Acute bladder outlet obstruction: due to severe prostate enlargement, blood clots, or urethral compression

Need for accurate measurements of urinary output in the critically ill

Assist healing of an open sacral or perineal wound in incontinent patients

End-of-life/comfort care

Strict, prolonged immobilization: potentially unstable thoracic or lumbar spine, multiple traumatic injuries (pelvic fracture)

Select perioperative conditions: urological surgery or other surgery near/adjacent to the genitourinary (GU) tract; prolonged duration of surgery (remove catheter at end of surgery or in PACU); large volumes of fluids or diuretics to be given during surgery; need for intraoperative urinary output monitoring

Stage III or IV pressure ulcer in the perianal area and the catheter is required for healing

PACU, postanesthesia care unit.
Adapted from the Centers for Disease Control and Prevention. (2009). *Guideline for prevention of catheter-associated urinary tract infections, 2009.* Retrieved from http://www.cdc.gov/hicpac/cauti/02_cauti2009_abbrev.html

no longer meets an indication for a urinary catheter, the catheter will be discontinued. ⊙ Nurse-driven protocols to remove urinary catheters are effective in reducing the number of CAUTIs and the amount of time catheters remain in place. Catheter monitoring is becoming standard practice, with many units initiating catheter rounds to assist nursing staff and providers in daily assessment of need. Many resources exist online for the interprofessional health care team and the public to learn about best practices for preventing CAUTI. Similar to central line infections, annual competencies for staff via simulation and educational programs to ensure up-to-date education are becoming a standard component of new hire programs and ongoing education.

Prevention of Complications and Patient Safety

A standard bundle of care for prevention of complications and patient safety has been developed for ICU care. Known as the *ABCDEs of Prevention and Safety*, the bundle includes awakening and breathing coordination, choice of sedation, delirium monitoring, and early mobility and exercise (Balas et al., 2014). The awakening and breathing trials are part of the sedation vacation, or stopping the sedation and restarting the sedation infusion at half of the previous dose. Daily awakenings in conjunction with daily breathing trials for vented patients has demonstrated effectiveness in shorter lengths of stay related to decreased time on the ventilator. ⊙ The nurse is the leader in implementing and coordinating this bundle to ensure interventions are initiated at the appropriate time during the recovery period and is the key in communicating between the members of the interdisciplinary team (Balas et al., 2014).

▇▇ ENDOVASCULAR AND SURGICAL CLIPPING TREATMENT OPTIONS

There are both endovascular options and surgical options available to treat patients with IAs. Selection of the best approach and timing of the intervention depend on a number of factors, including location of the IA, size of the IA, comorbidities, and severity of the SAH. Many studies have been conducted on the location of the IA and clipping or coiling. Evidence has shown that MCA IAs are easily accessed and respond well to treatment by surgical clipping. Giant IAs (>25 mm) are treated by clipping because the large number of coils needed may result in undue weight on the IA and cause the coils to dislodge. Long-term results of clipping versus coiling also have some influence over which treatment should be used. Studies have found clipping to be the most effective method for permanent treatment of an IA because most evidence indicates that regrowth of the IA seldom occurs (Fox & Choi, 2009). The International Subarachnoid Aneurysm Trial (ISAT) found that endovascular-coiled patients had a mortality or dependency rate of 23.7% as compared to 30.6% for a group that had undergone surgical clipping. There was significant evidence during this study to indicate that coiling was superior to clipping, and the study because of strong evidence supporting coiling of the aneurysm (Fox & Choi, 2009).

Regardless if an endovascular or a surgical approach is chosen, the priority treatment of a ruptured IA is focused on securing the vessel and obliteration of the IA either by direct means (surgical clipping) or indirect methods (endovascular embolization/coiling). Preprocedure workup of the patient may include laboratory testing, chest radiograph, and an ECG. ⊙ Nursing interventions may vary somewhat depending on organizational policy and procedures but generally include preoperative bathing with cloths impregnated with 2% CHG, oral care, and ongoing monitoring of the patients' vital signs and neurological assessments.

Endovascular Coiling

Endovascular treatment for IAs has been in existence for about 20 years. Advances in technology and materials have provided endovascular neurosurgeons several options for securing an IA. The decision whether to clip or coil generally depends on the location, the neck of the IA, and the availability of resources (i.e., experienced staff and equipment). Patients with higher grade SAH and with significant or multiple medical comorbidities tend to be treated with interventional coiling instead of intraoperative clipping. Posterior circulation IAs are more amenable to coiling based on location and the high risks associated with surgical clipping (Green et al., 2013).

Endovascular access to the IA is obtained via the same procedure as for cerebral angiogram. The patient is prepared as for a surgical procedure and undergoes general anesthesia. Microcatheters (<3 Fr) specifically designed for intracranial use are threaded from the groin insertion site upward to the cerebral vasculature and to the IA to be treated. Fluoroscopy is used during placement of the microcatheter and deployment of the coils into the IA (Fox & Choi, 2009).

Coils are usually made of very thin, tightly wound platinum wires. A wide variety of coil options are available, and the main criterion for choosing one type over another depends on the coil diameter, length, and its three-dimensional (3D) shape. The 3D shape of the coil should mirror the IA shape as much as possible (Boulos & Dalfino, 2012). Coils are packed into the IA until the neck is occluded and the full IA causes the blood inside the IA to clot, thereby decreasing the risk of hemorrhage or rebleeding. References to "packing" the IA with coils suggest that the IA is completely filled with coils. However, most IAs are embolized at a coil volume of 25% to 30% of the fundus, and the remaining volume is filled with a thrombus (Dalfino, Gandhi, & Boulos, 2012; **Fig. 8-4**).

Additional Endovascular Options

Other options and techniques for endovascular treatment of an IA include balloon-assisted embolization, liquid embolic agents, stent-assisted coil embolization, and

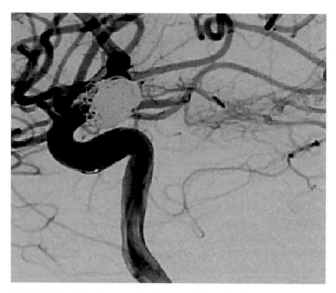

FIGURE 8-4 Angiogram showing completion of coil embolization with coils tightly packed within 1.1 cm left ophthalmic ICA aneurysm. *(Courtesy: Christopher S. Ogilvy, MD, Massachusetts General Hospital, Boston, MA. From Hickey, J. V. [2014]. The clinical practice of neurological and neurosurgical nursing [7th ed.]. Philadelphia, PA: Lippincott Williams & Wilkins.)*

employing a staged approach. Balloon-assisted IA embolization is a technique employed whereby a balloon is positioned and inflated in the parent vessel as the coils are deployed into the IA. Once the coils are in place, the balloon is deflated and the patency of the parent vessel is examined via angiography. This approach is useful for treating ruptured wide-necked IAs because no antiplatelet agents are needed, but there is a risk of ischemic complications related to balloon inflation and occlusion of normal blood flow to the brain through the parent vessel (Dalfino et al., 2012).

Liquid embolic agents (i.e., Onyx HD 500) are used with the balloon-assisted method. The Onyx is administered through the microcatheter after balloon inflation. Liquid embolic agents have not been routinely used as a first-line intervention for IAs; it is more commonly used for AVMs. However, Onyx has been effective as an adjunct therapy for IAs. Saccular aneurysms with broad-based necks are difficult to obliterate with clips or coils; however, they have been successfully treated with the liquid embolic agents (Vesek, Laughlin, Pazuchanics, Horton, & Cockroft, 2011). Stent-assisted embolization is beneficial as the stent helps to prevent coils from protruding into the parent vessel. In addition, the stent may serve as a scaffold and promote endothelialization over the IA neck and divert blood flow away from the IA. The staged approach may use a combination of stents, coils, and/or a liquid agent over a period of several days to months to obliterate the IA. When a stent is used in the staged procedure, the time between stent placement and coiling may be as long as 3 to 4 months while endothelialization takes place. The disadvantages to this approach are the IA remains unsecured for that duration and it may be difficult to impossible to reaccess the IA through the stent (Dalfino et al., 2012).

The risks associated with coiling may include an allergic reaction or renal failure related to contrast dye, bleeding at the puncture site, or infection. An uncommon occurrence is the perforation of the IA during embolization; consequently, bleeding may be difficult to control because there is no option for external pressure (Fox & Choi, 2009). Thrombo-embolism may occur due to the manipulation of the catheter or coil placement into the IA (Fox & Choi, 2009). Patients with *unruptured* IAs are given aspirin and clopidogrel in addition to IV heparin to reduce the risk of thromboembolism. Patients with a *ruptured* IA are also given anticoagulant therapy with a heparin infusion, but the timing and dose varies from one endovascular neurosurgeon to another (Boulos & Dalfino, 2012).

It should be noted that the overall risks associated with endovascular coiling and surgical clipping are comparable (Fox & Choi, 2009). Coiling is less invasive with a lower risk of infection. Patients often have shorter lengths of stay when compared to clipping, but it is important to note that the care of the patient postendovascular coiling for a ruptured IA is essentially the same as patients having open craniotomy and IA clipping. Immediate postprocedure care includes careful neurological assessments as well as close monitoring of the groin insertion site and lower extremity pulses. Patients with unrup-tured IAs treated with endovascular techniques often require only an overnight hospital stay (Fox & Choi, 2009).

Surgical Clipping

One of the first documented surgeries from 1885 reported that Sir Victor Horsley ligated an ICA of a patient with a giant aneurysm. In 1931, Dr. Norman Dott of Edinburgh performed the first surgery specifically for treating an IA by using a wrapping technique. In 1937, Dr. Walter Dandy first reported the use of an "aneurysm clip." The advances in IA clipping continued throughout the years, and over the last 20 years, clipping has been considered the standard of care (Washington et al., 2011).

The risk of rupture in an unsecured IA reportedly ranges from 0% to 2.3% per year. A recent meta-analysis found an overall risk of rupture to be about 0.9% per year; however, the risk of rupture can vary with the patient's age, gender, aneurysm characteristics such as size, location, and a previous history of IA. Studies have been conducted on the feasibility and cost-effectiveness of preventive treatment of IAs. Consideration must be given to the possibility of neurological injury and disability or death related to the preventive interven-tions. In 2003, the International Study of Unruptured Intracranial Aneurysms (ISUIA) re-ported prospective data on the management of unruptured IAs, but no conclusions could be drawn from the results (Greving, Rinkel, Buskins, & Algra, 2009). Research continues given the advancements in technology, treatment modalities, and genetic markers.

Randomized trials such as the Barrow Ruptured Aneurysm Trial (BRAT) screened 725 patients with SAH and enrolled 500 eligible patients over 3 years. Patients were assigned to either surgical intervention, (i.e., IA clipping) or to endovascular therapy (i.e., coiling). Overall, 238 patients were assigned to IA clipping and 233 patients to coil-ing. After a year, 403 of the patients were available for evaluation, and of this group, 358 patients had actually undergone treatment. The remainder of the patients either had no identifiable source of the SAH or they had died prior to treatment. The study found that a year after treatment, a policy of intent to treat favoring coil embolization resulted in fewer poor outcomes than clip occlusion (McDougall et al., 2012, p. 143). A large number of patients assigned to the coil embolization group crossed over to surgical clip-ping even though they were treated with coil embolization. The findings demonstrated fewer poor outcomes at 1 year with coil embolization; however, the study illustrated the importance and need for high-quality surgical clipping as an alternative treatment mo-dality (McDougall et al., 2012).

▌▙ THE CONTINUUM OF STROKE CARE

Stroke Prevention—The Beginning of the Continuum

Strategies to mitigate or prevent SAH-related complications are continually being evaluated, reevaluated, or undergoing revisions based on technological advances and evidence-based research. Primary prevention of stroke including stroke caused by aSAH has been discussed in Chapter 1. Secondary prevention and treatment have been discussed in this chapter. ⊙ All interprofessional team members have a major role to play in both primary and secondary prevention of stroke including aSAH.

The Stroke Care Continuum—Emergency Department

⊙ Standards for emergency medical services (EMS) have been established to include training of personnel to perform the prehospital stroke assessment. Data have shown that EMS personnel had an 86% to 97% stroke identification sensitivity with stroke assessment training compared to 61% to 66% without stroke training. Part of the EMS assessment is to determine the time when the patient was "last known well," check blood glucose levels, and transport the patient to the nearest stroke-certified facility, which may be a primary stroke center (PSC), comprehensive stroke center (CSC), or a Get With The Guidelines (GWTG)-Stroke hospital (American Heart Association/American Stroke Association [AHA/ASA], 2013). If a designated stroke center is within a reasonable range, the EMS personnel may bypass a hospital that does not have stroke resources and transport to the stroke center. EMS staff alert the receiving hospital of a "code stroke" that is comparable to the well-known "code blue" for cardiac events. The code stroke is part of the "Stroke Chain of Survival" composed of the "seven D's"—detection, dispatch, delivery, door, data, decision, and drug—and includes the patient, family members, and members of the interprofessional healthcare team (AHA/ASA, 2013).

Studies have shown that patients older than 80 years of age are more likely to have a delayed presentation to the ED. This elderly age group is at risk for strokes and is more likely to be living alone. Preexisting conditions may also prohibit the elderly patient from activating EMS. Cautious use of sedating medications in patients with aSAH is recommended to prevent masking subtle neurological changes (Ryan & Harbison, 2011). See Chapter 4 for more information on prehospital stroke care.

The Stroke Continuum of Care—Intensive Care Unit

⊙ Patients with aSAH are admitted to an ICU for close monitoring and ongoing assessments. A common thread among aSAH patients upon admission is a complaint of the "worst headache of my life." Minimizing stimulation for the patient (e.g., low light, quiet environment, sedation) and elevating the head of bed to 30 degrees to promote venous drainage are among the standard protocols of care. Physicians specially trained in critical care with additional specialization in the care of patients with neurological disorders are a growing trend in the interprofessional team caring for patients with SAH. The use of critical care physicians, also known as *neurointensivists*, has demonstrated improved outcomes and decreased lengths of stay for patients. RNs and advanced practice nurses with specialized knowledge and training in the care of neuroscience patients are also critical to the achievement of optimal patient outcomes.

Clinical Pearl: Nurses who specialize in caring for neurological/neurosurgical patients can demonstrate their expertise by becoming a certified neuroscience or stroke-certified nurse. The Certified Neuroscience Registered Nurse (CNRN) and Stroke Certified Registered Nurse (SCRN) are national board examinations offered by the American Board of Neuroscience Nursing (ABNN) for RNs with a minimum of 2 years' experience caring for neuroscience patients.

Upon arrival to the ICU, cardiac and continuous blood pressure monitoring is initiated. Accurate and hourly neurological assessments are vital and should include the National Institutes of Health Stroke Scale (NIHSS) and GCS. Patients with aSAH and evidence of hydrocephalus or a deteriorating condition may have an EVD device implanted. Standards vary per institution whether an EVD is placed in the patients' ICU room or in the operating room (OR).

Interventions to reduce the risk of rebleeding are implemented and maintained until the patient is taken to the OR or endovascular suites to secure the IA. Blood pressure management, as previously described, is essential in the care of the aSAH patient. Pain medication, anxiolytic agents, and sedation may be used as needed for patient comfort and assist with blood pressure control (Abate & Citerio, 2014). Nursing interventions to maintain a quiet environment are part of the preoperative care as well: keeping lights low, closing drapes or blinds, and maintaining strict bedrest. Although the current trend is to limit use of indwelling urinary catheters to avoid the risk of a CAUTI, placement of a urinary catheter as a temporary measure may be ordered with the accepted indications of "critically ill/strict intake and output" (Abate & Citerio, 2014). Recent trends in ICU care have seen a move toward family-centered care and open visitation. As an advocate for the patient, the nurse and members of the interprofessional health care team are expected to use clinical judgment based on the patient's condition whether the presence of one or two select family members or a significant other would be helpful and comforting to the patient or add to the risk of rebleed with stressful family dynamics.

Clinical Pearl: The trend for open visiting hours creates challenges at times for the bedside nurse for maintaining a quiet, restful environment particularly for the patient with aSAH. Advocating for the patient can provide safety for the patient while supporting the needs of loved ones.

For the patient undergoing neurosurgical clipping, postoperative nursing care includes assessment of the craniotomy site for bleeding or signs of infection. Postoperative considerations for the patient undergoing endovascular embolization or coiling include assessment of the catheter insertion site for bleeding, hematoma, or infection and careful assessment of lower extremity pedal pulses in the immediate recovery period. Patients with either intervention should have sufficient pain management using pharmacological and nonpharmacological interventions, prophylaxis for gastric ulcer prevention, bowel care, and early mobilization with the support of physical therapy (PT), occupational therapy (OT), and speech therapy. Institutions often have specific protocols for postoperative care that may include applying ice to the incision and guidelines for frequency of vital signs and assessments. The nurse should follow the approved unit protocols for ICP monitoring and documentation including the anatomic landmark for leveling an external ventricular drainage system, for example, the "zero" mark at two fingers above the ear to approximate the foramen of Monro or tragus of the ear (AANN, 2009).

⊙ Nursing responsibilities in the immediate postoperative period include accurate and frequent neurological assessments and monitoring vital signs and values generated by intracranial monitoring or cardiovascular monitoring devices, such as a noninvasive continuous arterial-based pressure monitor. Regardless of the method by which the IA is secured (clip or coil), focused neurological assessments are critical because subtle changes may occur related to postoperative edema with open craniotomy and surgical clipping or due to inflammation in response to coiling. Cranial nerve deficits have been reported postcoiling and thought to be caused by mechanical compression from the coils and acute inflammation caused by intra-aneurysm thrombosis (Nishino et al., 2009). Deterioration of neurological function as indicated by changes in the neurological assessments may indicate postoperative/postcoiling complications (i.e., stroke, clip or coil displacement, or increased ICP) and require immediate physician notification (Deshaies, Eddleman, & Boulos, 2012).

An external monitoring device for ICP monitoring may be placed in the ED or upon arrival at the ICU depending on the clinical condition of the patient. Many institutions place EVDs or intraparenchymal monitors in the ICU using specific protocols for maintaining sterile procedure within a nonsterile environment. Others may reserve placement of a monitoring device until the patient is in the OR. When the device is placed in the ICU, nursing responsibilities are focused on patient safety: monitoring vital signs; controlling blood pressure; administering sedation as ordered; and ensuring protocols for drug "time-out," verification of side/site, and adherence to infection control practices are maintained (Green et al., 2013). Monitoring devices vary in capability from monitoring ICP to a combination of ICP monitoring and CSF drainage to more complex measurements to assess brain tissue oxygenation (Licox catheter), cerebral microdialysis, venous oximetry (jugular bulb catheter), continuous EEG, or continuous TCD. Monitoring devices also provide a means to assess CPP and evaluate the ICP waveform (Rabenstein, Lanzino, & Wijdicks, 2010).

⊙ Other common complications that are seen in the critical care environment have been previously discussed. The unpredictable yet often probable side effects of aSAH may include seizures, sepsis, and neurogenic cardiac complications (Patel & Samuels, 2012). Supportive care and prophylactic measures are aimed at mitigating the incidence and severity of complications of SAH, but a key component is that accurate neurological assessments by the neuroscience nurse and other interprofessional team members are critical for the patient's well-being and the ability of the health care team to intervene in a timely manner.

The Stroke Continuum of Care—Acute Care

⊙ The acute phase of care requires continued monitoring for the development of any complications and preparation for transition to the next level of care. Once the patient is able to be transferred from the ICU, evaluation for posthospital placement begins. As with all hospitalized patients, discharge planning begins shortly after admission. Case managers and social workers are consulted while the patient is in the ICU in order to create a foundation of support for the patient and family for both before and after discharge. These members of the interprofessional team have a wealth of knowledge regarding insurance, Medicare/Medicaid programs, skilled nursing facilities, and their individual requirements for patient acceptance and payer sources. See Chapter 10 on rehabilitation and Chapter 11 on poststroke community integration.

▓▓ CERTIFICATION, QUALITY MEASURES, OUTCOMES, AND COST

Certification and Quality Measures

In 2003, The Joint Commission (TJC) began its primary stroke center certification program in collaboration with AHA and ASA. To date, there are over 1,000 certified primary stroke centers in all 50 states, including Puerto Rico. In 2012, TJC launched a new certification for CSCs. CSC certification is reserved for centers with advanced medical, surgical, and neurointerventional radiology capabilities. Therefore, many patients with SAH receive care at CSCs, although they may initially be stabilized at a PSC and then transferred accordingly. There are currently 68 CSC-certified centers in the United States. Stroke certification is only available to hospitals with TJC accreditation. TJC Certificate of Distinction for Primary and Comprehensive Stroke Centers recognizes organizations that follow best practices for stroke care. These organizations must meet the requirements for Disease-Specific Care Certification as well as clinically specific requirements that include the following: follow a standard method to deliver care based on the Brain Attack Coalition's "Recommendations for Primary Stroke Centers" or "Recommendations for Comprehensive Stroke Centers"; support activities for patient self-management; adapt treatments to individual patient needs; support communication between health care settings and providers while maintaining patient confidentiality; use standard performance measures to analyze and improve treatments; and demonstrate compliance with clinical practice guidelines established by the AHA/ASA (TJC, 2013).

PSCs must collect data and report on eight performance measures. The stroke core measures are VTE prevention, discharged on antithrombotic therapy, anticoagulation for atrial fibrillation/flutter, thrombolytic therapy, antithrombotic therapy by the end of day 2 of the hospital stay, discharged on a statin medication, stroke education, and rehabilitation assessment (TJC, 2013). TJC evaluates all PSCs every 2 years with a site visit that includes tracer methodology, conversations with staff nurses and management teams, and an assessment of ongoing staff education programs. CSCs must meet additional quality metrics—including timelines of care in ischemic stroke, ICH, and SAH management and mortality and complication measurement for surgical and endovascular management of aSAH—as well as continue to meet the PSC eight performance measures.

Det Norske Veritas Healthcare, Inc. (DNVHC), also known as *DNV Health care*, offers another avenue for hospitals that do not have TJC accreditation but wish to demonstrate excellence in stroke care and hold primary or comprehensive stroke center certification. Both the Primary Stroke Center Certification and Comprehensive Stroke Center Certification programs offered by DNVHC incorporate requirements that include participation in Medicare programs and adherence to the guidelines of the Brain Attack Coalition and recommendations of the ASA (DNV-GL, 2009).

Outcomes

A study by Jaja et al. (2013) examined socioeconomic status (SES) related to outcomes of acute life-threatening cerebrovascular and cardiovascular diseases among two nationally representative databases in the United States and Canada between 2005 and 2010 and 2004 and 2010, respectively. The Discharge Abstract Database (DAD) is operated by the Canadian Institute for Health Information and the National (Nationwide) Inpatient Sample (NIS), which is managed by the Healthcare Cost and Utilization Project (HCUP) by the Agency for Healthcare Research and Quality (AHRQ). The databases contain information on sociodemographic, diagnostic, therapeutic, and administrative information on hospital discharges at the patient level. In the United States, the NIS collects a representative subsample of 20% of all discharges from acute care hospitals whereby its counterpart, DAD, mandatorily collects information from all discharges in Canada. Patients with a secondary diagnosis of cerebral injury were excluded to minimize the chance of including those with traumatic SAH (Jaja et al., 2013).

Interestingly, the study found that SES is associated with aSAH mortality risk in the United States but not in Canada. The effect of insurance coverage was another factor in the U.S. results. Neurosurgical patients who were inadequately insured had worse outcomes; conversely, patients with better insurance tended to live in more affluent neighborhoods with better access to timely, and high-quality, specialized care. Clearly there were several limitations to this study; however, it does point to the need for further research on access to care and how care is provided (Jaja et al., 2013).

> *Clinical Pearl:* A measureventionist is an RN whose main function is to help reduce HACs, complications, and readmissions through quality and compliance monitoring of evidence-based patient safety standards. The measureventionist collaborates with bedside nurses to ensure adherence to quality measures through a review of nursing documentation and direct observation of the patients.

Cost

Between 2001 and 2008, the number of patients who have been treated for an unruptured IA has steadily risen with the increased use of endovascular coiling. The greater the number of procedures that are performed (e.g., clipping and coiling), the higher the costs associated with the treatments at a time when Medicare payments are lagging behind compared to the rate of inflation.

A study conducted by Brinjikji, Kallmes, Lanzino, and Cloft (2012) used the NIS discharge database to examine to the hospital costs associated with clipping and coiling of unruptured IAs. The NIS represents 20% of all inpatient admissions to nonfederal hospitals in the United States. The data are collected by the HCUP of the AHRQ. The correlation between age, gender, and discharge status (home, short-term facility, long-term facility, and in-hospital death) and costs were examined for 2008. The study found that coiling without complications was nearly $3,000 more expensive than surgical clipping. The higher costs were related to the high costs of the endovascular devices. However, factoring in hospital costs, intensive care, and longer lengths of stay for patients undergoing surgical clipping, there were no statistical differences between the costs of coiling or surgical clipping of IAs. The study noted that Medicare payments were substantially lower than the costs to treat unruptured IAs. Therefore, efforts must be made to increase hospital reimbursement or decrease hospital costs in order for the treatments to be economical for health care organizations (Brinjikji et al., 2012).

Hospitals are evolving in their care delivery systems due to changes in regulatory and documentation requirements, quality initiatives, and online reporting of outcomes. The biggest changes are coming with health care reform aimed at reducing health care costs and improving consistency of care. For example, the Institute of Medicine (IOM, 2013) estimated that 30% of health care spending in 2009 was wasted due to poor-quality care, fraud, organizational inefficiencies, and other issues. Part of the changes in stroke care as of 2014 is the "all-or-none" stroke quality bundle that requires all aspects of stroke care to be addressed prior to patient discharge. The quality bundle includes patient/family education on how to call 911, smoking cessation, modifiable risk factors, stroke warning signs and symptoms, and the need for follow-up care. In addition, providers must address VTE prophylaxis, antithrombotic medication and statin therapy prescribed at discharge, and rehabilitation evaluation. Quality audits are commonplace in hospitals, and often, staff nurses are involved in reviewing documentation for adherence to quality measures that may affect hospital reimbursements tied to patient outcomes (Fonarow et al., 2013).

Treating patients with aSAH requires a multitude of resources and an interprofessional team with expertise in stroke. The direct costs of aSAH are related to expenses for all aspects of care from prehospital to the ED admission, diagnostic workup, and medications and continuing on through rehabilitation to the skilled nursing facility or long-term care. Indirect costs are not as easy to measure yet have far-reaching effects on the community due to unemployment, depression, caregiver-related loss of work time, and decreased ability to maintain social relationships. Clearly, all costs are greater when a young patient suffers aSAH based on a longer life expectancy (Le Roux & Wallace, 2009).

▉ FUTURE TRENDS

Research in all aspects of SAH and associated complications is ongoing. Improvements in care are evidenced by advances in surgical and interventional techniques, mechanisms for early identification of vasospasm, attention to abnormal laboratory values, and an increased focus on "nonevents" to prevent other nonneurological complications. Evidence-based bundles of care have demonstrated effectiveness in reducing HAIs when the protocols and the components of the bundles are standardized and adhered to with diligence.

Intracranial Stents

Intracranial stents have been used for the past 10 years. Patients with wide-necked, fusiform, or lobulated IAs are considered for stenting when surgical clipping or endovascular coiling may not be possible or effective in securing the IA. Stenting requires pretreatment with aspirin and clopidogrel (Plavix), and patients with conditions that require treatment with warfarin are less ideal candidates given the risks of hemorrhage from the required anticoagulant and antiplatelet therapies. Patients also must demonstrate compliance with medication regimens because there is a long-term medication regimen post intracranial stent, and they must understand the risks of in-stent occlusion or stroke symptoms if antiplatelet therapy is discontinued. If the patient cannot be compliant or take antiplatelet medications, he or she should not have intracranial stent placement because of the high risk of postprocedure complications such as in-stent thrombosis.

The Pipeline Embolization Device (PED), a flow-diverting stent, is an option for patients who have an IA that is difficult or impossible to treat by surgical clipping or endovascular embolization. The design of the PED redirects blood flow, thereby decreasing the inflow and outflow forces of the IA that promotes stasis of blood flow and delayed thrombosis, which in turn leads to reconstruction of the parent vessel. The PED is a self-expandable device that occludes the IA neck while preserving the patency of the arterial branches covered by the device. The difference is that the PED provides delayed occlusion versus the immediate occlusion achieved via endovascular coiling or surgical clipping (Cruz et al., 2012) (**Fig. 8-5**).

The PED is not without risks (e.g., IA rupture, delayed parent vessel occlusion, or ipsilateral intraparenchymal hemorrhage); therefore, other interventions should be considered. Consideration must be given to the management of aSAH and vasospasm because the PED is thought to promote thrombosis of the covered small vessels (perforator arteries) because these vessels are more sensitive to a reduction in blood flow. In the event that endovascular treatment of vasospasm is needed, the stents may interfere or prevent balloon angioplasty if the affected branch is not accessible because of stent coverage. Intravascular therapy with intra-arterial injections (e.g., nicardipine, milrinone, papaverine) may be the only options remaining if medical interventions are insufficient (Cruz et al., 2012). The PED was approved for use by the U.S. Food and Drug Administration (FDA) in 2011 (Dalfino et al., 2012).

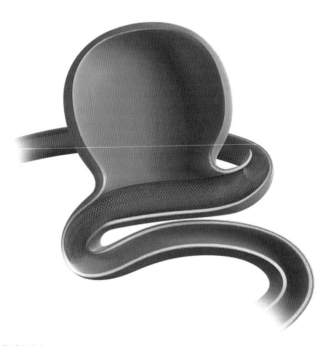

FIGURE 8-5 PED deployed across the neck of an aneurysm (*Image courtesy of Covidien Neurovascular, Mansfield, MA. From Hickey, J. V. [2014]. The clinical practice of neurological and neurosurgical nursing [7th ed.]. Philadelphia, PA: Lippincott Williams & Wilkins.*)

Early Brain Injury

Early brain injury (EBI) is a relatively new concept that examines the overall brain injury after aSAH. Several studies have indicated that the pathophysiological after-effects of aSAH are not limited to vasospasm but extend to a global ischemic injury to the brain. The ramifications of a global brain injury post-SAH may change treatment modalities and protocols that historically have been aimed at vasospasm. The question of EBI as the main cause of mortality in aSAH has been raised by these findings because the impact of aSAH on the brain includes increased ICP, decreased cerebral blood flow, reduction in CPP and brain tissue oxygenation, a breakdown in the blood–brain barrier, and neuronal cell death. Research on EBI is advancing and will continue to be brought into the forefront as more is learned about this concept. Current knowledge about reversal of vasospasm does not necessarily improve outcomes; the research may demonstrate that treating EBI is more effective (Cahill & Zhang, 2009).

Early Mobilization

Patients with SAH may be critically ill after the IA rupture and during the first 7 to 10 days when mobilization is not recommended due to vital sign instability, the presence of multiple invasive lines, or fluctuating neurological assessments. However, all patients should be mobilized as early as possible to decrease complications associated with critical illness. Early mobilization programs involve the interprofessional team in patient management and plan of care and have demonstrated effectiveness in improving functional outcomes, reducing lengths of stay, and decreasing costs. Both PT and OT can be particularly helpful in assisting the team with early mobilization. Early mobilization programs including those on mechanical ventilation have been shown to be safe and decrease intubated/ventilated days. For example, early mobilization within 24 hours of stroke onset was found to be reasonable and did not increase 3-month mortality. Other findings demonstrated that patients returned to walking 2.5 days faster; had improved function at 3 and 12 months; and, at 7 days post stroke, were less depressed.

Recent research has reported no significant effect on ICP or CPP with passive or active range of motion among patients with SAH in the ICU receiving PT (Kocan & Lietz, 2013). Bedrest is still recommended for patients with unsecured IA, but once surgical or endovascular interventions to clip or coil the IA are completed, the risk of rebleeding is minimal. Considerations to mobilize a patient with SAH depend on blood pressure stability and avoidance of hypotension. Patients with anterior communicating artery IA rupture may have problems with short-term memory, agitation, behavior, or personality changes; however, this should not preclude the nurse from obtaining orders for therapies including cognitive evaluation and work toward safe mobilization of the patient (Kocan & Lietz, 2013).

Oral Hygiene

Good oral hygiene dates back to Florence Nightingale, but the association of poor oral hygiene and increased respiratory infections including ventilatory-associated pneumonia (VAP) is new. Nursing organizations and individual nurses are consistent in their support of good oral hygiene and agree that this is an important part of the overall care of the patient. Research has shown that intubation may contribute to worsening oral health and increased bacterial load (Prendergast, Hallberg, Jahnke, Kleiman, & Hagell, 2009). Additional findings have determined that during hospitalization, the normal flora is replaced with pathogenic bacteria within 48 hours of admission. Endotracheal tubes (ETTs), bite blocks, and poor oral hygiene contribute to the development of VAP or ventilator-associated events (VAEs) (Prendergast et al., 2009). During this oral care study, vital signs including ICPs were recorded 30 minutes prior to, during, and 30 minutes after oral care was performed. In the nearly 1,000 data points of recorded ICP values, there were no overall differences in the three recorded ICP values. Other studies have supported these findings (i.e., Cutler & Davis, 2005); however; it should be noted that more research is needed (Prendergast et al., 2009).

Ongoing research has demonstrated the efficacy of an electric (battery-powered) toothbrush, tongue scraper, and oral care products (i.e., Biotene) in intubated patients to decrease bacterial load and improve overall oral hygiene (Prendergast et al., 2009). Bedside oral assessments with an associated oral care protocol based on assessment findings conducted by nurses is gaining support and progressing toward acceptance as a standard of care in the neuroscience patient population.

INTERPROFESSIONAL APPROACH TO CARE

Interprofessional rounds are an important part of the overall care of the patient with SAH. The patient often has multiple physical and cognitive problems that need attention from specialists to ensure the optimal recovery of the patient. SAH is a devastating event that takes a toll not only on the physical and cognitive capabilities of the patient but also has a huge impact on the financial and emotional stability of the family. Social services and case management should be involved in the plan of care from admission in order to develop a rapport and collaborative working environment with the patient and/or family. Chaplain services or other patient-requested spiritual care services should be available for comfort and support. Palliative care is essential for patients with severe SAH for family support and decision making, and the purpose of palliative care should be made clear at the outset. A misperception of palliative care persists that the services are equivalent to hospice care—even among the members of the health care team. Palliative care is an approach that improves the quality of life of patients and their families when faced with life-threatening events and is appropriate early in the course of an illness in conjunction with other therapies. See also Chapter 9 for discussion of palliative care.

SUMMARY

aSAH is a life-threatening, devastating, and complicated entity that requires specialized skill and expertise of physicians, surgeons, nurses, and other members of the interprofessional health care team to restore the patient to optimum functioning. A myriad of complications await the patient with aSAH; however, treatments and interventions exist to relieve or mitigate the effects of rebleeding, vasospasm, hydrocephalus, infections, thromboembolism, and other potential problems. Research is delving deeper into cerebral pathophysiology to determine the effects of cerebral hemorrhage on cellular physiology throughout the brain. Advances in surgical techniques and endovascular devices have contributed to the arsenal of treatment modalities available to patients. Standardization of interventions in the form of "bundles" has demonstrated efficacy in preventing HAIs and, as a result, decreasing the costs of care through shorter lengths of stay and fewer incidences of infection, VTE, and invasive line infections. Investigations are being conducted on early recognition and intervention for prevention and treatment of delirium in order to improve long-term outcomes. Technology has improved the capabilities and abilities of the interprofessional team to collaborate effectively to bring evidence-based practice and best practices to the care of patients with SAH so that patient will have the best outcomes possible.

REFERENCES

Abate, M. G., & Citerio, G. (2014). Management of subarachnoid hemorrhage. *Reanimation, 23*, S425–S432. doi:10.1007/s13546-013-0810-8

Ahmadian, A., Mizzi, A., Banasiak, M., Downes, K., Camporesi, E. M., Sullebarger, J. T., . . . Agazzi, S. (2013). Cardiac manifestations of subarachnoid hemorrhage. *Heart, Lung and Vessels, 5*(3), 168–178.

American Association of Neuroscience Nurses. (2009). Clinical practice guidelines: Subarachnoid hemorrhage. In H. J. Thompson & K. L. Lee (Eds.), *Care of the patient with aneurysmal subarachnoid hemorrhage* (pp. 1–30). Retrieved from http://www.aann.org/pubs/content/guidelines.html

American Heart Association & American Stroke Association. (2013). *Stroke training for EMS professionals.* Retrieved from http://www.strokeassociation.org/idc/groups/stroke-public/@wcm/@hcm/@sta/documents/downloadable/ucm_456069.pdf

Ando, G., Trio, O., & De Gregorio, C. (2010). Transient left ventricular dysfunction in patient with neurovascular events. *Acute Cardiac Care, 12*, 70–74. doi:10.3109/17482941003732758

Balas, M. C., Vasilevskis, E. E., Olsen, K. M., Schmid, K. K., Shostrom, V., Cohen, M. Z., . . . Burke, W. J. (2014). Effectiveness and safety of the awakening and breathing coordination, delirium monitoring/management, and early exercise/mobility bundle. *Critical Care Medicine, 42*(5), 1024–1036. Retrieved from http://www.icudelirium.org/medicalprofessionals.html

Bautista, C. (2012). Unresolved issues in the management of aneurysmal subarachnoid hemorrhage. *AACN Advanced Critical Care, 22*, 175–185. doi:10.1097/NCl.0b013e31824ebcfa

Becske, T., Lutsep, H. L., Jallo, G. I., Berman, S. A., Kirshner, H. S., & Talavera, F. (2013). *Subarachnoid hemorrhage treatment and management.* Retrieved from http://emedicine.medscape.com/article/1164341-treatment

Boulos, A. S., & Dalfino, J. C. (2012). Endovascular techniques for aneurysm therapy, arteriovenous malformation treatment, and carotid artery stent placement. In E. M. Deshaie, C. S. Eddleman, & A. S. Boulos (Eds.), *Handbook of neuroendovascular surgery* (pp. 158–185). New York, NY: Thieme.

Brinjikji, W., Kallmes, D. F., Lanzino, G., & Cloft, H. J. (2012). Hospitalization costs for endovascular and surgical treatment of unruptured cerebral aneurysms in the United States are substantially higher than Medicare payments. *American Journal of Neuroradiology, 33*, 49–51. doi:10.3174/ajnr.A2739

Cahill, J., & Zhang, J. H. (2009). Subarachnoid hemorrhage: Is it time for a new direction? *Stroke, 40*(3)(Suppl.), S86–S87. doi:10.1161/STROKEAHA.108.533315

Chalouhi, N., Hoh, B. L., & Hasan, D. (2013). Review of cerebral aneurysm formation, growth, and rupture. *Stroke, 44*, 3613–3622. doi:10.1161/STROKEAHA.113.002390

Claassen, J., Bernardini, G. L., Kreiter, K., Bates, J., Du, Y. E., Copeland, D., . . . Mayer, S. A. (2001). Effect of cisternal and ventricular blood on risk of delayed cerebral ischemia after subarachnoid hemorrhage: The Fisher Scale revisited. *Stroke, 32*, 2012–2020. doi:10.1161/hs901.095677

Crowley, R. W., Ducruet, A. F., McDougall, C. G., & Albuquerque, F. C. (2014). Endovascular advances for brain arteriovenous malformations. *Neurosurgery, 74*(Suppl. 1), 74–82. doi:10.1227/NEU.0000000000000176

Cruz, J. P., O'Kelly, C., Wong, J. H., Alshaya, W., Martin, A., Spears, J., & Marotta, T. R. (2012). Pipeline embolization device in aneurysmal subarachnoid hemorrhage. *American Journal of Neuroradiology, 34*, 271–276. doi:10.3174/ajnr.A3380

Cutler, C.J. & Davis, N. (2005). Improving oral care in patients receiving mechanical ventilation. *American Journal of Critical Care, 14*(5), 389–394. Retrieved from http://ajcc.aacnjournals.org/content/14/5/389.full

Dalfino, J. C., Gandhi, R. H., & Boulos, A. S. (2012). Introduction to endovascular equipment. In E. M. Deshaies, C. S. Eddleman, & A. S. Boulos (Eds.), *Handbook of neuroendovascular surgery* (pp. 114–157). New York, NY: Thieme.

Deshaies, E. M., Eddleman, C. S., & Boulos, A. S. (2012). Periprocedural patient evaluation. In E. M. Deshaies, C. S. Eddleman, & A. S. Boulos (Eds.), *Handbook of neuroendovascular surgery* (pp. 186–200). New York, NY: Thieme.

Diringer, M. N. (2009). Management of aneurysmal subarachnoid hemorrhage. *Critical Care Medicine, 37*(2), 432–440. doi:10.1097?CCM.0b013e318195865a

DNV-GL. (2009). Primary stroke center certification program requirements. Retrieved from http://dnvaccreditation.com

Dorhout, S. M., Algra, A., Vandertop, W. P., Van Kooten, F., Kuijsten, H. A., Boiten, J., . . . Van den Bergh, W. M. (2012). Magnesium for aneurysmal subarachnoid haemorrhage (MASH-2): Randomised, placebo-controlled trial. *The Lancet, 380*(9836), 44–49. doi:10.1016/S0140-6736(12)60724-7

Dumont, C., & Nesselrodt, D. (2012). Preventing CLABSI: Central line associated bloodstream infections. *Nursing, 42*(6), 41–46. doi:10.1097/01.NURSE.0000414623.31647.f5

Ferrara, A. R. (2011). Brain arteriovenous malformations. *Radiologic Technology, 82*(6), 543MR–560MR. Retrieved from http://phoenix.summon.serialssolutions.comezproxy.apollolibrary.com

Field, T. S., & Hill, M. D. (2011). Prevention of deep vein thrombosis and pulmonary embolism in patients with stroke. *Clinical and Applied Thrombosis/Hemostasis, 18*(5), 5–19. doi:10.1177/1076029611412362

Fonarow, G. C., Liang, L., Smith, E. E., Reeves, M. J., Saver, J. L., Xian, Y., . . . Schwamm, L. H. (2013). Comparison of performance achievement award recognition with primary stroke center certification for acute ischemic stroke care. *Journal of the American Heart Association, 2*(5), e000451. doi:10.1161/JAHA.113.000451

Fox, S., & Choi, D. (2009). To clip or to coil? Choosing the best treatment for cerebral aneurysms. *British Journal of Neuroscience Nursing, 5*(6), 264–269. Retrieved from ProQuest database.

Frangiskakis, J. M., Hravnak, M. H., Crago, E. A., Tanabe, M., Kip, K. E., Gorcsan, J. III., . . . London, B. (2009). Ventricular arrhythmia risk after subarachnoid hemorrhage. *NeuroCritical Care, 10*(3), 287–294. doi:10.1007/s12028-009-9188-x

Ganti, L., Jain, A., Yerragondu, N., Jain, M., Bellolio, M. F., Gilmore, R. M., & Rabinstein, A. (2013). Female gender remains an independent risk factor for poor outcome after acute nontraumatic intracerebral hemorrhage. *Neurology Research International, 2013*, 219097. doi:10.1155/2013/219097

Gerken, S. (2013). *Preventing positioning injuries: An anesthesiologist's perspectives.* Retrieved from http://www.aaos.org/news/aaosnow/jan13/managing7.asp

Green, D. M., Burns, J. D., & DeFusco, C. M. (2013). ICU management of aneurysmal subarachnoid hemorrhage. *Journal of Intensive Care Medicine, 28*, 341–354. doi:10.1177/0885066611434100

Greenburg, M. S. (2010). SAH and aneurysms. In M. S. Greenburg (Ed.), *Handbook of neurosurgery* (7th ed., pp. 1034–1097). New York, NY: Thieme.

Greving, J. P., Rinkel, G. J., Buskins, E., & Algra, A. (2009). Cost-effectiveness of preventive treatment of intracranial aneurysms. *Neurology, 73*(4), 258–265. Retrieved from http://www.neurology.org/content/73/4/258.long

Griffin, S., & Logue, B. (2009). Takotsubo cardiomyopathy: A nurse's guide. *Critical Care Nurse, 29*, 32–42. doi:10.4037/ccn2009907

Hight, H. C. (2010). *SCIP: Surgical care improvement project—A national quality partnership.* Retrieved from http://www.hsag.com/App_Resources/Documents/FMQAI_SCIP_VTE_LearningModule.pdf

Hunt, W. E., & Hess, R. M. (1968). Surgical risk as related to time of intervention in the repair of intracranial aneurysms. *Journal of Neurosurgery, 28*(1), 14–20.

ICU Delirium and Cognitive Impairment Study Group. (2014).*What is delirium?* Retrieved from http://icudelirium.org

Institute of Medicine. (2013). *Best care at lower cost: The path to continuously learning health care in America.* Washington, DC: The National Academies Press.

Jaja, B. N., Saposinik, G., Nisenbaum, R., Schweizer, T. A., Reddy, D., Thorpe, K. E., & Macdonald, R. L. (2013). Effect of socioeconomic status on inpatient mortality and use of postacute care after subarachnoid hemorrhage. *Stroke, 44*(10), 2842–2847. doi:10.1161/STROKEAHA.113.001368

Kocan, M., & Lietz, H. (2013). Special considerations for mobilizing patients in the neurointensive care unit. *Critical Care Nursing Quarterly, 36*(1), 50–55. doi:10.1097/CNQ.0b013e3182750b12

Labetalol. (2014). Retrieved from http://reference.medscape.com/drug/trandate-labetalol-342359

Le Roux, A. A., & Wallace, M. C. (2009). Outcome and cost of aneurysmal subarachnoid hemorrhage. *Neurosurgery Clinics of North America, 21*, 235–246. doi:10.1016/j.nec.2009.10.014

McDougall, C. G., Spetzler, R. F., Zabramski, J. M., Partovi, S., Hills, N. K., Nakaji, P., & Albuquerque, F. C. (2012). The Barrow Ruptured Aneurysm Trial Clinical Article. *Journal of Neurosurgery, 116*(1), 135–144. doi:10.3171/2011.8.JNS101767

McKeon, L., & Cardell, B. (2011). Preventing never events: What frontline nurses need to know. *Nursing Made Incredibly Easy!*, 44–52. Retrieved from http://www.nursingcenter.com/lnc/pdf?AID=1100852&an=00152258-201101000-00010&Journal_ID=417221&Issue_ID=1100706

Middleton, K., Esselman, P., & Lim, P. C. (2012). Terson syndrome. *American Journal of Physical Medicine & Rehabilitation, 91*, 271–274. doi:10.1097/PHM.0b013e3182328792

Murphy-Human, T., & Diringer, M. N. (2010). Sodium disturbances commonly encountered in the neurologic intensive care unit. *Journal of Pharmacy Practice*, *23*, 470–484. doi:10.1177/0897190010372323

Nishino, K., Ito, Y., Hasegawa, H., Shimbo, J., Kikuchi, B., & Fugii, Y. (2009). Development of cranial nerve palsy shortly after endosaccular embolization for asymptomatic aneurysm: Report of two cases and literature review. *Acta Neurochirurgica*, *151*(4), 379–383. doi:10.1007/s00701-009-0234-4

O'Grady, N. P., Alexander, M., Burns, L. A., Dellinger, E. P., Garland, J., Heard, S. O., . . . Saint, S. (2011). Guidelines for the prevention of intravascular catheter-related infections, 2011. *Healthcare Infection Control Practices Advisory Committee [HICPAC]*, 1–83. Retrieved from http://www.cdc.gov/hicpac/BSI/BSI-guidelines-2011.html

Oh, Y., Kim, D., Chun, H., & Yi, H. (2008). Incidence and risk factors of acute postoperative delirium in geriatric neurosurgical patients. *Journal of Korean Neurosurgical Society*, *43*(3), 143–148. doi:10.3340/jkns.2008.43.3.143

Patel, V. N., & Samuels, O. B. (2012). The critical care management of aneurysmal subarachnoid hemorrhage. In Y. Murai (Ed.), *Aneurysm*. InTech. doi:10.5772/48474

Penn, D. L., Komotar, R. J., & Connolly, E. S. (2011). Hemodynamic mechanisms underlying cerebral aneurysm pathogenesis. *Journal of Clinical Neuroscience*, *18*, 1435–1438. doi:10.1016/j.jocn.2011.05.001

Perry, J. J., Stiell, I. G., Sivilotti, M. L., Bullard, M. J., Hohl, C. M., Sutherland, J., . . . Wells, G. A. (2013). Clinical decision rules to rule out subarachnoid hemorrhage for acute headache. *The Journal of the American Medical Association*, *310*, 1248–1255. doi:10.1001/jama.2013.278018

Physician's Desk Reference: PDR Network, LLC. (2014). *Drug summary: Labetalol hydrochloride injection*. Retrieved from http://www.pdr.net/drug-summary/labetalol-hydrochloride?druglabelid=1568

Prendergast, V., Hallberg, I. R., Jahnke, H., Kleiman, C., & Hagell, P. (2009). Oral health, ventilator-associated pneumonia, and intracranial pressure in intubated patients in a neuroscience intensive care unit. *American Journal of Critical Care*, *18*, 368–376. doi:10.4037/ajcc2009621

Rabenstein, A. A., Lanzino, G., & Wijdicks, E. F. (2010). Multidisciplinary management and emerging therapeutic strategies in aneurysmal subarachnoid haemorrhage. *The Lancet Neurology*, *9*, 504–518. Retrieved from http://www.thelancet.com/journals/laneur/article/PIIS1474-4422(10)70087-9/fulltext

Raper, D. M., Starke, R. M., Komotar, R. J., Allen, R., & Connolly, E. S. (2012). Seizures after aneurysmal subarachnoid hemorrhage: A systematic review of outcomes. *World Neurosurgery*, *79*(5–6), 682–690. doi:10.1016j.wneu.2012.08.006

Rhoney, D. H. (2010). Introduction: Neurologic critical care. *Journal of Pharmacy Practice*, *23*(5), 385–386. doi:10.1177/0897190010372319

Rhoney, D. H., McAllen, K., & Liu-DeRyke, X. (2010). Current and future treatment considerations in the management of aneurysmal subarachnoid hemorrhage. *Journal of Pharmacy Practice*, *23*(5), 408–424. doi:10.1177/0897190010372334

Rincon, F., Rossenwasser, R. H., & Dumont, A. (2013). The epidemiology of admission of nontraumatic subarachnoid hemorrhage in the United States. *Neurosurgery*, *73*, 218–223. doi:10.1227/01.neu.0000430290.93304.33

Rinkel, G. J., Prins, N. E., & Algra, A. (1997). Outcome of aneurysmal subarachnoid hemorrhage in patients on anticoagulant therapy. *Stroke*, *28*(1), 6–9. Retrieved from http://stroke.ahajournals.org/content/28/1/6.full

Rosen, D.S. & Macdonald, R.L. (2005). Subarachnoid hemorrhage grading scale: A systematic review. *Neuro Critical Care*, *2*(2), 110–118. doi:10.1385/NCC:2:2:110

Ryan, D., & Harbison, J. (2011). Stroke as a medical emergency in older people. *Reviews in Clinical Gerontology*, *21*, 45–54. doi:10.1017/S095925981000033X

Schöller, K., Massmann, M., Markl, G., Kunz, M., Fesl, G., Brüchmann, H., . . . Schichor, C. (2013). Aneurysmal subarachnoid hemorrhage in elderly patients: Long-term outcome and prognostic factors in an interdisciplinary treatment approach. *Journal of Neurology*, *260*, 1052–1060. doi:10.1007/s00415-012-6758-1

Teasdale, G., & Jennett, B. (1974). Assessment of coma and impaired consciousness: A practical scale. *The Lancet*, *2*(7872), 81–84. doi:10.1016/S0140-6736(74)91639-0

Teasdale, G., Murray, G., Parker, L., & Jennett, B. (1979). Adding up the Glasgow Coma Score. *Acta Neuroschirurgica. Supplementum*, *28*(1), 13–16.

Teasdale, G. M., Drake, C. G., Hunt, W., Kassell, N., Sano, K., Pertuiset, B., & De Villiers, J. C. (1988). A universal subarachnoid hemorrhage scale: Report of a committee of the World Federation of Neurosurgical Societies. *Journal of Neurology, Neurosurgery, and Psychiatry*, *51*(11), 1457. doi:10.1136/jnnp.51.11.1457

The Joint Commission. (2013). *Facts about primary stroke center certification*. Retrieved from http://www.jointcommission.org/assets/1/6/Facts_About_Primary_Stroke_Center_Certification.pdf

Verma, R. K., Kottke, R., Andereggen, L., Weisstanner, C., Zubler, C., Gralla, J., . . . El-Koussy, M. (2013). Detecting subarachnoid hemorrhage: Comparison of combined FLAIR/SWI versus CT. *European Journal of Radiology*, *82*(9), 1539–1545. doi:10.1016/j.ejrad.2013.03.021

Vesek, J. M., Laughlin, M. M., Pazuchanics, S. J., Horton, T. G., & Cockroft, K. M. (2011). Onyx-500 HD liquid embolic agent for the embolization of broad-based saccular intracranial aneurysms: A case study. *Journal of Radiology Nursing, 30*(3), 96–102. doi:10.1016/j.jradnu.2011.07.001

Washington, C. W., Vellimana, A. K., Zipfel, G. J., & Dacey, R. G. (2011). The current surgical management of intracranial aneurysms. *Journal of Neurosurgical Sciences, 55*(3), 211–231.

Westermaier, T., Stetter, C., Wiles, G., Pham, M., Tejan, J. P., Eriskat, J., . . . Roosen, K. (2010). Prophylactic magnesium sulfate for treatment of aneurysmal subarachnoid hemorrhage: A randomized, placebo-controlled, clinical study. *Critical Care Medicine, 38*(5), 1284–1290. doi:10.1097/CCM.0b013e3181d9da1e

Wong, G. K. C., Ngai, K., Wong, A., Lai, S. W., Mok, V. C., Yeung, J., . . . Poon, W. S. (2012). Long-term cognitive dysfunction in patients with traumatic subarachnoid hemorrhage: Prevalence and risk factors. *Acta Neurochirurgica, 154*, 105–111.

Zebian, R. C., Kulkami, R., & Kazzi, A. A. (2013). *Emergent management of subarachnoid hemorrhage.* Retrieved from http://emedicine.medscape.com/article/794076-overview

CHAPTER 9

Management of Stroke-Related Complications

Mary Guhwe, Susan M. Chioffi, and Kelly Blessing

A myriad of complications can occur as a result of ischemic stroke, hemorrhagic stroke, and subarachnoid hemorrhage along the trajectory from onset through rehabilitation to outcomes. Some complications are common in the acute care phase, whereas others are more common in the rehabilitation and community care phase of recovery. This chapter discusses these common stroke-related problems from the perspective of description, pathophysiology, assessment/diagnosis, treatment, best practices, and evaluation. The roles of the various members of the interprofessional team are addressed as their roles relate to each complication.

▗▖ CEREBRAL EDEMA FROM STROKE

Cerebral injury from either hemorrhage or infarction after acute stroke can herald the development of cerebral edema around the affected vascular area. The mechanisms of infarction and ischemia are discussed in Chapter 5. Cerebral edema, if allowed to proceed unchecked, can result in a cascade in which the zones of infarct, ischemia and edema, widen. For some people who experience a stroke, cerebral edema will be a minor issue because of the smaller size and location of the area of injury, whereas for others, it will be a significant and possibly life-threatening problem. When considering neuroanatomy, it is clear that the development of even a small amount of edema can cause devastating problems in a patient with a pontine infarct or hemorrhage, whereas an elderly patient with a normal age-related cerebral atrophy could develop a significant amount of edema without manifesting severe physiological compromise.

The development of global edema is sometimes seen after subarachnoid hemorrhage (SAH) and is associated with poor outcome and increased mortality (Claassen et al., 2002). Patients who initially present with intracerebral hemorrhage (ICH) or SAH are at higher risk for poor outcomes from cerebral edema because their intracranial pressure is already elevated as a result of the space-occupying lesion that the hemorrhage represents. Further complicating the picture is that SAH patients are at risk for cerebral edema from both acute and delayed cerebral infarct (Schmidt et al., 2007). Perihematomal edema in the setting of ICH develops rapidly and increases significantly in a week to 10 days immediately following onset of ICH (Staykov et al., 2011). Some patients with ischemic stroke will experience the complication of hemorrhage into the area of infarct. This can range from asymptomatic petechial hemorrhages seen on imaging studies to large, life-threatening intracerebral hematomas. This hemorrhagic transformation of infarct increases the risk of cerebral edema.

Cerebral edema becomes a problem when it leads to intracranial hypertension, more commonly known as *increased intracranial pressure* (ICP). Cerebral edema can damage and displace brain structures not initially affected by the stroke and, in about 2% to 3% of cases, leads to central herniation and death. Although younger people with strokes have less comorbidity, which could complicate the management of cerebral edema, they have less intracranial space to accommodate swelling than do older patients with age-related atrophy of cerebral tissue. Patients with ICH are also at risk for delayed cerebral edema several days after the initial event as the breakdown of the extravasated red blood cells results in irritation of surrounding tissue and swelling (Thiex & Tsirka, 2007; Xi et al., 2001). Massive cerebral edema and the resulting herniation are the most feared consequences after acute stroke especially in younger patients who do not have brain atrophy.

Because cerebral edema is often a serious complication of stroke and can be associated with significant morbidity and mortality, discussions with the patient and/or their family about goals of care should be initiated early in the management and treatment of stroke. Even with maximal medical intervention, some patients with cerebral edema will not survive, and others may sustain permanent deficits because of new or increased infarct as a secondary effect of cerebral edema. Having discussions related to end-of-life care or establishing the existence of completed advance directives or living wills prior to the development of complications can facilitate decision making. It can be difficult for families to make decisions regarding either initiating or withdrawing care if they have not had an opportunity to consider their options earlier in the patient's hospital stay. In these cases, the palliative care specialists, if available, can be a vital support system and resource for the family and the interprofessional team in these cases.

Pathophysiology

Cerebral edema represents an abnormal increase of intracellular and/or extracellular water causing an increase in intracranial volume. The extent to which it is a local or generalized problem for a particular patient depends on the location of the original infarct or hemorrhage. Edema from a cerebellar lesion, for example, becomes a generalized problem when it obstructs the fourth ventricle and results in obstructive hydrocephalus. Swelling from cerebral edema is believed to peak between 2 and 4 days after initial injury, and there is a great deal of variation in the length of time it takes the edema to resolve. The greater the increase in ICP and the greater the number of interventions required to manage the increased ICP, the longer it usually takes for the edema to resolve.

Injury and ischemia trigger a harmful molecular cascade in which mediators such as free fatty acids, glutamate, or extracellular potassium are released or activated, leading to secondary swelling and nerve cell damage. The molecular cascade eventually encompasses the loss of membrane ionic pumps, which leads to cellular accumulation of water and eventually permanent damage to cellular functions (Jha, 2003). It is useful to keep in mind that there are three kinds of cerebral edema: cytotoxic, vasogenic, and interstitial. Cytotoxic and vasogenic edema often coexist in stroke patients (Rabinstein, 2006).

Vasogenic edema is seen most often in the white matter of the brain. It results from increased permeability of the endothelial cells in the capillary beds. As a result, a protein-containing filtrate leaks into the extracellular space. Vasogenic edema can develop around cerebral infarcts, brain tumors, and abscesses. Steroids have only been shown to be effective for edema related to brain tumors; osmotic therapy is more effective for other conditions (Rabinstein, 2006).

Cytotoxic edema occurs when there is an increase in fluids in neurons, glia, and endothelial cells as a result of adenosine triphosphate (ATP)–dependent sodium-potassium pump failure leading to the accumulation of sodium and fluid with the cells resulting in diffuse swelling. Both gray and white matter may be involved. Cytotoxic edema is often seen in relation to a hypoxic or an anoxic episode. It can also be seen with prolonged hypo-osmolar states such as water intoxication, hyponatremia, and syndrome of inappropriate secretion of antidiuretic hormone (SIADH). Steroids are not effective for this kind of edema, and therapy should be directed at restoration and maintenance of perfusion and oxygenation (Hickey, 2014; Rabinstein, 2006).

Interstitial edema is seen in prolonged hydrocephalus and is also known as *transependymal flow*. Cerebrospinal fluid (CSF) is not absorbed rapidly enough and is forced across ependymal tissue and into the periventricular white matter. It can be seen with both acute and subacute hydrocephalus. Patients with SAH are at high risk for interstitial edema because the location of the bleeding interferes with proper CSF drainage. Steroids are not an effective treatment for this type of edema, although acetazolamide can be used to decrease CSF production. Interstitial edema is initially best managed with temporary external drainage of the CSF. Some patients may require permanent alternative drainage through a surgical shunt placement (Rabinstein, 2006; Rincon & Mayer, 2008).

Assessment and Diagnosis

All clinicians involved in the patient's care should know the size and location of the original stroke as well as the time since the stroke occurred. This information will guide the frequency of the neurological examination as well as the focus of the examination. A patient with a brainstem stroke, for example, would benefit from especially close monitoring of cranial nerves, whereas a patient with a right middle cerebral artery (MCA) infarct should be closely monitored for the development of or worsening of a left-sided weakness. The bedside nurse conducting frequent serial neurological assessments will likely be the first to observe subtle early neurological changes, which could indicate the presence or worsening of edema or the risk of herniation. These findings should be reported to the physician or advanced practitioner. The comparison of the current neurological examination to the patient's baseline examination represents the most sensitive indicator of change.

A focal change in the neurological examination such as acute hemiparesis should prompt immediate concern about a localized intracranial event such as a hemorrhage or new infarct. A global change in the neurological examination such as deterioration from being completely intact to mildly confused, although it may herald cerebral edema, should also prompt evaluation of factors such as oxygenation, serum sodium, serum glucose, and body temperature, which can lead to neurological compromise. Computed axial tomography (CAT) scanning is an excellent tool for the rapid diagnosis of cerebral edema and can provide information to facilitate rapid intervention to limit patient deterioration. ICP monitoring can assist with the monitoring of cerebral edema and guide treatment (Jha, 2003). Although placement of an ICP monitor is still the "gold standard" for care, research is underway to investigate the various methods to allow non-invasive monitoring of ICP. Automated pupillometry, near-infrared spectroscopy, transcranial Doppler sonography, and optic nerve sheath diameter are some methods under investigation as ways of early identification of neurological deterioration (Rosenberg, Shiloh, Savel, & Eisen, 2011).

Treatment

Unstable stroke patients are best managed in a neurointensive care unit (NICU) staffed by a dedicated neurointensivist team. This model has been shown in studies to improve outcomes (Bershad, Feen, Hernandez, Suri, & Suarez, 2008; Diringer & Edwards, 2001). Initial basic management of all patients with stroke focuses on such measures as avoiding fever and hypoxemia, promoting cerebral venous drainage by keeping the head of the bed (HOB) elevated, and maintaining the head in a midline position. The overall goals of medical therapy are prevention of secondary complications through management of cerebral edema, maintenance of adequate blood and oxygen supplies, and optimization of cerebral metabolism (Singh & Edwards, 2013; Thiex & Tsirka, 2007). Proper management of hypertension, hyperglycemia, respiratory failure, and fever, as discussed elsewhere in this chapter, are integral to managing cerebral edema. Many of the factors associated with increased ICP have been identified and their management clarified through nursing research. Many of the interventions to manage patients at increased risk for problems related to ICP are collaborative problems and rely on astute nursing care rather than specific medical interventions (Olson, McNett, Lewis, Riemen, & Bautista, 2013; Olson, Thoyre, Bennett, Stoner, & Graffagnino, 2009).

The decrease in the level of consciousness often associated with cerebral edema frequently requires intubation and mechanical ventilation. Intubation and mechanical ventilation can make it easier and safer to manage pain, anxiety, and agitation because respiratory depression associated with pharmacological interventions is not a concern. Great care should be taken during intubation to avoid precipitous drops in blood pressure, which could worsen cerebral perfusion in the presence of elevated ICP. Propofol, in particular, can be associated with hypotension if not used judiciously during intubation (Mace, 2008). Continuous intravenous infusion of anxiolytics, amnestic agents such as propofol, and opioids can be helpful for the management of increased ICP, whereas other treatments are aimed at decreasing the edema (Finley Caulfield & Wijman, 2008). Stepwise protocols, originally designed for the management of traumatic brain injury, have been successfully applied to the management of cerebral edema after stroke. ICP monitoring has been routinely use for decades, but aggressive control of elevated ICP has not led to uniformly beneficial results. Nonetheless, ICP monitoring has been used to guide medical therapy and assist with the timing of possible surgical interventions. Osmotic therapy remains the bulwark of treatment of cerebral edema because of its rapid mode of action. Mannitol has been used for the longest time, but hypertonic saline has been gaining in popularity. The mechanisms by which mannitol works are not completely understood. It may work by a combination of decreasing brain volume through decreasing water content, decreasing CSF through the decrease in water content, improving perfusion through decreasing viscosity, and possibly acting as a neuroprotectant (Rabinstein, 2006).

Hypertonic saline in concentrations ranging from 2% to 23.5% is gaining in support as an osmotic diuretic with studies suggesting that it may be superior to mannitol (Mortazavi et al., 2012; Suarez, 2004). Hypertonic saline is believed to work by dehydrating brain tissue, reducing viscosity, increasing plasma tonicity, increasing regional brain tissue perfusion, diminishing inflammatory response to brain injury, and restoring normal membrane potentials (Suarez, 2004). Care of the patient receiving osmotic therapy requires vigilant monitoring of electrolytes and fluid balance. Fluid restriction has not been shown to directly affect cerebral edema and is to be avoided because of the potential for inducing hypotension and worsening the ischemic deficit. Controversy exists regarding the ideal level of blood carbon dioxide in the management of cerebral edema. In past years, hyperventilation was routinely used to maintain constant hypocarbia at around 25 mm Hg, but studies found that this practice was associated with cerebral vasoconstriction and increase in the size of the infarct (Broderick et al., 2007). More recently, laboratory investigations using animal models are studying permissive hypercarbia in neurological injury (Brambrink & Orfanakis, 2010; Glass, Fabian, Schweitzer, Weinberg, & Proctor, 2001). However, current best practices for the management of cerebral edema recommend maintenance of carbon dioxide levels in the normal range of 35 to 45 mm Hg for the stroke population. Induced hypothermia is also under investigation for the treatment of stroke-associated cerebral edema. Although various studies have reported encouraging preliminary results, larger trials are indicated because the therapy is not without risks or complications (De Georgia et al., 2004; Schwab et al., 2001).

Some subpopulations of patients require surgical intervention. For those with cerebellar lesions which are causing obstructive hydrocephalus, surgery is lifesaving. However, there is very limited research regarding the optimal management of patients with cerebellar infarct (Jensen & St. Louis, 2005). For patients with large MCA infarcts who are experiencing rapid neurological deterioration, decompressive hemicraniectomy should be considered. Several recent studies (e.g., DESTINY, HAMLET, and DECIMAL) have indicated that there is value in this procedure (Vahedi et al., 2007). However, the North American HEADFIRST trial, in which surgery was performed later in the course of the patient's illness, failed to show improved outcomes. Thus, the optimal timing of surgery is not yet known. As providers discuss prognosis with patients and families, it is vital to give serious consideration to the likelihood that increased survival is also associated with the increased likelihood of significant disability because of the severity of the underlying stroke.

The most common form of ICP monitoring currently involves the placement of a catheter, which can also be used for CSF drainage as a way of treating elevated ICP. Although the measuring of ICP is helpful, other modalities have been developed to look at other physiological parameters, which can impact cerebral edema. There are devices available which continuously monitor brain temperature, brain tissue oxygenation, and the biochemical milieu of brain parenchyma. These have initially been used in patients who have experienced traumatic brain injury, but their use is expanding into other neurological patient populations (Singh & Edwards, 2013). It is still not clear if more intensive monitoring correlates with improved patient outcomes in stroke patients (Dhawan & DeGeorgia, 2012).

Regardless of which therapeutic interventions are required for an individual patient, no treatment should be withdrawn abruptly. Medications should be weaned very slowly with close monitoring for worsening of the patient's condition. Mechanical ventilation should be carefully adjusted, as needed. If therapeutic hypothermia has been used, the patient should be gradually rewarmed, with close monitoring for indications of neurological deterioration (Diringer & Edwards, 2001). The clinical team should continue monitoring the ICP and other modalities in use to ensure that the patient is responding favorably to less intense treatment.

Given the likelihood of long-term disabilities associated with large-volume strokes, there are many studies underway that approach the issue from different perspectives. Some investigators are looking at early interventions designed to minimize the size of the initial stroke, whereas others are examining optimizing the timing of interventions by either improving monitoring techniques or developing new ones. Still, others are looking at ways to repair the damage wrought by the stroke by helping the body reverse the damage (Singh & Edwards, 2013). Most of these studies are in the very early stages of data collection. Ideally, given the morbidity and mortality associated with cerebral edema, all stroke patients at risk for this complication should be afforded the opportunity to participate in clinical trials.

Best Practices

As noted earlier, the unstable stroke patient is best managed in a NICU staffed by dedicated neurointensivists. Stroke patients outside of the ICU who are in the poststroke time frame, when they may still be at risk for the development of cerebral edema, are best managed by a dedicated stroke service (Jauch et al., 2013). Steroids have no role in the treatment of cerebral edema associated with stroke (Rabinstein, 2006). Hyperosmolar therapy remains a mainstay of treatment but requires appropriate monitoring modalities and gradual withdrawal once the clinical team feels that the patient no longer requires it (Rabinstein, 2006; Suarez, 2004). However, studies have not shown a clear link between the use of hyperosmolar therapy and improved long-term outcomes (Zazulia, 2009). ICP monitoring and drainage of CSF to relieve pressure remain mainstays of therapy. It remains controversial whether their use is associated with improved long-term outcomes (Jha, 2003). Mechanically ventilated patients should have their carbon dioxide levels maintained in the normal range of 35 to 45 mm Hg (Rabinstein, 2006). Hemicraniectomy is a valid treatment option for patients with life-threatening cerebral edema (Vahedi et al., 2007). Induced hypothermia is a promising therapy, which requires further study (Diringer & Edwards, 2001). Ongoing discussions about goals of care are integral to the management of the stroke patient with cerebral edema given the significant morbidity and mortality associated with its development. More studies to determine optimal management of cerebral edema in stroke patients are required (Singh & Edwards, 2013).

Evaluation

It is important to maintain a high index of suspicion for the development of cerebral edema in the first days or weeks after stroke. Should the patient develop cerebral edema, serial neurological examinations are used to evaluate the response to therapies, which are added in a step wise fashion. Serial neurological examinations coupled with normalization of data from various monitoring modalities show improvement. Once this occurs, therapies are withdrawn through a weaning process to ensure the patient no longer requires the interventions. Even with maximal medical therapy, some patients, particularly those with massive MCA infarctions, larger intraparenchymal hemorrhages, or the higher grades of SAH, will deteriorate, and the goals of therapy will switch to end-of-life care.

Clinical Pearl: A global change in the neurological examination such as deterioration from being completely intact to mildly confused, although it may herald cerebral edema, should also prompt evaluation of factors such as oxygenation, serum sodium, serum glucose, and body temperature which can lead to neurological compromise. Young patients who have a large stroke or SAH are at risk for developing cerebral edema and should ideally be transferred to a facility that has the ability for neurosurgical intervention in case the need arises.

ACUTE HYPERTENSIVE RESPONSE

An acute hypertensive response is defined by a systolic blood pressure (SBP) of 140 mm Hg or greater or a diastolic blood pressure of 90 mm Hg or greater in at least two recordings taken 5 minutes apart but within 24 hours of stroke symptom onset (Qureshi, 2008). This elevation of blood pressure (BP) occurs in about 75% of patients with ischemic stroke and in more than 80% of patients with ICH. Hypertensive response is independently associated with poor functional outcomes (Whitworth, 2003).

Because hypertension is a major risk factor for stroke, and many stroke patients have a past medical history of hypertension, it is usually difficult to distinguish inadequately treated or undetected chronic hypertension from acute hypertensive response in stroke. Distinct patterns, which suggest acute hypertensive response, include a reduction in the initial BP over a few days after admission without antihypertensive agents, or an initial requirement for more than one antihypertensive agent in the first few weeks post stroke followed by hypotensive events requiring rapid decreases in the patient's medication regimen. The SBP will usually trend down to normal or near normal values after vessel recanalization in patients with known ischemic stroke, strongly suggesting that there are mechanisms specific to acute stroke that cause an acute hypertensive response in stroke patients (Qureshi, 2008).

Pathophysiology

Depending on the area of a stroke, death of brain cells in areas of the brain involved in the regulation of cardiovascular function can occur. Cardiovascular functions affected can include heart rate and BP regulation. In both cerebral hemispheres, inhibitory and excitatory input is provided by the prefrontal and insular cortices. This input then connects to the nuclei in the brainstem. In addition to the brainstem, the cingulated cortex, amygdala, and hypothalamus also provide modulation of inhibitory and excitatory input (Nason & Mason, 2004). Because of the widespread distribution of these modulation areas, most stroke lesions involve these areas to a certain extent, which leads to a disruption in autoregulation of BP. The widespread nature of cardiovascular function control in the brain is also supported by studies reporting that irrespective of the location of cerebral ischemia, stroke patients showed a parasympathetic cardiac deficit. In addition, patients with a right-sided stroke have increased sympathetic cardiac activity (Dütsch, Burger, Dörfler, Schwab, & Hilz, 2007). These findings place stroke patients at an increased risk for cardiac arrhythmia and other cardiovascular events. For example, patients who present with SAH or ICH have a high risk of increased ICP, particularly in the presence of brainstem compression. This increase in ICP is associated with an increase in systemic BP. However, this increase in BP does not automatically resolve with treatment of the ICP, and instead, BP slowly trends down with resolution of mass effect or cerebral edema. This further supports evidence that the primary cause of an acute hypertensive response results from damage or compression of specific cerebral regions that mediate autonomic cardiovascular control.

Assessment and Diagnosis

⊙ In the setting of acute stroke, management of acute hypertensive responses is generally guided by evidence-based policies or protocols developed by the facility. BP can be monitored adequately with an inflatable cuff in most patients with acute hypertensive response. However, for patients with ICH or SAH, those who require frequent titration of medications, or those with deteriorating neurological status, intra-arterial monitoring should be considered for more accurate and timely measurement of BP. In patients with a suspected increased ICP, ICP monitoring may be necessary to monitor and manage cerebral perfusion pressure during systemic BP lowering. Patients with a decreased level of consciousness, midline shift, or compression of basal cisterns on computed tomography (CT) scan may also be considered for ICP monitoring. Although some acute care hospitals allow use of intra-arterial monitoring of BP and titration of some vasoactive medications in noncritical care settings, ICP monitoring requires an intensive care unit setting, preferably one which specializes in the care of neuroscience patients.

If the patient received thrombolytic therapy with tissue plasminogen activator (tPA), there are specific guidelines regarding how often vital signs including BP should be checked in addition to titration goals for BP management. Hypertension greater than 185/110 mm Hg in the first 24 hours after intravenous (IV) tPA administration for ischemic stroke is associated with higher rates of cerebral hemorrhage. Frequent vital sign and neurological assessments are necessary because of the risk of rapid neurological and vital sign changes. Current recommendations for patients treated with tPA are to check vital signs including BP every 15 minutes for 2 hours, then every 30 minutes for 6 hours, and then every 60 minutes for 16 hours for a total of 24 hours (Jauch et al., 2013).

⊙ Nurses are vital for assessing and monitoring of vital signs because they are the frontline providers and can quickly detect any changes or trends in vital signs that require intervention. Nurses who provide routine care for stroke patients should be trained in detailed neurological assessment including standardized scales such as the National Institutes of Health Stroke Scale. The scales assist in objectively quantifying changes in neurological status and prime the nurse and provider into action based on these neurological changes. Because increased BP is a common occurrence in stroke patients, the nurse should consistently be evaluating whether the elevated BP is physiological due to acute stroke or due to stroke complications such as hypoxia, increased ICP due to hemorrhagic transformation of an ischemic infarct or herniation due to cerebral edema, or pain. Although patients usually have an IV antihypertensive medication as needed (PRN) order as part of a protocol order set, it may be necessary to notify the medical provider if there is consistent use of a PRN antihypertensive medication in order to control BP that remains elevated above set targeted goals. The interprofessional team caring for the patient should clarify on daily rounds the point at which a physician or advanced practice provider should be made aware of the use of PRN antihypertensive agents.

When assisting a patient out of bed for the first time after stroke, the nurse should check vital signs because some patients may have an orthostatic response (e.g., rapid drop in BP on arising) as a result of being immobilized on bed rest. The use of beta-blockers such as labetalol for SBP control also puts patients at increased risk for orthostatic hypotension. If a patient becomes acutely hypotensive due to orthostatic hypotension, which is not immediately recognized or appropriately managed, it can exacerbate neurological deficits due to ischemia and extension of the stroke or due to damage to the viable tissue surrounding the area of ischemia.

Treatment

Treatment of acute hypertensive responses vary depending on the type of stroke and clinical picture of the patient. The different subpopulations of patients are further addressed in the following texts.

Patients with acute ischemic stroke: The area of injury in ischemic stroke can be divided into different regions depending on the risk for further damage. First, there is a region of severe reduction in blood flow referred to as the *core*; there is also an area of moderate reduction in blood flow referred to as the *penumbra* (Qureshi, 2008). The penumbra has viable brain cells due to sustained blood flow via collateral blood vessels. However, because of impaired autoregulation in the area of injury, this area is vulnerable to further ischemic injury with systemic BP reduction. This is because a decrease in systemic BP *and* cerebral perfusion pressure result in a reduction in blood flow. The greatest risk, however, is not just a drop in BP for ischemic stroke patients, but more importantly, it is the wide fluctuations in BP within the first few hours after the stroke due to the impaired autoregulation around the area of ischemia that causes an expansion of area of infarct. Current recommendations are against routine lowering of BP in acute ischemic stroke unless it repeatedly exceeds 220 mm Hg SBP or 120 mm Hg diastolic BP in the acute period (Jauch et al., 2013).

Patients with acute ischemic stroke receiving thrombolytic therapy: The acute hypertensive response among patients with ischemic stroke receiving thrombolytic therapy is frequently transient and usually resolves with recanalization of the affected blood vessel. However, these patients will usually need reduction in their BP prior to infusion of thrombolytic therapy because significantly elevated BP has been associated with an increased risk of ICH. Current stroke guidelines recommend the reduction of BP to the thresholds used for inclusion in the The National Institute of Neurological Disorders and Stroke rt-PA (NINDS rt-PA) Stroke Study Group efficacy trial before thrombolytic therapy is administered. In that trial, treatment of hypertension to less than 185/110 mm Hg did not adversely affect functional outcomes at 90 days ("Tissue Plasminogen Activator for Acute Ischemic Stroke," 1995).

Patients with ICH: About one third of patients presenting with ICH continue to demonstrate hematoma expansion with subsequent deterioration in the first few hours after onset of stroke symptoms, making BP control vital to reduce risk of hematoma expansion or rebleeding (Qureshi, 2008). An initial SBP greater than 150 mm Hg is associated with hematoma expansion and increased mortality among patients with ICH (Ohwaki et al., 2004).

Rapid reduction of BP in ICH patients is well tolerated likely because of reduced metabolism and preserved autoregulation in the perihematoma region unlike the disruption in autoregulation that occurs around the area of injury in ischemic stroke. The current guidelines recommend that for patients with SBP greater than 200 mm Hg or a mean arterial pressure (MAP) greater than 150 mm Hg, aggressive reduction in BP should be pursued using a continuous IV infusion of an antihypertensive agent with frequent BP monitoring. For those patients presenting with SBP greater than 180 mm Hg or MAP greater than 130 mm Hg and elevated ICP, consider reducing BP using intermittent or continuous infusion of medication while maintaining cerebral perfusion pressure greater than 60 mm Hg. If the patient presents with SBP greater than 180 mm Hg or MAP of greater than 130 mm Hg and no evidence of elevated ICP, then a modest reduction of BP (e.g., MAP of 110 mm Hg or target BP of 160/90 mm Hg) using intermittent or continuous IV medications to control BP is adequate (Morgenstern et al., 2010).

Patients with chronic hypertension: Chronic hypertension is a common diagnosis in stroke patients. Approximately 50% of patients who are admitted with a diagnosis of stroke have chronic hypertension requiring medication prior to admission (Qureshi, 2008). The abrupt discontinuation of antihypertensive medication to allow for permissive hypertension may lead to enhanced sympathetic activity, rebound hypertension, and a consequent increase in cardiovascular events in patients with coronary artery disease treated chronically on beta-blockers or those chronically on high doses of centrally acting drugs. The decision to continue or discontinue antihypertensive agents must be made on a case-by-case basis with the intent to avoid hypotension, excessive hypertension past SBP of 220 mm Hg, and myocardial ischemia, all of which can worsen neurological status resulting in prolonged hospitalization and adverse functional outcome. What may be less stressful to patients with cardiovascular disease is a reduction in the dose of the current agent or a change to a short-acting IV antihypertensive agent.

Patients with SAH: Most patients with aneurysmal SAH present with acute hypertensive response requiring IV infusion of antihypertensives prior to securing the aneurysm either by clipping or coiling procedures. About 4% to 17% of SAH patients will have a sudden episode of worsening neurological status that is suggestive of rebleeding within the first 12 hours of admission (Fujii et al., 1996; Ohkuma, Tsurutani, & Suzuki, 2001). Due to this risk of rebleeding, it is vital to control the BP to an SBP of less than 150 mm Hg (Ohwaki et al., 2004). Once the aneurysm has been secured, BP parameters can be liberalized even up to 200 mm Hg to allow for higher cerebral perfusion pressures. The higher cerebral perfusion pressure is vital especially for patient who have symptomatic cerebral vasospasm because the higher perfusion pressures can prevent secondary cerebral ischemia. The cerebral perfusion pressure is usually augmented using IV fluid boluses or high-volume infusions of IV fluids. No randomized trials of this intervention have been completed. However, clinical observations have revealed a rapid improvement in the neurological examination in many patients with this intervention and worsening when it is stopped prematurely (Connolly et al., 2012).

Best Practices

In patients with ICH, whose BP is not well managed with oral antihypertensive, continuous infusion of an antihypertensive agent should be used until the BP is controlled; once controlled, the patient can then be carefully transitioned to oral antihypertensives. In patients with ischemic stroke, continuous infusions of antihypertensive agents are rarely used for BP control to avoid quick reduction in BP and potentially resulting in worse neurological deficits. Practitioners are most likely to use a continuous infusion for BP control in ischemic stroke when the SBP is persistently elevated over 185 mm Hg in a patient who is eligible for thrombolytic therapy because there is need to control BP for thrombolytic therapy infusion to avoid ICH. The most common drug chosen for infusion is nicardipine because it has a rapid onset and short duration of action to allow for precise titration by the nurse at the bedside.

Based on the Joint National Committee (JNC) 8 recommendations, a targeted goal of a normal BP of less than 140/90 mm Hg for patients with diabetes mellitus or chronic kidney disease is reasonable after the acute stroke period. For the general population aged 59 years and younger, goal SBP is less than 140 mm Hg, whereas for those patients 60 years and older, the goal SBP is less than 150 mm Hg (James et al., 2014). Oral hypertensive agents can be initiated at 24 to 48 hours after symptom onset because most of the acute processes, such as risk to the ischemic penumbra and hematoma expansion, are uncommon after the first 24 hours. However, for some patients, permissive hypertension past an SBP of 140 mm Hg may be required even up to a week after acute stroke depending on neurological stability. The JNC 8 report does not address acute stroke management of BP; however, previous versions addressed this. The JNC 7 report recommended that the BP be maintained at intermediate levels (around 160/100 mm Hg) until neurological stability is achieved (Chobanian et al., 2003). The American Heart Association agrees that some patients may need higher BPs in the immediate period postischemic stroke with current recommendations to individualize therapy based on patient stability (Jauch et al., 2013). Special consideration includes patients with bilateral severe carotid stenosis, who may bear a high risk for stroke with aggressive BP lowering until carotid revascularization is performed. Other complications of stroke such as elevated ICP, progressive cerebral edema, ongoing cerebral ischemia due to occlusive vessel disease or symptomatic cerebral vasospasm, and postoperative cerebral changes require individualized management. When neurological stability is achieved, it is vital to pursue aggressive BP treatment to appropriate goal for secondary prevention of recurrent stroke because long-term benefits are noted in persons with and without a history of hypertension.

There is evidence that mortality is greater among patients in whom beta-blocker therapy is begun within 48 hours of symptom onset of stroke (Barer, Cruickshank, Ebrahim, & Mitchell, 1988). There is also evidence that long-term beta-blockers do not reduce risk of stroke and should not be used as first-line treatment for hypertension management. Thus, unless a patient has underlying cardiovascular disease, a beta-blocker should not be the first-line treatment for reducing BP (Wiysonge et al., 2007).

Traditionally, hemodynamic manipulation to allow for higher cerebral perfusion pressures has consisted of hemodilution, hypervolemia, and hypertensive therapy referred to as *triple-H therapy*. The focus now has shifted away from triple-H therapy to the maintenance of euvolemia and induced hypertension in select cases of symptomatic vasospasm (Connolly et al., 2012).

The American Heart Association/American Stroke Association (AHA/ASA) has published guidelines on how to manage stroke patients. Please see Chapters 6 to 8 on ischemic stroke, hemorrhagic stroke, and SAH for specific recommendations from these guidelines.

Evaluation

Ongoing evaluation of BP continues throughout the hospitalization. The primary care provider (PCP) is vital postdischarge for ongoing monitoring and management of BP. Medication regimens that include a once-a-day medication, or at most, twice-a-day regimen, are the most conducive to compliance by the patient. Every stroke patient should be evaluated by the PCP within a week to 2 weeks after discharge from an acute setting to ensure that no new stroke complications have occurred after discharge and to continue titration of antihypertensive therapy to the targeted goal BP.

The patient with hypertension should be encouraged to check his or her own BP routinely at home and keep a log that is reviewed with the provider to ensure that the BP goal is being maintained. Other secondary conditions such as obstructive sleep apnea should be considered in patients with chronic hypertension because there is evidence that sleep apnea is associated with an increased risk of stroke (Redline et al., 2010). Furthermore, use of continuous positive airway pressure (CPAP) for management of sleep apnea may be indicated to support BP control.

Clinical Pearl: Transition of care plays a critical role in the long-term clinical outcomes for patients and, when done well, can be significant in reducing readmission rates. Communication with the patient's PCP regarding hospital course and plans for long-term specialty care contributes to well-thought-out transition of care. Medication regimens that include a once-a-day medication, or at most, twice-a-day regimen, are the most conducive to compliance by the patient. It is often useful to preemptively assure male patients with hypertension that should they experience sexual dysfunction due to an antihypertensive agent, this is reversible and can be managed by switching to a different antihypertensive agent. This approach is important because if symptoms are experienced before this discussion, patients are likely to be noncompliant in the future for fear of medication side effects.

POSTSTROKE SEIZURES

Stroke is the most common cause of seizures and epilepsy in the elderly (Stefan & Theodore, 2012). Poststroke seizures occur in about 10% of the patients. There is a greater risk of seizures in patient with hemorrhagic stroke compared to ischemic stroke (Burneo, Fang, & Saposnik, 2010). Poststroke seizures are associated with poor functional outcome, higher mortality at 30 days and 1 year, longer hospitalization, and greater disability at discharge (Burneo et al., 2010). A higher rate in hospital mortality has also been associated with poststroke seizures (Vernino et al., 2003). This is likely related to worsening of preexisting neurological deficits at the time of seizure onset. This worsened clinical status can last anywhere from a week to several months (Hankey, 1993).

Patients with late-onset or remote symptomatic seizure are at highest risk of developing epilepsy than those with early-onset seizures. Although a small number of stroke patients actually develop epilepsy, studies have shown that late-onset seizures post stroke is an independent risk factor for the subsequent development of epilepsy. More than half of those patients with late-onset seizures develop epilepsy (Bladin et al., 2000). Risk factors for poststroke seizures include presence of cortical lesions (Bladin et al., 2000), large lesions involving more than one lobe or an entire lobe (Kilpatrick et al., 1990), male gender (Giroud et al., 1994), and lesions from cardioembolic phenomenon because this etiology tends to involve more than one lobe as well (Kilpatrick et al., 1990).

Pathophysiology

In those patients with ischemic strokes, early-onset seizures can be the result of regional metabolic dysfunction and neurotransmitter release secondary to ischemic hypoxia. Acute ischemia causes increased extracellular concentrations of glutamate. This is an excitatory neurotransmitter that may result in secondary neuronal injury particularly in the ischemic penumbra resulting in epileptogenic potential (Camilo & Goldstein, 2004). Other metabolic derangements at the time of stroke onset can increase the risk of forming an area of epileptogenic focus. Experimental models have demonstrated that hyperglycemia and alterations in sodium or calcium levels enhance the development of seizures (Uchino, Smith, Bengzon, Lundgren, & Siesjö, 1996). The ischemic penumbra may contain electrically irritable tissues that provide a focus for seizure activity. Thus, the size of ischemic penumbra also plays a potential role in the development of seizures. Studies have shown a correlation between the total amount and duration of depolarizing events with the penumbra size in ischemic stroke (Back, Ginsberg, Dietrich, & Watson, 1996; Camilo & Goldstein, 2004).

Contrary to early-onset poststroke seizures, late-onset seizures are most likely caused by structural changes to the brain tissue such as the formation of gliosis in the area of an old ischemic injury and the development of intracerebral scar tissue (Jennett, 1978). Poststroke changes to cell membranes and the subsequent development of collaterals during stroke recovery may also lead to the development of hyperexcitability of those areas, which leads to an epileptic focus that can then lead to seizures (Stefan & Theodore, 2012). In ICH and SAH, the cause of seizures is likely related to the presence of neurotoxic agents such as red blood cells and iron (Chusid & Kopeloff, 1962; Willmore, Sypert, & Munson, 1978). Late-onset seizures have a similar frequency in ischemic stroke and ICH, further suggesting a structural reason for seizures as that one provided by gliotic scarring (Jennett, 1978; Stefan & Theodore, 2012).

Assessment and Diagnosis

Seizure presentation can be clinical, in which case seizure activity is observed by providers or family. Presentation of seizures can also be subclinical, in which case the patient may have nonspecific physical assessment finding that prompts initiation of electroencephalographic (EEG) monitoring which then confirms seizure activity electrographically. Most often, EEG changes after stroke are nonspecific. However, when changes are present post stroke, they tend to be focal, especially in ischemic stroke, where there is usually focal slowing of EEG activity in the area of injury, loss of normal background activity, and reduction of overall amplitude (Cheung, Tsoi, Au-Yeung, & Tang, 2003). In ICH, slowing is not only focal but can also be diffuse or multifocal if vasospasm is present, which is often the case with SAH (Laino, 2007). Other possible findings include periodic lateralizing epileptiform discharges (PLEDs) and sharp activity and frontal intermittent delta activity (FIRDA) (Horner, Ni, Duft, Niederkorn, & Lechner, 1995; Niedzielska et al., 2001). The presence of PLEDs is usually indicative of recent infarction and has been associated with watershed infarcts (De Reuck, Goethals, Claeys, Van Maele, & De Clerck, 2006; Stefan & Theodore, 2012).

The registered nurse (RN) is vital in identifying subtle neurological changes to the patient's assessment, which may clue the interprofessional team that the patient may be having a waxing and waning neurological examination typical of seizure activity. The RN staff is also instrumental in keeping the patient safe should actual clinical seizures occur because many facilities have a protocol or plan of care related to seizure patients. This plan of care may involve padding bed rails and having the patient ambulate with assistance. The poststroke patient usually is admitted to a dedicated neuroscience unit with a neurologist directing his or her care. However, for those facilities without a dedicated neuroscience unit, collaboration with a neurologist may be warranted for assistance in identifying the appropriate therapy for the patient. Collaboration with the pharmacist is also vital to make sure of the selection of an appropriate pharmacotherapy agent with less side effects and interactions with other medications.

Treatment

There are no specific guidelines addressing the management of poststroke seizures because most of the studies addressing this condition have been observational or prospective studies. Most recommendations for the treatment of poststroke seizures are currently based on expert opinion or on consensus based on the available observational studies. The prophylactic initiation of anticonvulsants for patients with stroke who have not had a seizure is not recommended (European Stroke Organisation [ESO] Executive Committee & ESO Writing Committee, 2008; Stefan & Theodore, 2012). If a patient should have a poststroke seizure, there continues to be varying recommendations regarding how to manage the patient after that first seizure in the acute setting. Some experts recommend that in the case of a first time acute seizure onset, other causes of seizures should be ruled out; treatment should only be instituted if the patient has a second seizure or if the first seizure was prolonged or the patient was in status epilepticus with that first occurrence (Abbott, Bladin, & Donnan, 2001). However, given evidence of worse functional outcomes for patients with seizures, other experts recommend that once other causes of seizures have been ruled out, treatment with antiepileptic drugs (AEDs) should be started. This is because even if the occurrence was a first time seizure for the patient, the patient remains at increased risk of both status epilepticus and remote seizures as compared to other stroke patient (Ferro & Pinto, 2004).

Patients who develop status epilepticus should be appropriately treated with AEDs to be continued at discharge from the hospital. Although patients who develop epilepsy post stroke most often have a favorable outcome in terms of seizure freedom with monotherapy, a referral to a neurologist should be initiated for continued management postdischarge because treatment with AEDs does not reduce the risk of recurrent seizures after stopping AEDs (Gilad, Lampl, Eschel, & Sadeh, 2001; Stephen & Brodie, 2000).

Gabapentin and lamotrigine have the most efficacy and effectiveness as initial monotherapy for treatment of poststroke seizures in the elderly with partial seizures (Glauser et al., 2006). A study conducted by the Veterans Affairs (VA) confirmed this finding as well as with patient tolerance. Gabapentin and lamotrigine worked well as compared to carbamazepine (Rowan et al., 2005). Arif et al. (2010) retrospectively looked at effectiveness of AEDs in older adults with epilepsy, and they found that lamotrigine had the highest 12-month retention rate at 79%; levetiracetam, 73%; carbamazepine, 48%; gabapentin, 59%; oxcarbazepine, 24%; phenytoin, 59%; and topiramate 56%. Thus, first-line pharmacotherapies for poststroke seizures are lamotrigine, levetiracetam, and gabapentin (Arif et al., 2010).

Best Practices

◉ EEG, although very helpful in the diagnosis of seizures and epilepsy, does not rule out the presence of epilepsy if the results of testing are negative. It is always important for the interprofessional team to integrate clinical and assessment findings when making the decision about treatment or diagnosis of seizures. Before starting AEDs, the team should weigh the risk of anticonvulsant therapy with the individual patient especially as many will be elderly and particularly susceptible to drug reactions and interactions (Stephen & Brodie, 2000). Interaction with warfarin should especially be considered because many stroke patients are receiving warfarin for treatment of atrial fibrillation or other cardiovascular conditions. Drugs with a better tolerability profile and a favorable drug interaction profile may be more ideal especially for the elderly. Once-daily dosing can help to improve compliance as well. Newer agents may have improved tolerability profiles, but they may be most costly and thus could limit their use. It is also important to remember that medications such as carbamazepine and phenytoin which are classified as enzyme inducers have the potential to increase cardiovascular and cerebrovascular disease risk because they are potent inducers of the cytochrome P450 enzymes, which are involved in cholesterol synthesis (Mintzer & Mattson, 2009).

Evaluation

Ongoing monitoring for seizures is important for patients who have poststroke seizures, most especially as they recover and undergo community reintegration post stroke. If the patient had an acute seizure post stroke and treatment was initiated, then he or she may need to be reevaluated to determine if it is appropriate to wean off AEDs once he or she has advanced in his or her recovery. The patient who has seizures post stroke will also need monitoring by a neurologist to ensure a seizure-free period before he or she is permitted to drive again because many states have laws regarding how seizure patients use their privilege to drive. If patients are on other cytochrome P450 inducers, they may need ongoing monitoring for lipids and liver functions tests to ensure stability and tolerance of medical therapy.

Clinical Pearl: Patients who have a gaze preference or deviation on initial physical assessment after stroke should be evaluated for seizures if the gaze preference changes to the opposite side. This is usually informally referred to as wrong-way eyes. This is because when a patient has a stroke, the eyes look toward the side of the lesion. When a patient has a seizure, the eyes look away from the side of the lesion.

In the United States, there are laws related to people with seizures being able to drive while under treatment. Providers should be aware of the laws in their states so that they can help protect the public and advocate for their patients as well.

FEVER AND STROKE

Body temperature above 37.5°C is associated with a worse outcome and prognosis following acute stroke. Fever control is an important aspect of stroke patient care. Multiple retrospective studies published in the late 1990s and early 2000s confirmed experimental data linking fever, especially early in the course of acute stroke, to poorer outcomes (Hajat, Hajat, & Sharma, 2000; Phipps, Desai, Wira, & Bravata, 2011). Studies have demonstrated that close to 50% of patients will develop fever after acute stroke often from systemic infection. Patients who have experienced aneurysmal SAH are at higher risk for fever when there is intraventricular extension of the blood or a poorer overall clinical grade (Fernandez et al., 2007). Fever in stroke patients may result from infection, central fever from the stroke itself, side effects of medications, or a combination of factors. Early fever after stroke may be an indicator of the cause of the stroke such as infective endocarditis or of systemic infection such as urinary tract infection or early pneumonia (Jauch et al., 2013). Sinusitis from nasogastric tubes or naso- or oroendotracheal tubes should not be overlooked as a cause of fever (Aggarwarl, Azim, Baronia, & Kumar, 2012).

Patients at higher risk for infection and subsequent fever after stroke are older, have higher National Institutes of Health Stroke Scale (NIHSS) scores, and have a large-volume infarct. Pneumonia occurs in up to 22% of stroke patients and is the most common cause of death (Coplin, 2012; Wartenberg et al., 2011). Fever accelerates injury and normothermia preserves tissue; each 1-degree elevation in temperature on the Celsius scale raises the basal metabolic rate by 6% to 7%. A common observation in patients with neurological injury is that fever worsens the observed neurological examination, whereas control of fever improves it. One study reported a 3-month mortality rate of 1% in a normothermic group of stroke patients and a rate of 16% in the febrile group (Andrews et al., 2002). Fever in the neuroscience population has been shown to extend ICU stay and raise hospital costs (Diringer, Reaven, Funk, & Uman, 2004; Reaven, Lovett, & Funk, 2009).

Pathophysiology

Fever has been defined as an adaptive complex, coordinated autonomic, neuroendocrine, and behavioral response, which is often part of the acute-phase reaction to an immune challenge from both infectious and noninfectious causes (Saper & Breder, 1994). The mechanisms associated with fever's detrimental effect are thought to be the increase in metabolic demand, free radical production, and an increase in excitatory neurotransmitters. Reversing fever has been shown to cause multiple favorable cellular responses. Normothermia or hypothermia is associated with decreased release of the excitatory neurotransmitters glutamate and glycine, decrease release of calcium, decreased formation of free radicals, and decrease in AMPA-related delayed excitotoxic injury. This translates clinically into decreased cerebral metabolic rate and oxygen demand, decreased carbon dioxide production, and decreased ICP. The first concern in a hospitalized stroke patient with fever should be the development of acute infection, but noninfectious causes should simultaneously be considered.

Assessment and Diagnosis

◉ The bedside RN monitors serial temperatures and looks for subtle global changes in the neurological examination. Patients with more severe strokes would likely benefit from continuous rather than from intermittent temperature monitoring to enable more intensive management of impending fever. Continuous monitoring includes the ability to alert the nurse when a parameter is exceeded, allowing for more timely interventions. For stroke patients not admitted to the ICU, intermittent temperature monitoring should occur at least every 2 hours in the initial few weeks after stroke and whenever a change in patient status raises concern for fever as a contributing factor. The clinical team collectively and regularly assesses for adventitious breath sounds; monitors closely for signs of aspiration; inspects indwelling device sites for signs of inflammation, infection, or the development of skin breakdown; and assesses urine for signs of infection such as cloudiness or malodor. The interprofessional team monitors for evidence of leukocytosis and thrombocytosis with complete blood counts. Such clinical indications of infection should lead to a fever workup including pan cultures and possibly a chest radiograph. Serial chest radiographs to monitor for development, progression, and resolution of infiltrates or atelectasis can be ordered. Noninfectious causes of fever such as acute pulmonary embolism (PE), acute myocardial infarction (MI), acute pancreatitis, phlebitis, acute gout flare, or drug hypersensitivity reaction should be considered and ruled out, as appropriate. Based on medications which the patient may have recently received, neuroleptic malignant syndrome and malignant hyperthermia should also be considered.

Treatment

All methods of maintaining normothermia or inducing hypothermia are based on the principle that heat in the body is transferred from a higher to a lower temperature. The four methods of heat transfer are radiation, evaporation, conduction, and convection (Guyton & Hall, 2006). *Radiation* is the most passive method of heat transfer. Keep the environment cooler than the patient while avoiding shivering. *Evaporation* involves water on the skin evaporating and causing cooling as this occurs. Again, avoiding shivering is critical. *Conduction* involves the exchange of heat between two surfaces and is the principle underlying traditional cooling blankets. *Convection* involves the transfer of heat from a surface to a fluid and is the principle underlying intravascular cooling methods.

Surface cooling has always been an imperfect method of treating or avoiding fever. It is very difficult to achieve and maintain goal temperature. Shivering is a significant and difficult problem to manage; there is always concern about skin breakdown. Rewarming cannot be performed in a controlled manner, and it is very nursing labor intensive. Newer methods of surface cooling have been developed, which address these concerns and which can provide controlled cooling and rewarming (Mayer et al., 2004; Scaravilli, Tinchero, & Citerio, 2011). The difficulties inherent in these methods of cooling led to research into convection and the development of intravascular cooling devices. Intravascular cooling allows for rapid control of temperature with less shivering, maintenance of temperature in the desired range, controlled gradual rewarming, and is less nursing intensive.

Shivering, while a normal response attempts to induce hypothermia, is counterproductive in patients with neurological injury. It raises metabolic rate, increases oxygen consumption, and can lead to increased ICP (Mayer et al., 2004; Presciutti, Bader, & Hepburn, 2012). Attempts to control shivering often require increased sedation as well as the use of systemic paralytic agents. Deployment of these therapies increases the risk of pneumonia, increases time on mechanical ventilation, increases time in the ICU and interferes with neurological assessment, and places the patient at increased risk for critical illness myopathy or neuropathy (CIM or CIN). These are complications of critical illness seen in patients who have experienced severe multisystem organ dysfunction, often with sepsis (Kress & Hall, 2014). They are often seen in those who required prolonged use of IV paralytic agents. CIM and CIN present as muscle weakness and failure to wean from mechanical ventilation. Research is ongoing regarding the underlying cause; the diagnoses should be considered in patients experiencing difficulty in weaning with new bilateral weakness or paralysis (Ydemann, Eddelien, & Lauritsen, 2012). A simple bedside shivering assessment tool can be used to trend shivering in response to adjustments in therapies (Presciutti et al., 2012). Recommendations garnered from the available literature advocate for establishing and treating the underlying cause of the fever and the use of appropriate antipyretic measures (Gross, Sung, Weingart, & Smith, 2012; Jauch et al., 2013; O'Grady et al., 2008). However, consensus does not yet exist on optimal measures. It is not clear from studies if there is a definite improvement in long-term outcome if measures are taken to avoid fever through prophylactic use of either antipyretic medications or antibiotics.

⊙ If the patient is believed to be at high risk for hemorrhagic conversion of the stroke, some clinicians prefer the use of acetaminophen over ibuprofen or aspirin. Studies indicate that current antipyretic medications are only minimally effective, suggesting that escalation to other measures to manage fever should occur early in the course of management (Jauch et al., 2013). IV antipyretics have not been studied sufficiently to recommend routine use over available enteral forms of these medications (Coplin, 2012). Because there is data suggesting that acute stroke patients who are hypothermic on presentation have better outcomes, inducing normothermia or hypothermia with either surface or intravascular, cooling may be attempted. Great care must be taken with these methods to avoid shivering, which will only increase metabolic demand and hinder fever reduction. Ice packs and traditional cooling blankets have been shown to be ineffective and erratic in consistently reducing fever. Induced cooling is often very uncomfortable for the patient. Because it may require significant sedation and possibly intubation and mechanical ventilation to avoid shivering, induced hypothermia should only be undertaken in the ICU where the appropriate level of monitoring can occur. There is ongoing research, particularly in the area of inducing hypothermia, studying optimal temperature management post stroke (Coplin, 2012). When induced hypothermia is used as a therapy, the nurse and clinical team needs to be even more vigilant in monitoring for developing infections because fever will be suppressed. Aggressiveness in the treatment of fever should be tailored to the perceived risk of deterioration and worsened outcomes in specific patients.

⊙ Prevention of fever is the best method of avoiding the complications associated with fever in the stroke patient. Indwelling devices should be maintained, changed, or removed in accordance with institutional policies. Because pneumonia is the most likely infection in acute stroke, measures to prevent and combat pneumonia should be instituted. Several interventions can be implemented. The HOB should be maintained at 30 degrees or higher to prevent aspiration. Patients who are able to cough and deep breathe or participate in the use of incentive spirometry should be taught and encouraged to do so. Use of specialty beds which can provide rotation or chest physical therapy can be useful. Vest percussion to help loosen secretions can be helpful. If the patient is high risk for aspiration, nursing staff should scrupulously adhere to recommendations from speech therapy (ST). These recommendations include that meals adhere to the recommended consistency, liquids are appropriately thickened, and the patient either feeds himself or herself or is fed in the manner recommended by ST, which usually involves eating slowly and alternating small bites of food with small sips of liquids. Family members who wish to assist with feeding should be taught appropriate techniques and then monitored intermittently by the nurse to ensure they are consistently using the techniques.

Best Practices

Many national and international health care organizations have issued guidelines endorsing aggressive fever management in the neuroscience patient population. Pneumonia and urinary tract infections are the most common infections in stroke patients (Wartenberg et al., 2011). The use of the ventilator-associated pneumonia (VAP) bundle for prevention of pneumonia and compliance with standards on early removal of urinary catheters are supported in the literature (Institute for Healthcare Improvement, 2012). There are no widely accepted guidelines regarding frequency of obtaining cultures and chest radiographs for the evaluation of a new fever in a hospitalized patient. There is no agreement regarding the long-term benefits of inducing hypothermia in the acute stroke patient, although the success of the therapy with other patient populations is encouraging. Studies of the benefits of hypothermia are currently underway (Jauch et al., 2013).

Evaluation

Evaluation for fever is an ongoing process throughout the hospital stay of the stroke patient, although more frequent measurements of temperature and interventions to maintain normothermia are indicated in the first several days after acute stroke when it is most critical to protect ischemic tissue and hopefully limit the size of the infarct. The clinical team works together to implement therapies in a timely fashion and change therapy as indicated while monitoring closely for complications of therapy.

Clinical Pearl: Patients with drug-induced fever often look better clinically than patients with fever from an infectious cause. A diagnosis of drug-induced fever should be a diagnosis of exclusion, making sure that all other infectious etiologies have been well investigated first.

RESPIRATORY FAILURE AND STROKE

The incidence of respiratory failure associated with stroke varies, depending on the mechanisms underlying the stroke. The majority of patients who experience ischemic stroke will not require early intubation (Jauch et al., 2013). Patients at highest risk are those with a large-volume cerebral infarcts or infarctions involving the brainstem. Only 5% to 10% overall may require intubation, but up to 25% of those with ischemic MCA stroke may need intubation. The mortality rate for acute stroke patients requiring intubation is higher than seen in those who do not require intubation (Milhaud, Popp, Thouvenot, Heroum, & Bonafé, 2004; Santoli et al., 2001). Patients with ICH strokes have significantly higher rates of intubation and mechanical ventilation and significantly higher early mortality rates as well (Broderick et al., 2007; Towfighi, Greenberg, & Rosand, 2005). Patients who sustain an aneurysmal SAH may require intubation acutely, depending on the severity of the SAH, whereas others will only require it while undergoing the securing of the ruptured aneurysm (Seder & Mayer, 2009).

Unfortunately, emergent intubation and mechanical ventilation may be required before the likely stroke outcome is known or advanced directives have been addressed. Early and frequent discussions with family and patient, to the extent that the patient is able to participate, are critical in determining whether intubation will be part of maximal medical intervention or whether extubation and withdrawal of support will be more appropriate. Older patients who are comatose at the time of admission and intubated have the poorest outcomes even with aggressive therapy (Foerch, Kessler, Steckel, Steinmetz, & Sitzer, 2004). The reason for delayed intubation is often related to pneumonia from aspiration. Again, discussions with family and patient will determine whether the best course of action for that patient will encompass maximum therapy or if palliative care is more appropriate. The AHA/ASA has published guidelines on palliative and end-of-life care in stroke to guide practice (Holloway et al., 2014).

Development of acute respiratory distress syndrome (ARDS) is rare (2% to 4%) in acute ischemic stroke but is associated with higher mortality (Rincon et al., 2014). A recent study of patients with hemorrhagic stroke found a significantly higher incidence (25%) than was seen in ICH (Elmer et al., 2013), whereas another study found an incidence of approximately 27% in patients with SAH (Kahn et al., 2006).

◉ In some patients, it may be possible to manage airway problems in the short term with CPAP or bilevel positive airway pressure (BiPAP) and avoid intubation. Some studies have shown that stroke patients, especially those with cardiac or pulmonary disorders, are at high risk for developing hypoxemia in the days immediately following the stroke (Roffe et al., 2003; Sulter, Elting, Stewart, den Arend, & De Keyser, 2000). However, limited data exist about the use of supplemental oxygen in patients who have not demonstrated hypoxia through documented oxygen desaturations. Rather, the interprofessional clinical team, and in particular, the bedside nurse, should closely monitor the acute stroke patient for signs of partial airway obstruction, aspiration, incipient pneumonia, or the development of irregular breathing patterns, all of which can lead to hypoxia seen at the bedside as oxygen desaturation. *Incipient pneumonia* is based in a clinical judgment that a particular patient's difficulties with managing oral secretions, compromised ability to cough effectively, and impaired swallowing are beginning to manifest as abnormal breath sounds, subtle changes in respiratory effort, and low-grade fever which may herald a need to increase such measures as chest physiotherapy to avoid pneumonia. All members of the interprofessional team should be cognizant of applicable medical history such as the diagnoses of chronic obstructive pulmonary disease (COPD), congestive heart failure (CHF), or obstructive sleep apnea (OSA) (Jauch et al., 2013). If a patient arrives with the diagnosis of sleep apnea, he or she should be encouraged to use his or her home machine for management while hospitalized. If the patient has not been using a device, this should be discussed with the patient and family, and the importance of proper management of sleep apnea is stressed. If sleep apnea is noted in a patient not previously diagnosed, a sleep study and fitting of a proper device can be ordered. Given that sleep apnea is an independent risk factor for stroke, managing it properly is important for secondary prevention after stroke (Durgan & Bryan, 2012; Yaggi et al., 2005).

In patients in which intubation has resulted in placement of a tracheotomy tube, two considerations need to be addressed. The first is weaning from mechanical ventilation, and the second is weaning from the tracheostomy back to a natural airway. A study which investigated tracheostomy rates in patients with ischemic stroke found that less than 2% required a tracheostomy, but 33% of patients who underwent decompressive craniectomy required a tracheostomy (Walcott et al., 2014). The optimum timing for a tracheostomy in patients with acute ischemic or hemorrhagic stroke has not been well studied, but a large multicenter trial is underway (Bösel et al., 2013). Early tracheostomy is anecdotally favored for patient comfort and is associated with increased ease of weaning from mechanical ventilation.

Pathophysiology

Respiratory failure can result in both hypercapnia and hypoxemia, which can worsen stroke outcome by expanding ischemic injury and raising ICP. The three primary pathways leading to acute respiratory failure in acute ischemic stroke are disturbance of respiratory rhythm generation, interruption in descending respiratory pathways, or bulbar weakness leading to aspiration. If a patient has comorbidity such as OSA or COPD, is a current tobacco smoker, or is using illicit substances, he or she may develop respiratory failure earlier or more easily. Normal respirations are maintained by a balance of metabolic, autonomic, voluntary, and limbic inputs. The metabolic or autonomic pathways maintain acid–base balance and oxygenation. Lesions in the pons and medulla can disrupt these pathways leading to an inability to maintain adequate respirations particularly when the patient is sleeping. Impaired autonomic ventilatory control can be manifested in a variety of abnormal and inadequate breathing patterns. Apneustic and ataxic patterns of breathing require intubation in patients who are receiving aggressive medical therapy and may herald impending death in patients who are receiving palliative care.

The development of hiccups requires close monitoring because they may signal a medullary lesion and can be a precursor to the development of a pathologic breathing pattern. Primary central neurogenic hyperventilation is rare but problematic because of the resulting derangement in acid–base balance. Interruption of voluntary respiratory pathways can lead to respiratory apraxias such as the inability to cough voluntarily, initiate swallowing, or breath holding. Cheyne-Stokes respirations represent an alteration in voluntary control of breathing and can be seen in up to 50% of patients after unilateral supratentorial infarct but may also be seen in infratentorial infarct as well. **Table 9-1** shows the abnormal breathing patterns.

Such patients may require intubation to prevent episodic hypoxemia from compromising the ischemic penumbra and increasing the size of the infarct. Limbic or emotional respiration represents a descending pathway that preserves respiratory modulation to emotional stimuli including laughing, coughing, and anxiety. Patients with bulbar lesions are at increased risk for aspiration pneumonia because of a combination of impaired swallowing, abnormal respiratory patterns, reduced vital capacity, and reduced or absent triggering of the cough reflex. Pneumonia from a variety of pathogens is seen in approximately 20% of patients after acute stroke. Patients with ICH strokes are at high risk for respiratory failure given that they are more likely to have vomited at the time of stroke (Broderick et al., 2007). Patients with high-grade SAH may develop respiratory failure requiring intubation and mechanical ventilation for a variety of reasons, including poor neurological function, aspiration, or acute lung injury related to SAH (e.g., neurogenic pulmonary edema) (Davison, Terek, & Chawla, 2012; Seder & Mayer, 2009). Hypoxemia may worsen the effects of cerebral ischemia and should be avoided.

Assessment and Diagnosis

The initial assessment of patients with acute stroke will determine if they are at increased risk for respiratory failure. As noted earlier, some patients will be obviously distressed and require intubation at the scene or in the emergency department. The RN and other members of the interprofessional clinical team will need to collect an accurate clinical history, most often from records or from the patient's family, to determine if there are comorbidities and risk factors such as COPD, OSA, or use of tobacco or illicit substances. The NIHSS can be used to determine existence and severity of dysarthria. Dysarthria, which is often accompanied by dysphagia, indicates that the patient likely has difficulty managing secretions and is at high risk for aspiration and possibly pneumonia and respiratory failure. In many institutions, the bedside RN can administer a bedside swallow test according to a protocol to determine initial risk for aspiration. If the stroke patient is found to be at risk for aspiration, nothing by mouth (NPO) status is maintained until assessment is completed by an ST for recommendations to guide the timing of reintroduction and progression of oral intake.

TABLE 9-1 Respiratory Patterns Associated with Lesions at Varying Levels of the Brain

The following abnormal respiratory patterns are seen in conditions that affect the respiratory centers of the brainstem directly and indirectly. *Primary brainstem injury* occurs as a result of direct injury, ischemia, infarction, or a tumor located in the brainstem respiratory centers. *Secondary brainstem injury* can occur as a result of ischemia secondary to impending herniation from a supratentorial lesion (e.g., cerebral edema, space-occupying lesion) or, rarely, an infratentorial lesion or CNS depression from metabolic conditions or drug overdose. However, increased ICP with impending herniation is the major cause of abnormal respiratory patterns.

Pattern and Location	Description
Cheyne-Stokes respirations	
Lesion: may be associated with bilateral widespread cortical lesions but most often associated with bilateral thalamic dysfunction; may also result from bilateral damage anywhere along the descending pathway between the forebrain and upper pons; can also be associated with metabolic abnormalities as seen in uremia and heart failure patients	Rhythmic waxing and waning pattern Brief periods of hyperpnea alternating with short period of apnea Pattern due to two factors: (1) increased sensitivity to carbon dioxide resulting in change in depth and rate and (2) decreased stimulation from respiratory centers resulting in apnea
Central neurogenic hyperventilation	
Lesion: midbrain and upper pons	Prolonged and rapid hyperpnea from 40–70 breaths per minute Rare and must be differentiated from reactive hyperventilation related to metabolic abnormalities May lead to respiratory alkalosis
Apneustic breathing	
Lesion: lower pons	A prolonged inspiratory gasp with a pause at full inspiration in which the breath is held and then released.
Cluster breathing	
Lesion: lower pons or upper medulla	Clusters of periodic respirations that are irregular in frequency and amplitude, with varying periods of apnea between clusters of breaths.
Ataxic breathing	
Location: medulla	Completely irregular, unpredictable pattern in which inspiratory gasps of varying amplitude and length are interspersed with periods of apnea.

CNS, central nervous system; ICP, intracranial pressure.
From Hickey, J. V. (Ed.). (2014). *The clinical practice of neurological and neurosurgical nursing* (7th ed.). Philadelphia, PA: Lippincott Williams & Wilkins.

The bedside RN and other members of the interprofessional clinical team will monitor the work of breathing, assess for the development and/or progression of adventitious breath sounds, and evaluate the patient's ability to manage secretions. Respiratory therapists with experience in working with neurological patients are integral to managing ventilator settings, monitoring weaning parameters for either extubation or liberation from the ventilator, and providing input for weaning and removal of the tracheostomy tube as the patient improves. Throughout the weaning process, the interprofessional care team uses frequent and serial assessments of the work of breathing (e.g., respiratory rate and depth, use of accessory muscles), adequacy of cough effort, and ability to clear secretions to ascertain how well the patient is progressing with the weaning process. Ideally, the process will proceed smoothly and rapidly, but there are often setbacks and plateaus; the interprofessional team should be certain that the patient and family understand this aspect of the process.

Treatment

The nurse encourages the patient to participate in basic pulmonary toilet such as coughing and deep breathing and use of an incentive spirometry. If chest physiotherapy, with either a specialty bed or a chest vest, is prescribed by the interprofessional care team, the nurse ensures the therapy is carried out and monitors patient response. Some studies support the use of CPAP starting the first night after stroke in patients with OSA as a way to improve long-term outcome post stroke (Lévy & Pépin, 2011). If the patient has required intubation and mechanical ventilation, the nurse monitors response to therapy and works with the interprofessional care team to wean the patient from mechanical ventilation and to move toward extubation. The interprofessional care team works collaboratively to manage any anxiety related to the weaning process. Stroke patients often meet respiratory criteria for extubation, but the care team may hesitate because of concerns about ongoing ability of airway protection. Use of the Glasgow Coma Scale (GCS) score may be helpful in predicting successful extubation in patients with MCA stroke. However, some stroke patients who required intubation will require tracheostomy placement. Other stroke patients who were intubated initially will become candidates for transition into palliative care, and their extubation will be terminal and managed in conjunction with the palliative care team. The bedside nurse along with the entire interprofessional team works to establish and maintain a therapeutic relationship with the patient and family to facilitate decision making regarding intensity of care.

The ST and respiratory therapist (RT) work with the interprofessional team to implement the use of speaking valves or capping trials and determine the optimal timing of tracheostomy progression to decannulation (Christopher, 2005; Morris, McIntosh, & Whitmer, 2014). However, a lack of standardization exists regarding tracheostomy weaning, and nurses can be integral in the effort to develop and establish standardized protocols (Morris et al., 2014). The bedside nurse is key in assessing patient's readiness and tolerance to weaning, but a systematic approach to tracheostomy management provided by a dedicated team is likely to result in fewer complications during weaning.

It is not readily apparent from a review of the literature how often patients with acute stroke will not be able to be weaned either from mechanical ventilation or from dependency on an artificial airway. Patients whose stroke has resulted in a *locked-in* syndrome will often require tracheostomy and prolonged mechanical ventilation (Smith & Delargy, 2005). Unfortunately, tracheostomy increases the difficulty for out-of-hospital placement for stroke patients. Studies, which have investigated long-term outcome for all patients requiring long-term tracheostomy, have found high mortality rates in the first year (Engoren, Arslanian-Engoren, & Fenn-Buderer, 2004).

Artificial airway placement complicates the already impaired ability of a stroke patient to communicate with loved ones and his or her care team, and it increases the stress in an already stressful situation. Nonverbal communication methods such as facial expressions, gestures, pointing, eye movement or blinking, and possibly sign language are encouraged for patients with artificial airways, although the stroke may have already significantly compromised communication abilities. An ST can determine whether some sort of communication device such as letter or picture boards, flashcards, or more sophisticated devices may be appropriate for a particular patient. The bedside nurse ensures the implementation and appropriate use of communication tools by all members of the care team.

Best Practices

⊙ There are no prospective trials, which have established an optimal mode of ventilation for stroke patients. For those patients who have required intubation and mechanical ventilation, the mode of ventilation is often related to the reason for intubation and the sedation requirements of the patient. An RT with experience in the care of patients with neurological disease including stroke is invaluable in the appropriate management of stroke patients. Groups of interventions, or "bundles," have been introduced in the last decade for the prevention of common ICU complications. The VAP bundle, which includes HOB elevation, daily sedation vacations, assessment of extubation readiness, peptic ulcer disease prophylaxis, deep vein thrombosis prophylaxis, and proper oral care, has been shown to significantly reduce the incidence of VAP (Tolentino-DelosReyes, Ruppert, & Shiao, 2007; Wip & Napolitano, 2009). However, use of the VAP bundle is not definitively supported by large clinical trials so that controversy exists about the use of the bundle (O'Grady, Murray, & Ames, 2012). Sometimes, patients with stroke will require a tracheostomy but, as noted earlier, there is no clear data regarding timing of tracheostomy. Additionally, there is no clear data about the number of stroke patients who will be discharged from an acute care hospital to either a long-term care facility or home with a tracheostomy in place.

Evaluation

⊙ Evaluation of respiratory function in the stroke patient is a continuous process requiring frequent reassessments by all members of the care team for any evidence of change. Stroke patients who have required intubation and mechanical ventilation will require daily assessments of their ability to be weaned and liberated from mechanical ventilation. Those who have gone on to require tracheostomy placement will require daily reassessment of their ability to progress to decannulation. Those patients who did not initially require an artificial airway will require close monitoring in the days immediately following the stroke to identify any deterioration in their ability to continue to protect their airway or for the development of pneumonia. Patients in whom the decision has been made to transition to comfort measures only will require monitoring for signs of distress, which may require intervention for comfort such as glycopyrrolate to alleviate for copious secretion management. End-of-life care is discussed in more detail later in this chapter.

Clinical Pearl: If at all possible, patients able to tolerate a progression to decannulation prior to discharge should have a care plan that allows progression to decannulation at the care facility where they are placed. Long-term care facilities usually have a limited number of beds for patients with tracheotomies, so having a structured plan in place for tracheostomy tube removal can facilitate placement.

▓▓ HYPERGLYCEMIA

Hyperglycemia has been noted to be a common occurrence in acute stroke patients, especially during acute ischemic stroke, with more than 40% of patients presenting with hyperglycemia. Patient presenting with ICH and SAH also experience hyperglycemia with three out of four patients presenting with SAH having hyperglycemia on admission (Kruyt et al., 2009). There is evidence that hyperglycemia is associated with poorer neurological outcome at 3 months despite adjustments for age, stroke severity on admission, other vascular risk factors, and diabetes mellitus (DM) (Badjatia et al., 2005; Bruno et al., 2002; Kruyt et al., 2009). In ischemic stroke, there is evidence that hyperglycemia is only associated with nonlacunar strokes (Bruno et al., 1999). Among ischemic stroke patients treated with IV recombinant tissue plasminogen activator (rtPA), hyperglycemia has been associated with symptomatic ICH and subsequent poorer clinical outcomes (Bruno et al., 2002). The association between DM, hyperglycemia, poor glycemic control, and stroke outcomes remain controversial mainly due to the lack of controlled studies that specifically define optimal glucose control during acute brain ischemia.

Pathophysiology

Many studies have evaluated hyperglycemia in acute stroke, but there has been no consensus regarding a specific mechanism responsible for hyperglycemia not associated with DM encountered in stroke patients. In part, it is difficult to separate those patients with DM, whether known or unknown, from those patients experiencing hyperglycemia related to acute ischemic stroke. DM is a risk factor for ischemic stroke. It is much easier to identify hyperglycemia related to acute cerebral injury in SAH because DM is not a risk factor for SAH (Feigin et al., 2005). Another possible explanation for elevated glucose levels at admission is that many stroke patients present in a nonfasting state and therefore may have elevated glucose levels. Another mechanism implicated in hyperglycemia associated with acute stroke is a stress response mediated partly by the release of cortisol and norepinephrine (O'Neill, Davies, Fullerton, & Bennett, 1991). This stress response has also been implicated in SAH. It is believed that the activation of the sympathetic autonomic nervous system results in increased levels of cortisol and catecholamines, which persist even up to 10 days post-SAH (Naredi et al., 2000; Vergouwen et al., 2010). The increased levels of these hormones promote multiple process including glycogenolysis, gluconeogenesis, proteolysis, and lipolysis, all resulting in excessive glucose production and hyperglycemia (Barth et al., 2007; Seematter, Binnert, Martin, & Tappy, 2004).

Assessment/Diagnosis

Hyperglycemia is most often defined as blood glucose levels greater than 140 mg/dL via finger stick glucose check or serum glucose check. Many patients are placed on NPO until a formal speech evaluation is completed, which usually is within 24 hours of admission. Thus, in the time prior to this formal evaluation, the patient is only on non–dextrose-containing IV fluids unless there are contraindications such as dialysis-dependent renal failure. Routine blood sugar checks every 6 hours while NPO are recommended. In addition, it is recommended that every stroke patient be screened for DM by checking a glycosylated hemoglobin level. This will assist the interprofessional clinical team in determining whether hyperglycemia at admission is the result of under-treated or untreated DM or is associated with an acute reaction to the stress of the stroke.

The nursing staff is vital in recognizing patients who have elevated glucose levels because they are the interprofessional team members responsible for monitoring blood glucose at the bedside in addition to oral intake of food and fluids. Many patients with baseline diagnosis of DM will have their oral hypoglycemic medications held while on NPO status and during hospitalization due to unpredictable nutritional intake and risk of lactic acidosis if medications such as Glucophage are administered to patients who received contrast medium needed for some diagnostic studies. The pharmacist is also a vital interprofessional team member and is helpful in determining appropriate medication selection for those patients with newly diagnosed DM or for the patient presenting with hyperglycemia difficult to control in the acute setting either due to preexisting diabetes or due to ongoing critical illness.

Treatment

Currently, there is no clinical evidence that targeting blood glucose to a particular level during acute ischemic stroke will improve outcomes. The main risk from aggressive hyperglycemia correction in acute stroke appears to be possible hypoglycemia. It is reasonable to follow the current American Diabetes Association (2010) recommendation to maintain the blood glucose in a range of 140 to 180 mg/dL in all hospitalized patients. Dysphagia and dysarthria are complicating problems in the glucose management of acute stroke patients. Many stroke patients, after evaluation by ST, are initially placed on diets with modified textures and fluid viscosities. The nursing staff is vital in ensuring adequate patient intake of both food and fluids and reporting any difficulties to the rest of the interprofessional care team. The nutritionist/dietitian works with the patient and family to first identify food preferences, which will increase adherence to diets involving modified textures and viscosities and, secondly, to discuss ways to improve adherence to a healthy diet after discharge. The ST continues to engage the patient in therapy to assist with strategies to avoid aspiration resulting in complications such as pneumonia or pneumonitis. Scheduled home insulin regimens will likely require significant modification from home doses, and if the patient is a newly diagnosed diabetic, the assistance of a DM management specialist will be helpful especially in providing education regarding management, preventing of complications, and adherence to a diabetic diet.

Best Practices

Nutritional intake varies among stroke patients, and adjusting hyperglycemia treatment to suit oral intake is difficult in the few days to weeks following stroke, complicating efforts to maintain the targeted glucose level of 140 to 180 mg/dL. The current recommendation is to use regular insulin to treat hyperglycemia but to err on the side of mild hyperglycemia rather than hypoglycemia because mortality is increased for patients with hypoglycemia compared to those with hyperglycemia. This is why the goal for glucose is not less than 140 mg/dL but rather above the 140 mg/dL mark (Jauch et al., 2013). The care team should communicate this information to the patient and family so they understand this temporary deviation from what may or will become long-term management goals for the patient.

Once the patient's hyperglycemia is resolved and DM has been ruled out, routine glucose monitoring should be discontinued to avoid unnecessary testing, support cost savings, and avoid potential medical errors associated from administration of regular insulin to a patient who does not need insulin administration.

Evaluation

Patients who present with hyperglycemia should have their glucose levels followed, but unless diagnosed with DM, they should not have any oral hypoglycemic agents started in the acute setting. Patients with pre-DM should receive ongoing nutritional counseling to assist with lifestyle changes to prevent or slow progression of hyperglycemia. Patients whose hemoglobin A1C suggests poor blood glucose control should be referred to an endocrinologist for more aggressive control to prevent further complications from diabetes.

Clinical Pearl: If DM medications are started or changed during hospitalization, compliance can be increased if affordability is taken into consideration because some of the newer insulin preparations are expensive if the patient is uninsured or may carry higher copayments. It is especially important to take time to educate the patient in layman's terms regarding the disease process and nutrition, especially stressing that DM is a chronic condition that requires long-term follow-up and management.

▮▮ DEEP VEIN THROMBOSIS

The risk of deep vein thrombosis (DVT) in hospitalized patients is a well-recognized complication. It is even more vital to monitor for this serious complication in stroke patients than in other patient populations due to the increased likelihood of prolonged immobility. Some stroke patients are at greater risk due to a previous history of DVT, dehydration, malignant disease, or clotting disorders (Kappelle, 2011). DVT occurs in up to 50% of patients with ischemic stroke who did not receive pharmacological prophylactic therapy. These DVTs most often develop between days 2 and 7 after stroke onset (Brandstater, Roth, & Siebens, 1992) with about 80% of the DVTs occurring in the first 10 days post stroke (CLOTS Trials Collaboration, 2009). DVT is associated with increased mortality and morbidity in stroke patients. Patients with ICH tend to have an increased risk of DVT compared to ischemic stroke patients. This is likely due to the recommended delay in initiation of pharmacological prophylaxis in hemorrhagic stroke as well as more severe focal deficits.

Clinically, a DVT may be asymptomatic. The major concern associated with asymptomatic proximal DVT is the potential for PE. This is a major clinical concern because it is believed that PEs account for 13% to 25% of early deaths after stroke (J. Kelly, Rudd, Lewis, & Hunt, 2001). Fatal PEs are unusual in the first week post stroke or in the acute setting after stroke unless a patient has a prolonged acute setting stay. PEs are most frequent between the second and fourth weeks post stroke when patients have been discharged home or to a rehabilitation facility (Viitanen, Winblad, & Asplund, 1987). Nonfatal PEs usually result in significant morbidity due to impaired cardiorespiratory reserve adversely affecting rehabilitation and functional outcome.

Pathophysiology

Factors contributing to the development of venous thrombosis include venous stasis, activation of coagulation factors, and vein damage. These factors are commonly referred to as the *Virchow triad.* Venous stasis can occur in the presence of anything that slows or obstructs the flow of venous blood, resulting in an increase in viscosity of the blood and the subsequent formation of microthrombi. When microemboli are not washed away by normal blood flow, an accumulation of microemboli can form in an area resulting in a thrombus that propagates. Endothelial (intimal) damage, whether due to intrinsic factors or due to external trauma to a blood vessel, can also result in thrombus formation because once there is endothelial damage, a hypercoagulable state occurs due to a biochemical imbalance between circulating coagulation factors. After the initial damage, platelets adhere to the subendothelial surface due to the presence of von Willebrand factor or fibrinogen in the vessel wall. Neutrophils and platelets are activated, and they release inflammatory mediators. Resulting complexes that form on the surface of platelets increase the rate of thrombin generation and fibrin formation. As a result, a mature thrombus composed of platelets, leukocytes, and fibrin develops in the wall of the vein, resulting in a DVT (Kuijper et al., 1997).

Assessment and Diagnosis

◉ The nursing staff, physical therapist (PT), and the occupational therapist (OT) are critical team members in the prevention of DVTs. The nurse ensures that PT and OT have timely access to the patient so that they can complete an initial evaluation for ambulation safety and mobility. Recommendations from PT and OT provide direction for the safe and early mobilization and ambulation of the patient. The nurse can then assist the patient with mobility because PT and OT may not work with the patient on a daily basis in the acute care setting. The nurse is also the interprofessional team member best situated to regularly inspect the patient's leg for signs of DVT development and communicate such findings to the rest of the care team.

Doppler ultrasound is an effective and economical technique for detecting symptomatic proximal DVTs. However, there is evidence that the sensitivity of Doppler ultrasound for the diagnosis of asymptomatic proximal DVT is only 62%, and for asymptomatic below-knee DVTs, only 48% (Wells, Lensing, Davidson, Prins, & Hirsh, 1995). However, many studies reporting these findings were completed in high-risk postoperative patients. The stroke patient population may have other characteristics that complicate DVT diagnosis unlike the sample in the reported studies. Although thrombi missed with ultrasound screening tend to be smaller and nonocclusive, it has been suggested that the technique may be unsatisfactory as a routine screening tool because many DVTs will not be detected. Thus, other tests such as serum levels of D-dimers are used in conjunction with ultrasound technology for patients in whom DVT is strongly suspected but not confirmed by ultrasound.

An alternative to ultrasound is magnetic resonance imaging (MRI), which is noninvasive and allows simultaneous imaging of the venous system in both lower limbs. In addition, pelvic vein and inferior vena cava thrombosis are accurately identified, which presented an important advantage over other techniques (Fraser, Moody, Morgan, Martel, & Davidson, 2002). However, it is an expensive modality, and it is has limited availability.

D-Dimers are composed of cross-linked fibrin and are formed as a waste product in the degradation of the fibrin matrix of fresh venous thromboemboli (J. Kelly et al., 2001). Acute nonlacunar ischemic strokes increase D-dimer levels. An elevation in D-dimer will usually decrease to baseline over the first 30 days post stroke. This elevation has stimulated debate about use of D-dimers in stroke patients, resulting in multiple studies specifically investigating the use of a D-dimer assay as a screening test for subclinical DVT in stroke patients. There is evidence that in patients who are on average 25 days post stroke, a threshold of 1,092 ng/mL has a sensitivity of 100% and specificity of 66% for diagnosing DVT as detected by Doppler ultrasound (Harvey, Roth, Yarnold, Durham, & Green, 1996).

Although these findings support the use of D-dimer as a screening test to allow the provider to identify patients who should undergo targeted imaging with ultrasound or MRI, the results cannot be applied to patients in the first few days after stroke. The other important issue to remember is that several D-dimer assays are now available for commercial use, and they are not all interchangeable. The results from studies using one manufacturer's test cannot necessarily be applied to another manufacturer's test. Thus, when providers translate evidence related to D-dimer assay usage into practice, it is important to keep this in mind.

Treatment

Ischemic stroke patients should be started on pharmacological DVT prophylaxis upon admission, unless they received thrombolytic therapy with tPA in which case providers will need to wait for a full 24 hours prior to initiating pharmacological DVT prophylaxis (Jauch et al., 2013). For patients with ICH, pharmacological DVT prophylaxis can be started 3 to 4 days post onset of hemorrhage, as long as there is no evidence of ongoing rebreeding (Wu et al., 2011). Patients with aneurysmal SAH can be started on pharmacological DVT prophylaxis 3 to 4 days post aneurysm coiling or clipping. If it is a nonaneurysmal SAH, those patients are not started on pharmacological DVT prophylaxis due to risk of rebleeding. They are, however, given mechanical DVT prophylaxis, and early mobility is encouraged.

DVT prophylaxis in patients with stroke: low-molecular-weight heparin (LMWH): Despite a small but definite risk of major hemorrhage, LMWH is the preferred medication for the prevention of DVT in patients with ischemic stroke. There is evidence that enoxaparin, the most commonly used LMWH, when compared to unfractionated heparin, is more effective at reducing the risk of DVT and PE in stroke patients (Sherman et al., 2007).

Unfractionated heparin (UFH): Patients who, due to renal dysfunction or other medical reasons, cannot receive LMWH should receive UFH for DVT prophylaxis. Usually, this is defined as a 5,000 unit dose administered every 8 hours for the general medicine patient. However, for the patient with increased risk of bleeding, as in the case of patients with large ischemic stroke or those with SAH or ICH, the recommendation is an adjusted dose of 5,000 units every 12 hours. UFH should be used only if LMWH is contraindicated in that patient.

Graduated compression stockings: The routine use of stockings alone as prophylaxis for DVT is not adequate and should be avoided. There is evidence that full-length elastic stockings do not significantly reduce the risk of DVT, as compared with no stockings (CLOTS Trials Collaboration, 2009). Both knee-high stockings and thigh-high stockings are associated with an increase in the risk of skin breakdown. This is especially problematic in stroke patients who often have communication and cognitive deficits from their stroke which prevent them from reliably being able to report discomfort or skin breakdown.

Sequential compression devices: For patients who cannot receive pharmacological prophylaxis for DVT due to risk of bleeding, as is the case with ICH patients in the first few days post hemorrhage, use of mechanical methods of DVT prophylaxis is recommended. The method with the least skin irritation remains the sequential compression device. There is evidence that intermittent compression prevents DVT and prevents venous stasis (CLOTS Trials Collaboration, 2013). The major disadvantage of relying on a mechanical method for prophylaxis over pharmacological prophylaxis is that of proper application of the device, making sure the device is turned on, and compliance.

Treatment of DVT in stroke patients: Treatment of DVT requires initiation of anticoagulation. The choice of anticoagulant is largely based on clinician choice. The duration of treatment depends on multiple factors, including whether the DVT was provoked or not, whether this is a first time DVT versus recurrence, and whether genetic predisposition to hypercoagulability exists.

Acute treatment: Prior to the approval of the thrombin inhibitor, rivaroxaban, for DVT treatment by the FDA, treatment of DVT could only be accomplished with warfarin, which takes several days to achieve its desired therapeutic effect. For this reason, oral anticoagulant therapy alone without bridge therapy with either continuous IV heparin or therapeutic dosing with subcutaneous enoxaparin or another LMWH was unacceptable. Now, if patients are being treated with rivaroxaban, there is no need for bridge therapy because therapeutic anticoagulation is achieved with the initial dose. The advantage of rivaroxaban is that it does not require routine clinic visits or blood work for monitoring because dosing is standardized. The disadvantage is that it currently has no generic version and is expensive. Warfarin, on the other hand, is very affordable, although its use is frequently cumbersome for the patient. Dosing of warfarin is highly individualized because it interacts with many foods and medications and thus requires regular international normalized ratio (INR) monitoring of the blood to maintain a narrow therapeutic range and avoid either under or over anticoagulation.

For bridge therapy while initiating warfarin, most clinicians initiate treatment with LMWH rather than UFH. The ease of administration and efficacy of LMWH makes this the preferred anticoagulant because there is no need for titration or checking activated partial thromboplastin times (APTTs) as with UFH infusion. UFH infusion requires continued hospitalization until the patient achieves therapeutic anticoagulation with warfarin, whereas patients using LMWH can be discharged once they or a family member has received appropriate instruction and demonstrated the ability to safely and successfully administer the required subcutaneous injections. Appropriate follow-up for INR monitoring and medication adjustment should be arranged by the care team prior to patient discharge. Although LMWH is associated with a lower risk of hemorrhage in medical patients, data comparing LMWH and UFH in stroke patients are insufficient to draw conclusions about their relative safety in this context especially in relation to hemorrhagic conversion of infarct. However, most diagnoses of clinical venous thromboembolism are made several days after stroke onset, by which time, the risk of hemorrhagic stroke transformation is lower.

The recommendation is to administer weight-adjusted LMWH divided into two doses for 5 to 7 days as initial treatment while bridging to Coumadin therapy. Because LMWH is predominantly excreted by the renal route, it should not be used in patients with significant renal dysfunction for risk of drug accumulation resulting in hemorrhagic complications. For patients with history of heparin-induced thrombocytopenia (HIT), an acceptable agent is the synthetic pentasaccharide fondaparinux, which is at least as effective and safe as LMWH in the treatment of DVT.

For patients at high risk of bleeding or renal dysfunction, a continuous infusion of UFH may be more appropriate given that UFH, in the low doses delivered via continuous infusion, is eliminated from the bloodstream via a saturable mechanism in which it binds to the reticuloendothelial system and endothelium (Boneu, Caranobe, & Sie, 1990). The other advantage is that it has a shorter half-life compared to LMWH or fondaparinux. Some stroke patients who require anticoagulation for DVT may still potentially require placement of a tracheostomy or percutaneous gastric feeding tube or may still have an ICP monitoring device in place which will require removal; the ability to quickly and easily suspend anticoagulation is advantageous for them. The main disadvantage of using heparin infusion in stroke patients who are not expected to require surgical interventions or invasive diagnostic testing is that it prolongs hospitalization, resulting in increased patient costs. Using LMWH and fondaparinux injections while bridging to Coumadin therapy reduces the length of stay in the hospital because these patients can be managed in either rehabilitation facilities or the outpatient setting.

Long-Term Treatment of Deep Vein Thrombosis

First proximal DVT occurs in the context of a transient risk factor (e.g., surgery or trauma): In this situation, the risk of recurrence is very low and a limited duration of therapy of 3 months is adequate (Levine et al., 1995).

First DVT occurs in the context of active malignant disease: Malignancy, especially if newly diagnosed, is an ongoing risk factor. Patients with malignancy have a higher incidence of recurrent thrombosis and bleeding complications while receiving oral anticoagulation therapy (Prandoni et al., 2002). This is likely due to the prothrombotic state associated with cancer and to the difficulty of managing oral anticoagulant therapy with concomitant chemotherapy drugs, unpredictable oral intake, and liver dysfunction. Studies have shown that long-term anticoagulation therapy with LMWH is more effective than warfarin for preventing recurrent venous thrombosis without a statistically significant increase in bleeding risk in cancer patients (Meyer et al., 2002). It is recommended that all patients who have active malignant disease be treated with LMWH for at least 6 months if they have adequate renal function. Not only will it lead to lower risks of recurrent thrombosis but also it facilitates the management of patients who need to undergo multiple procedures (e.g., biopsy, line insertion) and who have periodic thrombocytopenia due to chemotherapy. Because the risk of DVT recurrence is higher among patients with cancer than among those without cancer, anticoagulation is recommended as long as the cancer is felt to be active. It is recommended to wait 6 months after cure or complete remission before discontinuing therapy (Prandoni et al., 2002).

First DVT occurs in the context of a thrombophilic defect: These defects include factor V Leiden; prothrombin gene mutation; deficiencies in protein C, protein S, and antithrombin; increased factor VIII levels; hyperhomocysteinemia; and elevated antiphospholipid antibody levels. Patients with persistently elevated antiphospholipid antibody levels have a higher relative risk of recurrence after stopping anticoagulation therapy for a first DVT than those without this thrombophilia. It has been reported that patients with an elevated factor VIII level have a 2-year risk of recurrence of 37% after stopping anticoagulant agents, compared with 5% among those with normal levels (De Stefano et al., 1999). However, many of the studies that looked at this as a risk factor included calf vein thromboses, which have a lower risk of recurrence. Currently, with the exception of patients with elevated antiphospholipid antibody levels or those with homozygous genetic defects, it is not routinely recommended to offer prolonged anticoagulation therapy after a first idiopathic DVT (Kearon, 2004). However, it is recommended to place the patient on aspirin for secondary stroke prevention if the patient has had a stroke and not placed on prolonged anticoagulation for other reasons such as atrial fibrillation.

Recurrent DVT: After a second recurrence of DVT, the risk of further thromboembolic events following the discontinuation of anticoagulation therapy is believed to be excessive if only 6 months of oral anticoagulation therapy is administered. Therefore, it is generally recommended that anticoagulation therapy be continued. However, no study has investigated the risk of recurrent DVT if both events occurred during a transient risk period. In this situation, a shorter duration of anticoagulation therapy may be adequate (3 to 6 months), but other factors may influence this decision. When considering prolonging anticoagulation therapy, the risks of bleeding must be individualized and weighed against the potential benefits of preventing recurrence of thrombosis.

Best Practices

Currently, there are no recommendations for routine surveillance for DVT in stroke patients. Currently, the focus is on prevention of DVT unless a patient becomes symptomatic, then further testing is warranted at that time to confirm diagnosis of DVT. Best practices in prevention of DVT are a combination of nonpharmacological and pharmacological therapies. These include early mobilization, hydration, intermittent pneumatic compression, UFH, or LMWH.

Avoiding dehydration post stroke is vital. Dehydration after ischemic stroke is independently associated with DVT (J. Kelly et al., 2004). In the context of DVT prophylaxis, fluid intake has not been evaluated in a clinical trial, but current guidelines recommend keeping patients well hydrated in the early stage of ischemic stroke. This is especially important for those patients with dysphagia or with communication deficits which affect their ability to ask for oral fluids or taking in enough oral fluids. Extremity swelling, especially in the hemiplegic extremity or in the extremity with a central catheter, should warrant further investigation for DVT in the hospitalized stroke patient.

Evaluation

The preferred method for reevaluation of resolution of DVT is currently Doppler ultrasound because it is widely available and affordable. Patients need reimaging in 3 to 6 months to evaluate resolution of DVT if the plan is to discontinue anticoagulation. However, if the patient is asymptomatic and requires long-term anticoagulation, there is no need for reimaging. For those patients needing long-term anticoagulation, bleeding risk can be assessed during yearly visits, which will enable a risk–benefit evaluation to determine if anticoagulation therapy should continue.

⊙ For patients with thrombophilic defects, it is important to refer them to a hematology specialist to ensure that a comprehensive hypercoagulability workup is completed because this determines long-term anticoagulation decision. Hypercoagulability studies completed in the acute setting may need to be repeated in the outpatient setting to ensure that inflammatory responses in the acute setting were not responsible for any positive results. Hypercoagulability testing tends to be expensive so the interprofessional care team uses careful judgment in deciding which patients should have this blood work initiated in the acute setting. If any of the test results raise concern for hypercoagulability, a referral to a hematologist is beneficial so that a decision regarding long-term anticoagulation can be made as well as determining the use of testing other family members to better assess their risk of stroke or other thrombotic events.

Clinical Pearl: Some of the hypercoagulability studies can be abnormal in the acute period and some cannot be completed while patients are on pharmacological DVT prophylaxis. Thus, prior to sending these patients for evaluation, the interprofessional care team will need to make sure only those tests appropriate for the inpatient setting are completed to avoid later repetition as these tests are expensive.

URINARY TRACT INFECTIONS

Urinary tract infection (UTI) is a recognized common complication of stroke with rates of up to 24% within the first week to first month (Langhorne et al., 2000). Factors that increase the likelihood of UTI after stroke include female gender, older age, functional dependence before stroke, higher baseline NIHSS score, poor cognitive function, and catheterization (Stott, Falconer, Miller, Tilston, & Langhorne, 2009). Urinary catheters remain the most cited and studied risk factor for health care–associated UTI, and their use may be more common in patients with stroke especially those with severe deficits at admission, thereby further increasing the risk of UTI. In 2010, the cost of a single catheter-associated UTI was estimated to be $775 to $1,500, with further increase in cost if secondary bacteremia occurred (Tambyah, Knasinski, & Maki, 2002).

When a UTI occurs during hospitalization for stroke, it may have serious consequences including longer length of stay, increased costs of care, exposure to IV antibiotics, and risk of the development of bacteremia. In addition, there is evidence that neurological outcome worsen with poststroke infections as indicated by this subset of patients scoring poorly on the modified Rankin Scale and an increase in the risk of death or disability at 3 months (Aslanyan, Weir, Diener, Kaste, & Lees, 2004). It is well documented that fever in patients with brain injury from any etiology, including stroke, correlates with poorer outcome in many measures including increased mortality, poor outcome on the modified Rankin Scale and the Barthel Index, and longer hospital length of stay. Infection is also a risk factor for delirium, which worsens functional outcome, mortality, and increases hospital stay in patients with stroke (Stott et al., 2009).

Pathophysiology

Catheter-associated urinary tract infections (CAUTIs) are the most studied problem. The CAUTI can stem from exogenous sources (health care workers' hands or equipment) or endogenous sources (meatal, rectal, or vaginal colonization). Pathogens from exogenous or endogenous sources enter the urinary tract extraluminally by migration along the outside of the catheter or intraluminally by migration along the internal lumen of the catheter. Many catheter drainage systems currently available have addressed the intraluminal migration of pathogens by use of sterile closed-drainage systems, although breaks in the system can still occur. As early as 1 day post initial catheterization, a biofilm forms on both the extra- and intraluminal surfaces of the catheter, increasing the ability of microorganisms to adhere to the surfaces and promoting colonization (Maki & Tambyah, 2001). Bacteria fixed to the biofilm are difficult to eradicate without removing the catheter.

Another mechanism that may contribute to the development of UTIs in the stroke patient is the relationship between the central nervous system and the immune system.

Brain injury may initially cause both local and systemic inflammation as evidenced by increased brain and plasma inflammatory cytokines immediately after stroke in animal models (Offner, Vandenbark, & Hurn, 2009). Many stroke patients may have a mildly elevated white blood cell count, which normalizes in the few days post stroke. After this initial systemic inflammation, a systemic immunosuppression can also occur. Although the underlying process driving immunosuppression after stroke is not clear, it is hypothesized that sympathetic signaling to the lymphoid organs is affected post stroke, resulting in activation of the locus coeruleus which releases norepinephrine. The stress response resulting from this release of norepinephrine causes an induction of immunologic changes (Chamorro, Urra, & Planas, 2007).

Assessment and Diagnosis

Urinalysis and urine culture remains the standard for diagnosis of UTI. Although urinalysis results can suggest the presence of a UTI, it is important to obtain a culture as well to narrow antibiotic coverage and also ensure there is no resistance to the chosen antibiotic. Ask the patient regarding any urinary symptoms because it may be necessary to start treatment in symptomatic patients prior to availability of culture results. Patients suspected of having a UTI who have a urinary catheter in place should be evaluated regarding ongoing need for an indwelling catheter. If the urinary catheter can be discontinued, a urinalysis and urine culture should be sent from a spontaneous void or subsequent in and out catheterization to avoid false-positive results from catheter colonization. Patients who have a continued need for catheterization should have their catheter changed and a urinalysis and urine culture collected from the new catheter.

⊙ The nurse plays a major role in preventing unnecessary catheterization. Use of bladder scanning techniques prior to use of urinary catheters for urinary retention may assist with avoiding urinary catheter use. If the patient does require a catheter, evaluate the continued need for a catheter on a daily basis. Many stroke patients who have received tPA have urinary catheters placed so that staff can avoid urgent placement post infusion of tPA when there is increased risk of bleeding. For these patients, it is vital that the catheters be discontinued once the 24-hour post-tPA time period is completed. Early mobility, especially in patient with baseline impaired urinary function, decreases risk of worsening urinary function while hospitalized. PT and OT, prior to getting the patient out of bed for their first therapy session, should ask the nurse or other member of the medical team about continued need for a catheter because this can affect participation in therapy as well.

Treatment

Uncatheterized patients who have a urinalysis indicating an active UTI and have symptoms or other indications of infection, such as an elevated white blood cell count (leukocytosis) or fever, should be treated with antibiotics without delay. The choice of antibiotic is individualized to the patient, depending on known allergies and whether he or she is on anticoagulants such as warfarin, which interact with many antibiotics. The initial treatment of the UTI is with a broad-spectrum antibiotic until culture results are available; once culture results are available, the antibiotic choice can be narrowed to treat the causative organism. Patients who only have a urinalysis suspicion for infection, but no symptoms or other indications of infection, should not be treated unless the culture shows growth of a pathogen. This practice avoids unnecessary exposure to antibiotic therapy and possible emergence of resistant organisms.

Patients who have a CAUTI should be treated for complicated UTI. All male patients, catheterized or not, who have a UTI diagnosed should also be treated for a complicated UTI. Female patients who had no catheter exposure are considered to have an uncomplicated UTI and should be treated for only 3 days.

Best Practices

There are interventions which could potentially decrease UTI after stroke, and further research is necessary to define the best strategies to minimize this important complication. Several studies have evaluated the use of prophylactic antibiotics in patients with stroke with mixed results. Questions regarding the risk of selected resistant organisms, defining the best antibiotic regimen, and determining which patients with stroke may benefit from prophylaxis remain unanswered, and so currently, it is not recommended to prophylactically treat stroke patients with antibiotics for UTI prevention. Because urinary catheters have an established link to UTI in the general medical population, reducing the use of urinary catheters likely lowers the incidence of UTI post stroke. Condom catheters are another alternative urinary collection system for men without urinary retention, which reduces the risk of UTI, but they do not eliminate the risk of UTIs completely.

Many medical facilities now use computer order entry, and thus stroke units can take advantage of this resource and use a computerized notification system, which triggers a decision by providers when their patients have urinary catheters placed especially in the emergency department. This trigger in the medical record forces a response to either continue or discontinue the catheter with a reason required for continuing the catheter. There is also evidence that instituting a nursing protocol to discontinue urinary catheters without a physician's order in patients without indications for continuation of an indwelling catheter assists in reducing CAUTIs (Meddings et al., 2014).

Evaluation

Once a UTI has been treated, there is usually no need for reevaluation. However, in patients with a history of drug-resistant pathogens, there may be need for a repeat urinalysis if the patient was asymptomatic at the time of diagnosis. If the patient was symptomatic at the time of diagnosis, asking the patient about resolution of symptoms is also sufficient to ensure adequate treatment.

Clinical Pearl: Some patients have positive urine culture without associated urinary symptoms such as dysuria, frequency, or urgency. The positive culture may be related to bladder colonization by pathogens and not indicative of an active infection. The interprofessional care team should consider urinary symptoms and other clinical signs such as an elevated white blood cell count prior to initiating treatment to avoid overuse of antibiotics, which can result in more antibiotic resistance. Furthermore, urinalysis and urine cultures should not be sent from catheters that have been indwelling for more than 24 hours.

URINARY INCONTINENCE

Urinary incontinence (UI) is a common and distressing problem after stroke for a number of patients. It affects 40% to 53% of admitted stroke patients, decreasing to 25% at discharge, but persists at 15% a year post stroke (Nakayama, Jørgensen, Pedersen, Raaschou, & Olsen, 1997). It is well established that UI is a strong marker of stroke severity and is associated with poor functional outcomes, increased institutionalization, and increased mortality. Despite evidence linking better outcomes to patients who regain continence, management of UI following stroke remains suboptimal, with less than two thirds of stroke units having a documented plan to promote continence (Mehdi, Birns, & Bhalla, 2013). What complicates the clinical problem is that UI carries a social stigma and patients are unlikely to discuss the problem with others including providers, choosing to endure the problem in silence.

Elderly patients are already at risk for UI, and stroke further increases this risk. Patients may also have prestroke conditions, such as benign prostatic hypertrophy (BPH), which increase their risk for urinary retention with subsequent UI especially if a urinary catheter is inserted during hospitalization. Patients can also have a UI due to language and communication deficits, which prevent them from letting caregivers know of their needs in a timely manner. Hemiparesis, which prevents patients from ambulating, also poses a risk for UI because the patient may refrain from asking for assistance with toileting because of concern of losing independence.

Pathophysiology

There are many ways in which UI can occur after stroke. One of the mechanisms involves disruption of the neural micturition pathways, resulting in bladder hyperreflexia and urgency incontinence. This is usually related to the location of the stroke because the regulation of bladder control requires connections between areas in the brain and tracts in the spinal cord that involve sympathetic, parasympathetic, and somatic systems (Fowler, Griffiths, & de Groat, 2008). Another mechanism involves UI due to stroke-related cognitive and language deficits with normal bladder function. When patients have aphasia or have other cognitive deficits, they tend to be incontinent because they are unable to ask for assistance with toileting. Finally, UI can occur because of concurrent neuropathy from comorbidities, such as DM or medication use, resulting in bladder hyporeflexia and overflow incontinence.

Studies, dating back to 1964 (Andrew & Nathan, 1964), found that the frontal lobe plays a significant role in bladder control. More recent studies have linked the frontal, frontoparietal, and temporal lobes and the internal capsule to UI after stroke. Other investigations report an association between patients with poststroke UI with large infarcts, aphasia, cognitive impairment, and functional disability (Gelber, Good, Laven, & Verhulst, 1993). Thus, emerging evidence points to the size of infarct as an indicator for UI rather than location of infarct.

Assessment/Diagnosis

The diagnosis of UI is sometimes overlooked by the interprofessional team. Some stroke patients have indwelling urinary catheters in the acute phase of stroke, and it can be difficult to distinguish catheter-related UI problems from those which might be stroke related. The team may assume that UI in the short term is a normal accompaniment to acute stroke and not focus on the possibility that it may become a long-term issue. In a review of the literature, there is no consensus on a clinically helpful definition of UI. Many definitions refer to UI as involuntary loss of urine or involuntary loss of urine perceived to be a problem. This definition does not include a quantified number of incontinent episodes to consider as a threshold for the diagnosis of UI. Such an objective measure could assist health care professionals by grading the severity of UI based on whether it occurs occasionally, weekly, daily, or with all urination.

When attempting to establish a diagnosis of UI, understanding what the problem means to the patient or his or her caregiver is important. Their perception about the severity of the UI will guide interventions. If the UI is occasional and not viewed as a significant problem, intervention might not be perceived as required. Additionally, they may not realize that UI is not a necessary sequela of stroke and that treatment may be available to resolve or improve UI. The interprofessional care team should include continence in discussions of long-term stroke management so that patients and their families will better understand problems they may face in the future. The patient's PCP should include UI in discussions about how the patient and caregiver are managing after the stroke. In the acute care setting, urodynamic studies are of little use (Pizzi et al., 2013) because some UI will resolve with recovery from the stroke and varies greatly from patient to patient. Thus, urodynamic studies should be reserved for patients who have persistent UI to assist with establishing the cause to guide treatment.

The bedside nurse is the best advocate for the patient to avoid unnecessary use of urinary catheters, which can result in urinary retention post catheter removal and result in over flow incontinence. There is evidence that favorable outcomes related to UI can be achieved through an interprofessional approach. Thus, OT and PT are in the best position to assist with identifying and instituting best practice interventions for poststroke UI especially in the postacute phase because they are in frequent contact with the patient when providing ongoing rehabilitation.

Treatment

Because there are multiple factors that can contribute to UI post stroke, it is not surprising that the treatment of UI has not been adequately addressed despite evidence indicating the magnitude and severity of the problem. Scheduled voiding is a useful first-line treatment in many cases of UI. However, this serves to alleviate the problem but does not eliminate it completely. There is evidence for treating nonstroke patients with incontinence using physiotherapy and bladder retraining programs. However, these programs have not been studied in stroke patients.

Best Practices

Many patients with UI will not report symptoms due to embarrassment, feeling that nothing can be done to resolve the problem or fear that surgery is the only option for management. It is important for the interprofessional team to specifically ask about UI while assuring the stroke survivor and caregivers that there are treatments available which may alleviate or resolve the problem. During hospitalization, the interprofessional team should establish whether a patient had preexisting UI.

Current recommendations are for a thorough assessment to categorize the type and severity of poststroke UI. Each patient with incontinence post stroke should have an individually tailored, structured management strategy to promote continence. This approach has been associated with better stroke outcomes and is usually successful if the patient's family or caregivers are included in this plan, especially for those patients with communication deficits or paresis.

UI patients should also have a urinalysis and culture, as necessary, to evaluate for the presence of infection because a UTI can present with UI particularly if it occurs in either patients who have not previously been incontinent or reemerges in patients who have become continent post stroke. Poststroke male patients should be assessed for underlying BPH that can complicate UI treatment. If diagnosed with BPH, the incontinence plan of care should also include treatment of underlying BPH and may require referral to the urologist.

Evaluation

In the acute and rehabilitation settings, the interprofessional team includes assessment of continence in daily care rounds. An individualized plan involves such interventions as scheduled toileting, and clear and timely communication about voiding needs should be in place and adjusted base on patient progress. The nursing staff members are the team members primarily responsible for instituting such a plan and keeping the team apprised of successes and setbacks. Stroke survivors who require long-term institutional placement should also have plans in place to address UI. Stroke survivors who are able to return home should be asked about continence during appointments with their PCP or stroke specialists. Ongoing evaluation involves skin assessment to ensure that incontinence dermatitis, if present, is treated early to avoid complications. Referral to a urologist for management of persistent UI may be needed in instances where UI is perceived as problematic by the patient or the caregiver.

Clinical Pearl: UI can be an embarrassing problem for most patients, so the interprofessional team needs to be sensitive about the questions asked and therapies offered to the patient. Cultural sensitivity is especially important because some cultures tend to classify genitourinary problems as very sensitive and taboo for discussion.

ACUTE AND CHRONIC PAIN AFTER STROKE

Pain syndromes after stroke are associated with increased functional dependence and cognitive decline. Poststroke pain can include, but is not limited to, headache, hemiplegic shoulder pain, and central poststroke pain. Some of these pain syndromes will clearly begin in the acute poststroke time period, whereas others will become evident months after discharge. The literature suggests that chronic pain is seen in 32% to 42% of stroke patients at 6 months post stroke but decreases to 11% to 21% by about 12 months post stroke (Yang, Grabois, & Bruel, 2009). Additionally, many older stroke patients have pain from osteoarthritis, which is a limiting factor in rehabilitation (Nguyen-Oghalai, Ottenbacher, Granger, & Goodwin, 2005).

Pathophysiology

Headache

The relationship of headache and stroke is complex. Several plausible mechanisms have been postulated to explain the relationship between headache and stroke. These include vascular dilation as a homeostatic response to ischemia and direct arterial irritation by a thrombus, embolism, or dissection. Chronic daily headaches or migraine headaches may be coincidental or consequential to stroke. There is evidence that headaches and migraines increase stroke risk and may actually mimic stroke symptoms. Hemorrhagic stroke may present with headache as the intracranial structures begin to become compressed by expanding blood products. Large vessel ischemic stroke may be associated with a preceding headache or a headache during or after the event. Some patients will have headaches only in the acute phase, but for others, it will become a chronic problem. Given the lengthy differential diagnosis for headache, it can be difficult to determine a clear relationship between stroke and subsequent chronic headache.

Hemiplegic Shoulder Pain

Hemiplegic shoulder pain (HSP) develops within weeks to months after stroke and occurs at increased rates in stroke survivors with higher degrees of motor impairment. It is thought to occur in 9% to 40% of stroke survivors, but studies have varied in their definition and assessment of shoulder pain (Lindgren, Jönsson, Norrving, & Lindgren, 2007). The clinical picture of HSP includes paralysis, glenohumeral subluxation, shoulder pain, and tenderness over the biceps brachii and supraspinatus tendons. Poststroke spasticity can play a significant role in HSP (Yang et al., 2009). Although the etiology of HSP is not clearly understood, it is suggested that there is initial injury to weak shoulder muscles, but changes in the peripheral and central nervous system may allow pain to persist or worsen beyond initial injury. In one small study, it was found that patients with HSP have lower local and distal pressure pain thresholds than subjects without HSP, suggesting that chronic pain may be associated with widespread central hypersensitivity (Soo Hoo, Paul, Chae, & Wilson, 2013).

HSP often increases with passive range of motion and/or dependent positioning. In addition, HSP is associated with reduction in functional use, interferes with rehabilitation, and increased hospital stays. At least one study suggests that it is possible to not only manage HSP but also resolve HSP in the poststroke patient (Gamble et al., 2002). The ways in which manipulation of the affected shoulder after acute stroke can contribute to chronic shoulder pain has not been well studied. However, it seems reasonable to assume that members of the interprofessional care team, such as nurses, PT, and OT as well as family members, learn how to safely provide assistance to the patient during exercise, including positioning and range of motion, to decrease the possibility of a rotator cuff injury. In particular, avoiding sudden traction on the limb can decrease the risk of unintentional injury (Yang et al., 2009).

Central Poststroke Pain

Central poststroke pain (CPSP) is a neuropathic pain syndrome that affects up to 12% of stroke survivors (Creutzfeldt, Holloway, & Walker, 2012). It usually develops within weeks to months after a stroke and is prevalent after infarction in cerebral areas responsible for pain perception and processing. CPSP is also known as *thalamic syndrome* or *thalamic pain syndrome* because it is thought to be exclusively associated with thalamic injury. The pain is described as constant, moderate, or severe pain from damage to the brain. Research has shown that CPSP can affect patients who did not have a stroke but with some form of involvement of the thalamic region of the brain. As a result, the syndrome is now commonly called *central poststroke pain* rather than thalamic syndrome. CPSP is believed to arise from a lesion in the spinothalamic-cortical pathway and is seen more often in stroke survivors with nonthalamic lesions. CPSP produces pain which is often described as burning, aching, or prickling. CPSP can be continuous or intermittent and may be spontaneous or elicited with activity with concurrent symptoms of dysesthesia, allodynia, and hyperalgesia (Creutzfeldt et al., 2012). Response to light touch and vibration remains normal (Yang et al., 2009). Because central pain does not usually occur until a month or more after the stroke, it may not be immediately recognized as a stroke-related problem. The likelihood of someone developing chronic central pain does not correlate with the severity of the stroke. CPSP is extremely distressing and has been known to be refractory to treatment.

Assessment/Diagnosis

Major challenges can be faced in assessing pain in the acute stroke patient. Self-reporting of pain is the most reliable method for pain assessment. Attempts should be made to provide patients with tools to assist with describing and rating their acute pain. Unfortunately, aphasia and other communication deficits can limit the use of self-reporting tools in acutely ill stroke patients, and this should be taken into consideration in planning patient care. The use of 0 to 10 rating scale should be offered to patients without obvious communication deficits. Additionally, there is some evidence of use of such scales even when used in critically ill intubated patients (Puntillo et al., 2009). Intubated patients and patients with expressive aphasia and severe dysarthria may be able to nod and point to numbers on 0 to 10 scale to report pain. When possible, patients who can communicate effectively should be asked for qualitative descriptors, location, and associated symptoms. For patients with whom communication is limited or impossible, careful observation should be made for pain-related behaviors such as grimacing, rigidity, wincing, eye closure, moaning, and clenched fists. ⊙ As pain can interfere with participation in therapeutic practices and lead to increased functional and cognitive decline, all members of the interprofessional care team must be aware of potential pain in the stroke patient population.

Treatment

⊙ *Headache*: Management of acute headache associated with stroke initially involves a combination of a nonsteroidal pain medication such as acetaminophen with a short-acting opioid analgesic with limited effects on mental status, such as fentanyl. Based on the patient's response to short-term management, the interprofessional team works collaboratively to institute a plan for long-term management in which opioid narcotics play a minimal role. The team should consider how such factors as stress, lack of sleep, or the stroke itself are contributing to the patient's headache. Ascertaining the patient's usual pattern of caffeinated beverage intake or prior use of over-the-counter pain medications may help establish the extent to which abrupt withdrawal of either or both may be contributing to the headache.

Long-term management of headaches in poststroke patients is not well studied, making it difficult to quantify the problem. Should a stroke survivor develop chronic headaches that do not respond to standard management techniques, referral to a headache specialist is appropriate. It is reasonable to consider preventive medications such as calcium channel blockers, anticonvulsants such as topiramate or gabapentin, or tricyclic antidepressants. Beta-blockers should not be used as initial prophylaxis because of the increased risk of cerebrovascular events. Medications that may cause vasoconstriction such as triptans, serotonin antagonists, and ergot alkaloids should be avoided in patients with ischemic stroke. In addition, patients with recent ICH stroke should avoid aspirin for acute headache treatment and avoid NSAIDs for prophylaxis of migraines or other headaches (Diener & Limmroth, 2004). The use of triptan medications should be avoided for several months in patients with SAH due to the risk of vasospasm (Diener & Limmroth, 2004; Weir, Grace, Hansen, & Rothberg, 1978).

⦿ *Shoulder pain*: Shoulder pain is the most common form of local pain that stroke survivors experience but, as noted earlier, studies have varied in the definitions used to study the problem. Although the management of musculoskeletal problems in the general adult population typically involves exercise and PT, these interventions are problems in stroke survivors because many have little to no voluntary movement in the affected arm and many also have spasticity. A sling can be used to stabilize the affected arm and improve comfort for the patient. Imaging studies should be ordered to evaluate for subluxation of the shoulder joint or rotator cuff injury because these injuries are common and contribute to pain in the affected shoulder (Yang et al., 2009). PT with range of motion is recommended based on proposed etiology, but there is currently no evidence that PT reduces pain or improves range of motion (Creutzfeldt et al., 2012). For resistant pain, the use of intra-articular or subacromial injections of corticosteroids or botulinum have been effective. The use of sonography and electrical stimulation are beneficial for treatment of HSP. Transcutaneous electrical stimulation has been used to reduce pain and improve glenohumeral subluxation (Price & Pandyan, 2001), and ultrasonic therapy has also been shown to decrease tenderness and improve mobility of the affected shoulder (Moniruzzaman, Salek, Shakoor, Mia, & Moyeenuzzaman, 2010). It is likely that the cause of chronic shoulder pain associated with stroke is multifactorial and further study is required to better define the problem so that more effective therapies can be developed and deployed. In some studies, a significant number of poststroke patients with shoulder pain experienced resolution with the therapies currently available (Lindgren et al., 2007; Gamble et al., 2002).

Chronic poststroke pain: There are no medications which have been consistently shown to help with central pain. The antidepressant amitriptyline and the AED lamotrigine have been found to be effective in many patients with CPSP, but further clinical trials to optimize pain management in this patient population are indicated (Frese, Husstedt, Ringelstein, & Evers, 2006). Mexiletine, fluvoxamine, and gabapentin have also been shown to be helpful (Kumar, Kalita, Kumar, & Misra, 2009). One small recent study suggested that a short course of methylprednisolone could be effective for stroke survivors with CPSP (Pellicane & Millis, 2013). Opioid analgesics have not been found to be effective for CPSP (Yang et al., 2009). PT, heat and massage, and electrical nerve stimulation are other therapies that may help with chronic pain. Some patients with severe central pain syndromes might benefit from surgical interventions. Deep brain stimulation and motor cortex stimulation have shown promise (Kumar et al., 2009). Sometimes, patients develop a cycle where they become depressed and anxious about their pain which worsens the pain and then exacerbates the depression and anxiety. Assistance from a mental health professional, with experience in helping people with chronic pain, can be invaluable.

Best Practices

Early recognition and management of pain is essential for patient comfort and optimal participation in rehabilitation. Pain assessments should be routinely conducted by all members of the health care team. Recognition of the underlying pain mechanism is essential in effectively managing poststroke pain. Self-reporting is the most accurate method for assessing pain; however, for patients with poststroke communication difficulties, alternative methods should be made available, and the patient should be observed for pain behaviors.

Evaluation

The PCP and neurologist monitor the patient at follow-up visits for either the development of chronic pain or resolution of chronic pain syndromes. If the patient continues to have unresolved or worsening pain, then a referral to a pain specialist is indicated. Patients with chronic pain should also be screened for depression because depression is likely to be present in patients with chronic pain (Jönsson, Lindgren, Hallström, Norrving, & Lindgren, 2006).

DYSPHAGIA

Dysphagia, abnormality in the oropharyngeal swallowing process, is common after stroke with 42% to 57% of stroke patients presenting with dysphagia within 3 days of stroke (Donovan et al., 2013). Fifty percent of stroke patients who present with dysphagia aspirate, and one third of patients who aspirate ultimately develop pneumonia severe enough to require treatment (Hinchey et al., 2005). There is limited research about the incidence of dysphagia and aspiration in the cerebral hemorrhage population. However, one small study by Suntrup et al. (2012) found that hematoma volume was not predictive of swallowing impairment. Aspiration without cough, also known as *silent aspiration*, is a serious problem that further increases the incidence of pneumonia by 54% (Nakajoh et al., 2000). Dysphagia is associated with increased length of stay, malnutrition, dehydration, and even death (Karatepe, Gunaydin, Kaya, & Turkmen, 2008).

Pathophysiology

Stroke lesions within the cerebral hemispheres can impair voluntary control and bolus transport during swallowing. Cerebral lesions can also result in impaired cognition, which further interferes with control of swallowing. Cortical lesions impair oral motor control and result in contralateral face, lip, and tongue weakness that impair the ability to effectively generate bolus transport. The left MCA is most often associated with impairment of swallowing. Lesions in the frontal lobes can create abulia, which can lead to pocketing of food, and therefore increase risk of aspiration. Brainstem lesions can alter sensation of the mouth and tongue and can affect the timing of swallow as well as laryngeal elevation, closure of the glottis, and cricopharyngeal relaxation. These impairments create risk for boluses of food, liquids, and even secretions to pass inadvertently into the bronchus and lungs.

Assessment/Diagnosis

Dysphagia or swallow screening tools help to identify patients at risk for swallowing difficulty and those in need of further in-depth assessment. These screening tools are the first steps in identifying patients who are at risk for aspiration. Early detection of swallowing difficulties allows for immediate intervention and reduces mortality, length of stay, and overall health care costs (Hinchey et al., 2005; Martino et al., 2005; Odderson & McKenna, 1993).

⦿ Suspected stroke aspirators should be kept strictly NPO until an ST, trained physician, or nurse can perform a screening evaluation. Unfortunately, there continues to be much debate regarding the best screening tool for dysphagia. A good screening tool should be valid, measure aspiration risk, assess for appropriateness of oral feeding, as well as identify patients who need further evaluation by a specialist. According to the American Speech Language Association, a "swallow screening is a pass/fail procedure used to identify individuals who require a comprehensive assessment of swallowing function or a referral for other professional or medical services" (American Speech-Language-Hearing Association, 2004). Furthermore, a clinical dysphagia screening test should be easy to administer as well as specific and sensitive for the condition.

⦿ One of the most reliable, sensitive, and clinically feasible dysphagia screening tools is a bedside water swallow trial that can be administered by the nursing staff (Donovan et al., 2013). The trained bedside nurse or medical staff may perform dysphagia screen and refer to ST, as needed. Hospital facilities that care for stroke patients should have immediate availability of clinical staff trained in the bedside dysphagia screening. Due to the high morbidity and mortality associated with undiagnosed dysphagia and aspiration, The Joint Commission's Comprehensive Stroke Center Certification Program require that one or more qualified STs be available 7 days a week to perform patient swallowing assessments during the acute stroke phase (The Joint Commission, 2013). A clinical swallowing evaluation is a behavioral evaluation of swallowing function. Generally performed by an ST, it consists of cranial nerve evaluation and direct observation of swallowing. If a swallowing dysfunction continues to be suspected after clinical evaluation, an instrumental dysphagia study by direct visualization with videofluoroscopy or fiberscope should be performed.

Dietary modifications or dysphagia diets are highly individualized and include modification of food texture and fluid viscosities. A registered dietitian serves as an invaluable resource when dietary modifications are required. Dietitians are able to assist both the care team and the patient in establishing foods and liquids that will be tolerated while also providing the nutritional value and fluid requirements needed.

Treatment

⦿ The goals for management of dysphagia are to reduce the mortality and morbidity associated with aspiration, improve nutritional intake, and progress patients to normal diet as quickly as possible. Approaches for the management of dysphagia include temporary enteral feeding, dietary modification, positioning for feeding, and behavioral techniques such as voluntary airway protection and effortful swallowing. Swallowing therapies, directed by an ST, focus on improving the swallowing physiology through oral exercises, temperature stimulation of the oropharynx, transcutaneous neuromuscular stimulation, or olfactory stimulation. Several randomized controlled trials support the use of therapy for dysphagia and have demonstrated favorable outcomes when these therapies are used (Martino, Martin, & Black, 2012).

Temporary placement of a nasogastric tube for medication and feeding may afford time for spontaneous recovery from dysphagia. However, temporary feeding tubes do not eliminate risk for silent aspiration of oral secretions. Members of the health care team should be mindful of positioning and oral hygiene to reduce the risk of aspiration.

Best Practices

All stroke patients should be screened for dysphagia as quickly as possible after stroke diagnosis, depending on the patient condition and stability. Due to risk of aspiration, stroke patients should remain NPO until dysphagia screening can be performed. Numerous dysphagia screening tools exist, and the choice of facility screening instruments should be based on validity, sensitivity, and specificity of the tool as well feasibility of implementation. One easily performed screening tool is the bedside water swallow test in which an individual is observed while drinking 3 oz of water without interruption; stopping, choking, or a wet-hoarse vocal quality for up to 1 minute following the test results in failure. If the poststroke patient fails the dysphagia screening, or if there is continued suspicion of dysphagia, referral should be made to ST for further evaluation and management. Referral to a registered dietitian should be made to assist with the development of a nutritional plan for those patients required dysphagia modified diets.

Evaluation

Patients should be monitored for swallowing difficulty throughout the acute and rehabilitative process. Although dysphagia is associated with higher morbidity and mortality, recovery is high and generally occurs within the first few days to weeks after stroke (Mann, Hankey, & Cameron, 1999; Singh & Hamdy, 2006). If through evaluation by ST of a poststroke patient is determined to be chronically or severely dysphagic, consideration of a surgical procedure for long-term enteral feeding device placement should be considered.

Clinical Pearl: Although dysphagia is often associated with brainstem strokes, remember that any cerebral lesion that affects oral muscle strength and coordination has the potential to produce swallowing difficulty. Cerebral lesions that create inattention, apraxia, or decreased concentration are also highly associated with dysphagia and aspiration (Martino et al., 2005). Patients who, experience dysphagia may also experience decreased nutritional intake. Monitor the patient for dehydration and change the hypoglycemic regimen to accommodate this decreased nutritional intake for patients with a diagnosis of diabetes prior to their stroke.

■■ COMMUNICATION DEFICITS AFTER STROKE

Aphasia is a disruption of the normal comprehension and formulation of language caused by dysfunction in specific brain regions and is often associated with acute stroke. Aphasia complicates 15% to 38% of ischemic strokes (Inatomi et al., 2008). ICH patients with aphasia have been reported to experience a slower recovery than patients with ischemic stroke (Sinanovic, Mrkonjic, Zukic, Vidovic, & Imamovic, 2011). Patients with SAH are more likely to have communication deficits related to problems with executive function, memory, and subtle dysfunction of comprehension and expression (Al-Khindi, Macdonald, & Schweizer, 2010). *Language* is the communication of thoughts and feeling through signals such as gestures, writing, or voice sounds and is subserved by a large complex neurocognitive network, usually located in the left cerebral hemisphere. More than 95%

of right-handed individuals are left hemisphere language dominant, and 31% to 70% of left-handed individuals are left-sided language dominant as well (Isaacs, Barr, Nelson, & Devinsky, 2006; Knetch et al., 2000). Patients affected by injury to brain structures that initiate processing and interpretation of language may present with loss of ability to speak, recognize names or objects, or understanding of verbal language and directions.

Dysarthria is defined as a motor-speech disorder resulting from acute injury to motor components of the motor-speech system and can be characterized by poor articulation. Dysarthria is observed in up to 30% of stroke patients (Jordan & Hillis, 2006).

Pathophysiology

Aphasia: The language network is defined by indiscrete regions within the perisylvian cortex, including Broca's area in the posterior inferior frontal gyrus, Wernicke's area comprising the posterior two thirds of the superior temporal gyrus, and the angular gyrus of the inferior parietal lobule. However, the formation and interpretation of language is highly complex. Research has shown that areas within the cerebrum contribute greatly to language including the insula for articulation; the frontal and temporal lobes for sentence-level processing; and regions of the temporal, occipital, and parietal cortex for awareness of words and meanings. Subcortical infarcts with subsequent aphasia have been associated with better prognosis than aphasias with cortical infarcts. However, imaging trials examining cerebral perfusion in subcortical aphasia patients indicate that subcortical aphasia is often associated with perfusion restrictions within the cortical language regions (de Boissezon et al., 2005; Hillis, Wityk, & Barker, 2002).

Aphasia can be classified as clinically defined syndromes that reflect observed deficits in fluency, content, repetition, naming, comprehension, reading, and writing; however, many patients experience a myriad of deficits that are not clearly defined by one aphasia subtype. Neuroanatomical models of aphasia classification offer general association of aphasia syndromes with neuroanatomical location. **Table 9-2** indicates the types of aphasia.

Dysarthria: Ischemic injury secondary to stroke may result in weakness, paralysis, or lack of coordination of the motor speech system resulting in dysarthria. With dysarthria, there are no problems with speech content, but there is simply an inability to produce and pronounce intelligible speech. Dysarthria can be generally classified as spastic, hyperkinetic, hypokinetic, ataxic, and flaccid, depending on presenting symptoms and structure pathology. Commonly, patients with acute stroke may have a mixed dysarthria syndrome. Patients with acute dysarthria may have decreased control over the tongue, throat, lips, and concurrent dysphagia may be present (**Fig. 9-1**).

Assessment/Diagnosis

⊙ Problems with poststroke communication difficulties often are apparent during the performance of the NIHSS and bedside examination, which is usually sufficient to assess for aphasia. Bedside RNs and other interprofessional team members should observe poststroke patients for their ability to comprehend, repeat, name, read, and write. Spontaneous speech should be assessed for fluency and content. The three most common tools used to evaluate and diagnose aphasia are the *Minnesota Test for Differential Diagnosis*, the *Porch Index of Communicative Ability*, and the *Boston Diagnostic Aphasia Examination* (Goodglass & Kaplan, 1983; Porch, 1981). These tools are extensive and comprehensive and are not well suited for the screening of language disorders in acute stroke. However, they may be used in long-term evaluation and management.

TABLE 9-2 Classification of Aphasias with Anatomic Correlations

Type	Description/Clinical Correlation	Anatomic Area or Lesion
Broca's aphasia	Unable to convert thoughts into meaningful language Agrammatism (inability to organize words into sentences) Telegraphic speech (use of content words without connecting words) Distorted production of speech sounds Impaired repetition Normal reception of language is intact.	Broca's area (frontal lobe areas 44 and 45), underlying white matter, or basal ganglia
Wernicke's aphasia	Fluent speech that is unintelligible because of pronunciation errors and use of jargon Impaired comprehension of verbal and written language but no focal motor deficit Impaired repetition	Wernicke's area (superior temporal gyrus, area 22)
Conduction aphasia	Impaired repetition	Connections between Broca's and Wernicke's areas
Anomic aphasia	Impaired naming ability with preservation of other language functions	Lesion outside the language areas; possibly lower temporal lobe lesion or of generalized cerebral dysfunction
Transcortical aphasia	Impaired expression or reception of speech, but *repetition is spared*	Arterial border zones
Subcortical aphasia	Fluent, dysarthric speech and hemiparesis	Left caudate nucleus or the left thalamus
Global aphasia	Combined features of Wernicke's aphasia and Broca's aphasia Impaired comprehension and expression of language Impaired repetition Commonly associated with a dense contralateral hemiplegia	Perisylvian or central regions; commonly seen with left middle cerebral artery infarction (in patients with left hemisphere dominance)

From Hickey, J. V. (Ed.). (2014). *The clinical practice of neurological and neurosurgical nursing* (7th ed.). Philadelphia, PA: Lippincott Williams & Wilkins.

There are many comorbid conditions that can be confused with aphasia and dysarthria. Patients with metabolic encephalopathy, dementia, and depression may exhibit abnormal speech content and have difficulty following commands. Patients with poor dentition or oropharyngeal defects may have baseline dysarthria. It is important for nurses, therapists, and medical providers to obtain thorough history to assess for other medical conditions that may obscure proper assessment of acute language impairments.

Treatment

Aphasia and dysarthria can be devastating to patients and their families; therefore, timely referral to ST is recommended. Speech language therapy (SLT) approaches to acute aphasia may focus on the language deficit itself or the use of compensatory communication techniques. Although research indicates benefit of SLT in poststroke aphasia regarding functional communication, reading, comprehension, expressive language, and writing, there is debate regarding the superiority of treatment strategies with

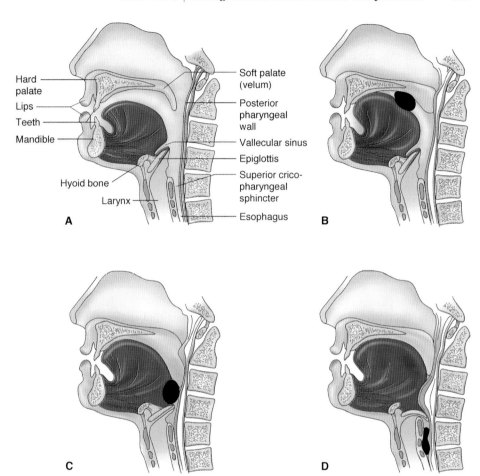

Hard palate
Lips
Teeth
Mandible
Hyoid bone
Larynx
Soft palate (velum)
Posterior pharyngeal wall
Vallecular sinus
Epiglottis
Superior crico-pharyngeal sphincter
Esophagus

A

B

C

D

FIGURE 9-1 **A–D:** Phases of normal swallowing. *(From Hickey, J. V. [Ed.]. [2014]. The clinical practice of neurological and neurosurgical nursing [7th ed.]. Philadelphia, PA: Lippincott Williams & Wilkins.)*

insufficient evidence to support one specific approach to deliver SLT for poststroke aphasia. Constraint-induced aphasia or language therapy, which is based on intensive therapy sessions that forced speech and avoidance of compensatory strategies, has shown modest benefit in chronic aphasia patients. However, the use of the constraint therapy in acute stroke is debated (Brady, Kelly, Godwin, & Enderby, 1996; Pulvermuller et al., 2001).

Data from clinical trials offer inconsistent results regarding the optimum start of therapy as well as duration. One review of 10 studies of 864 patients found that intense (mean 8.8 hours per week) speech and language therapy over a short period of time (mean 11.2 weeks) was more effective than less intense (mean 2 hours per week) therapy provided over longer periods of time (mean 22.9 weeks) (Bhogal, Teasell, & Speechley, 2003). However, a randomized controlled trial of 116 subacute patients found that patients who received therapy for 2 hours per week had similar results to those who received 5 hours of therapy per week (Bakheit et al., 2007).

Pharmacological therapies in poststroke aphasia patients are a newer area of treatment being investigated. A number of pharmacological agents have been studied in aphasia with the rationale of improving cerebral blood flow, replacing neurotransmitters, and enhancing neuroplasticity. However, results of these trials have shown limited benefits and require further investigation before the use of pharmacological agents can be recommended (Berthier et al., 2011; Greener, Enderby, & Whurr, 2010).

◉ Dysarthria treatment is generally managed through referral to ST and involves exercises to increase strength of articulator muscles and the use of alternate communication techniques. Alternate communication consists of flash cards or word boards to assist with conveying needs. Techniques for improving communication in the dysarthric patient include teaching a slower rate of speech, increasing volume of speech, frequent pausing, limiting conversation during periods of fatigue, and use of body language. Unfortunately, there is limited research with stroke patients to support their use. A review of the SLT literature for dysarthria secondary to nonprogressive brain damage found that there are no published controlled trials to support or refute the use of SLT in this patient population (Sellars, Hughes, & Langhorne, 2005).

Best Practices

◉ All stroke patients should be screened for communication deficits, and interprofessional team providers should be aware of the impact that communication deficits may have on the patient's participation in the plans of care. Patients suspected of communication deficits should be referred to ST for further assessment and management. Stroke patients with language deficits should be offered concentrated ST according to their deficits, objectives, and needs. Improved functional communication for aphasic patients may be achieved through the use of ST focusing on word production, word comprehension, reading and writing, and constraint-induced language therapy. Patients with poststroke dysarthria may benefit from SLT focused on strengthening articulator muscles and providing alternate methods of communication. There continues to be limited research regarding optimal treatment regimens for poststroke language therapies.

Evaluation

Prognosis of aphasia recovery often depends on underlying etiology and extent of injury. Most patients with poststroke aphasia have some improvement within the first few months. The severity of the initial aphasia strongly correlates with long-term prognosis. Often, those patients with minor aphasia at onset may recover completely. There is no evidence to suggest that handedness, gender, or age influence prognosis. Lazar et al. (2008) found that by 90 days, patients with significant aphasia after stroke improve by approximately 70% of the maximum potential recovery, as long as they receive at least some language therapy. Continued evaluation using facility-approved assessment tool should be carried out by speech language therapists and medical providers throughout the recovery process.

Clinical Pearl: Many patients with aphasia become frustrated due to their impaired communications. It is important for the interprofessional team to carve out time to interact with the patient so that the patient can feel included in decision making and plan of care, as this can be a stressful time for the patient with much uncertainty regarding recovery.

Patients with stroke, who may not have aphasia as a result of stroke, most often have some cognitive deficits including slowed information processing, which can affect their job performance when they return to work early after a stroke. It is important for ST to complete a language and cognitive assessment on all stroke patients to ensure that other cognitive and communication deficits besides aphasia are adequately addressed.

LONG-TERM COMMUNICATIONS DEFICITS

Some patients with stroke will have long-term communication problems. Dysarthria may not entirely resolve, making the stroke survivor difficult to understand, or there will always be some degree of aphasia. When considering communication deficits after stroke, the interprofessional team needs to consider the ways in which cognitive and perceptual sequelae after stroke will impact communication abilities. These sequelae may include such issues as impairments in memory, attention, initiation, problem solving, reasoning, apraxia, unilateral inattention or neglect, and agnosia. It has long been believed that much of language recovery occurs in the first weeks to months after stroke, with maximum recovery occurring within the first year. Newer studies suggest that with targeted therapies, more recovery of language may be possible in some patients even past the first 6 months after stroke (Miller, et al., 2010). The care team should also consider visual deficits, often seen in patients with right frontoparietal strokes, may be a form of communication deficit because it can lead to difficulties with such activities as goal-directed reaching, grasping, and pointing. Impaired communication abilities impact a patient's ability to function effectively in everyday life, and measures to improve communication can lead to improved well-being.

Pathophysiology

The area affected by the infarct determines the deficits which will be manifested by the patient. Theories are evolving regarding neuroplasticity and the ability of the brain to form new pathways to take over the functions of damaged areas (Musso et al., 1999; Shah, Szaflarski, Allendorfer, Hamilton, 2013; Thompson & den Ouden, 2008). Many patients have been known to spontaneously regain communication abilities long after the generally accepted time frame for recovery has passed.

Assessment/Diagnosis

ST is integral to diagnosis of problem and working with patients and families on solutions that include exercises, communication methods (picture or letter boards), and yes/no questions. There are many communication and cognition scales available to delineate the extent of the problem in order to tailor therapies which are discussed in the section on aphasia in this chapter. OT works with patients to enable them to overcome problems such as apraxia, inattention, and problem-solving deficits (Miller et al., 2010).

Treatment

Treatment of chronic communication problems centers on exercises to improve dysarthria and strategies to work around aphasia in order to maximize communication ability. An issue with long-term treatment may be the ability to pay for professional assistance because many insurance plans will only reimburse for a limited number of therapy sessions each year. Sessions involving physical, occupational, and speech therapy are considered as a whole, so it is important even over the long term that some of the therapy sessions involve communication. Although ST and OT can provide written materials and directions on how the patient and family can work independently, professional evaluation allows for objective assessment of progress as well as be helpful in modifying and progressing exercises. The National Aphasia Association, a nonprofit organization dedicated to helping those with aphasia, provides helpful information at their website and can be a valuable resource for patients and their families.

Best Practices

Five or more hours of weekly ST for those with chronic aphasia is considered standard management. There is a promising technique called *constraint-induced therapy*, which helps patients move beyond forms of communication that have come easily to them to those which may be more difficult but which will broaden their ability to interact with the world. The idea is to encourage patients to move beyond gesturing, drawing, or using a very limited number of words to return to speaking as their primary mode of communication. Look for community support groups for patient and significant others. The overall goal of therapy is to provide adaptive measures without encouraging learned non-use. Learned non-use occurs when a patient becomes so reliant on initial methods of communicating that he or she stops trying to acquire what might be better methods (Pulvermuller et al., 2001). There is ongoing research into the technique of transcranial magnetic stimulation as a noninvasive method of brain stimulation to improve language abilities in persons with aphasia.

Evaluation

On follow-up visits, providers working with the patient monitor both subjectively and objectively with communication scales to see how communication abilities have evolved between visits. Prescriptions for continued therapy are provided, as needed, for ongoing reimbursement of services.

POSTSTROKE DEPRESSION

Poststroke depression (PSD) is an important sequela of stroke that affects approximately one third to one half of stroke survivors within the first 2 years. Of patients affected by PSD, approximately 50% meet diagnostic criteria for major depression, whereas 50% of patients meet criteria for dysthymia/minor depression (Robinson, 1997, 2003). Onset of symptoms may occur within the acute or rehabilitative phase or may be delayed for months. Major depression is often associated with infarcts involving the left hemisphere. One study, which included patients with ICH, examined depression in patients with basal ganglia lesions (Herrmann, Bartels, Schumacher, & Wallesch, 1995). Studies investigating depression after SAH have estimated the frequency of depression to be from 5% to 50% (Al-Khindi, Macdonald, & Schweizer, 2010). Depression is also associated with increased hospital stays, increased morbidity and mortality, and decreased quality of life.

Pathophysiology

There is ongoing controversy regarding the underlying pathophysiology of PSD, and it is unlikely that PSD is a single disorder with one etiology. One commonly discussed hypothesis is that injury to the frontal cortex and basal ganglia disrupts the ascending noradrenergic and serotonergic projections, thus explaining the increased incidence of depression and mood disruptions in stroke patients with basal ganglia or frontal lobe infarcts (Robinson et al., 1984, 2000). Early onset of major depression after stroke is thought to be secondary to disruption of neural networks that support emotion, particularly those of the left hemisphere. Major depressive symptoms associated with PSD are often seen with larger lesions and increased functional impairment (Starkstein, Robinson, & Price, 1987; Starkstein, Robinson, Berthier, Parikh, & Price, 1988; Williams, Little, & Klein, 1986). There is some evidence that proinflammatory cytokines, including interleukin (IL)-1beta, 1L-18, tumor necrosis factor alpha, also serve to deplete serotonin after injury and may lead to development of depression (Spalletta et al., 2006). Finally, some researchers propose that PSD is not simply a result of injury to neural circuits and inflammation but is a result of social and psychosocial stressors that develop as a consequence of stroke. Studies in SAH patients with depression have suggested a link between the severity of the illness and fear of rebleeding; others have looked at the interplay between depression and cognitive issues post-SAH (Al-Khindi, Macdonald, & Schweizer, 2010).

Assessment/Diagnosis

Assessment of PSD may be complicated by aphasia and other cognitive and somatic stroke-related symptoms. Currently, there is no universally accepted screening or diagnostic tool for PSD, and health care facilities may vary in their approved instruments for screening. Traditionally, the *Diagnostic and Statistical Manual of Mental Disorders* (4th ed.; *DSM-IV*) criteria for depression have been used in research to establish a diagnosis of PSD. However, there is concern that *DSM-IV* does account for differences in symptom profiles between stroke patients and a general depression population and that the criteria do not weigh nonsomatic symptoms heavily enough to properly diagnose depression in a population of patients who are plagued by increased somatic symptoms due to natural stroke sequelae (Berg, Lonnqvist, Palomaki, & Kaste, 2009). The *DSM-IV* criteria also require a standardized psychiatric interview which can be burdensome for patients. Attempts continue to develop screening assessment tools for PSD that is clinically feasible to administer and offer high validity and reliability.

The *Beck Depression Inventory*, the *Hamilton Rating Scale for Depression* (HDRS), and the *Clinical Global Impression Assessment scales* in addition to the *DSM-IV* are useful in assessing depression, although none have shown superiority in assessing patients for PSD (Refer to Chapter 10 for a listing of depression scales). These assessment tools are not designed specifically for poststroke patients and often do not differentiate vegetative symptoms such as fatigue, psychomotor retardation, and insomnia that may be directly related to the stroke itself but are also part of the criteria of depression (Berg et al., 2009).The use of the *Visual Analogue Mood Scale* among patients with aphasia and cognitive impairment have not shown significant sensitivity and/or specificity to be recommended (Berg et al., 2009). The *Patient Health Questionnaires*, the *PHQ9* and *PHQ2*, are a 9-item and a two 2-item screening instruments that have reasonable validity and reliability and can be easily administered by nurses. The PHQ9 appears to perform reliably in a heterogeneous stroke population and is based on the nine *DSM-IV* symptoms of depression; therefore, it can be considered as a diagnostic tool as well as a screening instrument.

Treatment

Therapeutic strategies for the management and treatment of PSD are generally based in pharmacological therapy or psychotherapy. Antidepressant medications such as selective serotonin reuptake inhibitors (SSRIs), selective serotonin norepinephrine reuptake inhibitors (SSNRIs), or tricyclic antidepressants (TCAs) may be useful in treating PSD but should be used with caution particularly in the elderly because of known adverse event. Most of the research that has examined the use of pharmacotherapy in the treatment of PSD has focused on the SSRI and TCA medication classes with few studies to support the use of the newer SSNRIs. Psychotherapy includes direct patient–professional interactions that are targeted at assisting patients develop problem-solving skills and adjust to the emotional impact of stroke.

No one class of antidepressant medications have been shown to be superior in the treatment of PSD. Selection of pharmacological agent may be based on the depressive symptoms, side effect profile, and previous use of antidepressant medications, drug interactions, and concurrent medical conditions. A study by Jorge et al. (2003) examined the use of antidepressant medications for PSD and found that fluoxetine, an SSRI, and nortriptyline, a TCA, both significantly increased 9-year survival after stroke.

SSRIs have been used for many years in treating mood disorders and are generally well tolerated, making them the often preferred antidepressant agent. Fluoxetine is the most studied SSRI in the ischemic stroke patient population, although there has been much research on the use of sertraline as well. It should be noted that there has been concern that SSRI medications may theoretically increase bleeding risk due to effects on platelet aggregation; thus, the use of SSRIs in patients with hemorrhagic strokes or with concurrent use of antiplatelet or anticoagulants must be approached with caution.

In animal models, SSRIs have also been shown to have direct effect on the brain, encouraging new cell development; this has led to much research in the use of SSRIs in the treatment of PSD. Chollet et al. (2011) published the "Fluoxetine on Motor Rehabilitation after Ischemic Stroke" or "FLAME" trial, which reported improvement in motor deficits at 3 months for stroke patients who were treated with fluoxetine, even if they were not depressed.

Although the SSRI drugs have become the mainstay for the treatment of PSD, providers should be aware of other potential pharmacological options for treatment. Some patients may not tolerate or not have relief of the symptoms, and it is reasonable to attempt a course of a TCA. Nortriptyline is one of the most reported TCAs used in the effective treatment of PSD, although the inherent anticholinergic and muscarinic effects, as well as potential for cardiotoxicity, can limit their use in the elderly or cardiac patients.

Although psychotherapy continues to be used in adjunctive treatment of PSD, there are limited trials to support its use. In fact, a review of three trials including 455 participants showed no treatment effect in any of the end points measured (Hackett, Anderson, House, & Xia, 2008). As psychotherapy can be time-intensive, expensive, and requires professional expertise, it is often reserved for patients who are not tolerant or are resistant to antidepressant medication.

Best Practices

All patients with strokes should be screened for depressive symptoms using a validated tool throughout the continuum of stroke care. Patients with mild symptoms of depression may be initially managed by observant waiting. However, treatment of PSD has been associated with improved functional outcomes and may reduce mortality and morbidity and increase quality of life. SSRIs and TCA medications have been shown to improve PSD; however, there is more evidence to support the use of SSRIs due to improvement in functional recovery and more favorable adverse effect profile. There is little evidence to support routine psychotherapy in the PSD population, although it should be considered for patients intolerant or resistant to pharmacotherapy. Patients treated with antidepressant should be monitored regularly by professional and should include evaluation of severity of depression and adverse effects of treatment. Patients and their families should be instructed about risk of suicide and routinely asked about the presence of symptoms.

Evaluation

There continues to be much debate regarding the best screening and ongoing evaluation tools for PSD. Research has shown that patients may experience PSD symptoms acutely after strokes or may present with symptoms months after the event. Therefore, it is important to continue to monitor depressive symptoms using a valid, reliable, and easily administered rating instrument throughout the continuum of stroke care, including posthospital follow-up appointments and periodic health assessments with PCP.

⊙ Nurses and other care providers along with family members should be vigilant in monitoring poststroke patients for development of mood changes. Referral may be made to mental health professional with knowledge of depression following brain injury and appropriate pharmacotherapy should be considered. The American College of Physicians suggests that patients treated with antidepressants are to be continued on pharmacotherapy for at least 4 months beyond recovery, and treatment should be changed if there is no response within 6 weeks (Qaseem, Snow, Denberg, Forciea, & Owens, 2008). Patients and their families should be routinely questioned about worsening of depression, particularly after initiation or adjusting antidepressant medications.

Clinical Pearl: Because of the risk of suicide associated with antidepressant use, it is important to include family in the plan of care when first initiating antidepressants in poststroke patients. It is also important to allow time for the patient to go through the stages of grieving immediately post stroke prior to making a decision to treat for depression with pharmacological therapies. This is important because grieving the loss of independence or function is an important part of recovery.

▮▮ FALLS AND GAIT PROBLEMS

Many patients with stroke will have prolonged or permanent deficits, which increase the risk of falling post stroke. Falls are the most common poststroke complication, surpassing even urinary tract and pulmonary infections. According to studies, 15% to 65% of patients will experience a fall while still hospitalized, and nearly three quarters of stroke survivors will fall within the first 6 months after discharge (Batchelor, Hill, Mackintosh, & Said, 2010). Although more studies are required to better delineate the circumstances under which hospitalized stroke patients fall, many nurses may not realize that studies have shown that most falls occur during the daytime rather than at night (Weerdesteyn, de Niet, van Duijnhoven, & Geurts, 2008). One small prospective study found that near-falls while hospitalized and upper extremity disability were the two factors most correlated with postdischarge falls (Ashburn, Hyndman, Pickering, Yardley, & Harris, 2008). Although 5% of stroke patients will sustain a serious injury as a result of a fall, that injury, usually a hip fracture, could mean the difference between returning home and placement in a long-term care facility (Weerdesteyn et al., 2008). A hospitalized stroke patient will be found and helped up quickly, but a high percentage of those who fall at home will be unable to get up without assistance and may be down for a prolonged period of time, resulting in secondary injuries which may result in institutional placement. Complications resulting from falls are the fifth leading cause of death overall in adults. Fear of falling causes a significant number of older individuals to moderately or severely restrict their activities, which can paradoxically increase the likelihood of a fall from deconditioning.

Pathophysiology

Pathophysiology underlying fall risks varies by patient and stroke type. Some patients will have gait problems related to motor and/or sensory deficits which will create an increased risk for falls. Neglect syndromes, as well as cognitive deficits of judgment and impulsivity, must be taken into account when considering risk of falls. Long-term visual deficits from field cuts can contribute significantly to risk of falls. Older patients may have been high risk for falls prior to stroke from age-related changes in visual acuity, diabetic neuropathy retinopathy, or other chronic medical problems.

Assessment/Diagnosis

The interprofessional care team works together to delineate a patient's risk factors for falls. Risk factors other than the stroke itself include lower extremity weakness, advanced age, female gender, cognitive impairment, balance problems, arthritis, diabetes, orthostasis, alcohol use, and anemia. Older stroke patients are at higher risk for indoor falls than younger patients. The risk of falls increases with the number of risk factors present in an individual patient. PT and OT are keys in clearly delineating which stroke characteristics increase the risk of falls such as specific weakness, balance problems related to sensory disturbances, or poor visual acuity. ST can assist in establishing the presence and degree of cognitive impairment which also contribute to risk of falls.

Treatment

PT, OT, and ST can evaluate the patient and develop a multidisciplinary plan of care individualized to the patient. The plan is implemented while the stroke patient is hospitalized and continued after hospital discharge with reevaluation at appropriate intervals. The patient and family are provided with copies of the plan, and strategies are reviewed. The nurse provides reinforcement and encouragement prior to discharge. If the patient is to receive home health care visits after discharge, the home health nurse will review the plan and also provides reinforcement and encouragement while working with home or outpatient PT, OT, and ST.

It is helpful for all those involved in the poststroke care of a patient to remain cognizant of the fact that fatigue decreases the ability to manage deficits, and appropriate rest periods should be incorporated into any plan for the day. Families with computer access should be encouraged to access the AHA/ASA websites for helpful advice and information. The National Stroke Association has a brochure titled *Mobility after Stroke*, which patients and their families might find helpful. Should a fall occur, once appropriate care has been provided, the circumstances leading to the fall should be reviewed and strategies to prevent further falls be implemented.

Best Practices

A safety assessment of the home is helpful for many stroke survivors, although it is not clear if the decrease in falls is wholly attributable to environmental modifications made or to behavioral changes related to the therapist's visit. Surprisingly, bedrails seem to increase injuries and death without decreasing the risk of falls (Oliver, 2002; Parker & Miles, 1997). Some studies suggest that ensuring adequate vitamin D levels, particularly in women, may help decrease the risk of falls in older individuals, but further studies are warranted (Verheyden et al., 2013). A meta-analysis investigating falls did not identify any interventions which clearly and consistently reduced falls (Batchelor et al., 2010). Given the methodological variations in the studies reviewed, further studies are warranted, but because stroke survivors are a heterogeneous population, no one strategy will likely be found to be effective for all or even the majority. A recent prospective study confirmed the multifactorial nature of falls in stroke survivors (Tilson et al., 2012).

Evaluation

When patients are seen by their neurologist or PCP, they and their families should be queried about falls or near-falls, frequency of falls, and any changes in gait or balance. Diabetic patients should be monitored for development or worsening of peripheral neuropathy that could increase the risk of falls. The worsening of existing deficits can raise the question of a new stroke but should also lead to search for infection, particularly UTI.

Clinical Pearl: Falls in hospitalized stroke patients are more likely to occur during the day rather than at night. Most patients do not fall by accident; they fall because they have a difficult time giving up their independence and so attempt to ambulate on their own without first asking for help from the nursing staff. Others have neglect syndromes which prevent them from recognizing their own deficits. It is important for the care team to recognize how difficult it is for most patients to give up their independence and so they need frequent reassurance regarding their abilities.

▉ SPASTICITY/HEMIPARESIS AND HEMIPLEGIA

Loss of motor strength due to stroke is common with 88% of stroke patients affected (Gresham et al., 1995). *Hemiparesis* is the decrease in motor strength on one side of the body, whereas hemiplegia is paralysis or lack of motor strength on one side of the body. Patients affected by hemiparesis and hemiplegia have decreased muscle control, weakness, and decreased coordination and may develop increased muscle tone leading to spasticity.

Poststroke spasticity (PSS) is a leading cause of poststroke disability. Patients with severe weakness or paralysis are often affected. Observation cohort studies estimate that PSS may affect 17% to 43% of the 6.5 million American stroke survivors (Patel, 2011). Symptoms of spasticity depend on location of the affected muscles and joints but often include painful muscle spasms, hypertonicity, clonus, exaggerated deep tendon reflexes, scissor gait, and fixed joints. Spasticity may eventually result in contractures, joint deformities, and fixed postures. Recognizable posturing patterns can include shoulder adductions, elbow and wrist flexion, hip adduction, knee extension, and plantar flexion in the ankle.

Pathophysiology

Hemiparesis and hemiplegia are thought to be caused by ischemia and subsequent injury to the corticospinal tracts resulting in cell death. Although this is seen in ischemic stroke patients as a result of embolic or thrombotic blockage of vessels, it is mostly likely to be seen in SAH patients who develop delayed ischemic neurological deficits or as a complication of the procedure to secure the ruptured aneurysm. In patients with ICH, these deficits can result from compression of vessels or destruction of tissue by the hematoma. The severity of the hemiparesis and hemiplegia depends on the size of the resulting lesion as well as the location. Small cortical and subcortical lesions may result in little to no motor impairment. However, lesions in the internal capsule where there are dense motor fibers may result in devastating motor weakness and lead to loss of motor function even with smaller lesions.

Spasticity is characterized by velocity-dependent resistance of muscle to stretching. This type of muscle overactivity is known as *tonic stretch reflex*. The tonic stretch reflex is generally increased after lesions to the dorsal reticulospinal tract in the brainstem, where inhibition of motor activity occurs. However, lesions within the motor and the premotor cortexes can create spasticity due to increased phasic stretch reflex. However, spasticity is due not only to increased reflex activity but also to intrinsic changes of the muscles. Nonneuronal adaptive changes of the noncontractile and contractile units result in changes in the collagen tissues and tendons, stiffness of muscle fibers, loss of sarcomeres, and changes in mechanical muscle fiber properties (Sommerfield, Gripenstedl, & Welmer, 2012).

The time frame for the onset of spasticity after stroke depends on the underlying mechanism. Electromyographic (EMG) studies have shown that reflex-mediated increase in muscle tone reaches peak between 1 and 3 months after stroke. Intrinsic changes within the muscles are thought to initiate muscle resistance after 3 months (Fellows, Ross, & Thilmann, 1993; Thilmann, Fellows, & Garms, 1991).

Assessment/Diagnosis

Motor weakness and deficits are generally noted during the screening neurological examination of stroke patients. The NIHSS rates muscle strength using 4-point scale, although the sensitivity of NIHSS for identifying fine motor weakness is questioned (Brott, et al., 1989). The *Fugl-Meyer Assessment* is an extensive evaluation of motor function, but it is quite time intensive and impractical in the acute setting bedside assessment (Fugl-Meyer, Jaasko, Leyman, Olsson, & Steglind, 1975). The *Motor Assessment Scale* offers a briefer evaluation of motor strength and function, but it is generally limited to evaluation of stable motor deficits (Carr, Shepherd, Nordholm, & Lynne, 1988).

All stroke patients should be monitored for development of spasticity after stroke. There are several clinical instruments that can be used for determining spasticity, which are discussed further in the "Evaluation" section. As noted earlier, the timing of onset of spasticity is variable and therefore requires ongoing attention by all members of the team throughout the rehabilitation process.

Treatment

Treatment of poststroke hemiplegia and hemiparesis involved an interprofessional team including PT, OT, nurses, and other providers. Traditionally, treatment of hemiparesis and hemiplegia has been based on the neurophysiological theory or motor relearning, which emphasizes movements for task accomplishment. Constraint-induced movement therapy (CIMT), as well as mirror therapy, has also been used to assist in the rehabilitation of motor deficits with some benefit (Dohle et al., 2009; Thieme, Mehrhoz, Pohl, Behrens, & Dohle, 2012; Van der Lee et al., 1999, 2000). CIMT involves a combination of restraining of unaffected limb and intensive use of the paretic limb. Mirror therapy uses mirror images to superimpose correct movement of the unaffected limb over the hemiparetic or hemiplegic limb. Newer forms of treatment of stroke-associated motor deficits include neuromuscular and sensory stimulation of affected limbs (Chae et al., 1998). Referral to an orthotic specialist can assist in bracing of the affected limb to allow for maximum participation in activities of daily living (ADLs).

Therapy for PSS is typically targeted at reducing excessive muscle tone and providing patients with improved range of movement and better performance of ADLs. Treatment regimens for prevention and treatment of spasticity often involve a multiple-discipline approach that incorporates PT, OT, and systemic antispastic medication, local injections of botulism or phenol, and possibly surgical intervention (Thibaut et al., 2013).

Antispastic medication can be tried for troublesome spasticity, unless contraindicated. Baclofen, which inhibits both the monosynaptic and polysynaptic reflexes at the spinal level, is widely used. Other medications such as tizanidine and dantrolene as well as benzodiazepines can also be used but have more extensive side effect/risk profile. Common side effects of oral antispastic medication often carry risks of confusion and drowsiness, and there is weak evidence for use in stroke patients. Intrathecal baclofen, delivered by an implantable catheter, has shown to be effective in the generalized severe spasticity of cerebral origin (Sommerfield et al., 2012).

For patients with focal spasticity limited to one or two joints, botulinum toxin and intramuscular phenol injections have shown effectiveness in treating problematic focal spasticity. Botulinum toxin is a potent biologic toxin which acts by blocking neuromuscular transmission by inhibiting acetylcholine release, thereby reducing muscle tone. There is no evidence that suppression of spasticity by either PT or medication results in substantial improvements in motor function, and outcome studies have failed to demonstrate the superiority of any treatment approach in stroke rehabilitation.

When attempts are made to reduce spasticity, patients often use the increased tone in the limbs for strength and locomotion, and treatment outcomes may need to be titrated in order to maintain function. An example to consider would be a patient with severe lower extremity paresis who uses developed spasticity to provide support while walking.

Best Practices

An interprofessional team approach to rehabilitation of hemiparesis and hemiplegia should be undertaken as quickly as safely as possible after stroke. Therapy should be aimed at increasing active movement and functional use of affected limb. CIMT is generally not undertaken in the acute phase of stroke. Mirror therapy and the use of sensory stimulation of the affected limb should be considered for selected patients. Orthosis and adaptive devices should be used when possible to improve abilities to perform ADLs. Bedside nurses should be aware of safe positioning of affected limb within patients' visual field.

All patients with motor involved strokes should be observed and evaluated for development PSS. Treatment of PSS should be multidisciplinary and incorporate the use of prescribed pharmacological agents, therapeutic exercise, positioning, stretching, and splinting as needed. Intrathecal baclofen and injectable botulinum are reasonable treatment options for patients with distressing, resistant spasticity.

Evaluation

● Continued evaluation of motor deficits following stroke should be conducted during neurological examinations. Nurses, therapists, and other providers should evaluate ongoing need for assistive devices and for safety concerns. Patient and families should be questioned regarding abilities to perform ADLs.

Evaluation of spasticity can be difficult due to its multifactorial and complex nature. However, accurate evaluation of spasticity is needed to guide treatment decisions and measure patient progress. The *Ashworth and Modified Ashworth Scale* (MAS) are the most widely used methods of measuring clinical spasticity, due in a large part to the simplicity and reproducibility of findings. The MAS measures resistance to passive stretch and therefore can be criticized for measuring hypertonia of muscle rather than true spasticity (Bohannon & Smith, 1987). The Ashworth Scale assigns scores ranging from 0 (*no increased tone*) to 4 (*complete rigidity of joint on flexion or extension*) with 5 choices for each tested joints. The MAS, developed by Bohannon and Smith (1987), is similar to the Ashworth Scale but adds an additional score of $1+$ for joints that demonstrate resistance through less than half the movement.

Poststroke patients with spasticity require evaluation during the rehabilitation process and transition to community living. Ongoing evaluation by all members of the health care team for the development of comorbid conditions such as skin breakdown, pain, and depression is essential. Adequate support from family members and caregivers should be evaluated to ensure that problems with limited mobility can be safely addressed at home.

Clinical Pearl: The way in which a hemiplegic shoulder is manipulated during hospitalization may be related to the development of chronic shoulder pain. Acute traction on the affected arm should particularly be avoided. If in doubt about pain related to a hemiplegic shoulder, an orthopedic consultation should be pursued to rule out other complications.

▮▮ NEGLECT SYNDROMES

Hemispatial neglect, also known as *neglect, hemiagnosia*, and *hemineglect*, is a condition in which a lesion to one cerebral hemisphere creates inattention to the contralateral body or unilateral spatial neglect. Neglect is most widely described as failure "to report, respond or orient to novel or meaningful stimuli presented to the opposite side of the brain lesion" (Heilman & Valenstein, 1993). Stroke may affect the ability of an individual to direct attention in the visual, auditory, or tactile modalities. Terms such as *visual neglect, motor neglect, hemineglect, and inattention* are used to describe various types of neglect seen after stroke (The Cochrane Collaboration, 2008). Neglect syndromes are generally found after parietal lobe and, less common, frontal lobe lesions and affects a person's ability to look, listen, or make movement in one half of their environment (The Cochrane Collaboration, 2008). Interestingly, patients can even present with "representational neglect," in which they may ignore the left side of memories, dreams, and even visual hallucinations. The term *anosognosia* is often used to refer to a condition in which patients who suffer from hemineglect are unaware of their disability.

Extinction represents a common type of visuospatial inattention and is the impairment of the ability to perceive multiple stimuli of the same type presented to both sides of the body or environment. For example, a patient with extinction will not perceive touch to the left side of the body when touched on both sides, although the left side can detect the sensation of touch when each side is tested individually. Visual extinction arises from damage to parietal lobes and is characterized by difficulty in perceiving stimuli in the visual field contralateral to the brain lesion, although stimuli can be correctly identified when the visual fields are tested independent of one another.

Pathophysiology

There have been several proposed theories to explain the development of neglect syndrome; however, neglect syndromes reflect a group of heterogeneous disorders that possibly have varied pathophysiology. Thus, it is possible that there is no one theory that can fully explain its underlying mechanisms.

Kinsbourne's theory of hemispheric rivalry postulates that the contralateral attention is served by each hemisphere and mutual transcallosal inhibition keeps in check the overactivity in the opposing hemisphere to keep attention evenly allocated. Unilateral hemispheric injuries, such as cerebrovascular injury, disrupt the inhibitory process, thereby resulting in increased activity in the contralateral hemisphere. This overactivity in the contralateral hemisphere increases the inhibition to the injured hemisphere and creates an asymmetric attentional field exhibited as neglect (Kinsbourne, 1977). An alternate theory of neglect reflects the limited attentional ability of the right hemisphere after injury. The right cerebral hemisphere is considered to maintain attentional functions for both hemispatial fields; thus, right-sided neglect secondary to left hemispheric lesions is rare because of redundant processing of the right space by both right and left cerebral hemispheres (Heilman & Van Den Abell, 1980; Mesulam, 1981).

A third theoretical model for the development of neglect is proposed by Corbetta and Shulman (2002) and includes components from both the hemispheric rival theory and right hemispheric dominance theory of spatial processing. This model of neglect argues that partially segregated networks of brain areas carry out various attention functions and that dysfunction of distributed cortical networks, rather than structural damage to specific brain regions, is the underlying mechanism for the development observed neglect.

Assessment/Diagnosis

All patients with strokes should be assessed for visual and spatial neglects. Traditionally, the clinical assessment of unilateral neglect has involved the use of written tests such as line bisection tasks, cancellation tasks, and copying and drawing evaluations. Asking a patient to perform tasks such as combing the hair or dressing may reveal hemineglect if the patient fails to groom the hair or dress one half the body.

Treatment

⊙ Treatment for stroke patients with visual and/or spatial neglect often focuses on functional adaptation such as visual scanning, environmental adaptations, environmental cuing, limb activation, and patient and caregiver education. Nursing care and therapy sessions should be modified to cue attention to the impaired side in patients with neglect. Neglect rehabilitation studies have focused on techniques of prism adaptations, sensory stimulation, and virtual reality training. Some investigators have shown improvements in neglect following repetitive transcranial magnetic stimulation of the contralateral hemisphere (Oliveri et al., 2001). Unfortunately, rehabilitative techniques have shown limited success with little evidence that rehabilitative changes persist over time (Carter, Connor, & Dromerick, 2010).

Best Practices

⊙ All patients with suspected neglect syndromes should be assessed by OT. Neuro-optometry consult may also be beneficial in providing prism insert for eye glasses which direct images from a neglected field to the unaffected side. Treatment of neglect may include visual scanning techniques, cuing, imagery, virtual reality, limb activation, and positioning. Screening for falls and providing a safe environment for ambulation is of utmost importance.

Evaluation

Most research studies investigating neglect after stroke have shown that approximately 10% to 40% of patients demonstrating acute neglect will continue to exhibit symptoms at 3 to 12 months following injury (Black, Ebert, Leibovitch, Szalai, & Blair, 1995; Campbell & Oxbury, 1976; Cassidy, Lewis, & Gray, 1998; Colombo, De Renzi, & Gentilini, 1982; Samuelsson et al., 1997). Therefore, continued evaluation of neglect and improvement in functional outcomes should be performed. ADLs can be assessed by Barthel Index.

Clinical Pearl: It may be difficult to discern visual spatial neglect from homonymous hemianopia, which is the loss of visual fields secondary to damage within the visual pathways. This differentiation of pathologies may be particularly difficult in patients with large hemispheric lesions and those with communication deficits. It is important to test individual visual fields as well as to simultaneously test bilateral visual fields to distinguish between these two pathologies. Frequent reassessment may be needed as the patient's ability to communicate improves.

▉ STROKE-RELATED MORTALITY AND END-OF-LIFE CARE

Because stroke is primarily a disease of older people, patients will often have comorbidities which will affect outcomes (Sörös & Hachinski, 2012). One study found that advanced age and high NIHSS on presentation are associated with death soon after stroke (Nedeltchev et al., 2010). Another study found a correlation between need for mechanical ventilation and percutaneous endoscopic gastrostomy (PEG) placement with poor outcome (Golestanian, Liou, & Smith, 2009). In one retrospective study, patients whose stroke was determined to be from a cardioembolic source were found to have a higher risk of death than those whose stroke was from a different subtype (Stead et al., 2011). Atrial fibrillation, in particular, has been associated with increased morbidity and mortality (Steger et al., 2004). One prospective study investigating younger stroke survivors found lower mortality rates in this population (Leys et al., 2002). A recent Brazilian study found a higher risk of death in stroke patients who were diabetic or lacking in formal education (Goulart et al., 2013). Still another study found that about 75% of patients with a hemorrhagic stroke died within 5 years of the stroke (Kojic, Burina, Hodzic, Pasic, & Sinanovic, 2009). Although younger people who experience strokes will have a lower mortality rate than older people, stroke is associated with higher long-term mortality compared to their age cohort overall (Varona, 2010).

Pathophysiology

The pathophysiology underlying death from stroke is initially related to the size, location, and type of stroke. In the first week, death is most often attributed to direct effects of the stroke. With or without maximal medical intervention, the size of the stroke leading to herniation or the location of the stroke in a critical area such as the brainstem (control of vital signs) often result in early death. In one study of autopsies, PE was the most common cause of death in weeks 2 to 4, followed by pneumonia in weeks 2 to 3, and cardiovascular causes after the first 3 months (J. Kelly et al., 2001). It is not clear how many deaths in the days and months subsequent to stroke are related to withdrawal of life support. One small study suggested withdrawal of life support may represent a significant percentage of acute stroke deaths (A.G. Kelly, Hoskins, & Holloway, 2012). A prospective Korean study of 600 patients found that patients who experienced in-hospital complications had a higher risk of death in the first several years after stroke (Bae et al., 2005).

Assessment and Diagnosis

Given statistical data about mortality and major disability associated with stroke, it should be clear that palliative care programs for stroke are essential. It is important to have early discussions with families and, to the extent possible, patients regarding previously expressed wishes regarding to resuscitation status and advance directives. Ongoing discussions throughout hospitalization are important to be sure that all involved have realistic expectations regarding goals of care (Burton & Payne, 2012). The bedside nurse is available to answer questions for the patient and family along with assessing how well they have understood explanations of the patient's condition and likely outcomes. The case manager and social workers can be helpful to determine adequate family support and available resources for discharge to palliative care either at home or in a facility. If the institution has a specialized palliative care service, they should be formally consulted and available to work with the family and the patient (as possible). Palliative care appears to be most often used in decisions about withdrawal of the use of mechanical ventilation in acute stroke patients, but this is an area requiring further study (Burton & Payne, 2012). The AHA and ASA have released their first guideline of recommendations regarding palliative and end-of-life care for stroke patients. The guideline suggests that the interprofessional stroke team provide primary palliative care and involve a specialty palliative care team for especially complex problems. The aspects they consider essential to primary palliative care are the promotion and practice of patient and family centered care; the ability to effectively estimate prognosis; the development of appropriate goals of care; familiarity with common stroke decisions with end-of-life implications; the ability to assess and manage stroke symptoms; experience with palliative treatments; the ability to refer patients to a specialized palliative care service; allowing patients and families the opportunity for personal growth and access to bereavement services as appropriate; and, finally, participation in research and quality improvement (Holloway et al., 2014).

Although palliative care and stroke remains an understudied area, a British screening tool, the *Sheffield Profile for Assessment and Referral for Care* (SPARC), has been found to be helpful in deciding whether long-term stroke survivors should be referred to palliative care (Stevens, Payne, Burton, Addington-Hall, & Jones, 2007). The SPARC screening tool is holistic and can be used over time to gauge progression or improvement of various aspects of the lived experience of stroke survivors and their families, addressing problems in a timely manner. Many stroke survivors are older and have serious comorbidities which are likely to worsen over time, so palliative care should not be considered only in the acute phase. All patients and their families should be given opportunities over time to reaffirm their commitment to continued care or consider a change to palliative care and hospice.

Treatment

Treatment for the dying stroke patient is not necessarily just for the patient but must also focus on the family. Death of a loved one from stroke is especially life changing for families in which the patient was the main breadwinner or if young children are involved. Institutions vary in the practices focused on family support during the palliative care processes. Care for the patient and the family does not stop with palliative care. Goals of care often change over time, and an individualized patient-centered plan of care can be developed and modified as needs change over time that is consistent with the wishes of the patient and their family.

Best Practices

Although mortality is not preventable in the most severe strokes, stroke patients benefit from the implementation and adherence to standards for venous thromboembolism prophylaxis, removal of all indwelling catheters as soon as possible, use of VAP bundles, and other measures to decrease the incidence of complications which can lead to death. Working with the patient and family to increase the likelihood of adherence to measures intended to prevent future strokes is likely to decrease stroke-related deaths. Studies investigating death from stroke implicate inadequate secondary stroke prevention in both recurrent stroke and increased mortality (Cheung et al., 2007).

In those patients who die in the hospital, involvement of a palliative care team when withdrawal of support will occur is important. All members of the interprofessional care team should be equipped with the appropriate knowledge, skills, competence, and confidence to be able to work effectively to provide symptom management for patient comfort and to provide any other necessary support for the patient and family. End-of-life acute stroke care should be provided by a team with experience in the care of stroke patients. Understanding how underlying problems with cognition, dysphagia, and impaired communication related to stroke that can affect end-of-life care will enable the team to better support the patient and family. Given that stroke patients for whom end-of-life care is appropriate are unlikely to be able to express themselves, information should be obtained from the family and significant others regarding any wishes previously expressed by the patient in this regard. There is limited evidence about care for stroke patients and end-of-life issues, most notably airway/respiratory management, positioning, continence care, bowel management, pressure area care, and personal hygiene. The interprofessional team is also cognizant of the spiritual and religious needs of the patient and family and ensures that access to spiritual and religious support is provided.

Evaluation

For most dying stroke patients, evaluation both during the change from medical intervention to transition into palliative and end-of-life care leading to a peaceful death focuses on how well institutional policies and procedures supported the transition process. All members of the interprofessional care team are engaged in maintaining clear communication channels both within the team and with patients and their families. In instances where the death of the stroke patient is unexpected, the team reviews the care of the patient to ensure that all standards of care were met, especially preventable complications of stroke and hospitalization.

Case Study Mr. Multiple Falls (MF) is a 51-year-old, right-handed male with a past medical history of hypertension. He woke up on the morning of admission without deficits and went to work at Burger King, where at 9:20 a.m., he developed weakness on right arm and leg hemiparesis, drooling, and dysarthria. EMS was called and they took the patient immediately to the ED where initial vitals were BP, 193/119 mm Hg; HR, 90 beats per minute; RR, 39 breaths per minute; T, 37°C; O_2, 98% RA. Patient was initially alert, able to state name and location but was otherwise not oriented. He had a dense right-sided hemiparesis, left gaze deviation that could not be overcome by doll's maneuver, no blink to threat on right eye, copious secretions, and severe dysarthria. He was following commands initially, but after a stat CT scan, he was noted to be less responsive with increased secretions and so was intubated for airway protection. CT scan showed a large, left basal ganglia hemorrhage measuring 1.8 × 4.9 cm. BP continued to remain in 190s to 250s mm Hg despite nicardipine drip and a total of 40 mg IV labetalol. Patient's wife reportedly stated that patient is supposed to be on BP medications but does not take them. ∎

Hospital Course

Mr. MF was initially admitted to the NICU for stabilization and ongoing management. He was started on a clevidipine infusion for his malignant hypertension, which was weaned off 3 days later. He initially had a 4-mm left to right midline shift on CT which worsened to 7-mm shift in the first 24 hours after admission. Initially, he was treated with mannitol for 3 days. Mr. MF had an external ventricular drainage (EVD) device placed, which remained in place for 4 days. He had problems with agitation and delirium and was unable to be managed with redirection. He required Precedex infusion and initiation of Risperdal in NICU, and these were weaned off prior to transfer from NICU to the stepdown unit. Mr. MF required a bedside care attendant and wrist/hand restraints as well as oral anxiolytics and sleep aids to reestablish a normal sleep–wake cycle.

Complications

Mr. MP had a prolonged hospitalization of 73 days due to multiple factors complicating disposition planning including a continued requirement for a patient attendant for which many rehabilitation centers will decline admission due to inability to provide such services on a consistent basis. During his hospitalization, he worked with PT, OT, ST, and social work, and a discharge planner was involved in disposition planning. His right-sided spasticity required frequent passive range of motion. He had dysphagia requiring NG placement initially; however, it was discontinued once ST determined he was safe for oral intake. Mr. MF had multiple falls during his hospitalization, requiring a patient attendant at bedside at all times. Among his deficits were urinary and fecal incontinence, communication deficits, and decreased nutritional intake.

Outcome

Mr. MP was eventually discharged home with his wife with support of home health PT/OT/ST/nursing and nurse aide services. At the time of discharge, the patient did not have resources or insurance; he applied for Medicaid. His wife was able to take 2 weeks of Family and Medical Leave Act (FMLA) for the transition home. However, the patient needed 24-hour supervision and assistance related to his deficits for which his wife was unable to provide on her own. She had to find church members and other family members to assist. The patient had a modified Rankin Score of 4 or 5 for severe disability, which is consistent with inability to attend to personal bodily needs, thus requiring around-the-clock care.

Mr. MF had follow-up visit in the outpatient stroke clinic approximately 4 weeks after discharge. His wife reported that he had Medicaid pending. He was now working with PT, OT, or ST. Nursing services that had been providing home visits reported BP readings that were running less than 140/90 mm Hg. There had been no difficulties in taking his medications. Although he continued to have dense right-sided hemiparesis, he was able to make transfers from a bed to a chair with one-person assistance and had no falls since being home. Spasticity was under control with the use of oral baclofen, and Mr. MF had no complaints of pain. He was tolerating a regular diet, although he continued to have moderate dysarthria but no evidence of aspiration. UI continued to be a problem, causing Mrs. MF to sleep in another bed. Both the patient and his wife acknowledged Mr. MF's continued emotional lability with frequent crying and sadness. After a lengthy discussion regarding poststroke emotional disorders and depression, the decision was made to restart a low-dose fluoxetine. Risk and benefits were discussed including potential for worsening depression and suicidal ideations. The patient's wife was instructed to call the stroke clinic to discuss how Mr. MF was tolerating the fluoxetine, but both patient and wife understood that immediate results were not to be expected. Mr. MF was also scheduled to see his PCP within 2 weeks. A follow-up appointment was made for 3 months with the stroke clinic.

REFERENCES

Abbott, A. L., Bladin, C. F., & Donnan, G. A. (2001). Seizures and stroke. In J. Bogousslavsky & L. R. Caplan (Eds.), *Stroke syndromes* (2nd ed., pp. 182–191). Cambridge, United Kingdom: Cambridge University Press. doi:10.1017/CBO9780511586521.014
Aggarwarl, S. K., Azim, A., Baronia, A. K., & Kumar, R. (2012). Evaluation and management of nosocomial sinusitis in intensive care unit patients for pyrexia of unknown origin: Case report and review of literature. *International Journal of Medicine and Biomedical Research*, 1(2), 161–166.

Al-Khindi, T., Macdonald, R. L., & Schweizer, T. A. (2010). Cognitive and functional outcome after aneurysmal subarachnoid hemorrhage. *Stroke, 41*, e519–e536.

Ashburn, A., Hyndman, D., Pickering, R., Yardley, L., & Harris, S. (2008). Predicting people with stroke at risk of falls. *Age Ageing, 37*, 270–276.

American Speech-Language-Hearing Association. (2004). *Preferred practice patterns for the profession of speech-language pathology.* Rockville, MD: American Speech-Language-Hearing Association. Retrieved from http://www.asha.org/policy/PP2004-00191.htm

American Diabetes Association. (2010). Standards of medical care in diabetes—2010. *Diabetes Care, 33*(Suppl. 1), S11–S61. doi:10.2337/dc10-S011

Andrew, J., & Nathan, P. W. (1964). Lesions on the anterior front lobes and disturbances of micturiton and defaecation. *Brain, 87*, 233–262.

Andrews, P. J., Sleeman, D. H., Statham, P. F. X., McQuatt, A., Corruble, V., Jones, P. A., . . . Macmillan, C. S. A. (2002). Predicting recovery in patients suffering from traumatic brain injury by using admission variables and physiological data: A comparison between decision tree analysis and logistic regression. *Journal of Neurosurgery, 97*(2), 326–336.

Arif, H., Buchsbaum, R., Pierro, J., Whalen, M., Sims, J., Resor, S. R., Jr., . . . Hirsch, L. J. (2010). Comparative effectiveness of 10 antiepileptic drugs in older adults with epilepsy. *Archives of Neurology, 67*(4), 408–415. doi:10.1001/archneurol.2010.49

Aslanyan, S., Weir, C. J., Diener, H. C., Kaste, M., & Lees, K. R. (2004). Pneumonia and urinary tract infection after acute ischaemic stroke: A tertiary analysis of the GAIN International trial. *European Journal of Neurology, 11*(1), 49–53.

Back, T., Ginsberg, M. D., Dietrich, W. D., & Watson, B. D. (1996). Induction of spreading depression in the ischemic hemisphere following experimental middle cerebral artery occlusion: Effect on infarct morphology. *Journal of Cerebral Blood Flow and Metabolism, 16*(2), 202–213. doi:10.1097/00004647-199603000-00004

Badjatia, N., Topcuoglu, M. A., Buonanno, F. S., Smith, E. E., Nogueira, R. G., Rordorf, G. A., . . . Singhal, A. B. (2005). Relationship between hyperglycemia and symptomatic vasospasm after subarachnoid hemorrhage. *Critical Care Medicine, 33*(7), 1603–1609; quiz 1623.

Bae, H. J., Yoon, D. S., Lee, J., Kim, B. K., Koo, J. S., Kwon, O., & Park, J. M. (2005). In-hospital medical complications and long-term mortality after ischemic stroke. *Stroke, 36*(11), 2441–2445. doi:10.1161/01.STR.0000185721.73445.fd

Bakheit, A. M., Shaw, S., Barrett, L., Wood, J., Carrington, S., Griffiths, S., . . . Koutsi, F. (2007). A prospective, randomized, parallel group, controlled study of the effect of intensity of speech and language therapy on early recovery from poststroke aphasia. *Clinical Rehabilitation, 21*(10), 885–894.

Barer, D. H., Cruickshank, J. M., Ebrahim, S. B., & Mitchell, J. R. (1988). Low dose beta blockade in acute stroke ("BEST" trial): An evaluation. *British Medical Journal, 296*(6624), 737–741.

Barth, E., Albuszies, G., Baumgart, K., Matejovic, M., Wachter, U., Vogt, J., . . . Calzia, E. (2007). Glucose metabolism and catecholamines. *Critical Care Medicine, 35*(Suppl. 9), S508–S518. doi:10.1097/01.CCM.0000278047.06965.20

Batchelor, F., Hill, K., Mackintosh, S., & Said, C. (2010). What works in falls prevention after stroke?: A systematic review and meta-analysis. *Stroke, 41*(8), 1715–1722. doi:10.1161/STROKEAHA.109.570390

Berg, A., Lonnqvist, J., Palomaki, H., & Kaste, M. (2009). Assessment of depression after stroke: a comparison of different screening instruments. *Stroke, 40*(2), 523–529.

Bershad, E. M., Feen, E. S., Hernandez, O. H., Suri, M. F. K., & Suarez, J. I. (2008). Impact of a specialized neurointensive care team on outcomes of critically ill acute ischemic stroke patients. *Neurocritical Care, 9*(3), 287–292. doi:10.1007/s12028-008-9051-5

Berthier, M. L., Pulvermuller, F., Davila, G., Casares, N. G., & Gutierrez, A. (2011). Drug therapy of post-stroke aphasia: A review of current evidence. *Neuropsychology Review, 21*(3), 302-317.

Bhogal, S., Teasell, R., & Speechley, M. (2003). Intensity of aphasia therapy, impact on recovery. *Stroke, 34*, 987–993.

Black, S., Ebert, P., Leibovitch, F., Szalai, J. P., & Blair, N. (1995). Recovery in hemispatial neglect. *Neurology, 45*(Suppl. 4), A178.

Bladin, C. F., Alexandrov, A. V., Bellavance, A., Bornstein, N., Chambers, B., Coté, R., . . . Norris, J. W. (2000). Seizures after stroke: A prospective multicenter study. *Archives of Neurology, 57*(11), 1617–1622.

Bohannon, R. W., & Smith, M. B. (1987). Interrater reliability of a modified Ashworth scale of muscle spasticity. *Physical Therapy, 67*(2), 206–207.

Boneu, B., Caranobe, C., & Sie, P. (1990). Pharmacokinetics of heparin and low molecular weight heparin. *Baillière's Clinical Haematology, 3*(3), 531–544.

Bösel, J., Schiller, P., Hook, Y., Andes, M., Neumann, J. O., Poli, S., . . . Steiner, T. (2013). Stroke-related Early Tracheostomy versus Prolonged Orotracheal Intubation in Neurocritical Care Trial (SETPOINT): A randomized pilot trial. *Stroke, 44*(1), 21–28. doi:10.1161/STROKEAHA.112.669895

Bowen, A., Hazelton, C., Pollock, A., & Lincoln, N. B. (2013). Cognitive rehabilitation for spatial neglect following stroke. *Cochrane Database of Systematic Reviews*, (7), CD003586. Retrieved from http://summaries. cochrane.org/CD003586/STROKE_cognitive-rehabilitation-for-spatial-neglect-following-stroke

Brady, M. C., Kelly, H., Godwin, J., & Enderby, P. (1996). Speech and language therapy for aphasia following stroke. *Cochrane Database of Systematic Reviews*, 5, CD000425. Abstract retrieved from http://onlinelibrary.wiley.com/doi/10.1002/14651858.CD000425.pub3/abstract

Brambrink, A., & Orfanakis, A. (2010). "Therapeutic hypercapnia" after ischemic brain injury: Is there a potential for neuroprotection? *Anesthesiology*, *112*(2), 274–276. doi:10.1097/ALN.0b013e3181ca8273

Brandstater, M. E., Roth, E. J., & Siebens, H. C. (1992). Venous thromboembolism in stroke: Literature review and implications for clinical practice. *Archives of Physical Medicine and Rehabilitation*, *73*(Suppl. 5), S379–S391.

Broderick, J., Connolly, S., Feldmann, E., Hanley, D., Kase, C., Krieger, D., . . . Zuccarell, M. (2007). Guidelines for the management of spontaneous intracerebral hemorrhage in adults: 2007 update: A guideline from the American Heart Association/American Stroke Association Stroke Council, High Blood Pressure Research Council, and the Quality of Care and Outcomes in Research Interdisciplinary Working Group. *Stroke*, *38*(6), 2001–2023. doi:10.1161/STROKEAHA.107.183689

Brott, T., Adams, H., Olinger, C., Marler, J., Barsan, W., Biller, J., . . . Walker, M. (1989). Measurements of acute cerebral infarction: A clinical examination scale. *Stroke*, *20*, 864–870.

Bruno, A., Biller, J., Adams, H. P., Jr., Clarke, W. R., Woolson, R. F., Williams, L. S., & Hansen, M. D. (1999). Acute blood glucose level and outcome from ischemic stroke. Trial of ORG 10172 in Acute Stroke Treatment (TOAST) Investigators. *Neurology*, *52*(2), 280–284.

Bruno, A., Levine, S. R., Frankel, M. R., Brott, T. G., Lin, Y., Tilley, B. C., . . . Fineberg, S. E. (2002). Admission glucose level and clinical outcomes in the NINDS rt-PA Stroke Trial. *Neurology*, *59*(5), 669–674.

Burneo, J. G., Fang, J., & Saposnik, G. (2010). Impact of seizures on morbidity and mortality after stroke: A Canadian multi-centre cohort study. *European Journal of Neurology*, *17*(1), 52–58. doi:10.1111/j.1468-1331.2009.02739.x

Burton, C. R., & Payne, S. (2012). Integrating palliative care within acute stroke services: A developing a programme theory of patient and family needs, preferences and staff perspectives. *BMC Palliative Care*, *11*(1), 22. doi:10.1186/1472-684X-11-22

Camilo, O., & Goldstein, L. B. (2004). Seizures and epilepsy after ischemic stroke. *Stroke*, *35*(7), 1769–1775.

Campbell, D., Oxbury, J. (1976). Recovery from unilateral visuo-spatial neglect? *Cortex*, *12*, 303–312.

Carr, J., Shepherd, R., Nordholm, L., & Lynne, D. (1988). Investigation of a new motor assessment scale for stroke patients. *Physical Therapy*, *65*(2), 175–180.

Carter, A., Connor, L., & Dromerick, A. (2010). Rehabilitation after stroke: Current state of the science. *Current Neurology and Neuroscience*, *10*(3), 158–166.

Cassidy, T. P., Lewis, S., & Gray, C. S. (1998). Recovery from visuospatial neglect in stroke patients. *Journal of Neurology, Neurosurgery, and Psychiatry*, *64*(4), 555–557.

Chae, J., Bethoux, F., Bohinic, T., Dobos, L., Davis, T., & Friedle. (1998). A neuromuscular stimulation of for upper extremity motor and functional recovery in acute hemiplegia. *Stroke*, *29*, 975–979 doi: 10.1161/01.STR.29.5.975

Chamorro, A., Urra, X., & Planas, A. M. (2007). Infection after acute ischemic stroke: A manifestation of brain-induced immunodepression. *Stroke*, *38*(3), 1097–1103. doi:10.1161/STR.0000258346.68966.9d

Cheung, C. M., Tsoi, T. H., Au-Yeung, M., & Tang, A. S. Y. (2003). Epileptic seizure after stroke in Chinese patients. *Journal of Neurology*, *250*(7), 839–843. doi:10.1007/s00415-003-1091-3

Cheung, C. M., Tsoi, T. H., Hon, S. F. K., Au-Yeung, M., Shiu, K. L., Lee, C. N., & Huang, C. Y. (2007). Outcomes after first-ever stroke. *Hong Kong Medical Journal*, *13*(2), 95–99. doi:10.1161/01.STR.0000130989 .17100.96

Chobanian, A. V., Bakris, G. L., Black, H. R., Cushman, W. C., Green, L. A., Izzo, J. L., Jr., . . . Roccella, E. J. (2003). The Seventh Report of the Joint National Committee on Prevention, Detection, Evaluation, and Treatment of High Blood Pressure: the JNC 7 report. *The Journal of the American Medical Association*, *289*(19), 2560–2572. doi:10.1001/jama.289.19.2560.

Chollet, F., Tardy, J., Albucher, J. F., Thalamas, C., Berard, E., Lamy, C., . . .Loubinoux, I. (2011). Fluoxetine for motor recovery after acute ischaemic stroke (FLAME): A randomised placebo-controlled trial. *Lancet Neurology*, *10*(2), 123–130.

Christopher, K. L. (2005). Tracheostomy decannulation. *Respiratory Care*, *50*(4), 538–541.

Chusid, J. G., & Kopeloff, L. M. (1962). Epileptogenic effects of pure metals implanted in motor cortex of monkeys. *Journal of Applied Physiology*, *17*, 697–700.

Claassen, J., Carhuapoma, J. R., Kreiter, K. T., Du, E. Y., Connolly, E. S., & Mayer, S. A. (2002). Global cerebral edema after subarachnoid hemorrhage: Frequency, predictors, and impact on outcome. *Stroke*, *33*(5), 1225–1232.

CLOTS Trials Collaboration. (2009). Effectiveness of thigh-length graduated compression stockings to reduce the risk of deep vein thrombosis after stroke (CLOTS trial 1): A multicentre, randomised controlled trial. *Lancet*, *373*(9679), 1958–1965. doi:10.1016/S0140-6736(09)60941-7

CLOTS Trials Collaboration. (2013). Effectiveness of intermittent pneumatic compression in reduction of risk of deep vein thrombosis in patients who have had a stroke (CLOTS 3): A multicentre randomised controlled trial. *Lancet*, *382*(9891), 516–524. doi:10.1016/S0140-6736(13)61050-8

Colombo, A., De Renzi, E., & Gentilini, M. (1982). The time course of visual hemi-inattention. *Archiv Für Psychiatrie Und Nervenkrankheiten*, *231*(6), 539–546.

Connolly, E. S., Rabinstein, A. A., Carhuapoma, J. R., Derdeyn, C. P., Dion, J., Higashida, R. T., . . . Vespa, P. (2012). Guidelines for the management of aneurysmal subarachnoid hemorrhage: A guideline for health-care professionals from the American Heart Association/American Stroke Association. *Stroke*, *43*(6), 1711–1737. doi:10.1161/STR.0b013e3182587839

Coplin, W. M. (2012). Critical care management of acute ischemic stroke. *Continuum (Minneapolis, Minn.)*, *18*(3), 547–559. doi:10.1212/01.CON.0000415427.53653.1b

Corbetta, M., & Shulman, G. (2002). Control of goal-directed and stimulus-driven attention in the brain. *Nature Reviews Neuroscience*, *3*, 201–215.

Creutzfeldt, C. J., Holloway, R. G., & Walker, M. (2012). Symptomatic and palliative care for stroke survivors. *Journal of General Internal Medicine*, *27*(7), 853–860. doi:10.1007/s11606-011-1966-4

Davison, D. L., Terek, M., & Chawla, L. S. (2012). Neurogenic pulmonary edema. *Critical Care*, *16*(2), 212. doi:10.1186/cc11226

de Boissezon, X., Démonet, J. F., Puel, M., Marie, N., Raboyeau, G., Albucher, J. F., . . . Cardebat, D. (2005). Subcortical aphasia: A longitudinal PET study. *Stroke*, *36*(7), 1467–1473.

De Georgia, M. A., Krieger, D. W., Abou-Chebl, A., Devlin, T. G., Jauss, M., Davis, S. M., . . . Warach, S. (2004). Cooling for Acute Ischemic Brain Damage (COOL AID): A feasibility trial of endovascular cooling. *Neurology*, *63*(2), 312–317.

De Reuck, J., Goethals, M., Claeys, I., Van Maele, G., & De Clerck, M. (2006). EEG findings after a cerebral territorial infarct in patients who develop early- and late-onset seizures. *European Neurology*, *55*(4), 209–213. doi:10.1159/000093871

De Stefano, V., Martinelli, I., Mannucci, P. M., Paciaroni, K., Chiusolo, P., Casorelli, I., . . . Leone, G. (1999). The risk of recurrent deep venous thrombosis among heterozygous carriers of both factor V Leiden and the G20210A prothrombin mutation. *The New England Journal of Medicine*, *341*(11), 801–806. doi:10.1056/NEJM199909093411104

Dhawan, V., & DeGeorgia, M. (2012). Neurointensive care biophysiological monitoring. *Journal of Neurointerventional Surgery*, *4*(6), 407–413. doi:10.1136/neurintsurg-2011-010158

Diener, H. C., & Limmroth, V. (2004). Medication-overuse headache: A worldwide problem. *The Lancet Neurology*, *3*(8), 475–483. doi:10.1016/S1474-4422(04)00824-5

Diringer, M. N., & Edwards, D. F. (2001). Admission to a neurologic/neurosurgical intensive care unit is associated with reduced mortality rate after intracerebral hemorrhage. *Critical Care Medicine*, *29*(3), 635–640.

Diringer, M. N., Reaven, N. L., Funk, S. E., & Uman, G. C. (2004). Elevated body temperature independently contributes to increased length of stay in neurologic intensive care unit patients. *Critical Care Medicine*, *32*(7), 1489–1495. doi:10.1097/01.CCM.0000129484.61912.84

Dohle, C., Pullen, J., Naketen, A., Kust, J., Reitz, C., Karbe, H. (2009). Mirror therapy promotes recovery from severe hemiparesis: A randomized controlled trial. *Neurorehabilitation and Neural Repair*, *23*(3), 209–217.

Donovan, N. J., Daniels, S. K., Edmiaston, J., Weinhardt, J., Summers, D., & Mitchell, P. H. (2013). Dysphagia screening: State of the art: Invitational conference proceeding from the State-of-the-Art Nursing Symposium, International Stroke Conference 2012. *Stroke*, *44*(4), e24–e31. doi:10.1161/STR.0b013e3182877f57

Durgan, D. J., & Bryan, R. M. (2012). Cerebrovascular consequences of obstructive sleep apnea. *Journal of the American Heart Association*, *1*(4), e000091. doi:10.1161/JAHA.111.000091

Dütsch, M., Burger, M., Dörfler, C., Schwab, S., & Hilz, M. J. (2007). Cardiovascular autonomic function in poststroke patients. *Neurology*, *69*(24), 2249–2255. doi:10.1212/01.wnl.0000286946.06639.a7

Elmer, J., Hou, P., Wilcox, S. R., Chang, Y., Schreiber, H., Okechukwu, I., . . . Goldstein, J. N. (2013). Acute respiratory distress syndrome after spontaneous intracerebral hemorrhage. *Critical Care Medicine*, *41*(8), 1992–2001. doi:10.1097/CCM.0b013e31828a3f4d

Engoren, M., Arslanian-Engoren, C., & Fenn-Buderer, N. (2004). Hospital and long-term outcome after tracheostomy for respiratory failure. *CHEST Journal*, *125*(1), 220–227. doi:10.1378/chest.125.1.220

European Stroke Organisation Executive Committee & European Stroke Organisation Writing Committee. (2008). Guidelines for management of ischaemic stroke and transient ischaemic attack 2008. *Cerebrovascular Diseases (Basel, Switzerland)*, *25*(5), 457–507. doi:10.1159/000131083

Feigin, V. L., Rinkel, G. J. E., Lawes, C. M. M., Algra, A., Bennett, D. A., van Gijn, J., & Anderson, C. S. (2005). Risk factors for subarachnoid hemorrhage: An updated systematic review of epidemiological studies. *Stroke*, *36*(12), 2773–2780. doi:10.1161/01.STR.0000190838.02954.e8

Fellows, S., Ross, H., & Thilmann, A. (1993). The limitations of the tendon jerk as a marker of pathological stretch reflex activity in human spasticity. *Neurol Neurosurg Psychiatry*, *56*, 531–537.

Fernandez, A., Schmidt, J. M., Claassen, J., Pavlicova, M., Huddleston, D., Kreiter, K. T., . . . Mayer, S. A. (2007). Fever after subarachnoid hemorrhage: Risk factors and impact on outcome. *Neurology*, *68*(13), 1013–1019. doi:10.1212/01.wnl.0000258543.45879.f5

Ferro, J. M., & Pinto, F. (2004). Poststroke epilepsy: Epidemiology, pathophysiology and management. *Drugs & Aging*, *21*(10), 639–653.

Finley Caulfield, A., & Wijman, C. A. C. (2008). Management of acute ischemic stroke. *Neurologic Clinics*, *26*(2), 345–371. doi:10.1016/j.ncl.2008.03.016

Foerch, C., Kessler, K., Steckel, D., Steinmetz, H., & Sitzer, M. (2004). Survival and quality of life outcome after mechanical ventilation in elderly stroke patients. *Journal of Neurology, Neurosurgery, and Psychiatry*, *75*(7), 988–993. doi:10.1136/jnnp.2003.021014

Fowler, C. J., Griffiths, D., & de Groat, W. C. (2008). The neural control of micturition. *Nature Reviews. Neuroscience*, *9*(6), 453–466. doi:10.1038/nrn2401

Fraser, D. G. W., Moody, A. R., Morgan, P. S., Martel, A. L., & Davidson, I. (2002). Diagnosis of lower-limb deep venous thrombosis: A prospective blinded study of magnetic resonance direct thrombus imaging. *Annals of Internal Medicine*, *136*(2), 89–98.

Frese, A., Husstedt, I. W., Ringelstein, E. B., & Evers, S. (2006). Pharmacologic treatment of central post-stroke pain. *The Clinical Journal of Pain*, *22*(3), 252–260. doi:10.1097/01.ajp.0000173020.10483.13

Fugl-Meyer, A., Jaasko, L., Leyman, I., Olsson, S., & Steglind, S. (1975). The post stroke hemiplegic patient. I. A method for evaluation of physical performance. *Scandinavian Journal of Rehabilitation Medicine*, *7*, 13–31.

Fujii, Y., Takeuchi, S., Sasaki, O., Minakawa, T., Koike, T., & Tanaka, R. (1996). Ultra-early rebleeding in spontaneous subarachnoid hemorrhage. *Journal of Neurosurgery*, *84*(1), 35–42. doi:10.3171/jns.1996.84.1.0035

Gamble, G. E., Barberan, E., Laasch, H. U., Bowsher, D., Tyrrell, P. J., Jones, A. K. (2002). Post-stroke shoulder pain: A prospective study of the association and risk factors in 152 patients from a consecutive cohort of 205 patients presenting with stroke. *European Journal of Pain*, *6*(6), 467–474.

Gelber, D. A., Good, D. C., Laven, L. J., & Verhulst, S. J. (1993). Causes of urinary incontinence after acute hemispheric stroke. *Stroke*, *24*(3), 378–382.

Gilad, R., Lampl, Y., Eschel, Y., & Sadeh, M. (2001). Antiepileptic treatment in patients with early postischemic stroke seizures: A retrospective study. *Cerebrovascular Diseases (Basel, Switzerland)*, *12*(1), 39–43.

Giroud, M., Gras, P., Fayolle, H., André, N., Soichot, P., & Dumas, R. (1994). Early seizures after acute stroke: A study of 1,640 cases. *Epilepsia*, *35*(5), 959–964.

Glass, T. F., Fabian, M. J., Schweitzer, J. B., Weinberg, J. A., & Proctor, K. G. (2001). The impact of hypercarbia on the evolution of brain injury in a porcine model of traumatic brain injury and systemic hemorrhage. *Journal of Neurotrauma*, *18*(1), 57–71. doi:10.1089/089771501750055776

Glauser, T., Ben-Menachem, E., Bourgeois, B., Cnaan, A., Chadwick, D., Guerreiro, C., . . . Tomson, T. (2006). ILAE treatment guidelines: Evidence-based analysis of antiepileptic drug efficacy and effectiveness as initial monotherapy for epileptic seizures and syndromes. *Epilepsia*, *47*(7), 1094–1120. doi:10.1111/j.1528 -1167.2006.00585.x

Golestanian, E., Liou, J. I., & Smith, M. A. (2009). Long-term survival in older critically ill patients with acute ischemic stroke. *Critical Care Medicine*, *37*(12), 3107–3113. doi:10.1097/CCM.0b013e3181b079b2

Goodglass, H., & Kaplan, E. (1983). Boston Diagnostic Aphasia Examination (BDAE). Philadelphia: Lea and Febiger.

Goulart, A. C., Fernandes, T. G., Santos, I. S., Alencar, A. P., Bensenor, I. M., & Lotufo, P. A. (2013). Predictors of long-term survival among first-ever ischemic and hemorrhagic stroke in a Brazilian stroke cohort. *BMC Neurology*, *13*(1), 51. doi:10.1186/1471-2377-13-51

Greener, J., Enderby, P., & Whurr, R. (2010). Pharmacologic treatment for aphasia following stroke. Cochrane Collaboration. Published Online: 23 OCT 2001 Assessed as up-to-date: 4 JUL 001DOI: 10.1002/14651858. CD000424

Gresham, G., Duncan, P., Stason, W., Adams, H., Adelman, A., Alexander, D., et al. (1995). Clinical practice guidelines, Post stroke Rehabilitation, 16. US Department of Health and Human Services.

Gross, H., Sung, G., Weingart, S. D., & Smith, W. S. (2012). Emergency neurological life support: Acute ischemic stroke. *Neurocritical Care*, *17*(Suppl. 1), S29–S36. doi:10.1007/s12028-012-9749-2

Guyton, A. C., & Hall, J. E. (2006). *Textbook of Medical Physiology.* (11th ed.). Philadelphia: Elsevier Inc.

Hackett, M., Anderson, C., House, A., & Xia, J. (2008). Interventions for treating depression after stroke. *Cochrane Database of Systematic Reviews*, 4, Art. No.: CD003437. DOI: 10.1002/14651858.CD003437 .pub3

Hajat, C., Hajat, S., & Sharma, P. (2000). Effects of poststroke pyrexia on stroke outcome: A meta-analysis of studies in patients. *Stroke*, *31*(2), 410–414. doi:10.1161/01.STR.31.2.410

Hankey, G. J. (1993). Prolonged exacerbation of the neurological sequelae of stroke by post-stroke partial epileptic seizures. *Australian and New Zealand Journal of Medicine*, *23*(3), 306–306. doi:10.1111/j.1445-5994.1993 .tb01737.x

Harvey, R. L., Roth, E. J., Yarnold, P. R., Durham, J. R., & Green, D. (1996). Deep vein thrombosis in stroke. The use of plasma D-dimer level as a screening test in the rehabilitation setting. *Stroke*, *27*(9), 1516–1520. doi:10.1161/01.STR.27.9.1516

Heilman, K. M., & Van Den Abell, T. (1980). Right hemisphere dominance for attention: The mechanism underlying hemispheric asymmetries of inattention (neglect). *Neurology*, *30*(3), 327–330.

Heilman, K., & Valenstein, E. (1993). Neglect and related disorders. In *Clinical Neuropsychology* (3rd ed., pp. 279–336). Oxford: University Press.

Herrmann, M., Bartels, C., Schumacher, M., & Wallesch, C. W. (1995). Is there a pathoanatomic correlate for depression in the postacute stage of stroke? *Stroke, 26,* 850–856.

Hickey, J. V. (2014). *The clinical practice of neurological and neurosurgical nursing* (7th ed.). Philadelphia, PA: Lippincott Williams and Wilkins.

Hillis, A., Wityk, R., & Barker, P., et al. (2002). Subcortical aphasia and neglect in acute stroke: The role of cortical hypoperfusion. *Brain, 125,* 1094.

Hinchey, J. A., Shephard, T., Furie, K., Smith, D., Wang, D., & Tonn, S. (2005). Formal dysphagia screening protocols prevent pneumonia. *Stroke*, *36*(9), 1972–1976. doi:10.1161/01.STR.0000177529.86868.8d

Holloway, R. G., Arnold, R. M., Creutzfeldt, C. J., Lewis, E. F., Lutz, B. J., McCann, R. M., . . . Zorowitz, R. D. (2014). Palliative and end-of-life care in stroke: A statement for healthcare professionals from the American Heart Association/American Stroke Association. *Stroke*, *45*(6), 1887–1916. doi:10.1161 /STR.0000000000000015

Horner, S., Ni, X. S., Duft, M., Niederkorn, K., & Lechner, H. (1995). EEG, CT and neurosonographic findings in patients with postischemic seizures. *Journal of the Neurological Sciences*, *132*(1), 57–60.

Inatomi, Y., Yonehara, T., Omiya, S., Hashimoto, Y., Hirano, T., & Uchino, M. (2008). Aphasia during the acute phase in ischemic stroke. *Cerebrovascular Disease*, *25*(4), 316–323. doi: 10.1159/000118376.

Institute for Healthcare Improvement. (2012). *How-to Guide: Preventing Ventilator-Associated Pneumonia.* Cambridge, MA: Institute for Healthcare Improvement. Retrieved from http://www.ihi.org

Isaacs, K. L., Barr, W. B., Nelson, P. K., & Devinsky, O. (2006). Degree of handedness and cerebral dominance. *Neurology, 66,* 1855.

James, P. A., Oparil, S., Carter, B. L., Cushman, W. C., Dennison-Himmelfarb, C., Handler, J., . . . Ortiz, E. (2014). 2014 evidence-based guideline for the management of high blood pressure in adults: Report from the panel members appointed to the Eight Joint National Committee (JNC 8). *The Journal of the American Medical Association*, *311*(5), 507–520. doi:10.1001/jama.2013.284427

Jauch, E. C., Saver, J. L., Adams, H. P., Bruno, A., Connors, J. J., Demaerschalk, B. M., ... Yonas, H. (2013). Guidelines for the early management of patients with acute ischemic stroke: A guideline for healthcare professionals from the American Heart Association/American Stroke Association. *Stroke*, *44*(3), 870–947. doi:10.1161/STR.0b013e318284056a

Jennett, B. (1978). Post-traumatic epilepsy. *Scottish Medical Journal*, *23*(1), 102.

Jensen, M. B., & St. Louis, E. K. (2005). Management of acute cerebellar stroke. *Archives of Neurology*, *62*(4), 537–544. doi:10.1001/archneur.62.4.537

Jha, S. (2003). Cerebral edema and its management. *Medical Journal Armed Forces India*, *59*(4), 326–331. doi:10.1016/S0377-1237(03)80147-8

Jönsson, A. C., Lindgren, I., Hallström, B., Norrving, B., & Lindgren, A. (2006). Prevalence and intensity of pain after stroke: A population based study focusing on patients' perspectives. *Journal of Neurology, Neurosurgery & Psychiatry*, *77*(5), 590–595. doi:10.1136/jnnp.2005.079145

Jordan, L., & Hillis, A. (2006). Disorders of speech and language: Aphasia, apraxia, and dysarthria. *Current Opinion in Neurology*, *19*(6), 580–585.

Jorge, R., Robinson, R., Arndt, S., & Starkstein, S. (2003). Mortality and poststroke depression: A placebo-controlled trial of antidepressants. *American Journal of Psychiatry, 160,* 1823–1829.

Kahn, J. M., Caldwell, E. C., Deem, S., Newell, D. W., Heckbert, S. R., & Rubenfeld, G. D. (2006). Acute lung injury in patients with subarachnoid hemorrhage: Incidence, risk factors, and outcome. *Critical Care Medicine*, *34*(1), 196–202. doi:10.1097/01.CCM.0000194540.44020.8E

Kappelle, L. J. (2011). Preventing deep vein thrombosis after stroke: Strategies and recommendations. *Current Treatment Options in Neurology, 13*(6), 629–635. doi:10.1007/s11940-011-0147-4

Karatepe, A. G., Gunaydin, R., Kaya, T., & Turkmen, G. (2008). Comorbidity in patients after stroke: Impact on functional outcome. *Journal of Rehabilitation Medicine, 40*(10), 831–835. doi:10.2340/16501977-0269

Kearon, C. (2004). Long-term management of patients after venous thromboembolism. *Circulation, 110*(9 Suppl. 1), I10–I18. doi:10.1161/01.CIR.0000140902.46296.ae

Kelly, A. G., Hoskins, K. D., & Holloway, R. G. (2012). Early stroke mortality, patient preferences, and the withdrawal of care bias. *Neurology, 79*(9), 941–944. doi:10.1212/WNL.0b013e318266fc40

Kelly, J., Hunt, B. J., Lewis, R. R., Swaminathan, R., Moody, A., Seed, P. T., & Rudd, A. (2004). Dehydration and venous thromboembolism after acute stroke. *QJM: Monthly Journal of the Association of Physicians, 97*(5), 293–296.

Kelly, J., Rudd, A., Lewis, R., & Hunt, B. J. (2001). Venous thromboembolism after acute stroke. *Stroke, 32*(1), 262–267. doi:10.1161/01.STR.32.1.262

Kilpatrick, C. J., Davis, S. M., Tress, B. M., Rossiter, S. C., Hopper, J. L., & Vandendriesen, M. L. (1990). Epileptic seizures in acute stroke. *Archives of Neurology, 47*(2), 157–160.

Kinsbourne, M. (1977). Hemineglect and hemisphere rivalry. *Advances in Neurology, 18*, 41–49.

Knecht, S., Dräger, B., Deppe, M., Bobe, L., Lohmann, H., Flöel, A., . . . Henningsen, H. (2000). Handedness and hemispheric language dominance in healthy humans. *Brain, 123*(12), 2512–2518.

Kojic, B., Burina, A., Hodzic, R., Pasic, Z., & Sinanovic, O. (2009). Risk factors impact on the long-term survival after hemorrhagic stroke. *Medicinski Arhiv, 63*(4), 203–206.

Kress, J. P., & Hall, J. B. (2014). ICU-acquired weakness and recovery from critical illness. *New England Journal of Medicine, 370*(17), 1626–1635. doi:10.1056/NEJMra1209390

Kruyt, N. D., Biessels, G. J., de Haan, R. J., Vermeulen, M., Rinkel, G. J. E., Coert, B., & Roos, Y. B. (2009). Hyperglycemia and clinical outcome in aneurysmal subarachnoid hemorrhage: A meta-analysis. *Stroke, 40*(6), e424–e430. doi:10.1161/STROKEAHA.108.529974

Kuijper, P. H., Torres, H. I., Lammers, J. W., Sixma, J. J., Koenderman, L., & Zwaginga, J. J. (1997). Platelet and fibrin deposition at the damaged vessel wall: Cooperative substrates for adhesion under flow conditions. *Blood, 89*(1), 166–175.

Kumar, B., Kalita, J., Kumar, G., & Misra, U. K. (2009). Central poststroke pain: A review of pathophysiology and treatment. *Anesthesia and Analgesia, 108*(5), 1645–1657. doi:10.1213/ane.0b013e31819d644c

Laino, C. (2007). Periodic discharges on EEG linked to poor outcomes in ICH patients. *Neurology Today, 7*(18), 21–22. doi:10.1097/01.NT.0000295256.69427.ef

Langhorne, P., Stott, D. J., Robertson, L., MacDonald, J., Jones, L., McAlpine, C., . . . Murray, G. (2000). Medical complications after stroke: A multicenter study. *Stroke, 31*(6), 1223–1229.

Lazar, R., Speizer, A., Festa, J., Krakauer, J., & Marshall, R. (2008). Variability in language recovery after first-time stroke. *Journal of Neurology, Neurosurgery and Psychiatry, 79*(5), 530–534. doi:10.1136/jnnp.2007.122457

Levine, M. N., Hirsh, J., Gent, M., Turpie, A. G., Weitz, J., Ginsberg, J., . . . Powers, P. (1995). Optimal duration of oral anticoagulant therapy: A randomized trial comparing four weeks with three months of warfarin in patients with proximal deep vein thrombosis. *Thrombosis and Haemostasis, 74*(2), 606–611.

Lévy, P., & Pépin, J. L. (2011). CPAP treatment of sleep apnoea in the early phase of stroke: Growing evidence of effectiveness. *European Respiratory Journal, 37*(5), 997–999. doi:10.1183/09031936.00182810

Leys, D., Bandu, L., Hénon, H., Lucas, C., Mounier-Vehier, F., Rondepierre, P., & Godefroy, O. (2002). Clinical outcome in 287 consecutive young adults (15 to 45 years) with ischemic stroke. *Neurology, 59*(1), 26–33.

Lindgren, I., Jönsson, A. C., Norrving, B., & Lindgren, A. (2007). Shoulder pain after stroke: A prospective population-based study. *Stroke, 38*(2), 343–348. doi:10.1161/01.STR.0000254598.16739.4e

Mace, S. E. (2008). Challenges and advances in intubation: Rapid sequence intubation. *Emergency Medicine Clinics of North America, 26*(4), 1043–1068. doi:10.1016/j.emc.2008.10.002

Maki, D. G., & Tambyah, P. A. (2001). Engineering out the risk for infection with urinary catheters. *Emerging Infectious Diseases, 7*(2), 342–347. doi:10.3201/eid0702.700342

Mann, G., Hankey, G., Cameron, D. (1999). Swallowing disorders following acute stroke: prognosis and prognostic factors at 6 months. *Stroke, 30*, 744–748.

Martino, R., Foley, N., Bhogal, S., Diamant, N., Speechley, M., & Teasell, R. (2005). Dysphagia after stroke: Incidence, diagnosis, and pulmonary complications. *Stroke, 36*(12), 2756–2763. doi:10.1161/01.STR.0000190056.76543.eb

Martino, R., Matin, R., & Black, S. (2012). Dysphagia after stroke and its management. *Canadian Medical Association, 184*(10), 1127–1128.

Mayer, S. A., Kowalski, R. G., Presciutti, M., Ostapkovich, N. D., McGann, E., Fitzsimmons, B. F., . . . Commichau, C. (2004). Clinical trial of a novel surface cooling system for fever control in neurocritical care patients. *Critical Care Medicine, 32*(12), 2508–2515. doi:10.1097/01.CCM.0000147441.39670.37

Meddings, J., Rogers, M. A. M., Krein, S. L., Fakih, M. G., Olmsted, R. N., & Saint, S. (2014). Reducing unnecessary urinary catheter use and other strategies to prevent catheter-associated urinary tract infection: An integrative review. *BMJ Quality & Safety, 23*(4), 277–289. doi:10.1136/bmjqs-2012-001774

Mehdi, Z., Birns, J., & Bhalla, A. (2013). Post-stroke urinary incontinence. *International Journal of Clinical Practice, 67*(11), 1128–1137. doi:10.1111/ijcp.12183

Mesulam, M. (1981). Cortical network for directed attention and unilateral neglect. *Annals of Neurology, 10*, 309–325.

Meyer, G., Marjanovic, Z., Valcke, J., Lorcerie, B., Gruel, Y., Solal-Celigny, P., . . . Farge, D. (2002). Comparison of low-molecular-weight heparin and warfarin for the secondary prevention of venous thromboembolism in patients with cancer: A randomized controlled study. *Archives of Internal Medicine, 162*(15), 1729–1735.

Milhaud, D., Popp, J., Thouvenot, E., Heroum, C., & Bonafé, A. (2004). Mechanical ventilation in ischemic stroke. *Journal of Stroke and Cerebrovascular Diseases, 13*(4), 183–188. doi:10.1016/j.jstrokecerebrovasdis .2004.06.007

Miller, E. L., Murray, L., Richards, L., Zorowitz, R. D., Bakas, T., Clark, P., Billinger, S. A. (2010). Comprehensive overview of nursing and interdisciplinary rehabilitation care of the stroke patient: A scientific statement from the American Heart Association. *Stroke, 41*, 2402–2448.

Mintzer, S., & Mattson, R. T. (2009). Should enzyme-inducing antiepileptic drugs be considered first-line agents? *Epilepsia, 50*(Suppl. 8), 42–50. doi:10.1111/j.1528-1167.2009.02235.x

Moniruzzaman, M., Salek, K. M., Shakoor, M. A., Mia, B. A., & Moyeenuzzaman, M. (2010). Effects of therapeutic modalities on patients with post stroke shoulder pain. *Mymensingh Medical Journal, 19*(1), 48–53.

Morgenstern, L. B., Hemphill, J. C., Anderson, C., Becker, K., Broderick, J. P., Connolly, E. S., . . . Tamargo, R. J. (2010). Guidelines for the management of spontaneous intracerebral hemorrhage: A guideline for healthcare professionals from the American Heart Association/American Stroke Association. *Stroke, 41*(9), 2108–2129. doi:10.1161/STR.0b013e3181ec611b

Morris, L. L., McIntosh, E., & Whitmer, A. (2014). The importance of tracheostomy progression in the intensive care unit. *Critical Care Nurse, 34*(1), 40–48; quiz 50. doi:10.4037/ccn2014722

Mortazavi, M. M., Romeo, A. K., Deep, A., Griessenauer, C. J., Shoja, M. M., Tubbs, R. S., & Fisher, W. (2012). Hypertonic saline for treating raised intracranial pressure: Literature review with meta-analysis. *Journal of Neurosurgery, 116*(1), 210–221. doi:10.3171/2011.7.JNS102142

Musso, M., Weiller, C., Kiebel, S., Muller, S. P., Bulau, P., & Rijntjes, M. (1999). Training-induced brain plasticity in aphasia. *Brain, 122*(9), 1781–1790.

Nakajoh, K., Nakagawa, T., Sekizawa, K., Matsui, T., Arai, H., & Sasaki, H. (2000). Relation between incidence of pneumonia and protective reflexes in post-stroke patients with oral or tube feeding. *Journal of Internal Medicine, 247*(1), 39–42. doi:10.1046/j.1365-2796.2000.00565.x

Nakayama, H., Jørgensen, H. S., Pedersen, P. M., Raaschou, H. O., & Olsen, T. S. (1997). Prevalence and risk factors of incontinence after stroke: The Copenhagen Stroke Study. *Stroke, 28*(1), 58–62. doi:10.1161/01 .STR.28.1.58

Naredi, S., Lambert, G., Edén, E., Zäll, S., Runnerstam, M., Rydenhag, B., & Friberg, P. (2000). Increased sympathetic nervous activity in patients with nontraumatic subarachnoid hemorrhage. *Stroke; a Journal of Cerebral Circulation, 31*(4), 901–906.

Nason, M. W., Jr., & Mason, P. (2004). Modulation of sympathetic and somatomotor function by the ventromedial medulla. *Journal of Neurophysiology, 92*(1), 510–522. doi:10.1152/jn.00089.2004

Nedeltchev, K., Renz, N., Karameshev, A., Haefeli, T., Brekenfeld, C., Meier, N., . . . Mattle, H. P. (2010). Predictors of early mortality after acute ischaemic stroke. *Swiss Medical Weekly, 140*(17–18), 254–259. doi:smw-12919

Nguyen-Oghalai, T. U., Ottenbacher, K. J., Granger, C. V., & Goodwin, J. S. (2005). Impact of osteoarthritis on the rehabilitation of patients following a stroke. *Arthritis Care & Research, 53*(3), 383–387. doi:10.1002 /art.21166

Niedzielska, K., Barańska-Gieruszczak, M., Kuran, W., Rzeski, M., Romaniak, A., Ryglewicz, D., . . . Wołkow, L. (2001). EEG value in cases of epileptic seizures in early phase of stroke. *Neurologia i Neurochirurgia Polska, 35*(4), 595–603.

O'Grady, N. P., Murray, P. R., & Ames, N. (2012). Preventing ventilator-associated pneumonia: Does the evidence support the practice? *JAMA, 307*(23), 2534–2539.

O'Grady, N. P., Barie, P. S., Bartlett, J. G., Bleck, T., Carroll, K., Kalil, A. C., . . . Masur, H. (2008). Guidelines for evaluation of new fever in critically ill adult patients: 2008 update from the American College of Critical Care Medicine and the Infectious Diseases Society of America. *Critical Care Medicine, 36*(4), 1330–1349. doi:10.1097/CCM.0b013e318169eda9

O'Neill, P. A., Davies, I., Fullerton, K. J., & Bennett, D. (1991). Stress hormone and blood glucose response following acute stroke in the elderly. *Stroke*, *22*(7), 842–847.

Odderson, I. R., & McKenna, B. S. (1993). A model for management of patients with stroke during the acute phase. Outcome and economic implications. *Stroke*, *24*(12), 1823–1827.

Offner, H., Vandenbark, A. A., & Hurn, P. D. (2009). Effect of experimental stroke on peripheral immunity: CNS ischemia induces profound immunosuppression. *Neuroscience*, *158*(3), 1098–1111. doi:10.1016/j.neuroscience.2008.05.033

Ohkuma, H., Tsurutani, H., & Suzuki, S. (2001). Incidence and significance of early aneurysmal rebleeding before neurosurgical and neurological management. *Stroke*, *32*(5), 1176–1180. doi:10.1161/01.STR.32.5.1176

Ohwaki, K., Yano, E., Nagashima, H., Hirata, M., Nakagomi, T., & Tamura, A. (2004). Blood pressure management in acute intracerebral hemorrhage: Relationship between elevated blood pressure and hematoma enlargement. *Stroke*, *35*(6), 1364–1367. doi:10.1161/01.STR.0000128795.38283.4b

Oliver, D. (2002). Bedfalls and bedrails- what should we so? *Age and Ageing*, *31*, 415–418.

Oliveri, M., Bisiach, E., Brighina, F., Piazza, A., La Bua, V., Buffa, D., Fierro, B. (2001). rTMS of the unaffected hemisphere transiently reduces contralesional visuospatial hemineglect. *Neurology*, *57*(7), 1338–1340.

Olson, D. M., McNett, M. M., Lewis, L. S., Riemen, K. E., & Bautista, C. (2013). Effects of nursing interventions on cranial pressure. *American Journal of Critical Care*, *22*(5), 431–438. doi:10.4037/ajcc2013751

Olson, D. M., Thoyre, S. M., Bennett, S. N., Stoner, J. B., & Graffagnino, C. (2009). Effect of mechanical chest percussion on intracranial pressure: A pilot study. *American Journal of Critical Care*, *18*(4), 330–335. doi:10.4037/ajcc2009523

Parker, K., & Miles, S. H. (1997) Deaths caused by bedrails. *Journal of the American Geriatric Society*, *45*(7), 797–802.

Patel, A. (2011). Successful treatment of long-term, poststroke, upper-limb spasticity with onabutulinumtoxin A. *Physical Therapy*, *91*(11), 1936.

Pellicane, A. J., & Millis, S. R. (2013). Efficacy of methylprednisolone versus other pharmacologic interventions for the treatment of central post-stroke pain: A retrospective analysis. *Journal of Pain Research*, 6, 557–563. doi:10.2147/JPR.S46530

Phipps, M. S., Desai, R. A., Wira, C., & Bravata, D. M. (2011). Epidemiology and outcomes of fever burden among patient with acute ischemic stroke. *Stroke*, *42*(12), 3357–3362. doi:10.1161/STROKEAHA.111.621425

Pizzi, A., Falsini, C., Martini, M., Rossetti, M. A., Verdesca, S., & Tosto, A. (2013). Urinary incontinence after ischemic stroke: Clinical and urodynamic studies. *Neurourology and Urodynamics*, *33*(4), 420–425. doi:10.1002/nau.22420

Porch, B. (1981). *Porch Index of Communicative Ability (PICA)*. Palo Alto: Consulting Psychologists Press.

Prandoni, P., Lensing, A. W. A., Piccioli, A., Bernardi, E., Simioni, P., Girolami, B., . . . Girolami, A. (2002). Recurrent venous thromboembolism and bleeding complications during anticoagulant treatment in patients with cancer and venous thrombosis. *Blood*, *100*(10), 3484–3488. doi:10.1182/blood-2002-01-0108

Presciutti, M., Bader, M. K., & Hepburn, M. (2012). Shivering management during therapeutic temperature modulation: Nurses' perspective. *Critical Care Nurse*, *32*(1), 33–42. doi:10.4037/ccn2012189

Price, C. I. M., & Pandyan, A. D. (2001). Electrical stimulation for preventing and treating post-stroke shoulder pain: A systematic Cochrane Review. *Clinical Rehabilitation*, *15*(1), 5–19.

Pulvermuller, F., Neininger, B., Elbert, T., Mohr, B., Rockstroh, B., Koebbel, P., & Taub, E. (2001). Constraint-induced therapy of chronic aphasia after stroke. *Stroke*, *32*, 1621–1626.

Puntillo, K., Pasero, C., Li, D., Mularski, R. A., Grap, M. J., Erstad, B. L., . . . Sessler, C. N. (2009). Evaluation of pain in ICU patients. *CHEST Journal*, *135*(4), 1069–1074. doi:10.1378/chest.08-2369

Qaseem, A., Snow, V., Denberg, T., Forciea, M., & Owens, D. (2008). Clinical efficacy assessment subcommittee of the American College of Physicians using second-generation antidepressants to treat depressive disorders: A clinical practice guideline from the American College of Physicians. *Annals of Internal Medicine*, *149*(10), 725-733. doi:10.7326/0003-4819-149-10-200811180-00007

Qureshi, A. I. (2008). Acute hypertensive response in patients with stroke: Pathophysiology and management. *Circulation*, *118*(2), 176–187. doi:10.1161/CIRCULATIONAHA.107.723874

Rabinstein, A. A. (2006). Treatment of cerebral edema. *The Neurologist*, *12*(2), 59–73. doi:10.1097/01.nrl.0000186810.62736.f0

Reaven, N. L., Lovett, J. E., & Funk, S. E. (2009). Brain injury and fever: Hospital length of stay and cost outcomes. *Journal of Intensive Care Medicine*, *24*(2), 131–139.

Redline, S., Yenokyan, G., Gottlieb, D. J., Shahar, E., O'Connor, G. T., Resnick, H. E., . . . Punjabi, N. M. (2010). Obstructive sleep apnea-hypopnea and incident stroke. *American Journal of Respiratory and Critical Care Medicine*, *182*(2), 269–277. doi:10.1164/rccm.200911-1746OC

Rincon, F., Maltenfort, M., Dey, S., Ghosh, S., Vibbert, M., Urtecho, J., . . . Bell, R. (2014). The prevalence and impact of mortality of the acute respiratory distress syndrome on admissions of patients with ischemic stroke in the United States. *Journal of Intensive Care Medicine, 29*(6), 357–364. doi:10.1177/0885066613491919

Rincon, F., & Mayer, S. A. (2008). Clinical review: Critical care management of spontaneous intracerebral hemorrhage. *Critical Care, 12*(6), 237. doi:10.1186/cc7092

Robinson, R. G., Kubos, K. L., Starr, L. B., Rao, K., & Price, T. R. (1984). Mood disorders in stroke patients: importance of location of lesion. *Brain, 107*, 81-93.

Robinson, R. G. (1997). Neuropsychiatric consequences of stroke. *Annual Review of Medicine, 48*, 217–229. doi:10.1146/annurev.med.48.1.217

Robinson, R. G., Schultz, S. K., Castillo, C., Kopel, T., Kosier, J. T., Newman, R. M., . . . Starkstein, S. E. (2000). Nortriptyline versus fluoxetine in the treatment of depression and in short-term recovery after stroke: a placebo-controlled, double-blind study. *American Journal of Psychiatry, 157*, 351.

Robinson, R. G. (2003). Poststroke depression: prevalence, diagnosis, treatment, and disease progression. *Biological Psychiatry, 54*(3), 376–387.

Roffe, C., Sills, S., Halim, M., Wilde, K., Allen, M. B., Jones, P. W., & Crome, P. (2003). Unexpected nocturnal hypoxia in patients with acute stroke. *Stroke, 34*(11), 2641–2645.

Rosenberg, J. B., Shiloh, A. L., Savel, R. H., & Eisen, L. A. (2011). Non-invasive methods of estimating intracranial pressure. *Neurocritical Care, 15*(3), 599–608. doi:10.1007/s12028-011-9545-4

Rowan, A. J., Ramsay, R. E., Collins, J. F., Pryor, F., Boardman, K. D., Uthman, B. M., . . . Tomyanovich, M. L. (2005). New onset geriatric epilepsy: A randomized study of gabapentin, lamotrigine, and carbamazepine. *Neurology, 64*(11), 1868 1873. doi:10.1212/01.WNL.0000167384.68207.3E

Samuelsson, H., Jensen, C., Ekholm, S., Naver, H., & Blomstrand, C. (1997). Anatomical and neurological correlates of acute and chronic visuospatial neglect following right hemisphere stroke. *Cortex, 33*, 271–285.

Santoli, F., Jonghe, B. D., Hayon, J., Tran, B., Piperaud, M., Merrer, J., & Outin, H. (2001). Mechanical ventilation in patients with acute ischemic stroke: Survival and outcome at one year. *Intensive Care Medicine, 27*(7), 1141–1146. doi:10.1007/s001340100998

Saper, C. B., & Breder, C. D. (1994). The neurologic basis of fever. *The New England Journal of Medicine, 330*(26), 1880–1886. doi:10.1056/NEJM199406303302609

Scaravilli, V., Tinchero, G., & Citerio, G. (2011). Fever management in SAH. *Neurocritical Care, 15*(2), 287–294. doi:10.1007/s12028-011-9588-6

Schmidt, J. M., Rincon, F., Fernandez, A., Resor, C., Kowalski, R. G., Claassen, J., . . . Mayer, S. A. (2007). Cerebral infarction associated with acute subarachnoid hemorrhage. *Neurocritical Care, 7*(1), 10–17. doi:10.1007/s12028-007-0003-2

Schwab, S., Georgiadis, D., Berrouschot, J., Schellinger, P. D., Graffagnino, C., & Mayer, S. A. (2001). Feasibility and safety of moderate hypothermia after massive hemispheric infarction. *Stroke, 32*(9), 2033–2035.

Seder, D. B., & Mayer, S. A. (2009). Critical care management of subarachnoid hemorrhage and ischemic stroke. *Clinics in Chest Medicine, 30*(1), 103–122, viii–ix. doi:10.1016/j.ccm.2008.11.004

Seematter, G., Binnert, C., Martin, J. L., & Tappy, L. (2004). Relationship between stress, inflammation and metabolism. *Current Opinion in Clinical Nutrition and Metabolic Care, 7*(2), 169–173.

Sellars, C., Hughes, T., & Langhorne, P. (2005). Speech and language therapy for dysarthria due to non-progressive brain damage. *The Cochrane Database of Systematic Reviews*, (3), CD002088. doi:10.1002/14651858. CD002088.pub2

Shah, P. P., Szaflarski, J. P., Allendorfer, J., Hamilton, R. H. (2013). Induction of neuroplasticity and recovery in post-stroke aphasia by non-invasive brain stimulation. *Frontiers of Human Neuroscience*. doi: 10.3389/fnhum.2013.00888

Sherman, D. G., Albers, G. W., Bladin, C., Fieschi, C., Gabbai, A. A., Kase, C. S., . . . Pineo, G. F. (2007). The efficacy and safety of enoxaparin versus unfractionated heparin for the prevention of venous thromboembolism after acute ischaemic stroke (PREVAIL Study): An open-label randomised comparison. *Lancet, 369*(9570), 1347–1355. doi:10.1016/S0140-6736(07)60633-3

Sinanovic, O., Mrkonjic, Z., Zukic, S., Vidovic, M., & Imamovic, K. (2011). Post-stroke language disorders. *Acta Clinica Croatia, 50*(1), 79-94.

Singh, V., & Edwards, N. J. (2013). Advances in the critical management of ischemic stroke. *Stroke Research and Treatment, 2013*, e510481. doi:10.1155/2013/510481

Singh, S., & Hamdy, S. (2006). Dysphagia in stroke patients. *Postgraduate Medical Journal, 82*(968), 383–391.

Smith, E. & Delargy, M. (2005). Locked-in syndrome. *BMJ, 330*(7488), 406-409 doi: 10.1136/bmj.330.7488.406

Sommerfield, D., Gripenstedl, U., & Welmer, A. (2012). Spasticity after stroke: An overview of prevalence, test instruments, and treatments. *American Journal of Physical Medicine and Rehabilitation, 91*(9), 814–820.

Soo Hoo, J., Paul, T., Chae, J., & Wilson, R. D. (2013). Central hypersensitivity in chronic hemiplegic shoulder pain. *American Journal of Physical Medicine and Rehabilitation, 92*(1), 1–9.

Sörös, P., & Hachinski, V. (2012). Cardiovascular and neurological causes of sudden death after ischaemic stroke. *The Lancet Neurology, 11*(2), 179–188. doi:10.1016/S1474-4422(11)70291-5

Spalletta, G., Bossu, P., Ciaramella, A., Bria, P., Caltagirone, C., & Robinson, R. (2006). The etiology of post-stroke depression: A review of the literature and a new hypothesis involving inflammatory cytokines. *Molecular Psychiatry, 11*(11), 984–991.

Starkstein, S., Robinson, R., & Price, T. (1987). Comparison of cortical and subcortical lesions in the production of poststroke mood disorders. *Brain, 110,* 1045–1059.

Starkstein, S., Robinson, R., Berthier, M., Parikh, R., & Price, T. (1988). Differential mood changes following basal ganglia vs thalamic lesions. *Archives of Neurology,* 725–730.

Staykov, D., Wagner, I., Volbers, B., Hauer, E. M., Doerfler, A., Schwab, S., & Bardutzky, J. (2011). Natural course of perihemorrhagic edema after intracerebral hemorrhage. *Stroke, 42*(9), 2625–2629. doi:10.1161/STROKEAHA.111.618611

Stead, L. G., Gilmore, R. M., Bellolio, M. F., Jain, A., Rabinstein, A. A., Decker, W. W., . . . Brown, R. D. (2011). Cardioembolic but not other stroke subtypes predict mortality independent of stroke severity at presentation. *Stroke Research and Treatment, 2011,* 281496. doi:10.4061/2011/281496

Stefan, H., & Theodore, W. H. (2012). *Epilepsy part II: Treatment: Handbook of clinical neurology.* Amsterdam, The Netherlands: Elsevier.

Steger, C., Pratter, A., Martinek-Bregel, M., Avanzini, M., Valentin, A., Slany, J., & Stöllberger, C. (2004). Stroke patients with atrial fibrillation have a worse prognosis than patients without: Data from the Austrian Stroke registry. *European Heart Journal, 25*(19), 1734–1740. doi:10.1016/j.ehj.2004.06.030

Stephen, L. J., & Brodie, M. J. (2000). Epilepsy in elderly people. *Lancet, 355*(9213), 1441–1446. doi:10.1016/S0140-6736(00)02149-8

Stevens, T., Payne, S. A., Burton, C., Addington-Hall, J., & Jones, A. (2007). Palliative care in stroke: A critical review of the literature. *Palliative Medicine, 21*(4), 323–331. doi:10.1177/0269216307079160

Stott, D. J., Falconer, A., Miller, H., Tilston, J. C., & Langhorne, P. (2009). Urinary tract infection after stroke. *QJM: Monthly Journal of the Association of Physicians, 102*(4), 243–249. doi:10.1093/qjmed/hcp012

Suarez, J. I. (2004). Hypertonic saline for cerebral edema and elevated intracranial pressure. *Cleveland Clinic Journal of Medicine, 71*(Suppl. 1), S9–S13.

Sulter, G., Elting, J. W., Stewart, R., den Arend, A., & De Keyser, J. (2000). Continuous pulse oximetry in acute hemiparetic stroke. *Journal of the Neurological Sciences, 179*(1–2), 65–69. doi:10.1016/S0022-510X(00)00378-6

Suntrup, S., Warnecke, T., Kemmling, A., Teismann, I. K., Harnacher, C., Oelenberg, S., & Dziewas, R. (2012). Dysphagia in patients with acute striatocapsular hemorrhage. *Journal of Neurology, 259*(1); 93–99.

Tambyah, P. A., Knasinski, V., & Maki, D. G. (2002). The direct costs of nosocomial catheter-associated urinary tract infection in the era of managed care. *Infection Control and Hospital Epidemiology, 23*(1), 27–31. doi:10.1086/501964

The Cochrane Collaboration (Ed.). (1996a). *Cochrane Database of Systematic Reviews: Reviews.* Chichester, UK: John Wiley & Sons, Ltd. Retrieved from http://summaries.cochrane.org/CD008728/interventions-for-preventing-falls-in-people-after-stroke

The Cochrane Collaboration (Ed.). (1996b). *Cochrane Database of Systematic Reviews: Reviews.* Chichester, UK: John Wiley & Sons, Ltd. Retrieved from http://summaries.cochrane.org/CD003586/cognitive-rehabilitation-for-spatial-neglect-following-stroke

The Joint Commision. (2013). *Advanced disease-specific care certification requirements for Comprehensive Sroke Center (CSC).* Retrieved from http://www.jointcommission.org/certification/advanced_certification_comprehensive_stroke_centers.aspx

Thibaut, A., Chatelle, C., Ziegler, E., Bruno, M. A., Laureys, S., & Gosseries, O. (2013). Spasticity after stroke: Physiology, assessment and treatment. *Brain Injury,* 1–13. DOI: 10.3109/02699052.2013.804202

Thieme, H., Mehrhoz, J., Pohl, M., Behrens, J., & Dohle, C. (2012). Mirror therapy for improving motor function after stroke. *Cochrane Database of Systemic Reviews, 14,* 3:CD008449. doi: 10.1002/14651858.CD008449.

Thiex, R., & Tsirka, S. E. (2007). Brain edema after intracerebral hemorrhage: Mechanisms, treatment options, management strategies, and operative indications. *Neurosurgical Focus, 22*(5), E6.

Thilmann, A., Fellows, S., & Garms, E. (1991).The mechanism of spastic muscle hypertonus: variation in reflex gain over the time course of spasticity. *Brain, 114,* 233–244.

Thompson, C. K. & den Ouden, D. B. (2008). Neuroimaging and recovery of language in aphasia. *Current Neurology and Neuroscience Reports, 8,* 475–483.

Tilson, J. K., Wu, S. S., Cen, S. Y., Feng, Q., Rose, D. R., Behrman, A. L., . . . Duncan, P. W. (2012). Characterizing and identifying risk for falls in the LEAPS study: A randomized clinical trial of interventions to improve walking poststroke. *Stroke, 43*(2), 446–452. doi:10.1161/STROKEAHA.111.636258

Tissue plasminogen activator for acute ischemic stroke. The National Institute of Neurological Disorders and Stroke rt-PA Stroke Study Group. (1995). *The New England Journal of Medicine, 333*(24), 1581–1587. doi:10.1056/NEJM199512143332401

Tolentino-DelosReyes, A. F., Ruppert, S. D., & Shiao, S. Y. P. K. (2007). Evidence-based practice: Use of the ventilator bundle to prevent ventilator-associated pneumonia. *American Journal of Critical Care, 16*(1), 20–27.

Towfighi, A., Greenberg, S. M., & Rosand, J. (2005). Treatment and prevention of primary intracerebral hemorrhage. *Seminars in Neurology, 25*(4), 445–452.

Uchino, H., Smith, M. L., Bengzon, J., Lundgren, J., & Siesjö, B. K. (1996). Characteristics of postischemic seizures in hyperglycemic rats. Journal of Neurological Science, 139(1), 21–27.

Vahedi, K., Hofmeijer, J., Juettler, E., Vicaut, E., George, B., Algra, A., . . . Hacke, W. (2007). Early decompressive surgery in malignant infarction of the middle cerebral artery: A pooled analysis of three randomised controlled trials. *Lancet Neurology, 6*(3), 215–222. doi:10.1016/S1474-4422(07)70036-4

Van der Lee, J., Wagenaar, R., Lankhorst, G. et al. (1999). Forced use of the upper extremity in chronic stroke patients: Results from a single-blind randomized clinical trial. *Stroke, 30*, 2369–2375.

Van der Lee, J., Beckerman, H., Lankhorst, G., Bouter, L. (2000). Constraint-induced movement therapy. *Physical Therapy, 80*(7), 711–713.

Varona, J. F. (2010). Long-term prognosis of ischemic stroke in young adults. *Stroke Research and Treatment, 2011*, e879817. doi:10.4061/2011/879817

Vergouwen, M. D. I., van Geloven, N., de Haan, R. J., Kruyt, N. D., Vermeulen, M., & Roos, Y. B. W. E. M. (2010). Increased cortisol levels are associated with delayed cerebral ischemia after aneurysmal subarachnoid hemorrhage. *Neurocritical Care, 12*(3), 342–345. doi:10.1007/s12028-010-9331-

Verheyden, G. S.A. F., Weerdesteyn, V., Pickering, R. M., Kunkel, D., Lennon, S., Geurts, A. C. H., & Ashburn, A. (2013). Interventions for preventing falls in people after stroke. *Cochrane Database of Systematic Reviews*, (5), CD008728. Retrieved from http://summaries.cochrane.org/CD008728/STROKE_interventions-for -preventing-falls-in-people-after-stroke

Vernino, S., Brown, R. D., Jr, Sejvar, J. J., Sicks, J. D., Petty, G. W., & O'Fallon, W. M. (2003). Cause-specific mortality after first cerebral infarction: a population-based study. *Stroke; a Journal of Cerebral Circulation, 34*(8), 1828–1832.

Viitanen, M., Winblad, B., & Asplund, K. (1987). Autopsy-verified causes of death after stroke. *Acta Medica Scandinavica, 222*(5), 401–408.

Walcott, B. P., Miller, J. C., Kwon, C. S., Sheth, S. A., Hiller, M., Cronin, C. A., . . . Sheth, K. N. (2014). Outcomes in severe middle cerebral artery ischemic stroke. *Neurocritical Care, 21*(1), 20–26. doi:10.1007/s12028-013-9838-x

Wartenberg, K. E., Stoll, A., Funk, A., Meyer, A., Schmidt, J. M., & Berrouschot, J. (2011). Infection after acute ischemic stroke: Risk factors, biomarkers, and outcome. *Stroke Research and Treatment, 2011*, 830614. doi:10.4061/2011/830614

Weerdesteyn, V., de Niet, M., van Duijnhoven, H. J. R., & Geurts, A. C. H. (2008). Falls in individuals with stroke. *Journal of Rehabilitation Research and Development, 45*(8), 1195–1213.

Weir, B., Grace, M., Hansen, J., & Rothberg, C. (1978). Time course of vasospasm in man. *Journal of Neurosurgery, 48*(2), 173–178. doi:10.3171/jns.1978.48.2.0173

Wells, P. S., Lensing, A. W., Davidson, B. L., Prins, M. H., & Hirsh, J. (1995). Accuracy of ultrasound for the diagnosis of deep venous thrombosis in asymptomatic patients after orthopedic surgery. A meta-analysis. *Annals of Internal Medicine, 122*(1), 47–53.

Whitworth, J. A. (2003). 2003 World Health Organization (WHO)/International Society of Hypertension (ISH) statement on management of hypertension. *Journal of Hypertension, 21*(11), 1983–1992. doi:10.1097/01 .hjh.0000084751.37215.d2

Williams, J. M., Little, M. M., & Klein, K. (1986). Depression and hemispheric site of cerebral vascular accident. *Archives of Clinical Neuropsychology, 1*, 393–398.

Willmore, L. J., Sypert, G. W., & Munson, J. B. (1978). Recurrent seizures induced by cortical iron injection: a model of posttraumatic epilepsy. *Annals of Neurology, 4*(4), 329–336. doi:10.1002/ana.410040408

Wip, C., & Napolitano, L. (2009). Bundles to prevent ventilator-associated pneumonia: How valuable are they? *Current Opinion in Infectious Diseases, 22*(2), 159–166. doi:10.1097/QCO.0b013e3283295e7b

Wiysonge, C. S., Bradley, H., Mayosi, B. M., Maroney, R., Mbewu, A., Opie, L. H., & Volmink, J. (2007). Beta-blockers for hypertension. *The Cochrane Database of Systematic Reviews*, (1), CD002003. doi:10.1002/14651858.CD002003.pub2

Wu, T. C., Kasam, M., Harun, N., Hallevi, H., Bektas, H., Acosta, I., . . . Savitz, S. I. (2011). Pharmacological deep vein thrombosis prophylaxis does not lead to hematoma expansion in intracerebral hemorrhage with intraventricular extension. *Stroke, 42*(3), 705–709. doi:10.1161/STROKEAHA.110.600593

Xi, G., Hua, Y., Bhasin, R. R., Ennis, S. R., Keep, R. F., & Hoff, J. T. (2001). Mechanisms of edema formation after intracerebral hemorrhage effects of extravasated red blood cells on blood flow and blood-brain barrier. *Stroke, 32*(12), 2932–2938. doi:10.1161/hs1201.099820

Yaggi, H. K., Concato, J., Kernan, W. N., Lichtman, J. H., Brass, L. M., & Mohsenin, V. (2005). Obstructive sleep apnea as a risk factor for stroke and death. *The New England Journal of Medicine, 353*(19), 2034–2041. doi:10.1056/NEJMoa043104

Yang, S., Grabois, M., & Bruel, B. (2009). Post-stroke pain. *Practical Pain Management.* 1–5. Retrieved from http://www.practicalpainmanagement.com/pain/other/post-stroke-pain

Ydemann, M., Eddelien, H. S., & Lauritsen, A. Ø. (2012). Treatment of critical illness polyneuropathy and/or myopathy—a systematic review. *Danish Medical Journal, 59*(10), A4511.

Zazulia, A. R. (2009). Critical care management of acute ischemic stroke. *Continuum Lifelong Learning in Neurology, 15*, 68–82. doi:10.1212/01.CON.0000348810.14427.c5

CHAPTER 10

Stroke Rehabilitation

Terrie M. Black, Pamela S. Roberts,
Sarah L. Livesay, and Joanne V. Hickey

Stroke is the fourth major cause of disease burden worldwide and the fourth leading cause of death in the United States (Hoyert & Xu, 2012). Together, heart disease and stroke are among the most widespread and costly health problems facing the nation today, accounting for more than $500 billion in health care expenditures and related expenses in 2010 alone (Agency for Healthcare Research and Quality [AHRQ], 2010). Of the many individuals who survive a stroke, nearly 30% are admitted to an inpatient rehabilitation facility (IRF). IRFs provide intensive rehabilitation therapy to patients recovering from illness or injury, delivering at least 3 hours of therapy per day from physical, occupational, and speech therapy, along with 24-hour rehabilitation nursing care. In 2012, over 373,000 Medicare beneficiaries received care in IRFs, resulting in almost $6.5 billion dollars in Medicare payments. Medicare is the principal payer for IRF services, accounting for 62% of IRF discharges in 2011(Medicare Payment Advisory Commission [MedPAC], 2011).

This chapter provides an overview of stroke inpatient rehabilitation with emphasis on care provided by interprofessional teams. Additionally, it describes common residual impairments, disabilities, and limitations encountered by stroke patients and applies evidence-based assessment, treatment, and evaluation practices to stroke rehabilitation.

▮▮ AN OVERVIEW OF REHABILITATION

Physical medicine and rehabilitation, also known as *physiatry* or *rehabilitation medicine*, is a branch of medicine that aims to enhance and restore functional ability and quality of life to those with physical impairments or disabilities. The development of rehabilitation as a subspecialty, its underlying philosophy, current evidence-based science, and the approach to care have unique characteristics that are discussed in this section.

A Brief History of Rehabilitation

The history of rehabilitation dates back to ancient Egypt in which there are references to adaptive aids and artificial limbs. The first issue of *Archives of Physical Medicine and Rehabilitation* was published in 1919. World War I had a great impact on rehabilitation because many surviving soldiers sustained amputation injuries and needed care; the Veterans Administration was created to care for those with service-related injuries. In 1938, a small group of physicians lobbied for specialty recognition for physical medicine and rehabilitation. Their efforts resulted in the founding of the American Academy of Physical Medicine and Rehabilitation in 1947. In 1941, Dr. Frank Krusen published the first comprehensive textbook on physical medicine and rehabilitation. In 1943, the Vocational Rehabilitation Act was enacted, providing funds for professional training and research, while at the same time broadening the scope of rehabilitation. This Act was the catalyst for growth in rehabilitation practice. In 1946, the term *physiatrist* was first used to describe a physician with specialized knowledge in physical medicine and rehabilitation. The Worker's Compensation Act, which placed an emphasis on the workplace, passed in 1965. In 1973, the Rehabilitation Act passed, demonstrating an increased public awareness of the needs of individuals with disabilities. This act provided guidelines prohibiting discrimination and promoted equal opportunity with the removal of barriers for those with disabilities (Association of Rehabilitation Nurses [ARN], 2011).

In 1990, the Americans with Disabilities Act (ADA) increased accessibility options for individuals with disabilities in the community, employment, education, and health care settings. Finally, after many years of being paid under the Tax Equity and Fiscal Responsibility Act (TEFRA), the payment structure for rehabilitation facilities underwent a major transformation with the implementation of the Inpatient Prospective Payment System in 2002 (ARN, 2011).

A Philosophy of Rehabilitation

A philosophy is a set of broad statements about fundamental beliefs and values. The philosophy of rehabilitation offers a framework to guide the overall rehabilitation process and includes the following concepts.

Rehabilitation is a philosophy of care, not a setting. It is a continuous process that depends on a team approach. The rehabilitation philosophy is founded on the idea that all individuals have inherent worth and have the right to be experts in their own health care (ARN, 2008, 2011; Gender, 1998). The goal of rehabilitation is to assist individuals with a disability and/or chronic illness to restore, maintain, and promote optimal health. Overall health promotion is an important component of rehabilitation for persons with chronic disabling conditions. The rehabilitation process addresses major areas of focus that include prevention, recognition, and management of comorbid conditions; facilitation of maximum coping and adaptation by the patient and family; prevention of secondary disability by promotion of community reintegration including participation in home, family, recreational, and vocational activities; enhancement of quality of life in view of the disability; and prevention of recurrent stroke and other vascular conditions (Leifer et al., 2011; Miller et al., 2010).

Rehabilitation is often defined as the restoration of the person to the highest physical, mental, social, vocational, and economic capacity (World Health Organization [WHO], 2001). Rehabilitation endeavors to prevent further disability, to maintain the patient's remaining abilities, and to restore lost functions. In all aspects of a disabling injury or disease, a person moves through a period of adjustment and adaptation and then proceeds to restoration. Rehabilitation programs are centered on the philosophy that is geared toward helping the person obtain and maintain his or her optimal functional capability. The philosophy of care reinforces the person's abilities and motivation to retain the highest level of independence. Integration of restorative interventions is an ongoing process that uses input from the interprofessional team in order to establish the best way or method to optimize the person's underlying capability and functional performance. Goals are patient-centered and mutually determined between the interprofessional team and the patient and family, with an emphasis on community reentry and integration to minimize deficits, prevent complications, promote wellness, and optimize quality of life.

The Interprofessional Rehabilitation Team

A variety of team models exist in the rehabilitation setting, including multidisciplinary, interdisciplinary, transdisciplinary, and interprofessional models. These models are described in Chapter 3 and briefly in **Table 10-1**. The preferred model for the 21st century is the interprofessional practice model. This is the model that sets the framework for discussion of rehabilitation in this chapter. Regardless of the model used in rehabilitation, key characteristics of high-functioning teams include common goals, collaboration, collegiality, trust, mutual respect, cooperation, open communications, patient-centered care, and a commitment to quality outcomes. High-quality stroke care requires a dedicated team of professionals trained in the assessment and treatment of cerebrovascular disease. Evidence suggests that early referral and admission to an organized, interprofessional inpatient rehabilitation program within the first 4 weeks after stroke can result in a decrease in the absolute number of stroke-related deaths (Miller et al., 2010). Additionally, rehabilitation can reduce long-term disability and serve to enhance recovery post stroke (Miller et al., 2010). Many hospitals have developed stroke centers that provide stroke care from the acute hospital through the continuum of care using interprofessional teams who provide coordinated stroke services.

The interprofessional rehabilitation team provides care that is patient-centered, family-centered, effective, efficient, equitable, timely, safe, and evidence-based. A high level of cooperation, coordination, and collaboration characterize the relationships

TABLE 10-1 Team Models

Model	Description
Multidisciplinary	• Individuals from various disciplines contribute skills specific to their own discipline. • Goals are discipline-specific rather than in common.
Interdisciplinary	• Therapies are provided by team members from different disciplines to reach a common goal agreed upon by team members. • Problem solving extends beyond the individual disciplines.
Transdisciplinary	• One or two individual disciplines are responsible for implementing the treatment plan. • Duplication of efforts is minimized and sustains a blurring of discipline so that one team member can substitute for another. • Cross-training, ability to provide care across disciplines, and flexibility of the team members are critical to the success of goal attainment.
Interprofessional	• Cooperation, coordination, and collaboration • Collective identity and shared responsibility for a patient or group of patients

between professions in delivering patient-centered care. Interprofessional team–based care is care delivered by intentionally created, usually relatively small workgroups in health care who are recognized by others, as well as by themselves, as having a collective identity and shared responsibility for a patient or group of patients, such as stroke patients. Open communications among health providers, the patient, and family are a hallmark of patient-centered care in which the patient and family have an equal voice in care decisions. This concept of relying on the patient and family to have an active voice in care decision is the focus of current research initiatives such as the Patient-Centered Outcomes Research Institute (PCORI, 2014).

⦿ Interprofessional rehabilitation team members include a variety of health professionals working together to meet the comprehensive needs of a patient. **Table 10-2** provides a list of professionals commonly involved in the rehabilitative care of the stroke patient along with their roles. **Figure 10-1** depicts an expanded number of caregivers that may be required in comprehensive stroke rehabilitation. In order to practice effectively in interprofessional teams, a new model for educating health professionals is being implemented. The goal of interprofessional education is to "prepare all health professions students for *deliberatively working together* with the common goal of building a safer and better patient-centered and community/population oriented U.S. health care system" (Interprofessional Education Collaborative Expert Panel, 2011, p. 3). The focus on standards and competencies extends beyond initial professional education. The professional associations for rehabilitation practitioners set and publish standards of care and scope of practice for each specialty (**Table 10-3**). Many organizations also offer national certification examinations by which professionals demonstrate competency in their specialty area of practice. National certification may be required for legal authority to practice in a state. These organizations emphasize the need for developing and maintaining ongoing interprofessional practice competencies for contemporary practice.

⦿ The interprofessional team approach in rehabilitation has been identified as critical to achieving and maximizing patient outcomes for patients with stroke (Miller et al., 2010). **Table 10-4** lists the characteristics of a high-performance interprofessional team.

A Theoretical Framework for Rehabilitation

Because of the complexity and heterogeneity of stroke in the rehabilitation setting, a commonly applied framework in conceptualizing residual stroke deficits is provided by WHO. The *International Classification of Functioning, Disability and Health* is commonly referred to as the *ICF*. The *ICF* framework and its concepts have existed for over 25 years and use a biopsychosocial approach to human functioning and disability (WHO, 2001), as shown in **Table 10-5**. This framework transcends individual disciplines and provides a cross-cultural framework (Tempest & McIntyre, 2006). With the *ICF*, functioning is viewed as a distinct and separate concept. *Functioning* refers to "limitations and restrictions related to a health problem" (Cieza et al., 2005, p. 212). The *ICF* model is a means to view an individual and his or her interactions with the environment and everyday functioning (McIntyre & Tempest, 2007). The dynamic and interactive components of the model provide a viable, theoretical framework applicable to rehabilitation practice. According to Kearney and Pryor (2004), clinicians should prevent and minimize impairments, enable activities, prevent and minimize activity limitations, and enable participation. ⦿ In order to do this, the interprofessional team must first understand the social aspect of disability and the impact that health professionals can have in reducing stigmas and barriers to an individual's overall function.

TABLE 10-2 Major Interprofessional Rehabilitation Team Members

Discipline	World Wide Web Site	Description
Certified rehabilitation counselors	www.crccertification.com	Assist individuals with disabilities to maximize their vocational and avocational living goals in the most integrated setting possible through the application of the counseling process, including vocational and counseling, case management, referral, and service coordination; identifying and addressing employment and attitudinal barriers; and job analysis, development, and placement services.
Neuropsychologists	www.apa.org	Specialize in brain-behavior relationships and have extensive training in anatomy, physiology, and neuropathology. They identify and treat cognitive and neurobehavioral dysfunction and through assessment also monitor recovery and thereby enhance community reintegration.
Occupational therapists	www.aota.org	Focus on the "skills of living" necessary for independent and satisfying living. OT services include customized treatment programs to perform daily activities, comprehensive home and job site evaluations and adaptation recommendations, performance skills assessment and interventions, adaptive equipment recommendations and training, and family and caregiver education.
Rehabilitation nurses (RNs)	www.rehabnurse.org	Manage complex medical issues, provide ongoing patient and caregiver education, and establish care plans to maintain optimal wellness. RNs use a holistic approach to fulfill patients' medical, environmental, spiritual, vocational, and educational needs via principles from other disciplines and their own unique medical expertise (bowel, bladder, and skin management). In all care settings, RNs function as coordinators/case managers, collaborators, and counselors. An RN with at least 2 years of practice in rehabilitation who passes the Association of Rehabilitation Nurses examination can earn the Certified Rehabilitation Nurse distinction.
Physical therapists (PTs)	www.apta.org	Experts in examining and treating neuromuscular problems that affect the abilities of individuals to move. PTs practice in many settings and with all age groups.
Physicians	www.aapmr.org	Usually coordinate the rehabilitation team and manage medical conditions pertaining to stroke and comorbidities. A physician may be a physiatrist (i.e., specializing in physical medicine and rehabilitation and thus restoration of function in individuals with problems that range from simple physical mobility to more complex cognitive issues).
Recreational therapists	www.atra-online.com	Provide treatment services and recreation activities to individual with disabilities to facilitate independent physical, cognitive, emotional, and social functioning by enhancing individuals' current skills and assisting new skill development for daily living and community function. Besides discharge planning for community reintegration, they help individuals develop or redevelop social, discretionary time, decision-making, coping, self-advocacy, and basic skills to enhance overall quality of life.
Social workers	www.naswdc.org	Assist individuals, groups, or communities restore or enhance their capacity for social functioning, while creating societal conditions favorable to their goals. Requires knowledge of human development and behavior; social, economic, and cultural institutions; and interactions among these factors. Social workers help prevent crises; counsel individuals, families, and communities to facilitate coping with everyday stresses; and identify resources to allow individuals with disabilities to remain in the community.
SLPs	www.asha.org	Assess speech, language, and other cognitive functions, as well as swallowing, and provide interventions and counseling/education to address language and speech disorders (e.g., aphasia, apraxia of speech, dysarthria, and cognitive-communication impairment). SLPs also intervene when swallowing and cognitive disorders exist. They provide services to all age groups and in all care settings.

OT, occupational therapy; SLPs, speech-language pathologists.

From Miller, E. L., Murray, L., Richards, L., Zorowitz, R. D., Bakas, T., Clark, P., & Billinger, S. A. (2010). Comprehensive overview of nursing and interdisciplinary rehabilitation care of the stroke patient: A scientific statement from the American Heart Association. *Stroke, 41*(10), 2402–2448.

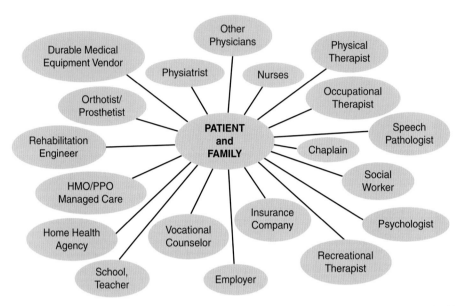

FIGURE 10-1 Multiple caregivers that may be required in comprehensive rehabilitation. HMO, health maintenance organization; PPO, preferred provider organization. (*From Frontera, W. R. [Ed.]. [2010]*. Delisa's physical medicine and rehabilitation: Principles and practice *[5th ed.]. Philadelphia, PA: Lippincott Williams & Wilkins.*)

Rehabilitation focuses on activities to optimize functioning and health. For example, an individual with a stroke may have dysphagia and hemiplegia. These impairments may result in activity limitations in bathing, dressing, and other self-care activities and impact on roles or participation within the family and society such as employment or being a church participant. The *ICF* framework is useful in rehabilitation because it can be used by the ⊙ interprofessional team to address the complex needs of stroke survivors and their reintegration into the community.

TABLE 10-3 Professional Associations

Discipline	Professional Organizations
Occupational therapist	American Occupational Therapy Association (AOTA)
Speech-language therapist	American Speech-Language-Hearing Association (ASHA)
Physical therapist	American Physical Therapy Association (APTA)
Recreational therapist	American Therapeutic Recreation Association (ATRA)
Rehabilitation registered nurse	Association of Rehabilitation Nurses (ARN)
Physiatrist	American Academy of Physical Medicine and Rehabilitation (AAPM&R)
Orthotist and prosthetist	American Academy of Orthotists and Prosthetists
Dietitian	Academy of Nutrition and Dietetics (formerly the American Dietetic Association)
Pharmacist	American Pharmacists Association
Respiratory therapist	American Association for Respiratory Care

From Miller, E. L., Murray, L., Richards, L., Zorowitz, R. D., Bakas, T., Clark, P., & Billinger, S. A. (2010). Comprehensive overview of nursing and interdisciplinary rehabilitation care of the stroke patient: A scientific statement from the American Heart Association. *Stroke, 41*(10), 2402–2448.

TABLE 10-4 *Characteristics of a High-Performance Interprofessional Stroke Team*

- Provide holistic care to the patient and the family.
- Establish collaborative goals with the team that results in best possible outcomes for patient and family.
- Maintain collegial, respectful, and supportive relationships with other team members.
- Communicate and interact effectively to facilitate group processes and team building.
- Reinforce care provided by other team members.
- Participate in team meetings and offer input.
- Coordinate team activities.
- Evaluate effectiveness of the treatment plan on an ongoing basis.
- Advocate for the patient, family, and caregiver.
- Act as resource for other professionals on rehab team, with each bringing specialized knowledge and skill set to the team.
- Provide education for other rehabilitation team members.
- Reinforce teaching provided by other disciplines and health care specialists.

Adapted from Miller, E. L., Murray, L., Richards, L., Zorowitz, R. D., Bakas, T., Clark, P., & Billinger, S. A. (2010). Comprehensive overview of nursing and interdisciplinary rehabilitation care of the stroke patient: A scientific statement from the American Heart Association. *Stroke, 41*(10), 2402–2448.

Rehabilitation professionals must adopt a social understanding of disability so that communication between disciplines can occur effectively. In addition, the *ICF* framework guides interventions, promotes collaboration among disciplines, and serves to guide future research. One of the strengths of the *ICF* is to help plan interventions to meet specific functional goals that are relevant for an individual to resume activities and become an active member within society. A common framework is needed for health professionals to communicate about function, health, and disability—both within a discipline as well as across disciplines. The *ICF* framework serves as such a model (Cieza et al., 2005).

Evidence-Based Practice and Clinical Practice Guidelines for Rehabilitation

Evidence-based practice (EBP) is defined as use of the best scientific knowledge and research evidence available to guide practice, along with expert opinion and patient and

TABLE 10-5 *The International Classification of Functioning, Disability and Health*

Classification	Definition
Impairment	Any loss or abnormality of psychological, physiological, or anatomic structure or function
Activity limitations (formerly *disability*)	Any restriction or lack resulting from impairment of ability to perform an activity in the manner or within the range considered normal for a human being
Participation (formerly *handicap*)	A disadvantage for a given individual, resulting from impairment or disability, which limits or prevents the fulfillment of a role that is normal for an individual

From World Health Organization. (2001). *International Classification of Functioning, Disability and Health.* Geneva, Switzerland: Author.

family values and preferences. EBP and clinical practice guidelines (CPGs) are used to support clinical decision making in the rehabilitation setting (Miller et al., 2010). CPGs are systematically developed statements to assist practitioners in making appropriate evidence-based decisions for specific clinical circumstances such as in the care of the patient with stroke. CPGs define the specific assessment parameters, diagnostic and treatment modalities, treatment options, and management strategies and contain recommendations based on evidence from a systematic review and synthesis of the published health care literature (Miller et al., 2010). The major organizations such as the American Heart Association (AHA) and the American Stroke Association (ASA) provide information about the rigor of the process involved in preparing their CPGs. ⊙ In 2010, the AHA/ASA published CPGs specific to interprofessional rehabilitative stroke care. Although a comprehensive summary of the guidelines is beyond the scope of this chapter, the guidelines serve as evidence-based framework for the interprofessional team caring for the patient with stroke across the entire continuum. CPGs are also useful in providing a framework to plan, implement, and evaluate stroke rehabilitation programs at a population level. For example, CPGs specific to urinary incontinence in stroke set a standard for stroke rehabilitation programs to conduct a comprehensive assessment of premorbid bladder function, identify the type of poststroke incontinence present, and initiate a behavioral bladder training program specific to the type of incontinence present (Miller et al., 2010).

The Stroke Care Continuum

⊙ The stroke care continuum begins with community outreach focused on screening for early detection of risk factors that can lead to a stroke. Educational programs teach patients, providers, and emergency response teams to recognize the symptoms of stroke. Many stroke teams use stroke protocols to facilitate rapid diagnosis and intervention (The Joint Commission [TJC], 2014). Emergency departments (EDs) work with emergency medical systems to ensure that stroke patients are identified when in route to the ED. Stroke teams facilitate rapid diagnosis and intervention to address acute stroke management and include early involvement of rehabilitation professionals. Stroke units with interprofessional care including early rehabilitation accelerate recovery and reduce complications. Rehabilitation management should be integrated throughout stroke recovery.

▮▮ FUNCTIONAL DEFICITS COMMONLY SEEN IN STROKE PATIENTS

Initiating rehabilitation early after the stroke is associated with improved function post stroke. A strategy for whole body rehabilitation consisting of minimizing or interrupting sedation and beginning physical and occupational therapy in the earliest days of critical illness is safe and well tolerated and results in better functional outcomes at hospital discharge, a shorter duration of delirium, and more ventilator-free days compared with standard care (Schweickert et al., 2009). Because of the heterogeneity and complexity of stroke, residual deficits are often observed in patients with a diagnosis of stroke. ⊙ In order to facilitate the recovery process, the interprofessional team must identify, assess, treat, and evaluate each individual patient's unique clinical deficits and build a treatment plan that is tailored to address these issues. Common deficits typically observed in stroke patients are described in greater detail in the following section.

Activities of Daily Living Deficits

Description and Assessment

An estimated 50 million stroke survivors have significant physical, cognitive, and emotional deficits; 25% to 74% of these survivors require some assistance or are fully dependent on caregivers for activities of daily living (ADL) (Anderson, Linto, & Stewart-Wynne, 1995; Kalra & Langhorne, 2007). ADL are activities that are conducted routinely in daily life such as eating, dressing, grooming, bathing, and toileting. They are commonly measured in rehabilitation using the Functional Independence Measure (FIM) instrument (Bottemiller, Bieber, Basford, & Harris, 2006; Keith, Granger, Hamilton, & Sherwin, 1987; Ottenbacher, Hsu, Granger, & Fiedler, 1996). In recent publications, functional status, particularly ADL, was found to have an effect on hospital readmissions. DePalma et al. (2013) reported that unmet ADL needs and transitions involving coping with functional disability are correlated with increased hospital readmissions. This finding is further supported by Arbaje et al. (2008) who found that patients with two hospitalizations within 60 days of discharge had reported at least one unmet ADL need prior to the first hospitalization.

Treatment and Evaluation

In many respects, all rehabilitation modalities and goals should aim to improve ADL. Functional status measured in ADL, including sleep routines and medication management into daily routines, should be integrated into the treatment plan for stroke patients beginning with the acute hospitalization and extending through rehabilitation into the postdischarge setting. Any plan to improve ADL function should be incorporated into the patient's daily routine along the continuum of care to the home environment. Rehabilitation interventions for ADL include use of adaptive equipment for dressing, bathing, and showering; use of durable medical equipment as applicable, including raised toilet seats and tub or bath chairs/benches; integration of dressing techniques such as one-handed method and/or use of adaptive equipment; and use of adaptive equipment for ADL such as feeding, hygiene, grooming, eating, and ambulation.

Clinical Pearl: Functional status, particularly unmet ADL needs, was found to have an effect on hospital readmissions. Addressing ADL needs is important during the rehabilitation process.

Skin Management

Description and Assessment

Stroke patients are at risk for problems with skin integrity from redness to pressure ulcers due to a number of contributing factors such as immobility, loss of sensation, poor circulation, and presence of pressure, friction or shear; incontinence; decreased sensory perception; hemiparesis or hemiplegia; older age; and altered awareness or consciousness (Miller et al., 2010). Frequent monitoring of skin integrity is imperative beginning in the acute hospital setting through rehabilitation and transition to the community setting. There are many scales available to assess skin integrity. The Braden Scale is frequently used across hospital and rehabilitation settings and may be helpful to determine patients at high risk for skin breakdown and target interventions to the high-risk patient (Miller et al., 2010).

Treatment and Evaluation

The key elements involved in perpetuating skin breakdown are pressure, friction, and shearing forces. Interventions aimed at decreasing skin breakdown should target minimizing pressure by altering positions frequently as well as minimizing friction and shearing forces on the skin. Intact skin integrity is critical for success of the rehabilitation process without secondary complications of reddened or open areas, which can impede the patient's rehabilitation and recovery. Characteristics of a successful skin management program includes intact skin with no reddened areas or broken skin and the patient or caregiver understanding the implications of a good skin management program and how to implement such a plan.

The following interventions can assist to maintain skin integrity (Miller et al., 2010): ◉ maintain adequate hydration and nutrition; teach patient skin care and weight-shifting strategies; reposition patient every 2 hours; avoid excessive friction, pressure, and shearing when moving patient; keep patient skin clean and dry; use pressure-relieving devices, such as gel mats or cushions, as applicable; educate family and caregivers on proper skin care prior to discharge; and consult with other interprofessional team members, as needed, such as the nutritionist to promote optimal healing if any broken area exists.

Clinical Pearl: Exercise vigilance in checking the skin integrity of stroke patients, especially those who are using devices such as splints and orthoses.

Cognitive Deficits

Description and Assessment

Cognitive impairment is a common problem for stroke survivors (Leys, Henon, Mackowiak-Cordoliani, & Pasquier, 2005; Linden, Skoog, Fagerberg, Steen, & Blomstrand, 2004). A study by Serrano, Domingo, Rodriguez-Garcia, Castro, and Del Ser (2007) found that in a sample of 327 stroke patients, 12.6% had cognitive impairment. The nature and degree of cognitive impairment that occurs after a stroke depends on the location and size of the stroke. Stroke resulting in damage to the left hemisphere may result in difficulty with language skills and loss of memory. Damage to the right hemisphere may result in difficulties with attention, thinking, and behavior. Damage to the frontal lobe of the brain may cause difficulty in the ability to control and organize thoughts and behavior, resulting in difficulty with executive function including thinking through the steps of a complex task (Cicerone, Levin, Malec, Stuss, & Whyte, 2006; Sohlberg et al., 2007). Cognitive impairment is associated with decreased ability to perform ADL and instrumental activities of daily living (IADL) (Salter, Teasell, Bitensky, Foley, & Bhogal, 2014). A number of tools are available to assess the extent and nature of cognitive impairment post stroke. **Table 10-6** provides a summary of communications and cognitive assessment tools.

TABLE 10-6 Communication and Cognitive Tests for Stroke Patients

Tool	Domain	Time to Administer (min)	Comments
Western Aphasia Battery–Enhanced*	Body function and structure: aphasia	~60	Widely used in research and clinical practice to assess spoken and written language production and comprehension, calculation, drawing, and visuoconstruction skills. Includes a shortened version for bedside administration or screening purposes.
Mini Inventory of Right Brain Injury–2*	Body function and structure: right hemisphere disorders	~30	Screening tool to identify cognitive and communicative deficits common after right hemisphere brain damage (e.g., impaired higher level language, affect processing, visual scanning).
Apraxia Battery for Adults–2*	Body function and structure: apraxia	~20	Six subtests to identify apraxia of speech and limb and oral apraxia. Classifies deficits as mild, moderate, severe, or profound. Acceptable psychometric qualities.
Dysarthria Examination Battery	Body function and structure: dysarthria	~60	Identifies presence and severity of dysarthria by evaluating respiration, phonation, resonation, articulation, and prosody via 21 quantitative tasks and 15 rating scales.
Reading Comprehension Battery–2*	Body function and structure: reading	~30	Ten subtests to assess reading at single-word to paragraph levels. Most appropriate for patients with aphasia. Acceptable psychometric qualities.
Boston Naming Test, 2nd Ed.*	Body function and structure: spoken word retrieval	~15–30	Confrontation naming test widely used in both research and clinical practice, primarily as part of an aphasia evaluation. Guidelines for normal and impaired performance in a variety of populations (e.g., other languages, high vs. low education) can be found in the empirical literature.
Assessment of Language-Related Functional Activities*	Activities and participation: communication	30–90	Includes functional activities (e.g., check writing, telephone tasks) to assess listening, reading, speaking, and writing and some cognitive and basic motor skills. Standardized on a large sample of individuals with and without neurological damage.
ASHA Functional Assessment of Communication Skills for Adults*	Activities and participation: communication	~20	HCP or family caregiver rates 43 items pertaining to patient's social communication, communication of basic needs, reading, writing, and number concepts as well as daily planning. Reliable, valid, and sensitive measure for individuals with aphasia due to left-hemisphere stroke.
Quality of Communication Life Scale*	Activities and participation: quality of life	~15	Eighteen statements that reflect social participation and quality-of-life issues specific to communication are rated by the patient on a 5-point vertical scale. One of the few quality-of-life tools designed for patients with aphasia.

(continued)

TABLE 10-6 Communication and Cognitive Tests for Stroke Patients *(continued)*

Tool	Domain	Time to Administer (min)	Comments
Cognitive Linguistic Quick Test*	Body function and structure: cognition and language	15–30	Available in English and Spanish to assess attention, memory, executive function, language, and visuospatial perception. Suitable for individuals with diverse neurological diagnoses.
Test of Everyday Attention	Body function and structure: attention	~60	Although more widely used with traumatic brain injury survivors, can also be administered to stroke patients to assess auditory and visual sustained, selective, and divided attention as well as attention switching.
Color Trails Test*	Body function and structure: attention	~5–15	Assesses sustained attention and attention switching, with nominal language or cultural bias. Good psychometric qualities.
Behavioral Inattention Test*	Body function and structure; activities: neglect	15–30	Identifies presence and severity of unilateral visual neglect via traditional paper-pencil tasks (e.g., letter cancellation, line bisection) and everyday activities (e.g., making a phone call).
Wechsler Memory Scale–IV	Body function and structure: memory	Depends on whether part or whole test given	Comprehensive test of auditory and visual immediate and delayed memory and visual working memory. Includes an older adult (65–90 years) and adult (16–69 years) battery. Has strong psychometric qualities and software to assist with scoring.
Location Learning Test	Body function and structure: memory	~15–25	Assesses visuospatial learning and recall in older adults (50–96 years), particularly those with suspected dementia. Involves learning and recalling the location of pictured everyday objects in array.
Dells-Kaplan Executive Function System	Body function and structure: executive functions	Depends on whether part or whole test given	Nine subtests designed to assess a number of executive functions (e.g., cognitive flexibility, inhibition, planning, problem solving) in individuals 8–89 years of age. Strong psychometric qualities.
Rivermead Behavioral Memory Test–I	Activities and participation: memory	~30	Evaluates everyday memory abilities (e.g., remembering a person's name, story retelling, route recall) with four parallel versions to allow reliable, repeated administrations. Not recommended if patient has significant visuoperceptual deficits.
Behavioral Assessment of the Dysexecutive Functioning Syndrome	Activities and participation: executive function	~60	Seven subtests to evaluate several executive skills (e.g., planning, temporal judgment) using everyday activities (e.g., key search task). Includes a questionnaire that can be completed by both the patient and caregiver to evaluate their perceptions of the patient's executive abilities.

ASHA, American Speech-Language-Hearing Association; HCP, health care provider.

*Indicates that subtests or the entire test may be suitable for patients with language production or comprehension impairments.

From Miller, E. L., Murray, L., Richards, L., Zorowitz, R. D., Bakas, T., Clark, P., & Billinger, S. A. (2010). Comprehensive overview of nursing and interdisciplinary rehabilitation care of the stroke patient: A scientific statement from the American Heart Association. *Stroke, 41*(10), 2402–2448.

Treatment and Evaluation

The primary goal of cognitive rehabilitation is to improve deficits in order to optimize safety, daily functioning, independence, and quality of life. In developing a cognitive rehabilitation program, it is important to identify all areas of cognitive impairment and to develop a coordinated plan to address each deficit area. Therefore, multiple assessment tools may be necessary to complete a cognitive evaluation. Additionally, patients may be referred to a neuropsychologist for a formal evaluation of cognitive deficits.

Cognitive rehabilitation involves a systematic, functionally oriented provision of therapeutic activities that is based on assessment and understanding of the patient's cognitive deficits (Cicerone et al., 2000). Interventions should reinforce or strengthen previously learned patterns, establish new patterns of cognitive activity through compensatory cognitive mechanisms or establish new patterns of activity through external compensatory mechanisms through environmental structuring and support, and finally enable patients to adapt to their cognitive deficits.

Cognitive rehabilitation is associated with three stages of treatment: acquisition, application, and adaptation (Sohlberg & Mateer, 2001). Acquisition involves teaching the purpose and treatment strategy that were chosen. This phase helps patients recognize and accept deficits as well as understand the benefits of treatment. Problem orientation and awareness is addressed in this stage and allows patients to recognize and understand the deficits and rationale for receiving cognitive treatment. The next phase, application, is aimed to improve the effectiveness and independence in compensating for deficits as well as promotion of internalizations of strategies, that is, reduced reliance on external cues. This stage is associated with provision of practice and gradual removal of cues to help the patient learn to apply the strategy. That is, the therapist provides structure, practice, and repetition to help optimize the patient's ability to use external aids or other strategies in functional tasks. The final stage is adaptation, which promotes transfer of training to tasks including those that are less structured, more novel, complex, and/or distracting. This stage promotes the generalization of skills from a structured therapy approach to less structured environments such as home, community, and work.

⊙ Within rehabilitation teams, it is important to establish which interprofessional team member will administer cognitive tests because these deficits fall under the expertise of various team members (Turkstra, Coelho, & Ylvisaker, 2005). Neurocognitive rehabilitation may include the expertise of psychology, neuropsychology, speech-language pathology, and occupational therapy. For stroke patients, rehabilitation interventions aimed at improving cognitive impairment may include assisting with designing a routine, such as doing activities or tasks at specified times during the day; breaking down tasks into steps; putting things away in the same place or in a familiar place; integrating compensatory strategies such as a memory book or journaling; and integrating internal versus external cues into daily activities.

Clinical Pearl: Development of a cognitive rehabilitation program should identify all areas of cognitive impairment in order to develop a coordinated plan to address each deficit area.

Communications Deficits

Description and Assessment

Communication includes the ability to receive, send, process, and comprehend concepts including verbal, nonverbal, and graphic symbol systems. Communication disorders may be seen in the process of hearing, language, and/or speech (American Speech-Language-Hearing Association [ASHA], 1993). Speech disorders are impairments of the articulation of speech sounds, fluency, and/or voice. Language disorders are impairments in comprehension, both verbal and nonverbal. Language disorders involve the forms of language including the sound system (phonology), the structure of words (morphology), the order and combination of words (syntax), the content of language (semantics), and the function of language used in communication (pragmatics). Common communication disorders seen after stroke include aphasia and dysarthria, although the pathophysiological basis for each is different.

Aphasia is a disturbance in the comprehension and formulation of language and results from damage to the language centers of the brain, usually located in the left hemisphere. Aphasia is seen in 16% to 37% of patients with an acute stroke (Engelter et al., 2006; Kauhanen et al., 2000; Tsouli, Kyritsis, Tsagalis, Virvidaki, & Vemmos, 2009; Wade, Hewer, & David, 1986) which accounts for approximately 100,000 new cases of aphasia in the United States each year (Damasio, 1992). Aphasia is one of the most common poststroke disorders because the middle cerebral artery (MCA) supplies the language centers and is a common site of ischemic stroke. **Figure 10-2** shows the neuroanatomy associated with aphasia. Aphasia significantly impacts quality of life in patients and is associated with decreased socialization, depression, and impairment in overall communications (Kauhanen et al., 2000; Wade et al., 1986). Severity of aphasia is a strong predictor of long-term mortality and need for assistance in stroke patients (Tsouli et al., 2009).

Clinical aphasia, as a central neurological disturbance of language, is an impairment of language that is characterized by paraphrasing, word-finding difficulty, and impaired comprehension. It affects the production or comprehension of speech including the ability to read and write (National Aphasia Association, 2014). A classification system, called the *Boston classification system*, is often used to classify the types of aphasia. The *Boston Diagnostic Aphasia Examination* 3rd edition (BDAE-3) is a collection of tools that assist the practitioner to identify and determine disorders of language function and neurologically recognized aphasia syndromes. The BDAE is a neuropsychological battery that is used to evaluate adults who have suspected aphasia and evaluates language skills that are based on auditory, visual, and gestural modalities; processing functions including comprehension, analysis, and problem solving; and response modalities including writing, articulation, and manipulation (Spreen & Risser, 2003).

Most common types of aphasia include Wernicke's aphasia, Broca's aphasia, and global aphasia. **Table 10-7** shows a classification of aphasia and descriptions. *Broca's aphasia or expressive aphasia* is difficulty in expressing thoughts into words and involves difficulty stringing words together to form complete sentences (Beeson & Robey, 2006). *Wernicke's aphasia or receptive aphasia* involves difficulty with understanding spoken language (Beeson & Robey, 2006). *Global aphasia* includes difficulty in both understanding and forming words and sentences and is associated with a large left hemispheric stroke. Global aphasia is more common in the acute period after a stroke and affects

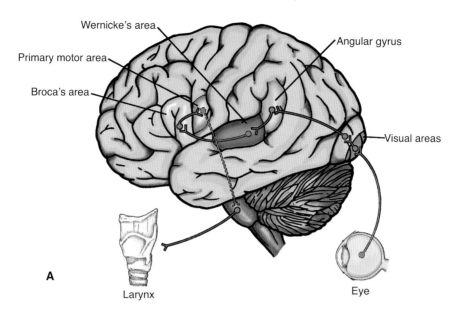

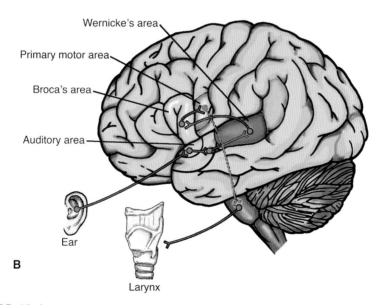

FIGURE 10-2 Neuroanatomical pathways for aphasia. (*From Hickey, J. V. [Ed.]. [2014]. The clinical practice of neurological and neurosurgical nursing [7th ed.]. Philadelphia, PA: Lippincott Williams & Wilkins.*)

TABLE 10-7 Classification of Aphasias with Anatomic Correlations

Type	Description/Clinical Correlation	Anatomic Area or Lesion
Broca's aphasia	Unable to convert thoughts into meaningful language Agrammatism (inability to organize words into sentences) Telegraphic speech (use of content words without connecting words) Distorted production of speech sounds Impaired repetition Normal reception of language is intact.	Broca's area (frontal lobe areas 44 and 45), underlying white matter, or basal ganglia
Wernicke's aphasia	Fluent speech that is unintelligible because of pronunciation errors and use of jargon Impaired comprehension of verbal and written language but no focal motor deficit Impaired repetition	Wernicke's area (superior temporal gyrus, area 22)
Conduction aphasia	Impaired repetition	Connections between Broca's and Wernicke's areas
Anomic aphasia	Impaired naming ability with preservation of other language functions	Lesion outside the language areas; possibly lower temporal lobe lesion or of generalized cerebral dysfunction
Transcortical aphasia	Impaired expression or reception of speech, but *repetition is spared*	Arterial border zones
Subcortical aphasia	Fluent, dysarthric speech and hemiparesis	Left caudate nucleus or the left thalamus
Global aphasia	Combined features of Wernicke's aphasia and Broca's aphasia Impaired comprehension and expression of language Impaired repetition Commonly associated with a dense contralateral hemiplegia	Perisylvian or central regions; commonly seen with left middle cerebral artery infarction (in patients with left hemisphere dominance)

From Hickey, J. V. (Ed.). (2014). *The clinical practice of neurological and neurosurgical nursing* (7th ed.). Philadelphia, PA: Lippincott Williams & Wilkins.

approximately 25% to 32% of patients with stroke (Laska, Hellblom, Murray, Kahan, & Von Arbin, 2001). Patients with *anomic or amnesic aphasia* have difficulty in using the correct names for particular objects, people, places, or events.

A growing body of research indicates a significant relation between neuroplastic changes and language recovery (Johansson, 2000; Thompson, 2000). Neuroplasticity is the ability of the nervous system to respond to intrinsic or extrinsic stimuli by reorganizing its structure, function, and connections (Cramer et al., 2011). This research suggests that a major purpose of rehabilitation is to maximize neural plasticity and lead to functional communication gains. The degree and rate of recovery from aphasia varies based on the type and severity of the aphasia, with initial severity associated with poorer outcome (Ferro, Mariano, & Madureira, 1999; Laska et al., 2001). Recovery patterns for aphasia may vary from resolution within the first few days to months or years. Patterns of recovery include spontaneous recovery within the first few days, weeks, and months. This is improvement that occurs as the brain heals from a stroke. Improvement in aphasia recovery can be characterized by progression in communication skills, with the majority of improvement in the areas of auditory comprehension and spontaneous word production. In the first 6 months following a stroke, fluent aphasia patients made the most gains, whereas those with global aphasia made the least amount of gains. In the same study, in the second part of the first year, fluent aphasia showed the least amount of improvement, whereas the most improvement was in the global aphasia group (Sarno & Levita, 1979). Some studies suggest that improvement in language abilities may occur years later following the neurologic injury (Holland, Greenhouse, Fromm, & Swindell, 1989; Kendall et al., 2006), that is, neuroplasticity of the brain enhances the ability of the brain to rewire itself and provides the ability of recovery to extend for months or years. Intensity of therapy over a short period of time may improve the outcomes of speech and language therapy for stroke patients with aphasia (Bhogal, Teasell, & Speechley, 2003).

Other neurogenic speech disorder includes apraxia and dysarthria. *Speech apraxia* is characterized by an erroneous production of speech sounds, reduced rate of speech, and disorders of prosody, also known as the *rhythm and intonation of speech* (Wambaugh, Duffy, McNeil, Robin, & Rogers, 2006). *Dysarthria* is characterized by slurred, slow, and difficult-to-understand speech (Yorkston, Hakel, Beukelman, & Fager, 2007). It accounts for nearly a quarter of outpatient consults to the speech-language pathologist (Mackenzie, 2011). Even though dysarthria is a common symptom in cerebral ischemia, minimal information on its anatomic specificity and associated characteristics as well as etiologic mechanisms is known (Urban et al., 2000). Recently, Canbaz, Celebisoy, Ozdemirkiran, and Tokucoglu (2010) found that the majority of lesions associated with dysarthria were located in the corona radiata followed by pontine lesions. Further, dysarthria prognosis in this study was greatest in the infratentorial lesions on the right side (Canbaz et al., 2010).

Treatment and Evaluation

Aphasia rehabilitation is often led by a speech-language pathologist, also known as a *speech therapist* and should be provided as early as possible.

Constraint-induced therapy, most frequently used in motor weakness rehabilitation, has also been applied to aphasia rehabilitation. In this case, constraint means avoiding the use of compensatory strategies and forcing the use means communication by talking only (Cherney, Patterson, Raymer, Frymark, & Schooling, 2008). Effectiveness of low-frequency repetitive transcranial magnetic stimulation (rTMS) and intensive speech therapy in poststroke patients with aphasia is a potentially useful neurological rehabilitation technique (Abo et al., 2012). Transcranial magnetic stimulation (TMS) is a noninvasive procedure that used magnetic fields to create electric currents in discrete brain areas (Wasserman et al., 2008). Application of rTMS with the appropriate frequency, intensity, and duration can lead to increases or decreases of excitability of the affected cortex (Pascual-Leone, Davey, Wasserman, Rothwell, & Puri, 2002); in chronic stroke patients, left hemisphere activation has been associated with improved language, and new right hemisphere activation has been observed following speech-language pathology intervention (Cornelissen et al., 2003; Richter, Miltner, & Straube, 2008). Other strategies for rehabilitation professionals to integrate into interventions for patients who have communication difficulties include the following: have patients speak in short sentences; have patients use gestures in addition to speaking; if unable to speak, use communication board strategies or other alternative technology applications; use writing or pictures to ensure that the patient has understood the message; allow additional time for the patient to speak; and be sensitive to the frustration or sense of loss the patient may experience.

Clinical Pearl: Use a normal voice tone when speaking to the patient with aphasia.

Visual Deficits

Description and Assessment

Vision impairments occur frequently after stroke across a spectrum of domains and severities. As many as 87% of stroke patients will manifest some variation of oculomotor dysfunction (Ciuffreda et al., 2007). Oculomotor dysfunction includes nystagmus; abnormalities of vision including saccades, with vergence abnormalities the most common; convergence insufficiency; accommodation; and eye alignment. Other symptoms include difficulty tracking objects (Ciuffreda et al., 2007). Oculomotor-based vision intervention includes oculomotor learning, which is a more specific aspect of motor learning; visual attention and visual field deficits that involve saccadic tracking across midline; remapping of visual space; and localization (Kapoor, Ciuffreda, & Suchoff, 2001; Karnath, Himmelbach, & Kuker, 2003). Hemianopsia, or loss of a visual field on one side of the visual field, is detected in 36% of patients with right hemisphere lesions and in 25% of patients with left hemisphere lesions (Stone, Halligan, & Greenwood, 1993). Binocular vision dysfunction is common after stroke (Wolter & Preda, 2006). Binocular vision involves coordination of the eye muscles that control eye movement. When eye muscles are not properly aligned, the eyes must allow significant corrections to maintain fusion and minimize diplopia (Wolter & Preda, 2006).

The functional implications of visual system malfunction may significantly limit recovery. Visual dysfunction limits progress during the standard rehabilitation continuum of care and decreases overall quality of life (Papageorgiou et al., 2007; Riggs, Andrews, Roberts, & Gilewski, 2007). Stroke-related visual problems include eye movement disorders such as eye deviation, visual field deficits such as hemianopsia or quadrantanopia, reduced visual acuity, and visual inattention or neglect (Pollack et al., 2012). Visual neglect usually occurs after right temporal or parietal stroke.

Treatment and Evaluation

The need for visual rehabilitation is increasingly recognized as a critical element of post-stroke rehabilitation. Neurovisual rehabilitation focuses on restitution, compensation, and/or substitution for the visual deficit (Kerkhoff, 2000). Compensation provides a system that will expand the visual field but does not improve internal function. Rehabilitation focuses on the development of abilities through a visual motor–oriented approach that will stimulate the internal neurological system to interact more efficiently with the environment. Visual field deficits may be treated using compensation techniques including head turning or the use of prism glasses. The use of optical devices such as hemianoptic prisms can improve outcomes in patients with homonymous hemianopsia. Hemianoptic prism spectacles enhance peripheral awareness by projecting the picture from the decreased visual field into the functioning visual field (Gottlieb & Miesner, 2004). Prisms affect spatial representation by causing the optical deviation of the visual field; that is, prisms produce changes in orientation with corresponding shifts in both eye movements. Optically, prisms bend light rays toward the base, causing an apparent shift of the image toward the apex from the viewpoint of the observer. The most common type of prism is the Fresnel membrane lenses or prisms that are cemented onto the lens surface. The prism is located outside the residual field of view when the person looks straight ahead. Prism segments are used to expand the upper and lower quadrants. To expand the upper quadrant of the field, the base-out prism segment is placed at the upper part of the glasses on the side of the field loss (e.g., left lens for left hemianopia) (Gottlieb & Miesner, 2004).

Partial or total visual occlusion is an option to eliminate the symptoms of double vision for treatment of binocular dysfunction. Total occlusion is accomplished with a patch by either alternating the patch between the two eyes, covering the eye that has a decrease in visual acuity, or covering the eye with better vision to increase the function of the more limited eye. Partial occlusion is accomplished using the patient's prescription glasses or on a pair of frames without lenses. Opaque tape is placed over the lens of the nondominant eye starting on the nasal side of the lens and moving laterally until the patient is no longer seeing double. Elimination of double vision through either partial or full occlusion can assist with a patient's ability to perform ADL (Wolter & Preda, 2006).

Perceptual deficits include the ability to organize, process, and interpret incoming visual information. Perceptual deficit rehabilitation includes the "transfer of training approach" and the "functional approach" (Edmans, Webster, & Lincoln, 2000). The transfer of training approach asserts that practice during ADL on a perceptual task will improve performance. The functional approach strives to promote functional independence through the use of repetitive practice in ADL. Visual impairment is common in stroke patients and is a major factor in one's ability to conduct daily functions. It is important to increase awareness about visual problems because vision and vision-related deficits are often underassessed and undertreated (Wolter & Preda, 2006). An association between vision impairment and ADL has been established.

A treatment plan should be developed by the interprofessional team. Occupational therapists have specialized knowledge in visual rehabilitation and visual adaptive devices (Horowitz, 2004; Wolter & Preda, 2006). Interventions include the following: integration of compensation or rehabilitation in ADL including repetition; incorporation of scanning activities including heading turning and the use of verbal or tactile cues; visual inattention or neglect treatment; and integration of prisms and/or patching into daily tasks, as prescribed by a vision specialist, often carried out by the occupational therapist or other interprofessional team members.

The rehabilitation needs of patients with vision deficits vary considerably. The level of care and disciplines required are based on the complexity of the problems, goals, and attributes of the patient. The first step is to identify patients with vision-related difficulties after a stroke and to quantify their visual deficits. Specific elements that should be included in the evaluation of vision rehabilitation are visual function, assessment of the patient's ability to perform tasks requiring vision, assessment of cognitive and psychological status, assessment of risks to the patients due to their visual loss or impairment combined with any other comorbid conditions, and assessment of the potential to benefit from rehabilitation. This includes understanding of the vision impairments and impact on daily activities, safety, and environmental barriers such as lighting or home safety (American Academy of Ophthalmology Vision Rehabilitation Committee, 2012). The overall goal of vision intervention is to eliminate or lessen visual problems in order to reduce the frequency and severity of the patient's signs and symptoms limiting participation in daily activities due to vision-related problems (Wolter & Preda, 2006).

Clinical Pearl: Early identification of vision deficits and integration into the rehabilitation program assists with ADL performance.

Dysphagia

Description and Assessment

Stroke is one of the most common causes of dysphagia in the adult population, with 42% to 67% of patients presenting with dysphagia within 3 days of a stroke. Fifty percent of these patients aspirate, and about one third who aspirate develop pneumonia (Hinchey et al., 2005). Dysphagia is a disorder of swallowing. Dysphagia and other swallowing dysfunctions may range from physical difficulty of bringing the food to the mouth to manipulation of food in the mouth. Dysphagia may also result from cognitive deficits from surgical intervention, neurological impairments, structural problems, and positioning problems that impact feeding, eating, and swallowing (Cox et al., 2006; Roberts, Cox, Schubert, & Gentry, 2009).

Dysphagia is a problem that is often seen and addressed by the interprofessional team. The consequences of dysphagia include dehydration, aspiration pneumonia, and airway obstruction (Palmer, Drennan, & Baba, 2000). In assessing the patient for dysphagia, a clinical swallowing evaluation is often completed by a swallowing therapist or speech therapist at the bedside. Many clinical swallowing evaluations rely on the patient to have overt signs of potential aspiration such as coughing or a wet sound when phonating (Terre & Mearin, 2006). The primary drawback of the clinical swallowing evaluation is not being able to detect silent aspiration (Daniels et al., 1998; Smith, Logemann, Colangelo, Rademaker, & Pauloski, 1999). Instrumental evaluations of swallowing are used to provide additional information to assist in the management of dysphagia. The most common tests include the modified barium swallow (MBS), which is a specialized test using a moving x-ray to evaluate a swallowing disorder. This information is used to select the safest diet and any specific compensatory modifications that may be needed. Fiberoptic endoscopic evaluation of swallowing (FEES) is a specialized test using a small camera inserted through the nose to the throat to evaluate swallowing. As with the MBS, the information is used to determine the best diet and compensatory modifications for safe oral intake.

There are four main phases in the swallowing process. See **Figure 9-1**. The first phase is the oral preparatory phase in which the food is chewed, mixed with saliva, and then formed into a cohesive bolus. The second phase is the oral phase in which the food is moved in the mouth from the front to the back with a squeezing action performed primarily with the tongue. The third phase is the pharyngeal phase, which begins with the trigger of the swallow. In this phase, when the food enters the upper throat area, the soft palate elevates, and the epiglottis seals off the trachea. The tongue moves backward and the pharyngeal wall moves forward. These actions assist with moving the food downward to the esophagus. The final phase is the esophageal phase in which the food bolus enters the esophagus and transports the food directly to the stomach through a squeezing action of the throat muscles (Logemann, 1998).

Treatment and Evaluation

It is important to address swallowing problems because they impact on quality of life and place the patient at risk for complications from aspiration. Eating and drinking are key functions to basic survival and are part of daily activities including social events that relate to relationships, acceptance, entertainment, and ADL. Disordered swallow function is associated with aspiration pneumonia and increased mortality rates (Miller et al., 2010). Evidence is lacking regarding interventions to improve swallow, and research is needed to further guide this field of rehabilitation. Interventions commonly employed by the interprofessional team to address dysphagia include (Miller et al., 2010) ongoing swallow assessment, as discussed earlier; encouragement of self- feeding; employment of low-risk feeding strategies such as modified diet consistency, reduced distractions while eating, eating while seated, and slow eating with small bites of food; employment of airway protection strategies such as chin tuck or head rotation while swallowing; electric stimulation; and electromyography biofeedback.

Clinical Pearl: Be aware that for the patient with stroke who has a wet or gurgled voice, leftover food in mouth or coughing during eating may indicate the presence of dysphagia.

Paresis, Paralysis, Incoordination, and Decreased Mobility

Description and Assessment

Disability after stroke often includes difficulty with balance and mobility due to loss of muscle control as a result of paresis or paralysis, poorly timed and uncoordinated movements (ataxia), increased or decreased muscle tone, and the inability to coordinate, perform, or carry out specific movements. Motor relearning following a stroke is a focus of research, especially brain plasticity or the ability of the brain to reorganize and develop new pathways. Weakness is associated with postdischarge falls, and it is a significant risk factor for compromised safety in stroke survivors. Decreased mobility increases the risks of deep vein thrombosis (DVT), falls, pressure ulcers, and other medical complications (Kelly, Rudd, Lewis, & Hunt, 2001). There are a number of assessment tools available to quantify and trend motor dysfunction in poststroke survivors (**Table 10-8**).

Treatment and Evaluation

Weakness and decreased mobility is a significant area of research in poststroke rehabilitation. Several rehabilitation modalities address evolving approaches that target the ability of the individual to regain movement (Shumway-Cook & Woollacott, 2011). Motor learning is the acquisition or modification of learned movement patterns over time (Shumway-Cook & Woollacott, 2011). Motor learning is one common theory applied to movement rehabilitation. This theory involves practice of motor movement and experience, which leads to permanent changes in the person's ability to produce quality movement. Motor control is the outcome of motor learning and involves the ability to produce purposeful movements of the extremities and postural adjustments in response to task and environmental demands (Carr & Shepherd, 1998).

Other approaches used in the treatment of motor weakness include neurodevelopmental treatment (NDT), Neuro-Integrative Functional Rehabilitation and Habilitation (NEURO-IFRAH), and proprioceptive neuromuscular facilitation (PNF). NDT is a therapeutic approach that was developed for the treatment of individuals with

TABLE 10-8 Examples of Upper Extremity and Lower Extremity Motor Assessment

Tool	Domain	Time to Administer	Comments
Grip dynamometry	Unilateral hand strength	10 min	A commonly used single-item assessment that correlates with function, morbidity, and mortality. Reliability and validity data are available. It can be painful for people with arthritis, and it only measures static strength.
Handheld dynamometry	Unilateral muscle strength	Depends on no. of motions tested; ~2 min/motion	Quick and uses inexpensive equipment. The no. of items depends on the no. of muscle groups tested. Some reliability and validity are available. Results can depend on the strength of the therapist to resist the movements of the person with stroke.
Fugl-Meyer Motor Assessment–UE subscale	Unilateral UE and LE gross motor coordination, balance, sensation, and ROM	45–50 min	A 113-item scale divided into UE, LE, sensation, ROM, pain, and balance scales. UE and LE subscales are most commonly used in the literature. Stroke rehabilitation guidelines recommend this tool. Data are available on reliability, validity, sensitivity to change, and item functioning. Weaknesses include that it is lengthy, has ceiling effects in more mild stroke patients, offers limited assessment of object manipulation and finger individualization, and has inconsistency in its administration across the literature.
Action Research Arm Test	Unilateral arm and hand coordination	30 min	A 20-item, quick assessment commonly used in literature; however, because items are presented in ascending difficulty and each subtest stops when the patient cannot perform an item, not all items are necessarily given. Data on reliability, validity, and sensitivity to change are available. It does not measure tasks that require finger individualization, and only task completion is scored.
Box and Block Test	Unilateral gross finger coordination	10 min	A quick, single-item, commonly used assessment that is available commercially. Reliability and validity data are available. Its weakness is that it only measures one task.
Motor Assessment Scale	UE, LE, general mobility, sitting balance, and coordination	10–15 min	This 9-item test offers a quick assessment of motor function. Reliability and validity have been reported.
Chedoke-McMaster Stroke Assessment*	Unilateral gross motor coordination	1 hr	Created for stroke assessment and contains two subscales: Impairment Inventory (22 items) and Activity Inventory (15 items). It is commercially available, and training workshops are offered. Reliability and validity data are available. Its weakness is its length.
Wolf Motor Function Test*	Arm and hand coordination; combination of single joint movements and simulated unilateral functional activities	20–30 min	A 15-item assessment created for stroke rehabilitation that uses inexpensive materials. Assesses time to perform items and quality of item performance. Little test administration training is required. Some reliability and validity data are available. Weaknesses are that it is lengthy, it consists of a mixture of body function and activity-level items, and the tester needs to fabricate the test because it is not available commercially.

Assessment	Measures	Time	Description
Stroke Rehabilitation Assessment of Movement (STREAM)	LE movement and mobility	15 min	Has 30 items equally distributed among two subscales: upper limb movements, lower limb movements, and basic mobility. Movements are scored on a 3-point scale. Mobility items are scored on a 4-point scale, with one additional category to allow for independence with the help of a mobility aid. The STREAM is quick to administer, and reliability and minimal clinically important difference data are available.
Activity Level			
Wolf Motor Function Test*	See above	See above	See above
Chedoke-McMaster Stroke Assessment*	See above	See above	See above
Jebsen Test of Motor Function	Arm and hand coordination; simulated unilateral functional activities	20–30 min	A 7-item assessment that is available commercially and commonly used. Some reliability and validity data are available. Weaknesses are that it is lengthy, and only time to perform is assessed.
Chedoke Arm and Hand Inventory	Arm and hand coordination; simulated bilateral functional activities	25–35 min	A 13-item tool with some reliability and validity data available. The only UE assessment consisting of all bilateral real-life tasks; however, it requires some fabrication, only quality of performance is measured, and training is required to use the rating scale.
Motor Activity Log	Self-report measure of arm and hand use in daily activities	15 min	Has several versions but most commonly has 30 items divided into unilateral and bilateral tasks. A quick, self-report assessment of hand use in real life. Some reliability and validity data are available. It cannot be used with people with aphasia or cognitive problems that limit comprehension.
Rivermead Mobility Index	General mobility	5–10 min	A 15-item tool that quickly quantifies mobility function. Except for 1 item (standing unsupported) observed by the therapist, the rest are the individual's self-report (yes/no). Some reliability and validity data are available. A weakness is the uncertainty regarding its sensitivity to change, and because of self-report items, it may be inappropriate for some individuals with aphasia.

UE, upper extremity; LE, lower extremity; ROM, range of motion.

*The Wolf Motor Function Test and the Chedoke-McMaster Stroke Assessment are both body structure and function and activity level assessments because they have items that are purely movements and some items that are simulated activities.

From Miller, E. L., Murray, L., Richards, L., Zorowitz, R. D., Bakas, T., Clark, P., & Billinger, S. A. (2010). Comprehensive overview of nursing and interdisciplinary rehabilitation care of the stroke patient: A scientific statement from the American Heart Association. *Stroke, 41*(10), 2402–2448.

pathophysiology of the central nervous system. The NDT, also known as the *Bobath approach*, uses direct handling and guidance to optimize function through the initiation and completion of tasks (Lennon & Ashburn, 2000). NEURO-IFRAH is a technique that is integrative of all systems of the person. This integrates many aspects of therapy in order to restore a patient to the fullest physical, mental, social, vocational, and economic status by reacquiring and learning new skills (NEURO-IFRAH Organization, n.d.).

PNF has been used since the late 1930s and 1940s when Herman Kabat began using PNF concepts to stimulate distal segments so that the proprioceptors in the more proximal segments became stimulated (Burton & Brigham, 2013). His techniques were based on Sherrington's principles of irradiation, reciprocal innervation, and inhibition (Voss, Ionta, & Myers, 1985). These principles describe the rhythmic and reflexive actions that lead to coordinated motion. Today, a variety of these motor theories and techniques are used in rehabilitation to improve stroke mobility.

Additional stroke movement deficits may include difficulty with sitting or standing balance, safely moving weight from one side of the body to the other, and moving the body forward while walking (Geiger, Allen, O'Keefe, & Hickes, 2001). Walking requires balance, motor control, sensation, coordination, and the ability to shift weight. Treatment interventions are aimed at improving mobility between different surfaces such as from the bed to chair or getting on and off a chair, walking, wheelchair mobility, and stair management. Regaining mobility is considered a primary goal of the stroke patient early in the rehabilitation process (Craig, Wu, Bernhardt, & Langhorne, 2011). The involvement of physical therapy in stroke rehabilitation with a focus on gait activities is associated with the most significant improvement in mobility post stroke (Latham et al., 2005).

The literature describing the best method for safe, efficient, and progressive ambulation is varied. Some literature supports task-specific gait training, which may have beneficial effects on functional gait (Hesse et al., 1995; Laufer, Dickstein, Chefez, & Marcovitz, 2001). Locomotor training using body weight support on a treadmill is an example of task-specific gait training that uses a harness to provide partial body weight support in conjunction with a treadmill. This allows the body weight support harness to provide assistance for postural control, the treadmill to provide control and progression of walking speed, and the repetitive training of the complete gait cycle allows for an appropriate pattern of input in order to simulate locomotor pattern (Cernak, Stevens, Price, & Shumway-Cook, 2008). The mechanisms and techniques used to impact mobility and stroke are only partially understood. One of the most important aspects of any type of gait training is to have the patient as active as possible. Having the patient as active as possible may be related to improvements in motor learning as well as reduce secondary complications.

The use of robotics in gait training provides an important opportunity, and further research is needed to fully understand the potential therapeutic benefits of this therapy (Pennycott, Wyss, Vallery, Klamroth-Marganska, & Riener, 2012). Mobility devices such as braces, canes, walkers, and/or wheelchairs may assist stroke patients with mobility. It is another treatment modality gaining popularity in motor control research. Virtual reality is the inclusion of realistic stimulation of an environment using three-dimensional graphics with the use of a computer system and interactive software and hardware (Keshner, 2004). It allows for the creation of a synthetic environment with precise control over many physical variables that influence behavior while recording physiological and kinematic responses. Virtual reality provides real-time feedback regarding the accuracy of task performance as well as the ability to simulate activities that might have excessive risk to the patient. It is often implemented in the form of a game in which there are specific goals and some form of reward for success. The use of virtual reality in stroke rehabilitation is undergoing rapid development and testing and is increasingly integrated into stroke rehabilitation within clinical settings as well as for home programs (Boian et al., 2002; Rizzo, 2002). In addition to motor control research, virtual reality may be applied to rehabilitation for impaired cognition and altered ADL (Gourlay, Lun, Lee, & Tay, 2000; Weiss, Bialik, & Kizony, 2003; Weiss, Naveh, & Katz, 2003).

Constraint-induced movement therapy (CIMT) is a rehabilitation intervention designed to promote the increased use of a weak or paralyzed arm. CIMT is most commonly used in patients post stroke. This theoretical approach involves constraining the unaffected arm in a sling, mitt, or a combination of both, thus forcing the use of the weaker or paralyzed arm in ADL. Patients using CIMT use their affected upper extremity on an intensive basis for several consecutive weeks. CIMT has a long history as a therapeutic intervention for paresis following stroke. Taub et al. (1993) conducted much of the original research in this area and initially described the phenomenon as *learned non-use*. Taub's work was conducted by constraining the intact forelimb of primates, which provided the first evidence of the learned non-use phenomenon. Taub and Wolf (1997) demonstrated significant improvements with the use of CIMT in a randomized clinical trial of nine individuals post stroke. Wolf, LeCraw, Barton, and Jann (1989) also found that forced use of hemiparetic upper extremities could reverse the effect of learned non-use among chronic stroke and brain-injured patients. This work was further expanded by Kunkel et al. (1999) who found an increase in the amount of use of the affected upper extremity in real-world environments. In a pilot study, Roberts, Vegher, Gilewski, Bender, and Riggs (2005) studied CIMT in an individual's home environment and how it was incorporated into meaningful ADL. The investigators found that the use of meaningful activities in the naturalistic environment may demonstrate improved patient satisfaction of functional outcomes.

Patients with stroke are at high risk for falls. A study evaluating poststroke fall risk demonstrated that 37% of stroke survivors fall within 6 months of their stroke. Of those who fell, 12% experienced frequent falls, falling more than five times (Miller et al., 2010). The study also revealed that many stroke survivors fall in their own home. Therefore, assessing for balance and coordination and counseling stroke patients about fall risk, during and after the rehabilitation phase, is a high priority. Fall or near-fall events during the acute care hospitalization and inability to use upper extremity at the time of hospital discharge or trunk instability are associated with postdischarge falls in stroke survivors (Miller et al., 2010).

In summary, the interprofessional rehabilitation team may employ a number of interventions to assist with regaining mobility after stroke, including use of supportive footwear when moving from surface to surface, removal of obstacles to avoid tripping or falling, integration of braces and/or mobility devices (as prescribed), integration of the therapeutic techniques for transferring and moving stroke patients, implementation of evidence-based rehabilitation therapies to regain function in paretic limb, and integration of supported gait training and the use of robotics to assist with gait training.

Clinical Pearl: CIMT is a task-oriented approach that focuses on constraining the use of the unaffected or stronger extremity to facilitate motor recovery in the affected or weaker extremity while engaged in activities.

Shoulder Subluxation and Positioning

Description and Assessment

Assessing for shoulder and scapular alignment in stroke patients to detect for any abnormalities that will interfere with shoulder and arm full range of motion and strength is very important. Proper positioning of the shoulder during ADL is critical for the prevention of subluxation and additional shoulder complications. The shoulder complex is a unique joint because it has mobility in all planes of motion. The glenohumeral joint relies on the integrity of muscular and capsuloligamentous structures for stability. Glenohumeral subluxation is a secondary complication of hemiplegia or paresis caused by stroke and occurs when the head of the humerus is dropped away from the joint. This occurs in 17% to 66% of stroke patients (Griffin & Bernhardt, 2006; Peters & Lee, 2003).

Treatment and Evaluation

Although there is no conclusive evidence for positioning or other forms of prevention, a quality rehabilitation plan incorporates strategies to mitigate secondary shoulder injury. When the patient is in bed, the upper extremity should be supported by a pillow (Bobath, 1970). While sitting in a wheelchair, a number of positioning devices or supports have been recommended, including lapboards and arm troughs (Bohannon, Thorne, & Mieres, 1983; Gresham et al., 1995; Moodie, Bresbin, & Grace Morgan, 1986). Other supports such as slings have also been described in the literature (Cailliet, 1980; Claus & Godfrey, 1985; Rajaram & Holtz, 1985).

There are various therapeutic approaches for treating shoulder subluxation. The literature suggests that taping or strapping of the affected shoulder and neuromuscular electrical stimulation (NMES) are effective interventions to address a weakened shoulder joint. Shoulder taping or strapping is used to support the shoulder joint structure, reduce or prevent pain, as well as maintain shoulder and scapular alignment. Shoulder strapping or taping has been shown to be useful during the early phases of a stroke (Griffin & Bernhardt, 2006; Morin & Bravo, 1997; Walsh, 2001). NMES has been used to treat shoulder subluxation. NMES uses electrical current to improve motor recovery, reduce pain and spasticity, strengthen muscles, and increase range of motion following stroke. The clinical applications of NMES for treatment of subluxation include muscle reeducation to stabilize muscle tone, cortical feedback, reduction of spasticity, continuous protection of the shoulder capsule, and meticulous joint alignment to expedite recovery of upper extremity function post stroke (Baker & Parker, 1986; Chae et al., 1998; Sheffer & Chae, 2007; Stokes-Turner & Jackson, 2002).

◉ Rehabilitation professionals should be aware of the various treatments for shoulder subluxation and upper extremity control and be advocates for implementation of shoulder protection techniques. Further, rehabilitation plays a critical role in providing education to the patient and family on the protection and prevention of secondary complications of the paretic arm. Interventions to support the affected limb and minimize pain and subluxation include the following: support the paretic arm with a pillow even when reclining in bed; support the paretic arm in a sling or use taping to support the affected shoulder; use additional supportive positioning devices such as an arm trough or lapboard, as appropriate; and apply evidence-based rehabilitation therapies such as NMES, CIMT, and others to regain function of the paretic limb.

Clinical Pearl: Shoulder taping or strapping that is used to support the shoulder joint structure, reduce and/or prevent pain, as well as address shoulder/scapular alignment has been shown to be useful during the early phases of a stroke.

Urinary Bladder Dysfunction

Description and Assessment

Bladder and bowel dysfunction occurs in approximately 25% to 50% of stroke survivors (Cournan, 2012; Miller et al., 2010). Urinary retention and incontinence is common in patients with a stroke and is associated with additional complications. Urinary retention can lead to a urinary tract infection or renal impairment in extreme cases. Women are about two times more likely to have urinary incontinence post stroke compared to men (AHA, 2014). In addition, bladder impairment may influence rehabilitation outcomes and ultimate return home or placement in a long-term care facility.

Before any plan of care is developed, it is important to first assess the patient to identify the patient's premorbid level of function, identify current altered patterns of dysfunction, and understand the mechanism of the bladder dysfunction. General interventions applied to all stroke patients struggling with incontinence will be discussed. However, bladder management programs must be tailored to the underlying etiology.

Functional incontinence occurs when factors such as immobility, confusion, and the inability to recognize the urge to void can lead to incontinence. *Stress incontinence* occurs when a small amount of urine leaks as a result of an incompetent urinary sphincter. *Urge incontinence* results in difficulty retaining urine, typically as a result of a hyperactive detrusor muscle, inability of the brain to inhibit or postpone voiding, or an increase in bladder sensitivity. *Overflow and retention incontinence* results from of an outlet obstruction with a decrease in detrusor activity. This may result in the following signs and symptoms: a palpable bladder; small, frequent voiding; and general fluid retention as evidenced by oral intake that exceeds urinary output. Often, the patient will have large postvoid urinary residuals.

Treatment and Evaluation

There are some general considerations in establishing a successful bladder management program; however, there may be additional suggestions based on the specific type of poststroke incontinence (Miller et al., 2010). It is essential for the rehabilitation team to individualize and implement a comprehensive bladder management program to facilitate both independence and quality of life. A baseline bladder assessment is conducted upon admission to rehabilitation. Daily monitoring of bladder status is necessary to determine the effectiveness of a bladder program. In order to successfully manage voiding activities, the patient must access the bathroom, manage clothing, use assistive devices, and perform perineal hygiene when needed (Cournan, 2012). Activities learned and practiced in rehabilitation can allow the patient to become more functional in the skills needed to successfully complete bladder management tasks.

Interventions for bladder dysfunction initiated by the interprofessional rehabilitation team are categorized as general interventions and specific interventions based

TABLE 10-9 Sample Bladder Management Program

Goal: Patient will be continent of bladder upon discharge from inpatient rehabilitation.

Interventions:
- Determine bladder history.
- Assess current bladder status.
- Remove Foley per orders within 48 hr of admission.
- Conduct bladder scan $\times$ 3 post voids; if bladder scan is greater than 100 mL or if patient does not void in 8 hr, perform intermittent catheterization.
- Toilet patient every 2 hr while awake.
- Limit fluids after 6 p.m.
- Maintain an accurate intake and output (I&O) record.
- Encourage the patient to participate in bladder retraining program.
- Maintain a bladder diary of voiding pattern.
- Evaluate bladder program each week to identify progress and/or barriers.
- Use a toilet or a bedside commode to promote complete emptying; avoid use of bedpan.
- Administer bladder medications as ordered.
- Urology consult, if indicated.

on underlying etiology. The general principles of a bladder management program include the following: determine the continence history; assess for evidence of urinary tract infection; maintain adequate hydration; establish bladder program; implement a timed voiding program initiated by the caregiver which is typically on an every 2-hour (while awake) basis; use prompted voiding which is initiated by the patient; use a bladder scan and catheterize, as needed, for postvoid residual (PVR); administer medications such as anticholinergics and desmopressin, as indicated; use a toilet versus bedpan to promote complete emptying; maintain the patient's dignity; and educate the patient about bladder management program. **Table 10-9** shows a sample bladder management program. In addition, incontinence pads may be used to keep the patient dry, prevent leakage, and protect the skin. For *stress incontinence*, consider teaching pelvic floor exercises, such as Kegel's exercises, to the patient. For patients with *overflow and retention incontinence*, schedule timed voiding with intermittent catheterizations; implement double voiding whereby the patient voids, waits a brief amount of time, and attempts to void again; and insert a Foley bladder catheter if the patient fails a trial voiding program.

Clinical Pearl: It is important to distinguish the underlying impairment when urinary incontinence is present so that an appropriate, individualized bladder management program can be implemented.

Bowel Dysfunction

Description and Assessment

As previously noted, bowel dysfunction occurs in approximately 25% to 50% of stroke survivors (Cournan, 2012; Miller et al., 2010). Before any interventions are initiated, first assess the patient's premorbid level of function as well as the underlying etiology of the bowel dysfunction. Clinicians must recognize key concepts and elements of a successful bowel management program to develop a plan based on the patient's individual needs. Bowel dysfunction may include constipation as well as fecal incontinence. Constipation has a high prevalence in patients with stroke and may be indirectly related to decreased mobility, decreased fluid and/or fiber intake, and overall increased dependence (Teasell et al., 2013). Constipation may result in pain, paralytic ileus, or obstruction, if left untreated. A reported 30% to 40% of stroke patients suffer from fecal incontinence while hospitalized for the acute stroke event, and up to 10% of stroke survivors suffer from fecal incontinence as a long-term complication after stroke (Miller et al., 2010). Often, fecal incontinence is related to an inability to mobilize to the toilet.

Intervention and Evaluation

Similar to management of bladder dysfunction, all stroke patients should be assessed for bowel dysfunction and daily bowel patterns on admission to rehabilitation. Interventions should be tailored to address the underlying etiology of constipation or fecal incontinence. Interventions to address bowel dysfunction may include the following: facilitate proper nutrition and hydration; increase fiber intake, either through diet or the use of bulk-forming stool softeners or laxatives; assess bowel status based on the patient history to establish an individualized bowel management program; establish and monitor the bowel program on a weekly basis; administer medications such as stool softeners or suppositories; use toilet-assistive devices such as bedpan or bedside commode, although the toilet is preferred versus a bedpan to facilitate proper emptying; and maintain the patient's dignity. **Table 10-10** shows a sample bowel management program.

Clinical Pearl: When implementing a bowel management program, change or modify only one intervention at a time to determine effectiveness/impact of that intervention on bowel status.

TABLE 10-10 Sample Bowel Management Program

Goal: Patient will be continent of bowel upon discharge from inpatient rehabilitation.

Interventions:
- Determine bowel history.
- Assess current bowel status.
- Encourage fluids to prevent constipation.
- Encourage a high-fiber diet.
- Encourage patient to participate in bowel management program.
- Maintain a record of bowel pattern.
- Evaluate the bowel program each week to identify progress and/or barriers.
- Use a toilet or a bedside commode to facilitate complete emptying; avoid use of bedpan.
- Administer stool softener and suppositories, as ordered and p.r.n.

Sexuality

Description and Assessment

Although sexual dysfunction is a problem reported by patients after stroke, little research has been conducted to define this problem or determine evidence-based interventions to assist with poststroke sexual dysfunction. Despite the lack of literature, sexual functioning should be assessed by the rehabilitation team. The assessment should include the patient's premorbid functioning and a sexual history. Issues surrounding emotional lability, libido, ability to communicate, and fatigue may impact sexual function in the patient with stroke. In addition, referral to other specialists such as a psychologist who specializes in sexual dysfunction may be indicated.

The acronym PLISSIT is an acronym for **P**ermission, **L**imited **I**nformation, **S**pecial **S**uggestions, **I**ntensive **T**herapy, a model of sex therapy that was developed by Annon (1976). The model is based on the assumption that the majority of people can resolve their sexual problems by following a program. The comprehensive four-step program provides the patient with education and behavioral strategies to integrate sexuality into their rehabilitation program in order to address sexual problems.

The steps include the following:

- **P**ermission provides patients with permission to speak about their sexual concerns and helps to validate the issue as a legitimate health concern (Ohl, 2007).
- **L**imited **I**nformation focuses on informative education including, but not limited to, anatomic and physiological information about how their body and their partner's body work and what is considered normal during sex (Haeberle, 2003).
- **S**pecific **S**uggestions provides specific tips, directions, and exercises to treat sexual problems (Haeberle, 2003).
- **I**ntensive **T**herapy step involves determining which patients have an additional factor contributing to sexual dysfunction and may need additional referrals to medical professionals (Wallace, 2008).

Assessment and Interventions

When sexual dissatisfaction or dysfunction is expressed by stroke survivors, interventions may include the following: incorporate sexual dysfunction models such as PLISSIT into rehabilitation program; discuss positioning techniques to manage paresis or paralysis; encourage use of alternative positioning techniques based on motor ability; discuss birth control options, if indicated; and refer to a psychologist with expertise in sexuality or sexual dysfunction, as needed.

Poststroke Depression

Description and Assessment

Depression is a common complication after stroke and is often underdiagnosed (Miller et al., 2010; Salter et al., 2013). Addressing the psychosocial, spiritual, and coping needs of the patient with stroke is critical to optimal recovery. Major risk factors for poststroke depression include female gender, premorbid history of depression, social isolation, and functional and cognitive impairment. Poststroke depression has been associated with higher mortality, poorer functional recovery, and decreased social activity (Miller et al., 2010).

Despite the recognition of poststroke depression as a significant complication, evidence regarding appropriate assessment and intervention is lacking. Much of the research on depression assessment and treatment has not been validated in stroke survivors. Regardless, attempts to identify and treat depression in stroke survivors should be a priority for the interprofessional rehabilitation team. Team members should consult and collaborate with one another to identify and address any potential concerns with patient exhibiting depression. A review of instruments currently used in practice to assess for depression is provided in **Table 10-11.**

Intervention and Evaluation

Patients with stroke may have concerns about self-image, role function, and depression. The rehabilitation team should facilitate adaptive coping strategies. Poststroke depression is associated with functional ability and may have a negative impact on recovery. Functional impairment and poststroke depression appear to interact with one another, with each influencing the recovery of the other. Active engagement and participation in the rehabilitation program is vital for patients with stroke. Motivation and psychosocial well-being can support this endeavor (Miller et al., 2010). A psychologist may be consulted for some patients as indicated by need for more coping and adjustment skills. In addition, a psychiatrist may be an adjunct team member for patients requiring medication management for coping, anxiety, or depression. Early identification of poststroke depression is imperative for success of maximizing functional ability. Treatment typically revolves around pharmacotherapy and psychotherapy. For more detailed interventions and evaluation of poststroke depression, please refer to Chapter 9.

All stroke patients should be screened and assessed upon admission for depression with a consult to either a psychologist or psychiatrist as needed. Basic rehabilitation team interventions from a psychosocial and spiritual approach may include the following assessment/intervention strategies: provide time for the patient to verbalize concerns; reflect and clarify patient's feelings; reinforce patient strengths; provide and encourage socialization opportunities; allow patient control when making care decisions; reduce stress whenever possible; use relaxation techniques, if applicable; provide time for patient to meet spiritual needs; schedule and facilitate patient and family conferences, as needed; facilitate pharmacologic treatment of depression as appropriate; provide resources for patient and caregivers post discharge; and refer to support group or peer support, if available.

THE POSTACUTE CARE STROKE CONTINUUM

The journey in postacute care stroke continuum begins with a comprehensive assessment using a standardized instrument. The Continuity Assessment Record and Evaluation (CARE) instrument measures health and functional status, changes in severity, and other outcomes for Medicare beneficiaries at admission and discharge from postacute care settings. The CARE item set includes the four domains of medical, functional, cognitive impairment, and social/environmental factors. These domains were chosen to either measure case-mix severity differences within medical conditions or predict outcomes (e.g., discharge to home or community, rehospitalization, and changes in functional or medical status). The CARE item set is designed to standardize assessment of a patient's medical, functional, cognitive, and social support status across acute and

TABLE 10-11 Instruments to Screen for Depression

Tool	Domain	Time to Administer (min)	Comments
Beck Depression Inventory	Body function; contextual factors	10	A 21-item instrument with a 4-point scale that is widely used, easy to administer, and good at assessing somatic symptoms but less useful with the elderly. It has established internal consistency and construct validity. Sensitivity and specificity are best with a cutoff score of 10 or greater.
Center for Epidemiologic Studies of Depression	Body function; contextual factors	<15	A 20-item, self-report, 4-point Likert measure that assesses depression symptoms in the general population. Easy to administer and has established internal consistency and construct validity. Not appropriate for aphasic patients.
Geriatric Depression Scale	Body function; contextual factors	10	A 30-item, self-report tool with yes/no responses. It is easy to administer with the elderly, the cognitively impaired, or those with visual and/or physical problems or low motivation. Has established reliability and validity but yields high false-negatives for minor depression. There is also a short form of 15 items.
Hamilton Depression Scale	Body function; contextual factors	<30	A 17-item tool with a 5-point scale used to assess depression severity in children and adults, including those with stroke. There is also a 21-item version, but the shorter version is more commonly used. Has established reliability and validity and correlates highly with other clinician-rated and self-report depression measures.
Patient Health Questionnaire 9-item Depression Scale	Body function; contextual factors	<5	A 9-item, easy-to-administer tool based on the 9 *Diagnostic and Statistical Manual of Mental Disorders* 4th edition (*DSM-IV*) depression criteria. A score ≥10 has excellent sensitivity and specificity with stroke survivors, and it performs equally well regardless of client age, gender, or ethnicity. A score ≥3 on the 2-item version of this questionnaire also has excellent sensitivity and specificity as a brief screening tool, but for diagnosis and a more complete depression evaluation, the additional 17 items should be given.

From Miller, E. L., Murray, L., Richards, L., Zorowitz, R. D., Bakas, T., Clark, P., & Billinger, S. A. (2010). Comprehensive overview of nursing and interdisciplinary rehabilitation care of the stroke patient: A scientific statement from the American Heart Association. *Stroke, 41*(10), 2402–2448.

postacute care settings, including long-term care hospitals (LTCHs), IRFs, skilled nursing facilities (SNFs), and home health agencies (HHAs). The CARE item set includes core items of setting regardless of condition and supplemental items that are used for certain conditions and measure severity and degree of need for specific conditions. The Centers for Medicare and Medicaid Services (CMS) has developed different versions of the CARE item set, which are being used in various initiatives including quality metrics for postacute care (CMS, 2014a; Gage, 2009).

There are several care options and levels of care that exist in the postacute care stroke continuum other than inpatient rehabilitation. Licensure and Conditions of Participation (CoP) may vary depending on the site. In addition, regulations and reimbursement vary depending on the setting and services provided. Studies show that up to 35% of Medicare patients are discharged annually to a postacute care stroke setting. Over a third of all beneficiaries discharged from acute hospitals will use other that services provided in an inpatient rehabilitation setting (Gage, 2009). Specifically, 41% are discharged to an SNF, 37.4% are discharged to their home with home health services, and 9% are discharged to outpatient therapy services. The remaining 10% to 12% leave the hospital for continued services at a specialized hospital such as an acute-level IRF (10.3%) or LTCH (2%) (Gage, 2009). The following briefly discusses these other levels of services and care. It is imperative that the stroke patient receives care in the appropriate setting and in the right amount, intensity, and duration of rehabilitation services (Camicia et al., 2014).

Skilled Nursing Facilities

SNFs are also known as *nursing homes*. These facilities may or may not offer rehabilitation services. However, if physical or occupational therapy services are offered to patients, it is provided at a much lower intensity, usually about an hour per day. For those SNFs that offer some rehabilitation services, they are referred to as *subacute level of care facilities*. Although CMS does not formally recognize *subacute* as a distinct level of care for payment purposes, it is a term used in the industry.

Long-Term Acute Care

LTCHs are licensed as hospitals but admit only patients who have an average length of stay of 25 days or more. Rehabilitation services may be offered in LTCHs; however, patients are generally more medically complex with multiple acute or chronic conditions. Therapy interventions include, but are not limited to, assessment and interventions for improvement in mobility, ADL, communication, and cognition. Furthermore, LTCHs are reimbursed under their own prospective payment system in which the requirements are based on the need for 24-hour care, functional recovery, and need for complex medical care.

Outpatient Rehabilitation

Outpatient rehabilitation may be part of a hospital, freestanding rehabilitation center, satellite clinic of a health care institution, or an independent and privately owned clinic. Requirements for admission include need for skilled intervention to address functional limitations that interfere with abilities to participate in ADL, IADL, mobility, communication, and cognition. The goal is to improve functional status and includes integration into the home and community activities (CMS, 2014b).

Home Health Care

Home health care is provided to patients in a home setting. Home health services include medical or psychological assessment; wound care; medication management; pain management; disease education and management; skilled nursing; physical therapy, occupational therapy, and speech-language therapy; medical social services; as well as home health aide services. Patients must require skilled care to improve a medical condition, to maintain the current condition, or to prevent or slow further deterioration. For a patient to qualify for home health services, a Medicare beneficiary must be confined to the home, be under the care of a physician, be receiving services under a plan of care which is established and periodically reviewed by a physician, and be in need of skilled care on an intermittent basis (CMS, 2014c).

Transition in Care: From an Inpatient Facility to Home

Lutz (2004) posits that discharge plans should consider caregiving resources and patient needs early on in the rehabilitation process, and recommendations from a CPG of stroke care and coordination also confirm this (Miller et al., 2010). Discharge planning should begin during the prescreening process or upon referral to rehabilitation. The goal of rehabilitation is to ideally discharge the patient home and to reintegrate the patient into the community of choice. Assessment of discharge needs and recommendations should be made in conjunction with the patient and all interprofessional team members; the social worker and case manager often assume a leadership role in coordinating the assessment and recommendation process and implementation of the plan. If the plan is to return the patient to the home environment, patient medical needs, necessary adaptive equipment or structural alternations, and available financial resources must be considered.

The family caregivers and social support systems must also be evaluated to ensure an environment conducive to optimal recovery. Interventions may include the following: discuss discharge goals with the patient and family; identify and eliminate barriers to discharge; complete home evaluation; explain all discharge instructions; reconcile all medications and arrange for medication prescriptions; obtain durable medical equipment; identify community support resources; schedule follow-up appointments and services; make referrals for additional services, if needed; assist patient and family with financial and community resources; and refer to other services or individuals, as needed, including vocational rehabilitation or driver evaluation.

Safety is a paramount concern for all patients, but it is of particular concern for the stroke patient with deficits in mobility and balance. Managing a safe environment whether in an institution or at home is important in order to prevent secondary complications. Safety interventions may include making clear paths to the bathroom as well as other rooms during acute hospitalization and rehabilitation and in home environments; modifying the physical environments with the use of assistive equipment such as raised toilet seat, tub chair/bench, handheld shower, plastic strips at the bottom of the tub and/or shower, safety bars, and other safety items; using nonskid shoes and avoiding slippery or slick surfaces; removing loose carpets or runners or fastening them down with nonskid tape; installing handrails in key areas (e.g., stairs); using adaptive equipment as prescribed; and using mobility devices as prescribed.

Clinical Pearl: *Identification of environmental barriers is important for a safe environment in order to prevent secondary complications.*

ACCREDITATION AND CERTIFICATION

There are accreditation and certification considerations that are specific to rehabilitation facilities and programs. The Commission on Accreditation of Rehabilitation Facilities (CARF) and The Joint Commission (TJC) programs will be discussed.

The CARF was established in 1966 as an independent, nonprofit organization that promotes quality and value of rehabilitation services through a consultative accreditation process. CARF's mission is to promote the quality, value, and optimal outcomes of services through a consultative accreditation process that centers on enhancing the lives of the patient, family, and other stakeholders (CARF, 2013). CARF accredits rehabilitation programs throughout the United States and internationally through established customer-focused standards to assist organizations to measure and improve the quality of rehabilitation programs and services. In 2003, CARF acquired the Continuing Care Accreditation Commission (CCAC), which accredits aging services continuums, including continuing care retirement communities and other organizations (CARF, 2014). In 2007, CARF began accrediting suppliers of certain Durable Medical Equipment, Prosthetics, Orthotics, and Supplies (DMEPOS).

CARF annually accredits thousands of programs across the continuum of care, serving children through seniors. Most common to stroke rehabilitation are the medical rehabilitation programs. Medical rehabilitation programs are provided in a variety of settings and specialty areas including inpatient rehabilitation, outpatient rehabilitation, home and community services, residential, vocational, brain injury, spinal cord system of care, stroke specialty, amputation specialty, interdisciplinary pain rehabilitation, occupational rehabilitation programs, case management, pediatric specialty programs, independent evaluation services, and cancer rehabilitation (CARF, 2014).

TJC was founded in 1951 and accredits more than 17,000 health care organizations and programs throughout the United States. Its mission is to "continuously improve the safety and quality of care to the public through the provision of healthcare accreditation and related services that support performance improvement in healthcare organizations" (TJC, 2014). Beginning in 2002, disease-specific care (DSC) certification was offered and includes stroke. Both accreditation and certification require an on-site review by TJC. Certification is designed to evaluate hospitals, disease management service companies, and other health care settings that provide disease management and chronic care services. Standards are a cornerstone of the components of DSC certification; others include CPGs and performance measures. Programs are expected to select and implement CPGs that best meet the patient populations served. For rehabilitation facilities and units, specialty certification is available for a variety of programs, including that of stroke rehabilitation. For programs seeking stroke rehabilitation certification, the preparation and attainment of certification is an organized team effort in which the interprofessional rehabilitation team has a vital role.

■ REGULATIONS AND REIMBURSEMENT

Section 4421 of the Balanced Budget Act of 1997 (Public Law 105-33) modified payment for rehabilitation hospitals by creating section 1886(j) of the Social Security Act, which authorized the per-discharge prospective payment system for inpatient rehabilitation hospitals and units for all Medicare Part A as of January 1, 2002. The Inpatient Rehabilitation Facility Prospective Payment System (IRF PPS) is the mechanism in which Medicare reimburses rehabilitation facilities. In order to be recognized as a rehabilitation hospital or unit, established criteria must be met (U.S. Department of Health and Human Services [DHHS], 2013). Rehabilitation hospitals use information from the Inpatient Rehabilitation Facility Patient Assessment Instrument (IRF-PAI) to classify patients into distinct groups based on clinical characteristics and expected resource needs. (See CMS website for the complete IRF-PAI instrument [CMS, 2014a]). Individual cases (patients) are grouped into Rehabilitation Impairment Categories (RICs) according to the primary condition for admission into the rehabilitation facility. These cases are then further grouped into Case-Mix Groups (CMGs) that group cases that are similar according to functional motor and, in some instances, cognitive and age scores (DHHS, 2013). In order to be recognized as a rehabilitation provider, the IRF must have the following components: a provider agreement; a medical director ($\geq$20 hours per week for units and full time for freestanding facilities); all patients admitted must meet the rehabilitation coverage (admission) criteria; and inpatient rehabilitation beds must be physically separate, not comingled, with other hospital beds. In order for a patient to be admitted to acute rehabilitation, the patient must require multiple therapy disciplines, an intensive level of rehabilitation services, the ability to participate in the intensive therapy program, physician supervision, and an interdisciplinary team approach to care (CMS, 2010).

To be considered reasonable and necessary by the CMS, the required documentation for rehabilitation admissions must include a preadmission screening, postadmission physician evaluation, an individualized overall plan of care, physician orders, and the IRF-PAI (see the following discussion) included in the medical record (CMS, 2010). In addition, weekly interprofessional team conferences must be held and reflect team communications. This communication should include (CMS, 2010) the following: the patient's progress toward goals or problems impeding progress and barriers to discharge; a functional status review for each problem area relevant to the patient; rehabilitation goals including any modifications in the treatment plan or goals; appropriate carryover training for the patient and/or caregiver; any discrepancies in the plan of care between disciplines explained; the current discharge plan including any modifications; and recommendations for the next level of care including follow-up information.

The IRF-PAI is the data collection instrument for the IRF PPS. The IRF-PAI is required by CMS to be completed for all Medicare Part A patients admitted to IRFs. The basis of the IRF-PAI includes the FIM instrument as a core component for rating patients (e.g., 12 motor items, 5 cognitive items; tub and shower transfer is excluded in determining the CMG). The IRF-PAI is completed upon admission and discharge; however, it is the admission rating that determines the CMG to which the patient is assigned. Currently, there are 87 CMGs with four tiers and another 5 CMGs that account for very short stays and patients who die in the IRF. The tiers are represented by comorbid conditions whereby an A = no comorbidities; B = tier 1 (highest); C = tier 2 (medium); and D = tier 3 (lowest). Each year, CMS updates the CMG relative weights and average lengths of stays (ALOS) with the most recent available data (CMS, 2014a).

Another component of the IRF PPS is the Quality Reporting Program (QRP). The IRF QRP was mandated by section 3004 of the Affordable Care Act (2010). A final rule announcing the IRF QRP was published in the *Federal Register* on August 5, 2011 (Vol. 76, No. 151). The QRP has various quality indicators, which are reported to CMS. Any IRFs that fail to successfully participate in the IRF QRP will receive reduced payments to the market basket update (DHHS, 2013). Reporting for the IRF QRP began on October 1, 2012. Initially, IRFs were required to submit data for two quality measures: IRF Measure #1: Percent of Residents or Patients with Pressure Ulcers That Are New or Worsened (Short Stay) (National Quality Forum [NQF] #0678); and IRF Measure #2: National Healthcare Safety Network (NHSN) Catheter-Associated Urinary Tract Infection (CAUTI) Outcome Measure (NQF #0138).

In the fiscal year (FY) 2014 IRF PPS final rule, CMS finalized the addition of three new measures and one revised quality measures to the IRF QRP. CMS made several key policy decisions in the FY 2014 IRF PPS final rule that will impact the way that IRFs report their quality measure data. IRFs that do not comply with the reporting requirements of the IRF QRP will see their annual payment update (for the applicable payment year) reduced by two percentage points beginning with FY 2014. The following measures are finalized in the FY 2014 IRF PPS final rule (DHHS, 2013): IRF QRP proposed Measure #1: Influenza Vaccination Coverage among Healthcare Personnel (NQF #0431); IRF QRP proposed Measure #2: Percent of Residents or Patients Who Were Assessed and Appropriately Given the Seasonal Influenza Vaccination (NQF #0680); and IRF QRP proposed Measure #3: All-Cause Unplanned Readmission Measure for 30 Days post IRF Discharge.

Accountable Care Organizations

The key to health care reform is in the transformation to an efficient, affordable health care delivery system that is based on patient-centered, coordinated, team-based care that is supported by health information technology. Accountable care organizations (ACOs) offer a payment reform approach designed to address the increasing health care costs, inefficiencies, and poor outcomes within the current health care delivery system. The goal of an ACO is to create an integrated network of providers in order to improve individual and population level health outcomes and control costs. Care delivered across the continuum of care will need to be integrated and coordinated, and providers will need to jointly be accountable for patients' outcomes (Lowell & Bertko, 2010; McClellan, McKethan, Lewis, Roski, & Fisher, 2010). Changes related to the ACO will surely impact the delivery of rehabilitation services.

Value-Based Purchasing

The CMS released its Hospital Value-Based Purchasing (VBP) final rule, which was required under the Patient Protection and Affordable Care Act (DHHS, 2011). VBP is a key element of the act and is described as a system of Medicare reimbursement based on quality achievements that links payment to performance. Higher quality achievements will receive higher payment. There are four main components to Medicare VBP. These include reporting hospital quality data for annual payment update (RHQDAPU), which is based on specific quality indicators; VBP with a penalty and reward system based on metrics from the RHQDAPU; a payment penalty occurs for certain negative conditions that are hospital acquired; and a payment penalty for high readmission rate as compared to peers (DHHS, 2011). The transition of the VBP initiative is for CMS to develop a closer link between Medicare payments and improvement in health care quality. The aim is to transform Medicare from a passive payer of claims based on volume of care to an active purchaser of care that is based on quality of services.

Bundling

Bundling payment, defined as bundling acute and postacute payment into one payment, is a proposed reimbursement structure to facilitate improved transitions after an acute stroke event and to improve quality of the stroke continuum of care. Bundled payment also holds acute care hospitals accountable for hospital readmissions as well as bringing greater efficiencies and cost savings to an entire episode of care. Bundling is complex, involving multiple elements, including the following: the scope of services to be bundled, duration of the episode, selection of patient assessment method, selection of bundler or accountable entity, selection of quality and outcome metrics, and selection of risk or case-mix adjusters. Bundling for services across providers offers the opportunity for better coordination and ensures continuity of care across settings. Improvement in coordination of care may reduce unnecessary duplication of services and potentially decrease medical errors and cost. Bundling payment, which seems conceptually simple, is complex and will require testing and demonstrations that will allow health systems to experiment with various models (MedPAC, 2008). This model will have a profound impact on stroke care.

Future Trends in Reimbursement for Rehabilitation Services

Health care policies, regulations, and laws influence the nature of rehabilitation services, especially in an inpatient setting. The payer and reimbursement environment according to health care settings drives the availability of tools and methods in which rehabilitation occurs. Continual changes to the health care delivery system will shape the future payer–reimbursement context. The Patient Protection and Affordable Care Act of 2010 will bring the most significant changes to American health care since the prospective payment reform in 1983. Health reform law introduces important changes for health care providers that will continue to unfold over the next decade. Regulation and coverage changes have continued to change between 2010 and 2013 and will continue to change. Changes in 2014 are expected to further change cost and reimbursement in coming years. The health care landscape will continue to evolve as innovation with new models and work to achieve integration through ACOs, VBP, and/or bundling. Bundled payments, performance-based reimbursement, transparency, and patient-driven outcomes are on the health care horizon.

S U M M A R Y

Rehabilitation standards and scopes of practice, along with pertinent CPGs, can serve as a framework for the provision of interprofessional rehabilitation care. A well-organized, evidence-based, interprofessional rehabilitation approach that includes the patient and family can further serve as a guide to delivering individualized rehabilitation care for the patient with a stroke. These components in combination can serve to provide a structure for provision of evidence-based care as well as a foundation for practice in the field of rehabilitation care of the patient with stroke.

Case Study: Rehabilitation Care of the Patient with Stroke

Mr. Ed is a 65-year-old male admitted to the rehabilitation unit at your facility. He had a left-sided ischemic stroke to the temporal lobe with right-sided hemiparesis. He is alert and oriented. His wife tells you that he had "spells" of weakness prior to his stroke, never lasting more than a few hours. He has a history of smoking, does not exercise, and is an insulin-dependent diabetic. He is slightly overweight. Although Mr. Ed is continent of his bowels, he states he has a history of constipation. He appears to have a neurogenic bladder as evidenced by his urinary incontinence. He exhibits occasional mild coughing when eating. Mr. Ed exhibits mild aphasia.

Mrs. Ed tells you that she wants to be supportive, but she is overwhelmed. She wants her husband to return home but is not quite sure how to care for him. She wonders how her husband can prevent having another stroke.

Questions

1. Name at least four risk factors associated with a stroke.
2. Which risk factors did/does Mr. Ed have?
3. Name at least three potential problems for the team to address with Mr. Ed.
4. Establish a bladder management program for Mr. Ed based on what you have learned about a neurogenic bladder.
5. Name at least three signs and symptoms of dysphagia. Would you suspect dysphagia in Mr. Ed's case? Why or why not?
6. What interventions would you implement for dysphagia?
7. What type of aphasia would you suspect Mr. Ed to have?
8. List two interventions for this type of aphasia.

After 1 week of rehabilitation, Mr. Ed complains of right shoulder pain.

9. What might you suspect? Why?

Mr. Ed progresses over the next 2 weeks and is now ready for discharge to home. The therapists have recommended continued therapy on an outpatient level.

10. What education would you have provided to Mr. Ed and his wife during this stay? What referrals would you suggest for a smooth transition to the community? ■

REFERENCES

Abo, M., Kakuda, W., Watanabe, M., Morooka, A., Kawakami, K., & Senoo, A. (2012). Effectiveness of low-frequency rTMS and intensive speech therapy in poststroke patients with aphasia: A pilot study based on evaluation by fMRI in relation to type of aphasia. *European Neurology, 68,* 199–208.
Agency for Healthcare Research and Quality. (2010). *2010 national healthcare quality and disparities reports.* Retrieved from http://www.ahrq.gov/research/findings/nhqrdr/nhqrdr10/qrdr10.html
American Academy of Ophthalmology Vision Rehabilitation Committee. (2012). *Preferred practice pattern® guidelines. Vision rehabilitation for adults.* San Francisco, CA: American Academy of Ophthalmology. Retrieved from http://www.aao.org/ppp
American Heart Association. (2014). *Heart disease and stroke statistics: 2014 update: A report from the American Heart Association.* Retrieved from http://circ.ahajournals.org/content/129/3/e28

American Speech-Language-Hearing Association. (1993). *Definitions of communication disorders and variations*. Retrieved from http://www.asha.org/policy/RP1993-00208/

Anderson, C. S., Linto, J., & Stewart-Wynne, E. G. (1995). A population-based assessment of the impact and burden of caregiving for long-term stroke survivors. *Stroke, 26*, 843–849.

Annon, J. (1976). *The behavioral treatment of sexual problems*. New York, NY: Harper & Row-Medical.

Arbaje, A., Wolff, J., Yu, Q., Powe, N., Anderson, G., & Boult, C. (2008). Postdischarge environmental and socioeconomic factors and the likelihood of early hospital readmission among community-dwelling Medicare beneficiaries. *The Gerontologist, 48*, 495–504.

Association of Rehabilitation Nurses. (2008). *Standards and scope of rehabilitation nursing practice*. Glenview, IL: Author.

Association of Rehabilitation Nurses. (2011). *The specialty practice of rehabilitation nursing: A core curriculum* (6th ed.). Glenview, IL: Author.

Baker, L. L., & Parker, K. (1986). Neuromuscular electrical stimulation of the muscles surrounding the shoulder. *Annual Biomedical Engineering, 66*(12), 1930–1937.

Balanced Budget Act of 1997, Pub. L. No. 105-33, 111 Stat. 251 (1997).

Beeson, P. M., & Robey, R. R. (2006). Evaluating single-subject treatment research: Lessons learned from the aphasia literature. *Neuropsychological Review, 16*, 161–169.

Bhogal, S. K., Teasell, R., & Speechley, M. (2003). Intensity of aphasia therapy, impact on recovery. *Stroke, 34*, 987–993.

Bobath, B. (1970). *Adult hemiplegia: Evaluation and treatment*. London, United Kingdom: William Heinemann Medical Books.

Bohannon, R. W., Thorne, M., & Mieres, A. (1983). Shoulder positioning device for patients with hemiplegia. *Physical Therapy, 63*, 49–50.

Boian, R., Sharma, A., Han, C., Merians, A., Burdea, G., Adamovich, S., . . . Poizner, H. (2002). Virtual reality-based post-stroke hand rehabilitation. *Studies in Health Technology and Informatics, 85*, 64–70.

Bottemiller, K. L., Bieber, P. L., Basford, J. R., & Harris, M. (2006). FIM score, FIM efficiency, and discharge disposition following inpatient stroke rehabilitation. *Rehabilitation Nursing, 31*(1), 22–25.

Burton, L., & Brigham, H. (2013). *Proprioceptive neuromuscular facilitation: The foundation of functional training*. Retrieved from http://www.functionalmovement.com/articles/Screening/2013-07-04_proprioceptive_neuromuscular_facilitation_the_foundation_of_functional_training

Cailliet, R. (1980). *The shoulder in hemiplegia* (3rd ed.). Philadelphia, PA: FA Davis.

Camicia, M., Black, T., Farrell, J., Waites, K., Wirt, S., & Lutz, B. (2014). The essential role of the rehabilitation nurse in facilitating care transitions: A white paper by the Association of Rehabilitation Nurses. *Rehabilitation Nursing, 39*, 3–15.

Canbaz, D. H., Celebisoy, M., Ozdemirkiran, T., & Tokucoglu, F. (2010). Dysarthria in acute ischemic stroke: Localization and prognosis. *Journal of Neurological Sciences (Turkish), 27*(1), 20–27.

Carr, J. H., & Shepherd, R. B. (1998). *Neurological rehabilitation: Optimizing motor performance*. Oxford, United Kingdom: Butterworth-Heinemann.

Centers for Medicare and Medicaid Services. (2010). *Medicare benefit policy manual*. Baltimore, MD: Author.

Centers for Medicare and Medicaid Services. (2014a). *IRF-PAI Assessment Instrument effective October 2014*. Retrieved from http://cms.gov/Medicare/Medicare-Fee-for-Service-Payment/InpatientRehabFacPPS/Downloads/IRF-PAI-FINAL-for-Use-Oct2014-updated-v4.pdf

Centers for Medicare and Medicaid Services. (2014b). *Medicare benefit policy manual. Coverage of home health services. Chapter 7, Sections 10-40*. Retrieved from https://www.cms.gov/Regulations-andGuidance/Guidance/Manuals/downloads/bp102c07.pdf

Centers for Medicare and Medicaid Services. (2014c). *Medicare benefit policy manual. Covered medical and other health services. Chapter 15, Section 220*. Retrieved from https://www.cms.gov/Regulations-and-Guidance/Guidance/Manuals/downloads/bp102c15.pdf

Cernak, K., Stevens, V., Price, R., & Shumway-Cook, A. (2008). Locomotor training using body-weight support on a treadmill in conjunction with ongoing physical therapy in a child with severe cerebellar ataxia. *Physical Therapy, 88*(1), 88–97.

Chae, J., Bethoux, F., Bohinc, T., Dobos, L., Davis, T., & Friedl, A. (1998). Neuromuscular stimulation for upper extremity motor and functional recovery in acute hemiplegia. *Stroke, 29*, 975–979.

Cherney, L. R., Patterson, J. P., Raymer, A., Frymark, T., & Schooling, T. (2008). Evidence-based systematic review: Effects of intensity of treatment and constraint-induced language therapy for individuals with stroke-induced aphasia. *Journal of Speech, Language, and Hearing Research, 51*, 1282–1299.

Cicerone, K. D., Dahlberg, C., Kalmar, K., Langenbahn, D. M., Malec, J. F., Bergquist, T. F., . . . Morse, P. A. (2000). Evidence-based cognitive rehabilitation: Recommendations for clinical practice. *Archives of Physical Medicine and Rehabilitation, 81*(12), 1596–1615.

Cicerone, K., Levin, H., Malec, J., Stuss, D., & Whyte, J. (2006). Cognitive rehabilitation interventions for executive function: Moving from bench to bedside in patients with traumatic brain injury. *Journal of Cognitive Neuroscience, 18*, 1212–1222.

Cieza, A., Geyh, S., Chatterji, S., Kostanjsek, N., Ustun, B., & Stucki, G. (2005). ICF linking rules: An update based on lessons learned. *Journal of Rehabilitation Medicine, 37*, 212–218.

Ciuffreda, K. J., Kapoor, N., Daniella Rutner, D., Suchoff, I. B., Han, M. E., & Craig, S. (2007). Occurrence of oculomotor dysfunctions in acquired brain injury: A retrospective analysis. *Optometry, 78*, 155–161.

Claus, S. W., & Godfrey, K. J. (1985). A new distal support sling for the hemiplegic patient. *American Journal of Occupational Therapy, 39*, 536–537.

Commission on Accreditation of Rehabilitation Facilities. (2013). *Standards manual and interpretive guidelines for medical rehabilitation.* Tucson, AZ: Author.

Commission on Accreditation of Rehabilitation Facilities. (2014). *Medical rehabilitation.* Retrieved from http://www.carf.org/Programs/Medical/

Cornelissen, K., Laine, M., Tarkiainen, A., Jarvensivu, T., Martin, N., & Salmelin, R. (2003). Adult brain plasticity elicited by anomia treatment. *Journal of Cognitive Neuroscience, 15*, 444–461.

Cournan, M. (2012). Bladder management in female stroke survivors: Translating research into practice. *Rehabilitation Nursing, 37*(5), 220–230.

Cox, M. S., Roberts, P. I., Holm, S. E., Kurfuerst, S., Lynch, A., & Schuberth, L. (2006). Feeding, eating, and swallowing specialty certification: Benefiting clients and occupational therapists. *OT Practice, 11*(8), 20–23.

Craig, L. E., Wu, O., Bernhardt, J., & Langhorne, P. (2011). Predictors of poststroke mobility: Systematic review. *International Journal of Stroke, 6*(4), 321–327.

Cramer, S. C., Sur, M., Dobkin, B. H., O'Brien, C., Sanger, T. D., Trojanowski, J. Q., . . . Vinogradov, S. (2011). Harnessing neuroplasticity for clinical applications. *Brain, 134*(Pt. 6), 1591–1609.

Damasio, A. R. (1992). Aphasia. *The New England Journal of Medicine, 326*(8), 531–539.

Daniels, S. K., Brailey, R., Priestly, D. H., Herrington, L. R., Weisberg, L. A., & Foundas, A. L. (1998). Aspiration in patients with acute stroke. *Archives of Physical Medicine and Rehabilitation, 79*, 14–19.

DePalma, G., Xu, H., Covinsky, K. E., Craig, B. A., Stallard, E., Thomas, J., III, & Sands, L. P. (2013). Hospital readmission among older adults who return home with unmet need for ADL disability. *The Gerontologist, 53*, 454–461.

Edmans, J. A., Webster, J., & Lincoln, N. B. (2000). A comparison of two approaches in the treatment of perceptual problems after stroke. *Clinical Rehabilitation, 14*(3), 230–243.

Engelter, S. T., Gostynski, M., Papa, S., Frei, M., Born, C., Ajdacic-Gross, V., . . . Lyreer, P. A. (2006). Epidemiology of aphasia attributable to first ischemic stroke: Incidence, severity, fluency, etiology, and thrombolysis *Stroke, 37*, 1379–1384.

Ferro, J. M., Mariano, G., & Madurcira, S. (1999). Recovery from aphasia and neglect. *Cerebrovascular Disease, 9*(Suppl. 5), 6–22.

Gage, B. (2009). *Post-acute care: Moving beyond the silos.* Retrieved from http://www.rti.org/files/fellowseminar/fellowseminar_longtermcare_gage.pdf

Geiger, R. A., Allen, J. B., O'Keefe, J., & Hickes, R. R. (2001). Balance and mobility following stroke: Effects of physical therapy interventions with and without biofeedback/force plate training. *Physical Therapy, 81*(4), 995–1005.

Gender, A. (1998). Scope of rehabilitation and rehabilitation nursing. In P. A. Chin, D. Finocchiaro, & A. Rosebrough (Eds.), *Rehabilitation nursing practice* (pp. 2–5). New York, NY: McGraw-Hill.

Gottlieb, D. D., & Miesner, N. (2004). Innovative concepts in hemianopsia and complex visual loss low vision rehabilitation for our older population. *Topics in Geriatric Rehabilitation, 20*(3), 212–222.

Gourlay, D., Lun, K. C., Lee, Y. N., & Tay, J. (2000). Virtual reality for relearning daily living skills. *International Journal of Medical Informatics, 60*, 255–261.

Gresham, G. E., Duncan, P. W., Stason, W. B., Adams, H. P., Adelmen, A. M., Alexander, D. N., . . . Trombly, C. A. (1995). *Post-stroke rehabilitation: Clinical practice guidelines number 16* (AHCPR Publication No. 95-0662). Rockville, MD: U.S. Department of Health and Human Services, Public Health Service, Agency for Health Care Policy and Research.

Griffin, A., & Bernhardt, J. (2006). Strapping the hemiplegic shoulder prevents development of pain during rehabilitation: A randomized controlled trial. *Clinical Rehabilitation, 20*(4), 287–295.

Haeberle, E. J. (2003). *Sexual dysfunctions and their treatment.* Retrieved from http://www2.hu-berlin.de/sexology/ECE5/index.htm

Hesse, S., Bertelt, C., Jahnke, M. T., Schaffrin, A., Baake, P., Malezic, M., & Mauritz, K. H. (1995). Treadmill training with partial body weight support compared with physiotherapy in nonambulatory hemiparetic patients. *Stroke, 16*, 976–981.

Hinchey, J. A., Shephard, T., Furie, K., Smith, D., Wang, D., & Tonn, S. (2005). Stroke practice improvement network investigators. Formal dysphagia screening protocols prevent pneumonia. *Stroke, 36*, 1972–1976.

Holland, A., Greenhouse, J., Fromm, D., & Swindell, C. (1989). Predictors of language restitution following stroke: A multivariate analysis. *Journal of Speech and Hearing Research, 32,* 232–238.

Horowitz, A. (2004). The prevalence and consequences of vision impairment in later life. *Topics in Geriatric Rehabilitation, 20*(3), 185–195.

Hoyert, D. L., & Xu, J. (2012). Deaths: Preliminary data for 2011. *National Vital Statistics Reports, 61*(6), 3.

Interprofessional Education Collaborative Expert Panel. (2011). *Core competencies for interprofessional collaborative practice: Report of an Expert Panel.* Washington, DC: Interprofessional Education Collaborative.

Johansson, B. B. (2000). Brain plasticity and stroke rehabilitation. *Stroke, 31,* 223–230.

Kalra, L., & Langhorne, P. (2007). Facilitating recovery: Evidence for organized stroke care. *Journal of Rehabilitation Medicine, 39,* 97–102.

Kapoor, N., Ciuffreda, K. J., & Suchoff, I. B. (2001). Egocentric localization in patients with visual neglect. In I. B. Suchoff, K. J. Ciuffreda, & N. Kapoor (Eds.), *Visual and vestibular consequences of acquired brain injury* (pp. 131–144). Sta. Ana, CA: Optometric Extension Program Foundation Press.

Karnath, H.-O., Himmelbach, M., & Kuker, W. (2003). The cortical substrate of visual extinction. *Neuroreport, 14,* 437–442.

Kauhanen, M. L., Korpelainen, J. T., Hiltunen, P., Maatta, R., Mononen, H., Brusin, E., . . . Myllyla, V. V. (2000). Aphasia, depression, and non-verbal cognitive impairment in ischemic stroke. *Cerebrovascular Disease, 10,* 455–461.

Kearney, P., & Pryor, J. (2004). The International Classification of Functioning, Disability and Health (ICF) and nursing. *Journal of Advanced Nursing, 46*(2), 162–170.

Keith, R. A., Granger, C. V., Hamilton, B. B., & Sherwin, F. S. (1987). The functional independence measure: A new tool for rehabilitation. *Advances in Clinical Rehabilitation, 1,* 6–18.

Kelly, J., Rudd, A., Lewis, R., & Hunt, B. J. (2001). Venous thromboembolism after acute stroke. *Stroke, 32,* 262–267.

Kendall, D., Nadeau, S., Conway, T., Fuller, R., Riestra, A., & Roth, L. J. G. (2006). Treatability of different components of aphasia: Insights from a case study. *Journal of Rehabilitation Research and Development, 43,* 323–336.

Kerkhoff, G. (2000). Neurovisual rehabilitation: Recent developments and future directions. *Journal of Neurology, Neurosurgery, and Psychiatry, 68,* 691–706.

Keshner, E. A. (2004). Virtual reality and physical rehabilitation: A new toy or a new research and rehabilitation tool? *Journal of Neuroengineering Rehabilitation, 1,* 8.

Kunkel, A., Kopp, B., Muller, G., Villinger, K., Taub, E., & Flor, H. (1999). Constraint-induced movement therapy for motor recovery in chronic stroke patients. *Archives of Physical Medicine Rehabilitation, 80*(6), 624–628.

Laska, A. C., Hellblom, A., Murray, V., Kahan, T., & Von Arbin, M. (2001). Aphasia in acute stroke and relation to outcome. *Journal of Internal Medicine, 249,* 413–422.

Latham, K., Jette, D. U., Slavin, M., Richards, L. G., Procino, A., Smout, R. J., & Horn, S. D. (2005). Physical therapy during stroke rehabilitation for people with different walking abilities. *Archives of Physical Medicine and Rehabilitation, 86*(Suppl. 2), 234–239.

Laufer, Y., Dickstein, R., Chefez, Y., & Marcovitz, E. (2001). The effect of treadmill training on the ambulation of stroke survivors in the early stages of rehabilitation: A randomized study. *Journal of Rehabilitation Research and Development, 38,* 69–78.

Leifer, D., Bravata, D. M., Conners, J. J., III, Hinchey, J. A., Jauch, E. C., Johnston, S. C., . . . Zorowitz, R. (2011). Metrics for measuring quality of care in comprehensive stroke centers: Detailed follow-up to brain attack coalition comprehensive stroke center recommendations: A statement for healthcare professionals from the American Heart Association/American Stroke Association. *Stroke, 42,* 849–877.

Lennon, S., & Ashburn, A. (2000). The Bobath concept in stroke rehabilitation: A focus group study of the experienced physiotherapists' perspective. *Disability and Rehabilitation, 22*(15), 665–674.

Leys, D., Henon, H., Mackowiak-Cordoliani, M. A., & Pasquier, F. (2005). Poststroke dementia. *The Lancet. Neurology, 4,* 752–759.

Linden, T., Skoog, I., Fagerberg, B., Steen, B., & Blomstrand, C. (2004). Cognitive impairment and dementia 20 months after stroke. *Neuroepidemiology, 23,* 45–52.

Logemann, J. (1998). Anatomy and physiology of normal deglutition. In J. Logemann (Ed.), *Evaluation and treatment of swallowing disorders* (2nd ed.). Austin, TX: Pro-Ed.

Lowell, K. H., & Bertko, J. (2010). The accountable care organization (ACO) model: Building blocks for success. *Journal of Ambulatory Care, 33*(1), 81–88.

Lutz, B. (2004). Determinants of discharge destination for stroke patients. *Rehabilitation Nursing, 29*(5), 154–163.

Mackenzie, C. (2011). Dysarthria in stroke: A narrative review of its description and the outcome of intervention. *International Journal of Speech-Language Pathology, 13*(2), 125–136.

McClellan, M., McKethan, A. N., Lewis, J. L., Roski, J., & Fisher, E. S. (2010). A national strategy to put accountable care into practice. *Health Affairs, 29*(5), 982–990.

McIntyre, A., & Tempest, S. (2007). Two steps forward, one step back? A commentary on the disease-specific core sets of the International Classification of Functioning, Disability and Health (ICF). *Disability and Rehabilitation, 29*(18), 1475–1479.

Medicare Payment Advisory Commission. (2008). *A path to a bundled payment around a hospitalization.* Retrieved from http://post-acute.org/bundling/index_files/Page885.htm

Medicare Payment Advisory Commission. (2011). *Report to the Congress: Medicare and the health care delivery system.* Washington, DC: Author.

Miller, E. L., Murray, L., Richards, L., Zorowitz, R. D., Bakas, T., Clark, P., & Billinger, S. A. (2010). Comprehensive overview of nursing and interdisciplinary rehabilitation care of the stroke patient: A scientific statement from the American Heart Association. *Stroke, 41*(10), 2402–2448. Retrieved from http://stroke.ahajournals.org/content/41/10/2402.long

Moodie, N. B., Bresbin, J., & Grace Morgan, A. M. (1986). Subluxation of the glenohumeral joint in hemiplegia: Evaluation of supportive devices. *Physiotherapy Canada, 38,* 151–157.

Morin, L., & Bravo, G. (1997). Strapping the hemiplegic shoulder: A radiographic evaluation of its efficacy to reduce subluxation. *Physiotherapy Canada, 49,* 103–108.

National Aphasia Association. (2014). *Aphasia definitions.* Retrieved from http://www.aphasia.org/content/aphasia-definitions

NEURO-IFRAH Organization. (n.d.). *FAQ's.* Retrieved from http://www.neuro-ifrah.org/faq.aspx#What_is_Neuro-IFRAH

Ohl, L. E. (2007). *Essentials of female sexual dysfunction from a sex therapy perspective: The P-LI-SS-IT model for sexual counseling.* Retrieved from http://www.medscape.com/viewarticle/555706_12

Ottenbacher, K. J., Hsu, Y., Granger, C. V., & Fiedler, R. C. (1996). The reliability of the Functional Independence Measure: A quantitative review. *Archives of Physical Medicine and Rehabilitation, 77,* 1226–1232.

Palmer, J. B., Drennan, J. C., & Baba, M. (2000). Evaluation and treatment of swallowing impairments. *American Family Physician, 61,* 2453–2462.

Papageorgiou, E., Hardiess, G., Schaeffel, F., Wiethoelter, H., Karnath, H. O., Mallot, H., . . . Schiefer, U. (2007). Assessment of vision-related quality of life in patients with homonymous visual field deficits. *Graefe's Archive for Clinical and Experimental Ophthalmology, 245*(12), 1749–1758.

Pascual-Leone, A., Davey, N., Wasserman, E. M., Rothwell, J., & Puri, B. (Eds.). (2002). *Handbook of transcranial magnetic stimulation.* London, United Kingdom: Arnold Press.

Patient-Centered Outcomes Research Institute. (2014). *Vision & mission.* Retrieved from http://www.pcori.org/content/vision-mission

Patient Protection and Affordable Care Act of 2010, Pub. L. No. 111-148, 124 Stat. 119 (2010). Retrieved from http://www.gpo.gov/fdsys/pkg/PLAW-111publ148/content-detail.html

Pennycott, A., Wyss, D., Vallery, H., Klamroth-Marganska, V., & Riener, R. (2012). Towards more effective robotic gait training for stroke rehabilitation: A review. *Journal of Neuroengineering and Rehabilitation, 9,* 65.

Peters, S. B., & Lee, G. P. (2003). Functional impact of shoulder taping in the hemiplegic upper extremity. *Occupational Therapy in Healthcare, 17*(2), 35–46.

Pollack, A., Hazelton, C., Henderson, C. A., Angilley, J., Dhillon, B., Langhorne, P., . . . Shahani, U. (2012). Interventions for age-related visual problems in patients with stroke. *The Cochrane Database of Systematic Reviews, 3,* CD008390.

Rajaram, V., & Holtz, M. (1985). Shoulder forearm support for the subluxed shoulder. *Archives of Physical Medicine and Rehabilitation, 66,* 191–192.

Richter, M., Miltner, W. H., & Straube, T. (2008). Association between therapy outcome and right-hemispheric activation in chronic aphasia. *Brain, 131,* 1391–1401.

Riggs, R. V., Andrews, K., Roberts, P., & Gilewski, M. (2007). Visual deficit interventions in adult stroke and brain injury. *American Journal of Physical Medicine and Rehabilitation, 86*(10), 853–860.

Rizzo, A. A. (2002). Virtual reality and disability: Emergency and challenge. *Disability Rehabilitation, 24,* 567–569.

Roberts, P., Cox, M., Schubert, L., & Gentry, K. (2009). Dysphagia intervention across the lifespan. *OT Practice, 14*(8), 12–17.

Roberts, P., Vegher, J., Gilewski, M., Bender, A., & Riggs, R. (2005). Client-centered occupational therapy using constraint-induced therapy. *Journal of Stroke and Cerebrovascular Diseases, 14*(3), 115–121.

Salter, K., Mehta, S., Bhogal, S., Teasell, R., Foley, N., & Speechley, M. (2013). Post stroke depression. In *Evidence-Based Review of Stroke Rehabilitation.* Retrieved from http://www.ebrsr.com

Salter, K., Teasell, R., Bitensky, J., Foley, N., & Bhogal, S. K. (2014). Cognitive disorders and apraxia. In *Evidence-Based Review of Stroke Rehabilitation.* Retrieved from http://www.ebrsr.com

Sarno, M. T., & Levita, E. (1979). Recovery in treated aphasia in the first year post-stroke. *Stroke, 10,* 663–670. doi:10.1161/01.STR.10.6.663

Schweickert, W. D., Pohlman, M. C., Pohlman, A. S., Nigos, C., Pawlik, A. J., Esbrook, C. L., . . . Kress, J. P. (2009). Early physical and occupational therapy in mechanically ventilated, critically ill patients: A randomized controlled trial. *Lancet, 373,* 1874–1882. Retrieved from http://www.thelancet.com/journals/lancet/article/PIIS0140-6736(09)60658-9/fulltext

Serrano, S., Domingo, J., Rodriguez-Garcia, E., Castro, M. D., & Del Ser, T. (2007). Frequency of cognitive impairment without dementia in patients with stroke: A two-year follow-up study. *Stroke, 38,* 105–110.

Sheffer, L. R., & Chae, J. (2007). Neuromuscular electrical stimulation in neuro-rehabilitation. *Muscle & Nerve, 35*(5), 562–590. doi:10.1002/mus.20758

Shumway-Cook, A., & Woollacott, M. H. (2011). *Motor control: Translating research into clinical practice* (4th ed.). Baltimore, MD: Lippincott Williams & Wilkins.

Smith, C. H., Logemann, J. A., Colangelo, L. A., Rademaker, A. W., & Pauloski, B. R. (1999). Incidence and patient characteristics associated with silent aspiration in the acute care setting. *Dysphagia, 14,* 1–7.

Sohlberg, M. M., Kennedy, M., Avery, J., Coelho, C., Turkstra, L., Ylvisaker, M., & Yorkston, K. (2007). Evidence-based practice for the use of external aids as a memory compensation technique. *Journal of Medical Speech-Language Pathology, 15,* xv–li.

Sohlberg, M. M., & Mateer, C. (2001). *Cognitive rehabilitation: An integrative neuropsychological approach.* New York, NY: Guilford Press.

Spreen, O., & Risser, A. H. (2003). *Assessment of aphasia.* New York, NY: Oxford University Press.

Stokes-Turner, L., & Jackson, D. (2002). Shoulder pain after stroke: A review of the evidence based to inform the development of an integrated care pathway. *Clinical Rehabilitation, 16,* 248–260.

Stone, S. P., Halligan, P. W., & Greenwood, R. J. (1993). The incidence of neglect phenomena and related disorders in patients with an acute right or left hemisphere stroke. *Age Ageing, 22*(1), 46–52.

Taub, E., Miller, N. E., Novack, T., Cook, E., Feming, W., Nepomuceno, C., & Connell, J. S. (1993). Technique to improve chronic motor deficit after stroke. *Archives of Physical Medicine and Rehabilitation, 74,* 347–354.

Taub, E., & Wolf, S. L. (1997). Constraint induced movement therapy techniques to facilitate upper extremity use in stroke patients. *Topics in Stroke Rehabilitation, 3,* 38–61.

Teasell, R., Foley, N., Salter, K., Hussein, N., Viana, R., & Campbell, N. (2013). Medical complications post-stroke. In *Evidence-Based Review of Stroke Rehabilitation.* Retrieved from http://www.ebrsr.com

Tempest, S., & McIntyre, A. (2006). Using the ICF to clarify team roles and demonstrate clinical reasoning in stroke rehabilitation. *Disability and Rehabilitation, 28,* 663–667.

Terre, R., & Mearin, F. (2006). Oropharyngeal dysphagia after the acute phase of stroke: Predictors of aspiration. *Neurogastroenterology Motility, 18,* 200–205.

The Joint Commission. (2014). *Advanced certification comprehensive stroke centers.* Retrieved from http//www.jointcommission.org/certification/advanced_certification_comprehensive_stroke_centers.aspx

Thompson, C. K. (2000). Neuroplasticity: Evidence from aphasia. *Journal of Communication Disorders, 33*(4), 357–366.

Tsouli, S., Kyritsis, A. P., Tsagalis, G., Virvidaki, E., & Vemmos, K. N. (2009). Significance of aphasia after first-ever acute stroke: Impact on early and late outcomes. *Neuroepidemiology, 33,* 96–102.

Turkstra, I., Coelho, C., & Ylvisaker, M. (2005). The use of standardized test for individuals with cognitive-communication disorders. *Seminars Speech Language, 26,* 215–222.

Urban, P. P., Wicht, S., Vukurevic, G., Fitzek, C., Fitzek, S., Stoeter, P., . . . Hopf, H. C. (2000). Dysarthria in acute ischemic stroke. *Neurology, 56*(8), 1021–1027.

U.S. Department of Health and Human Services. (2011). Medicare program: Hospital inpatient value-based purchasing program; final rule. *Federal Register, 76*(88), 26490–26547.

U.S. Department of Health and Human Services. (2013). 42 CFR Part 412 Medicare Program; Inpatient Rehabilitation Facility Prospective Payment System for Federal Fiscal Year 2014; Rules. *Federal Register, 78*(151), 47860–47934. Retrieved from http://www.gpo.gov/fdsys/pkg/FR-2013-08-06/pdf/2013-18770.pdf

Voss, D. E., Ionta, M. K., & Myers, B. J. (Eds.). (1985). *Proprioceptive neuromuscular facilitation: Patterns and techniques.* Philadelphia, PA: Harper & Row.

Wade, D. T., Hewer R. L., & David, R. M. (1986). Aphasia after stroke: Natural history and associated deficits. *Journal of Neurology Neurosurgery Psychiatry, 49,* 11–16.

Wallace, M. A. (2008). Assessment of sexual health in older adults. *American Journal of Nursing, 8*(7), 52–60.

Walsh, K. (2001). Management of shoulder pain in patients with stroke. *Postgraduate Medical Journal, 77*(912), 645–649.

Wambaugh, J., Duffy, J., McNeil, M., Robin, D., & Rogers, M. (2006). Treatment guidelines for acquired apraxia of speech: Treatment descriptions and recommendations. *Journal of Medical Speech-Language Pathology, 14*(2,), xxxv–lxvii.

Wasserman, E. M., Epstein, C. M., Ziemann, U., Walsh, V., Paus, T., & Lisanby, S. H. (2008). *Oxford handbook of transcranial stimulation*. New York, NY: Oxford University Press.

Weiss, P. L., Bialik, P., & Kizony, R. (2003). Virtual reality provides leisure time opportunities for young adults with physical and intellectual disabilities. *Cyberpsychology & Behavior, 6*, 335–342.

Weiss, P. L., Naveh, Y., & Katz, N. (2003). Design and testing of virtual environment to train stroke patients with unilateral spatial neglect to cross a street safely. *Occupational Therapy International, 10*, 39–55.

Wolf, S. L., LeCraw, D. E., Barton, L. A., & Jann, B. B. (1989). Forced use of hemiplegic upper extremities to reverse the effect of learned nonuse among chronic stroke and head-injured patients. *Experimental Neurology, 104*, 125–132.

Wolter, M., & Preda, S. (2006). Visual deficits following stroke: Maximizing participation in rehabilitation. *Topics in Stroke Rehabilitation, 13*(3), 12–21.

World Health Organization. (2001). *International Classification of Functioning, Disability and Health*. Geneva, Switzerland: Author.

Yorkston, K. M., Hakel, M., Beukelman, D. R., & Fager, S. (2007). Evidence for effectiveness of treatment of loudness, rate, or prosody in dysarthria: A systematic review. *Journal of Medical Speech-Language Pathology, 15*(2), xi–xxxvi.

CHAPTER 11

Poststroke Reintegration into the Community

Lindy Suarez

There are currently more than 7 million American stroke survivors and nearly 33 million worldwide (Feigin et al., 2014). Although some people who survive a stroke are able to return home and resume their normal routines in a relatively short period of time, the vast majority of survivors, up to 75%, require some level of postacute rehabilitation in order to reintegrate back into their community (Mosunmola, Adler, & Barrett, 2014). It is imperative that a comprehensive reintegration plan be established as early in the acute phase as possible to facilitate this transition.

Compassionate, respectful, patient-centered care is central to any successful patient discharge provided by the health care team. In a poll conducted by The Schwartz Center, both physicians and patients agreed that providing compassionate care plays a key role in how well the patient recovers from their illness (The Schwartz Center, 2010). Some of the key elements that patients identified when describing compassionate care were showing respect for the patient and his or her family members, listening to the concerns of the patient/family, spending adequate time with the patient/family, and understanding the patient as a person. A psychosocial assessment is a key tool to aid the interprofessional team to provide a comprehensive understanding of the patient and family/caregiver, psychosocial functioning, environment, resources, goals, and expectation for return to the community (Duncan et al., 2005).

This chapter will discuss the processes integral to a safe transition from the acute care setting back into the community for patients who have suffered a stroke. Topics addressed include postacute care and treatment options, the importance of the interprofessional approach to patient care, effective patient and family preparation for discharge, transitioning from the hospital or subacute facility to home, challenges that the patient will face after leaving the hospital, challenges faced by caregivers and strategies to avoid burnout, and community resources.

◾ AN INTERPROFESSIONAL APPROACH TO PATIENT CARE

Numerous studies have indicated that the most successful model for reintegration into the community for stroke patients is one that incorporates a multidisciplinary/interprofessional team approach (Stroke Unit Trialists' Collaboration, 2013). The review concluded that patients who received care from an organized stroke unit team had a higher likelihood of surviving the stroke, regaining their prestroke independence, and returning home than those who did not receive care from a team approach. Beginning on day 1 of admission, the role of the interprofessional team is to evaluate the stroke patient's functional status and determine the best fit for postacute rehabilitation treatment (Clarke, 2013). Key members of the team include physicians such as neurologists; internist, physiatrist, along with any other consulting physicians; advanced practice nurses (APNs) (nurse practitioners [NPs], clinical nurse specialists [CNSs]) and physician assistants (PAs); nurse case manager; social worker; therapists (occupational, physical, and speech therapy); bedside nurses; pharmacist; and other ancillary disciplines represented on the interprofessional stroke team. Each team member must assess the patient and identify both strengths and barriers in the patient's current condition and communicate the findings to the other team members. Ongoing communication regarding the patient's status is most effectively coordinated through the use of team meetings, daily rounds, or chart documentation (electronic medical record [EMR] or paper chart).

Clinical Pearl: The most successful model for reintegration into the community incorporates an interprofessional team approach.

Team Member Roles

Each member of the interprofessional team has both individual and collaborative roles within the team to contribute to the timely and efficient transition of the patient along the postacute care continuum. The following briefly describes these roles.

Physician. The physician's role in evaluating the appropriate postacute care plan is to determine what poststroke conditions will impact the patient's ability to safely return to the community. It is necessary to identify what cognitive and behavioral deficits the patient has because these deficits will impact on decisions regarding selection of rehabilitation treatments that will be most appropriate for the patient.

NPs, CNSs, and PAs. The role of the NP, CNS, and PA is to provide ongoing comprehensive care and coordination for the patient while in the acute setting and ensure that physicians and other team members are kept abreast of the patient's status. Additionally, they provide detailed assessments of the patient's strengths and barriers to successful reintegration to the community. In many acute care settings, it is the NPs, CNSs, or PAs who provide stroke education to patients and families.

Pharmacist. The pharmacist plays an important role on the team. Many stroke patients are already on medications prior to admission or will require medication management going forward. Patients may be prescribed a variety of medications including anticoagulation therapy, cholesterol-lowering medication, blood pressure medications, anticonvulsants, and diabetes management medications. Pharmacists may also participate in patient/family caregiver education on dosing instructions, side effects, and drug interactions of the medications the patient will be taking. Particular attention to discussions regarding medication compliance is important component of patient education and critical to avoidance of secondary stroke.

Nurse case manager. The role of the nurse case manager is to evaluate the appropriate options available to the patient based on insurance/resources in order to move the patient to the next appropriate level of care. There are a number of options available including a skilled nursing facility (SNF), acute rehabilitation facility (ARF), long-term acute care hospital (LTAC), or home with appropriate durable medical equipment and ongoing outpatient therapy. Appropriateness or best fit of any of these facilities will be determined by the team. The nurse case manager has to consider cost-effectiveness for the hospital while also considering the family's wishes and the best interest of the patient, keeping safety in mind at all times. The nurse case manager must work closely with the patient's insurance company to determine what benefits are covered.

Social worker. The role of the social worker, often in conjunction with the nurse case manager, is to explore the psychosocial impact of the illness on the patient and family and determine what resources, both financial and emotional, will be necessary for the patient to successfully transition back into the community. The social worker has three primary responsibilities: to assess the patient for psychosocial factors that could impact discharge plans, to help connect families with relevant community resources, and to provide emotional support and guidance to patients and their families.

Therapists. Occupational therapists, physical therapists, and speech therapists play a key role in the discharge planning process by communicating the patient's capabilities and deficits to the discharge planner and physician. These skilled therapists will also play an important role in the posthospitalization care process. They are able to assess the progress made in functional recovery from the rehabilitation activities completed during the acute care hospitalization. The goal of rehabilitation is to improve function so that the stroke survivor can become as independent as possible. This must be accomplished in a way that preserves dignity and motivates the survivor to relearn basic skills and activities of daily living that the stroke may have taken away. The individual therapists can determine what functional goals have been achieved and what will need to be addressed at the next level of care so that these needs are addressed in the plan of care at discharge.

Occupational therapist: The occupational therapists' role in the discharge process is to assess the patient's ability to perform activities of daily living, such as feeding, bathing, dressing, and toileting. They also perform assessments for wheelchairs and other adaptive devices to improve the patient's functional status when leaving the hospital.

Physical therapist: Physical therapists perform assessments of the patient's gait, balance, mobility, and sensory deficits. Based on their assessment of the patient, they design individualized programs aimed at regaining control over motor functions.

Speech therapist: Speech therapists evaluate the patient for language deficits and identify methods to communicate using alternative means of communication. They also help patients improve their ability to swallow, and they work with patients to develop problem-solving and social skills needed to cope with the aftereffects of a stroke (National Institute of Neurological Disorders and Stroke [NINDS], 2014). See Chapter 10 for further details on rehabilitation and transitions.

Bedside nurses: The bedside nurses' role is extremely important. They develop an understanding of the person's medical condition while in the hospital and see the family and caregiver interactions. The nurses' regular observations of the patient's conditions provide valuable information to medical staff in determining how well the patient will function when returning to the community. Nurses work closely with the patient and family/caregivers to provide education and training regarding the risk factors for secondary stroke and recognition of stroke signs and symptoms.

Postacute Rehabilitation Options

There are a variety of postacute models of care that may be appropriate for the discharging stroke patient. Determining which level of care that will best meet the needs of an individual patient begins very quickly upon admission to the hospital. ⊙ The case manager will most often contact the patient's insurance company immediately to determine the specific benefits to which of the patient is entitled. This is important to do early because often the insurance company case manager will need to assess the patient independently to approve benefits. It is also necessary to have the insurance company involved early because the approval process for the next level of care can be time-consuming. It is the responsibility of the case manager to ensure the timely discharge of the patient to next level. The case manager will also coordinate all of the assessments from the interprofessional team to make a recommendation on behalf of the team to the insurance company for their approval.

The determination of the level of care postacute is made based on a number of criteria, most of which are based on the team's recommendation along with guidelines set out by the Centers for Medicare and Medicaid Services (CMS). Depending on the extent of rehabilitation services still required to best meet the needs of the patient, the following options may be available:

- LTACs
- ARFs
- SNFs
- Home with support from home health services
- Home with outpatient therapy
- Palliative care or hospice care

In some cases, the patient may eventually require care offered in a long-term care facility. Unfortunately, in most cases, the cost of long-term care is not covered by insurance and is considered to be self-pay or self-funded. At the other end of the spectrum, many patients experience no lingering effects from the stroke and are able to return home with no postacute rehabilitation needs. They are advised to follow up with their primary care provider, which should include secondary prevention of stroke through the identification and management of stroke risk factors.

Clinical Pearl: The goal of rehabilitation is to improve function so that the stroke survivor can become as independent as possible.

The highest level of care available after discharge from the acute care hospital is a long-term acute care hospital known as an *LTAC*. This level of care is appropriate for those patients who no longer require an acute care setting but whose functional status has not improved enough to move to a lower level of care. Most often, patients are discharged to an LTAC when they require more complex medical care than is provided in an SNF but less care than is needed in an acute care setting. The patient's need for nursing and rehabilitative services are complex enough that only an inpatient LTAC setting can meet the requirements, and the expected length of stay is greater than 25 days (for shorter stays, consider SNP or an inpatient rehabilitation facility). Many LTAC-appropriate patients have primary medical or respiratory problems that are complex, requiring daily intervention by a physician, NP, or PA with intensive treatment.

The next level of care available to the stroke patient is the SNF. In this setting, the patient is required by Medicare (and in turn, private insurers) to be able to participate in a minimum of 3 hours of skilled therapy (occupational therapy [OT]/physical therapy [PT]/speech therapy [ST]) per day. Individuals in SNFs also still require nursing care and limited physician care. This level of care is ideal for patients who are not yet capable of managing the endurance required for the inpatient rehabilitation hospital setting. Fewer hours of therapy are offered at SNFs compared to inpatient rehabilitation units. SNFs are an excellent choice for patients who have endurance issues. The average length of stay for a stroke patient in an SNF is 7.15 days (American Health Care Association, 2011). Medicare patients must have spent three overnights (72 hours) in an acute care hospital in order to meet criteria for SNF benefit. Medicare part A (hospitalization) benefits provide a total of 100 days of skilled nursing. The breakdown of out-of-pockets costs to the patient is as follows (Medicare, 2014):

- Days 1 to 20: $0
- Days 21 to 100: $152 coinsurance per day of each benefit period
- Days 101 and beyond: all costs associated with care

For those patients with private insurance, benefits vary significantly by policy.

Another level of care that is commonly used for stroke patients is ARFs, either in a freestanding rehabilitation facility or within the acute hospital setting. Studies have shown that providing rehabilitation services in an ARF improves the quality of life and functional status of stroke patients significantly.

Patients typically stay in the facility for 2 to 3 weeks and participate in a coordinated, comprehensive, intensive program of rehabilitation. These programs involve at least 3 hours of active therapy daily, 5 or 6 days a week. Inpatient facilities offer a comprehensive range of medical services, including full-time physician supervision and access to a full range of therapists specializing in poststroke rehabilitation (NINDS, 2014). The average length of stay for stroke patients in a rehabilitation facility is typically 28 days and is considered a covered benefit under Medicare part A (hospitalization) along with acute hospital coverage. Again, private insurance coverage varies by policy and often covers a much more limited number of days than Medicare.

For those patients who are able to return home, whether directly from the acute care setting or from an SNF, rehabilitation hospital, or LTAC, the use of home health services is an additional source of ongoing rehabilitation. Home health service is a covered benefit under Medicare which requires that the patient be homebound and unable to leave the home to obtain outpatient therapy. Additionally, the patient must have at least one skilled need consisting of nursing care, OT, PT, or ST

In some cases, it is possible for the patient and family to also receive the services of a home health aide to provide a few hours a week of care for the patient or respite for the caregiver. The aide typically assists the patient with bathing and grooming activities. A social worker is also available as needed to provide supportive counseling for the patient and caregivers as well as provide resources in the community such as support groups.

Home health services are a covered benefit under Medicare and typically involve three visits per week by the individual therapist or nurse as needed. Those patients with private insurance may carry a home health benefit although, due to lower reimburse-ment rates by insurers, it is more difficult to find providers who will accept private in-surance patients. In these cases, it is often helpful to contact the insurance company directly for assistance. If the patient has been assigned a case manager with the insurance company, this is the best place to start.

For those patients with minimal skilled therapy needs and the ability to travel for services, outpatient therapy is an excellent option. Outpatient therapy services (OT/PT/ST) are often provided through the larger rehabilitation hospitals but are also available at many locations within a community, making it more accessible for the patient and his or her caregivers. It is often part of a continuum of therapy services that began while in the acute care setting. Patients typically attend therapy sessions 2 to 3 days a week (Mosunmola, Adler, & Barrett, 2014). Depending on individual needs, the patient may require OT/PT or ST, often all three. Many stroke survivors use outpatient therapy services for many years following a stroke. As plateaus are reached, the patient is often discharged to "take a break." The patient can always be reevaluated by his or her physiatrist to assess to determine whether the patient is ap-propriate to restart therapy in the future.

Services are provided through Medicare under part B (medical), which covers 80% of costs. It is recommended that the patient obtain Medicare gap coverage, which typi-cally covers the 20% not covered by Medicare. There are "caps" imposed on outpatient therapy. For 2014, the cap is $1,920 for PT and speech-language pathology (SLP) ser-vices combined and $1,920 for OT services (Medicare, 2014). With appropriate docu-mentation from the various therapists, it is possible to exceed the caps up to $3,700 for PT and ST combined and $3,700 for OT. Private insurers most often provide outpatient therapy as a covered benefit, although each policy varies as to the number or visits provided.

Palliative care or hospice services are another option for the stroke patient. This is reserved for those patients who have suffered the most severe stroke and are not ex-pected to survive longer than 6 months. Patients who have suffered a massive stroke may qualify for hospice care either during the acute phase of the stroke or as a chronic condi-tion many years after the stroke. Criteria for admission onto hospice care (Group Health Cooperative, 2014) include the following:

- Comatose patients with any four of the following on day 3 of a stroke have 97% mortality by 2 months:
    - Abnormal brainstem response
    - Absent verbal response
    - No response to pain
    - Serum creatinine of more than 1.5 mg/dL
    - Age 70 years or older
    - Dysphagia severe enough to prevent them from receiving food or fluids
    - Karnofsky score of poor performance status 40% or less
    - Poor nutritional status

Hospice is a 100% Medicare-covered benefit and provides a comprehensive network of services intended to provide comfort care and support for the patient and the fam-ily. In addition to the medical services provided by the hospice nurse, the patient and family also receive supportive services from chaplains and social workers and 1 year of bereavement services following the death of the patient. Hospice benefits are covered at 100% by Medicare and most private insurers. See Chapter 9 for further discussion of palliative care.

◼ PREPARING FOR DISCHARGE

Preparing both the patient and the caregivers for discharge should begin immediately upon admission to the hospital. There are many factors to consider when preparing the patient for discharge to the next level of care (Duncan et al., 2005). In the early stages, it may not be possible to identify which level of care will be appropriate at the time of discharge; however, there are a number of steps that can be implemented early in the acute hospitalization.

● One of the first steps in preparing the family for discharge is to conduct a formal psychosocial assessment, typically completed by the social worker. The assessment should address both the patient as well as the family/caregivers and include areas such as history of prestroke functioning (e.g., demographics, past medical and social history, emotional functioning, mental health history, education and employment history, veteran status, and legal aspects including any advance directives, powers of attorney, support systems, and coping mechanisms).

Additional elements of a comprehensive psychosocial assessment will include a thorough exploration of the relationships within the family system and what spiritual and cultural preferences are important to the patient and family that may impact successful transition to the community. An understanding of the family's resource needs is crucial to identify early in the process. Financial considerations have a huge impact on the patient's eligibility for various types of postacute rehabilitation services. If the patient is going home, it is critical to determine if the home is safe and accessible for someone who is disabled. This assessment can be provided through the services of a home health agency. With a physician referral, the home health nurse can conduct an in-home assessment and provide feedback and recommendations to the family/caregivers on how to equip the home to the meet the needs of individual patient. Examples of ways to make the home safe are moving area rugs out of the way to avoid risk for falls, installation of ramps to get in and out of the home using a wheelchair, and grabbing bars near toilets and showers.

Most importantly, the assessment needs to identify what the patient/family/caregiver perceptions are of the condition, treatment plan, and prognosis and what the hopes and expectations are for ongoing care of the patient (Duncan et al., 2005). The importance of family involvement in the care and planning cannot be emphasized enough. Patients with high levels of family support have been shown to increase the likelihood of return to home after hospital admission and a decreased chance of unscheduled readmission (Tsouna-Hadjis, Vemmos, Zakopoulus, & Stamatelopoulos, 2000).

Family/caregiver education includes programs that promote lifestyle changes and identify barriers to implementing these changes along with providing strategies to overcome the obstacles. In addition, education addresses the needs of the patient regarding his or her specific condition and care, treatment, and prevention. Caregivers are also provided with information regarding services that are available in the community including support group information, respite care, and social service support (The Joint Commission, 2013).

Clinical Pearl: Preparing both the patient and the caregivers for discharge should begin immediately upon admission to the hospital. Education and training must be provided in both written and interactive formats.

⦿ It is imperative that the interprofessional team document within the patient's medical record to reflect the patient and family/caregiver education. Formal documentation of all interventions, education, and training that are provided to the patient and family/caregivers must be completed, including an assessment of the family's level of understanding of the information that was provided.

⦿ The case manager will evaluate the financial resources and insurance benefits that will be available to the patient. In addition, if the patient is discharging directly home, the case manager will determine what, if any, durable medical equipment will be necessary such as a hospital bed, walker, wheelchair, and speech aides. To identify what PT and OT equipment will be necessary, collaboration with the physiatrist and OT/PT/ST team is important.

Family training and assessing the patient and the family caregiver's readiness to provide caregiving for the patient, once discharged from the acute setting, should begin as early as possible after the patient's admission. This task is often challenging because the family is typically in shock and overwhelmed by the circumstances and uncertainty surrounding the event and unable to process the extent of the ongoing challenges that the family will face. Caregivers may still be dealing with the unexpected challenge of balancing family and work commitments with visitations at the hospital. There may be young children at home who require care. For older stroke patients and their families, the spouse may have serious health problems and thus be unable to participate in the ongoing care needs of his or her disabled spouse. In this case, additional family support is crucial to getting the patient on the road to rehabilitation.

As part of the initial assessment, gathering an understanding of who will be involved in the ongoing care of the patient and ensuring they are included in all training activities and family meetings will assist in facilitating a successful discharge to the next level of care. It is important that family/caregivers are included in all decision making and treatment planning for the patient. In addition, it is essential to determine who the family decision maker is and if there is a different family member who may act as the spokesperson because they may not always be the same person. In cases where the patient is unable to make his or her own decisions, the team should determine whether the patient has completed a power of attorney document and who is legally designated to make decisions on behalf of the patient.

Clinical Pearl: Patients with high levels of family support have been shown to increase the likelihood of return to home after hospital admission and a decreased chance of unscheduled readmission.

⦿ All staff should monitor for signs of stress in the family caregivers especially as it relates to the patient's residual impairments such as speech and physical limitations, cognitive loss, personality changes, and incontinence issues (Duncan et al., 2005). Caregivers are often heard to say "There is no way I will be able to manage the needs of my loved one at home. He or she needs to stay here at the hospital until he or she gets back to normal." Of course, this is not realistic, and it is the responsibility of the care team to ensure that the family/caregivers are given the emotional support and resources to build confidence so that they will indeed be able to care for the patient upon discharge to next level of care.

Special attention must be paid to the "walking wounded," those patients who are physically well enough to return home but may be suffering from significant cognitive impairment. Assessment using the Mini-Mental State Examination and other testing methods can assist in making a determination of whether the patient can safely discharge home alone or if he or she will require some level of supervision in the home. See Chapter 10 for further discussion of cognitive assessment.

Clinical Pearl: Don't neglect the "walking wounded"; although they may seem highly functional, they may have significant cognitive impairment that will impact on recovery.

As part of the process of preparing the patient for discharge, helping the caregivers understand the needs of the patient and providing training and education to address these needs has been shown to be extremely valuable in ensuring the family's readiness for leaving the hospital. The training must incorporate how to manage the physical and speech limitations of the stroke survivor. Understanding how to safely transfer the patient and learning how to communicate with a patient with aphasia are two examples of real issues that families struggle with upon discharge. Ensuring that the family has learned how to use transfer boards and communication devices or strategies prior to discharge will increase the likelihood that the patient will reintegrate well into the community. Education should also be focused around learning about the causes and importance of compliance with recommended treatments; potential complications; and the goals, process, and prognosis of rehabilitation (Duncan et al., 2005).

Several recommendations have been suggested by Duncan et al. (2005) in the *Stroke Rehabilitation Clinical Practice Guidelines* concerning training and education for family/caregivers. The first recommendation is that the education be provided in both written and interactive formats. The use of return demonstration is an additional way to verify knowledge acquisition and allows the family/caregiver to practice the skills they have learned in a safe environment. Studies have shown that there is a higher degree of improved patient outcomes when family/caregivers are given written material combined with one-on-one interaction with the family to discuss the material and allow the caregivers to ask questions, share their concerns, and receive feedback from the clinician (Smith et al., 2008).

Another best practice recommendation was to identify a specific team member within the hospital who is responsible for providing the training and education to the family. This person, possibly a stroke educator or stroke nursing professional, can meet with each family and provide appropriate one-on-one training to explain the nature of the stroke, the goals of rehabilitation, long-term expectations, and the family's role in the process. In some hospital settings, a stroke binder is issued to each family which contains comprehensive information about the causes, risk factors, prevention, treatment, recovery path, blood pressure logs, and medication sheets.

Other helpful information that may be included in the binder is information about the role of nutrition in prevention of secondary stroke. Another critical content area is a section to provide resources available to the patient and families such as local support group meetings (refer to section on resources at the end of the chapter), Meals on Wheels, adult day care options, and in-home personal care assistants. At a minimum, materials and brochures are available through the American Stroke Association and the National Stroke Association that can be given to the patient and family. Additional information that should be given to the patient and caregivers includes follow-up appointment information and contact information of interprofessional team members in case questions arise after discharge. Caregivers are more comfortable with the discharge if they know they will be able to contact team members after they have left the hospital.

■ UNDERSTANDING THE NEW CHALLENGES FOR THE SURVIVOR

Every stroke survivor will have a different set of challenges post stroke, which can range from minor deficits to severe disabilities. The types of disabilities fall into several categories. Some level of paralysis is one of the most common and typically affects the side of the body opposite to the side of the brain damaged by the stroke. Motor deficits can present in varying degrees from partial to complete paralysis and can impact the survivor's ability to ambulate, transfer, grasp objects, and write. Some survivors have difficulty with swallowing or dysphagia, which makes eating regular food difficult or require use of a feeding tube. Activities of daily living such as self-feeding and toileting and bathing may require the help of a caregiver. Survivors feel a loss of dignity and independence related to the need for help in these situations. Sensitivity to these feelings is necessary when providing care for stroke patients.

Some stroke survivors experience sensory changes as a result of the stroke. They may lose the ability to feel pain or experience numbness in their affected limbs. One of early poststroke problems faced is urinary incontinence due to the inability to sense the need to urinate and in addition lack the ability to reach the bathroom in time. This is particularly emotional for stroke survivors, but in most cases, it is a temporary situation.

Chronic pain syndromes are another common disturbance for stroke survivors and can manifest itself in many ways—some of it may be related to damage to pathways in the brain (NINDS, 2014). Pain may also be present due to mechanical problems resulting from weakness or lack of use such as a "frozen shoulder." Occupational and physical therapists will assess for these issues on an ongoing basis. Identifying the causes and providing treatment for pain is critical for the comfort of the patient but also pain increases the likelihood that poststroke depression will develop. Regularly assessing for pain both in the acute phase and on an ongoing basis is recommended.

Another challenge that may result from sensory changes is sexual dysfunction. This is often a temporary situation but may cause long-term difficulties. Sexual disorders after stroke are thought to be due to multiple etiologies, including both organic and psychosocial causes. Sexual function in poststroke patients is often disregarded by health care professionals although sexuality is a fundamental part of quality of life. Beside pharmacological treatment, one of the most important but underestimated success factors of sexual dysfunction therapy is undeniably proper counseling, which is mandatory to provide correct information on poststroke sexuality, helping the patients and their partners to regain intimacy (Calabro & Bramanti, 2013). Language problems affect as many as 25% of stroke patients and involve the ability to speak, write, and understand spoken and written language (NINDS, 2014). Loss of language or aphasia can take on different forms depending on what part of the brain the stroke occurred. Whether the survivor suffers from Broca's or expressive aphasia, Wernicke's or receptive aphasia, or in the worst possible case global aphasia, the inability to communicate needs and feelings and the ability to socially interact is extremely frustrating. Language impairment affects everyone involved from the patient to the caregiver and causes significant emotional distress.

For those survivors with aphasia, feelings of isolation and the inability to express one's self create an environment where poststroke depression is likely. Survivors with aphasia often feel that others see them as "stupid." One stroke survivor with significant expressive aphasia who was a professor of English at a top university wears a large name badge wherever he goes that says "My name is John Smith, PhD, I have aphasia which is loss of language, not intelligence." ST is essential for persons with any form of aphasia on an ongoing basis. Improvements in the ability to communicate whether through speech or with the help of assisted speech devices can occur many years out from stroke—well past the previously thought first year post stroke. Connecting with a support group for both stroke survivors and caregivers of those with aphasia can be very helpful and rewarding and alleviate some of the feelings of isolation and provide opportunities to practice their language skills around others in a nonjudgmental forum. See Chapter 9 for further discussion of poststroke complications.

▐▋ UNDERSTANDING THE ROLE OF THE CAREGIVER

For the family member who is caregiver for the stroke patient, it is very challenging to adjust to the change in roles. When a family member becomes disabled due to a stroke or other chronic illness, it is common for others within the family to assume some of the roles that were performed by the stroke survivor. Caregivers have to take on new responsibilities, in addition to their own, and the stroke survivor quite often feels a sense of loss due to his or her disability as well as the loss of independence to former roles. This results in a strain on the relationship. The stroke survivor may feel as if he or she is not contributing to the family and the caregiver may feel distress over the new responsibilities that he or she may be ill equipped and unprepared to perform.

An example of how role changes affect the family is the stroke survivor may not be able to return to work, whether it is immediately or long term, resulting in the loss of his or her occupational role and possibly the role of sole family breadwinner. This in turn changes the role of the spouse who may have to juggle caregiving responsibilities with that of financial responsibilities. The spouse may also have responsibility now for the housework, meal preparation, and paying bills that was formerly managed by the stroke survivor.

For children of stroke survivors, there are role changes as well. Often, the adult children as well as younger children still living in the home will need to assume caregiver responsibilities. For adult children with families of their own and living away from parents, challenges of geography, financial, and their own family responsibilities are pushed aside to take on the caregiving tasks and can create conflict within the family system. If the stroke survivor was living alone prior to the stroke, going back home may not be an option, and decisions must be made regarding where the person will live. Some survivors move into their adult children's homes to ensure their safety.

For younger children living at home, additional responsibilities are expected and sacrifices are often required because the well parent may be overwhelmed with the primary caregiver/breadwinner role. The emotional and social needs of the children may be neglected. Special care must be taken to ensure that the needs of younger children are addressed. It may be helpful to suggest a support group that provides support for families. In all cases where the primary caregivers are children of the stroke survivor, one of the most significant challenges is that of role reversal. The child is now providing care to the parent. It can be challenging for children to "tell" their parent what to do, provide personal hygiene care, or feed and dress the parent. Again, support groups can provide a tremendous opportunity for child caregivers to provide mutual support and "lessons learned" from others experiencing similar situations.

Clinical Pearl: The stress of having a family member with a stroke is significant and can affect family members in different ways. Be vigilant to signs of stress that need intervention.

Depression and Stroke

The risk of depression is significant for stroke survivors. Although statistics vary in terms of prevalence, somewhere between 25% and 75% of stroke survivors will suffer from poststroke depression at some point. Numerous studies support the importance of identifying depression in poststroke patients and consider it to be the strongest predictor of quality of life for stroke survivors (Paolucci, 2008). Poststroke depression is associated with increased disability, increased mortality, and overall worse rehabilitation outcomes (Paolucci, 2008). It has also been shown that an absence of depressive symptoms or improvement of symptoms is associated with better functional recovery.

Typical assessment tools used for identifying depression are more difficult to administer to stroke patient because stroke patients often have cognitive and/or physical impairments that make assessment difficult. For the patient with aphasia, it becomes nearly impossible to determine whether the patient is experiencing depression or just unable to communicate his or her feelings. Most depression inventories or scales are designed to assess patients for primary depressive disorders and not patients for whom the depression in comorbidity. Despite the challenges in assessing the patient, every stroke patient should be evaluated using clinical criteria from the *Diagnostic and Statistical Manual of Mental Disorders* 5th edition (*DSM-5*). Common symptoms that have been found in stroke patients are weight loss, insomnia, fatigue, and reduced ability to concentrate (Carod-Artal, 2010). See Chapter 9 for a list of common depression assessment instruments.

Clinical Pearl: Stroke patients are at high risk for developing depression. Monitor the patient for signs and symptoms of depression and need for treatment during all visits.

The optimal choice of treatment options for depression in the acute setting is antidepressant medication. In a systematic review of randomized controlled trials comparing antidepressant therapy versus no therapy, those patients who received antidepressant drug treatment showed improvement in their depressive symptoms (Flaster, Sharma, & Rao, 2013). Ongoing assessment of the patient should be conducted at each follow-up appointment with the patient. Referrals for psychotherapy should be considered for patients in addition to antidepressant therapy when it becomes apparent that medication alone is not sufficient to reduce the depressive symptoms.

▮▮ TRANSITION FROM HOSPITAL SETTING TO HOME

Most stroke survivors will return home either after their acute hospitalization or after a stay at an extended care facility. This can be a very emotional time for both patients and family or caregivers. Fear and anxiety about what happens once the patient returns to the community is a common phenomenon. The safety net of the inpatient setting is taken away as the survivor and caregiver prepare to transition to the next phase in the recovery process. If the treatment team has provided the family with the information and resources that will be essential once the patient is discharged, the probability for a smooth transition home is more likely. It has been estimated that 18% of Medicare patients are readmitted within 30 days, and in many cases, this could be avoided by careful planning before discharge (Family Caregiver Alliance, 2014).

Clinical Pearl: Stroke recovery is a lifelong process for most survivors.

As part of the discharge plan, there are some topics that should be discussed with the family that will assist in the transition. Ensuring that medications are ordered and the family understands how/when/why each medication is necessary is an essential element of the discharge plan. Unfortunately, it has been estimated that 40% of patients older than the age of 65 years had medication discrepancies identified after discharge (Family Caregiver Alliance, 2014). Another area to discuss is contact information should an emergency arise and information about what actually constitutes an emergency. Contact information for nonemergency questions should be provided as well (preferably 24-hour telephone number) and follow-up appointments with physicians should be scheduled prior to leaving the hospital if at all possible. Refer to community resources at the end of the chapter.

If home health service has been recommended for the patient, the family/caregiver should have contact information for the agency providing the service and a date/time scheduled for the agency representative to come and complete the in-home assessment. If the patient will be receiving outpatient therapy upon discharge, the family should be provided with the medical order for treatment and be given several options for providers that meet the geographic and insurance needs of the family. Ideally, the location will be identified prior to discharge and the order faxed directly to the provider with an initial visit scheduled prior to discharge. Home health services are an excellent resource to ensure the course of rehabilitation continues. In addition, aides and social workers are available as part of the home health service.

Life at Home: Preparation and Transition

If durable medical equipment will be required for the patient at home, it is important to address what will the patient need: a hospital bed, wheelchair, walker, and transfer boards? These are all possible aids that the patient and family will need. Every detail that is completed ahead of time will build confidence in the patient and caregiver that they will not be left stranded and alone once they get home. Ideally, all durable medical equipment should be ordered and delivered to the home prior to or as close to the patient's discharge from the hospital as possible.

Many stroke centers have added new roles to the discharge planning process and may include the case manager, stroke coordinator, or stroke nurse navigator to provide a comprehensive approach to facilitate the discharge. The discharge planner should discuss with the family any limitations that affect their ability to provide care in the home. These may include physical, financial, or logistical limitations. If the patient will require 24-hour care, does the family have the resources to provide this care at home? If the spouse must continue to work full time, who will be available to provide around-the-clock care? Are there family members or friends who can assist with staying with the patient? The family may need to consider hiring private caregivers which is not a covered expense under Medicare, or most private insurance plans, and will be out of reach financially for many families. If the patient has a long-term care insurance plan, benefits may apply to in-home caregiving. Identifying family or friends to supplement caregiving needs may be necessary to provide full support for the patient. These are just a few examples of questions that need to be addressed as the patient returns home. Helping families look for options to overcome limitations will allow for a smooth transition. Identifying family or friends to supplement caregiving needs may be necessary to provide full support for the patient.

When the stroke survivor is discharged home, the family as a whole begins a new journey in life. Financial concerns often create the most stress for the family. If the survivor was the sole provider and is now unable to work, this becomes the number one concern. If the patient is not able to return to work, application for Social Security Disability Insurance or Supplemental Security Income (SSI) for low/no income individuals should be completed as quickly as possible. Application for these programs has become easier over the years and may be completed online at http://www.ssa.gov, in person at a social security office, or over the phone via a telephone interview. Application for Social Security Disability Insurance may be managed in conjunction with the survivor's short/long-term disability plans through his or her employer. It is important that the family work closely with the employer to make sure all applicable information is provided in a timely manner.

For those survivors who may be able to return to work but need a change in their position or adaptive equipment to continue to work, connection with the state vocational and rehabilitative services agency provides valuable resources to ensure that the survivor is able to successfully return to gainful employment. Every state has such agency and contacting them early to schedule an appointment is recommended to ensure the services are provided as quickly as possible.

For caregivers who work, taking time off to care for the survivor can be difficult and stressful. The Family and Medical Leave Act (FMLA) is a federal law that allows family members taking care of an ill family member to take up to 12 weeks in a 12-month period. This can be taken all at once or intermittently as needed. The employee's job is protected during the time that they are on FMLA (U.S. Department of Labor, 2014). This benefit is also available to the stroke survivor and is typically used in conjunction with short-term disability, ensuring the stroke survivor's job will be protected for 12 weeks. For seniors who are already receiving social security benefits and are living on a limited income, the additional costs of caregiving can become increasingly difficult. Financial support from children may become necessary or moving the survivor to live with other family members may become the only option to meet the demanding financial and physical needs of the stroke survivor.

An area that is often difficult for seniors is the cost of medications. Working with both the primary care physician and the neurologist, medication assistance programs are often available to provide free or low-cost medications for those with limited income. If a patient is prescribed an expensive medication with a high insurance copay, there is increased risk of noncompliance with medications, resulting in further health complications. It is important to understand the patient's financial barriers when prescribing medications. In some cases, it may be advisable to prescribe an alternate medication that is either on the patient's insurance plan or is available in generic form.

In cases where there is no family to care for the survivor, long-term placement in a nursing facility may be the only option available. In these cases, the stroke survivor will use existing financial resources to pay for custodial care in a facility. When personal resources are exhausted, state Medicaid nursing home benefits may be used. When possible, it is beneficial to meet with an elder care attorney to plan for the future needs.

When the survivor goes home, environmental modifications to the home may be necessary. This can be very costly, and in most cases, there are few if any financial assistance programs to fund these projects. Valuable information is available to survivors and families through the National Stroke Association series *Living after Stroke*. It provides online videos and webinars on how to do your own home modifications, and it lists resources to assist in the process (Mosunmola, Adler, & Barrett, 2014).

Many home modifications can be completed rather inexpensively ranging from $200 to $1,500. For more extensive remodeling, it is recommended that families contact a Certified Aging in Place consultant. Typically, they will offer a free or low-cost consultation and will provide the family with an overview of what modifications is necessary and the cost involved. These specialists are experts in the area of remodeling for seniors and those with disabilities to allow them to remain in their homes.

Being at home can feel very isolating for both the survivor and the family/caregivers and ensuring that they remain connected to the community is key to establishing a new sense of "normal" for the family. Finding support from others can help the survivor and family prevent this isolation. Reaching out to friends and other family members is a way to stay connected. This can be done through in-home visits, telephone, e-mails, and more recently, through video conferencing such as Skype. Other ways for the family to stay connected with the community is by building a support system through a stroke support group. Many families find support through their church/synagogue. Church communities may offer respite services to their members and also offer family counseling services. In larger cities, there are often many community resources that are available to patients and families. If at all possible, it is beneficial to participate in person; however, if this is not feasible, there are support options available online through national stroke organizations. If adjustment becomes too difficult for either the survivor or the family, it is recommended that they seek professional counseling for assistance. Counselors can provide emotional support to the family in dealing with this challenging adjustment and teach coping skills for all involved.

Quality of Life for Stroke Survivors

For the stroke survivor, a change in quality of life is inevitable. Many studies have been conducted to determine what indicators are most significant when assessing for quality of life. Four dimensions stand out as essential to evaluating quality of life for stroke survivors: physical, functional, psychological, and social health (Jonsson, Lindgren, Hallstrom, Norring, & Lindgren, 2005). The physical dimension relates to the survivor's overall health, disease process, and symptom-related aspects of quality of life. Functional health assesses the survivor's ability to provide self-care, mobility, physical abilities and activities, and capacity to perform various roles relative to family and work life. The psychological dimension is composed of cognitive functions including emotional status and a general sense of well-being, life satisfaction, and overall happiness. The social functioning dimension encompasses the survivor's ability both qualitatively and quantitatively to interact and conduct social interactions (Jonsson et al., 2005).

In one study conducted by Luengo-Fernandez et al. (2013), the investigators found that stroke survivors lost an average 2 out of 5 quality life years. The study also found that those survivors who were married had a significantly higher level of quality of life than did those who were single, divorced, or widowed. Higher educational levels were also shown to have a positive impact on quality of life. Interventions that increase the ability to perform in the four dimensions raise the quality level for the survivor. Participation in rehabilitation therapy aids the survivor in recovering some of his or her independence which in turn improves quality of life. Social interactions with family, friends, and support group members decreases the likelihood of feelings of isolation and helps decrease the chance of poststroke depression. Most importantly, finding new meaning and purpose in life post stroke greatly improves the survivor's quality of life.

Clinical Pearl: Social interaction decreases the likelihood of feelings of isolation and helps reduce the chance of poststroke depression.

Care of the Caregiver

Providing informal care for the stroke survivor at home is both physically and emotionally challenging. Caregivers may include spouses, children, siblings, and friends of the survivor. Often, a combination of new responsibilities, in addition to existing ones, creates new challenges that caregivers are most often ill-prepared to deal with. Caregivers find themselves thrust into an unexpected new role with little or no training and often with limited support for themselves.

Caregivers need information on all aspects of stroke. They need to be aware of the risk factors for secondary stroke, warning signs that a stroke is occurring, and information on how to care for their loved one at home (see Chapter 1 for discussion of secondary stroke prevention). Additionally, they may need to learn how to communicate with someone with aphasia and learn to dress, feed, toilet, and manage physical limitations of their loved one. They may need to assume the responsibilities of paying bills and other financial obligations with no prior experience. For example, one family caregiver spent months trying to resolve issues with the Internal Revenue Service regarding filing late income tax returns. Another family caregiver had no access to online payment or banking information because the stroke survivor could not remember the passwords to any of the accounts nor had he recorded them in any retrievable format anywhere. All of these new responsibilities, along with continuing to manage the responsibilities they had prior to their loved ones stroke, can and often does lead to caregiver burnout. Numerous studies have concluded that caregiver burden takes a tremendous toll on the physical and mental health of the caregiver (Brandon, 2013). In a study conducted by Schultz and Beach (1999), the authors concluded that caregivers providing long-term care had a 63% higher risk of dying than noncaregiver controls.

Key factors in preventing caregiver burnout are the caregiver's access to a support system, whether that be family assisting with the caregiving, participation in a support group, in-home care providers, or respite/day programs for the survivor. Those caregivers with assertive coping skills do best in providing long-term caregiving. Beneficial skills including taking charge, asking questions, willingness to ask for help, accepting help, and taking care of self had the most positive outcomes. Those with passive coping skills did more poorly and were more likely to isolate themselves from others, worry about the past/future, and focus on negative emotions (Brandon, 2013). Encouraging caregivers to take care of themselves is as important as caring for the stroke survivor.

Referrals for respite care should be provided to all patients and family/caregivers upon discharge. Respite encompasses a wide variety of services including home-based care as well as adult day care, skilled nursing, home health, and short-term institutional care. Respite can also be provided by volunteers from the community, churches, and family and friends of the patient.

Financial Implications

The financial burden associated with caregiving is significant. Although little research is available regarding the actual financial cost of long-term caregiving, studies have shown that family caregivers provide over $1.6 billion annually in care for stroke survivors (American Heart Association, 2013). Families may need to cash in savings account and retirement plans, borrow money from family members, and max out credit cards in order to care for a family member at home. For a stroke survivor who was previously working and may be forced to use the Consolidated Omnibus Budget Reconciliation Act of 1985 for health insurance, the cost can be as high as $1,500 per month. If the spouse is working, it is sometimes possible through a "change in status" clause in group insurance plans for the survivor to be added to the spouse's employee-sponsored insurance.

Follow-Up Care Post-Discharge

Ensuring that the patient has a follow-up plan in place is critical to reducing the readmission rate and keeping the patient safely at home during rehabilitation and recovery. Upon discharge, the patient should have appointments scheduled for follow-ups with his or her primary care physician, neurologist, and physical medicine and rehabilitation specialists along with any other health care providers that the patient may need. Typically, patients are seen for follow-up by neurologist within the first month of discharge, and a plan for future appointments is scheduled at that time. When possible, it is advisable to contact the patient and family caregiver by telephone or e-mail after discharge to answer any questions or concerns and monitor recovery. At a minimum, contact information is made available to the family should the need arise.

Support Groups

For stroke survivors and their families, the many changes that impact daily life can be extremely difficult and challenging for everyone involved. Stroke survivors may feel uncomfortable around their old circle of friends and feel as if they do not fit in. For survivors and caregivers alike, there is a high risk of becoming isolated. Research has shown that social isolation is a risk factor for poor outcome after a stroke (Boden-Albala, Litwak, Elkind, Rundek, & Sacco, 2005).

First and foremost, a strong support group of people who have shared a similar experience gives each participant hope that although life may not be the same as it was prior to the stroke, there is hope of developing a "new normal." Sharing similar experiences and concerns with others who may have already experienced the same situation unites members around their common experiences and helps them identify positive solutions. Support groups also empower group members to learn to help themselves and help each other and thus create meaningfulness in their lives. Meeting together in a safe place with common experiences creates a new sense of community for survivors and family/caregivers. New friendships are created and members are encouraged to become independent and not "let the stroke take over your life." As one support group facilitator noted to the group, "You're not allowed to call it 'your' stroke. You had it, but it doesn't have you."

For caregivers, support groups offer an opportunity to vent built-up frustration. Caregiving is exhausting and no one can understand better what that is like than another caregiver. A support group gives caregivers a chance to relieve stress, learn more about their family member's illness, gather information that can make life easier, and, most importantly, build a new support system. For caregivers, seldom do they have the opportunity to focus on themselves, and caregivers' support group allows them to focus on their own well-being. In one caregiver's group, it is said that if you aren't caring for yourself first, you can't take care of your family member. Support group members who have been in the group for some time, providing education, support, and accounts of experience with new members creates an opportunity for them to share their "expertise" and allows them to feel valued, an important element in maintaining a good quality of life.

Support groups also provide an opportunity for stroke survivors and their families/caregivers to receive ongoing education about the causes, treatments, and, most importantly, how to prevent secondary stroke. Often, support groups invite speakers to the meetings to talk about the importance of compliance with medications, how to control diabetes mellitus, and nutrition education. Many support groups are structured so that an educational component is provided during the first hour, and traditional support group activities occur during the second hour. Although it can be challenging to maintain a strong support group, the benefits are great for those who are able to participate.

There are many stroke survivors and family/caregivers who are not able to attend traditional support group meetings because of the complexity of their situation or logistical issues. Another way for stroke families to be able to connect with other families is through online support systems offered through various stroke organizations worldwide. Some organizations offer weekly "stroke chat" online or "call in" support groups, whereas others offer online forums where members can post questions and solicit feedback from others about how to handle a particular situation, gather information on treatment methods, or just share feelings with others. These groups draw from a larger population because many of them are national or international groups so that many people find these groups to be more beneficial than attending local support groups. Some people who use these groups also appreciate the anonymity that an online setting provides.

The good news is there are options available to meet a variety of needs. In addition to support groups, educational programs are available in many communities through the American Heart Association, senior centers, and often at local hospitals. Survivors and families should be encouraged to seek out opportunities to stay informed about stroke prevention and to stay abreast of new treatment modalities for rehabilitation.

Long-Term Impact

Stroke recovery is a lifelong process for most survivors. With new treatment modalities and rehabilitative equipment becoming available every day, it is important for stroke survivors to be aware of resources that are available to them. For example, a 90-year-old stroke survivor who attends a support group had been using the same motorized wheelchair for 10 years. This chair had not been meeting his needs for some time, but he didn't know that he was entitled to a new one every 5 years through Medicare. After a support group meeting with an OT who spoke about wheelchairs, he was able to be reevaluated for a new chair that was covered by Medicare and one that was much better suited to his needs. He shed tears of joy the day he received his new chair. Another survivor with significant aphasia had given up on ever being able to communicate since his stroke 7 years ago. After being reevaluated by a speech therapist, he now has a communication tablet that has given him a new opportunity to communicate with family and friends. As a result, it has decreased his sense of isolation. ◉ For interprofessional team members who see stroke survivors in the community, it is very important to continue to address the ongoing needs on a regular basis and recognize that recovery is an ongoing process with no end point.

As survivors and their families/caregivers adjust to life after stroke, a new sense of "normal" arises, and challenges that seemed insurmountable in the first few months after stroke become the normal routine and more manageable. For example, a family man who was a husband/father had suffered a massive hemorrhagic stroke with little chance of surviving. The family attended a support group meeting while the patient was in the intensive care unit. His wife was sure life would never be the same and was very distraught about the future. He did survive the stroke and 6 months later, he attended a support group meeting. He was with his wife and in a wheelchair and still having difficulty with aphasia and physical limitations, but they were both in the best of spirits. She was thrilled that he survived, and they had adapted relatively well to their new situation. It is amazing to see how far a person can come in a relatively short period of time. The wife had researched many aspects of stroke and was sharing her tips for managing, thus helping give hope to new members of the group. It was very encouraging for everyone to see the progress they had made.

Plasticity of the brain is being addressed in stroke recovery. Plasticity refers to the process that enables the brain to repair and reorganize cells. This means having healthy cells of the brain taking over jobs that were previously carried out by brain cells that were destroyed (Johansson, 2011). With the use of intense ongoing therapy, the brain can remap itself to work around dead and damaged areas through neuroplasticity processes, often with dramatic benefits. Therapies that use the brain's power to adapt have helped people overcome damage caused by strokes. Ongoing evaluation and treatment for the residual deficits should be assessed by the poststroke treatment team at each follow-up. In addition, assessment of psychosocial functioning should be included as a formal component of the poststroke treatment plan.

SUMMARY

When someone suffers a stroke, the lives of the patient and his or her family/caregivers are significantly impacted. Recovery is a lifelong process, and learning to adapt to the new challenges and developing a new normal needs to take place from early on after the stroke occurs. ⊙ Interprofessional team members play a significant role in laying the foundation for the patient and family to cope with the changes ahead. By providing comprehensive care, treatment, education, and access to support, the team not only promotes the safe transition to the community but also advances the skills to allow stroke survivors to lead healthy, meaningful lives with a sense of hope and purpose.

RESOURCES FOR STROKE SURVIVORS AND THEIR FAMILIES

American Heart Association/American Stroke Association
7272 Greenville Ave.
Dallas, TX 75231
1-888-4STROKE (478-7653)
http://www.strokeassociation.org/STROKEORG/

National Stroke Association
9707 East Ester Lane Suite B
Centennial, CO 80112
303-649-9299 800-STROKES (787-6537)
http://www.stroke.org/site/PageNavigator/HOME

National Institute of Neurological Disorders and Stroke
P.O. Box 3006
Bethesda, MD 20824
800-352-9424
http://www.ninds.nih.gov/index.htm

State Vocational Rehabilitation Agencies
http://wdcrobcolp01.ed.gov/Programs/EROD/org_list.cfm?category_cd=SVR

Social Security Administration, Disability
1-800-772-1213 (TTY 1-800-325-0778)
http://www.ssa.gov/disabilityssi/

Support Group Information
American Stroke Association
http://www.strokeassociation.org/STROKEORG/strokegroup/public/zipFinder.jsp

National Stroke Association
http://www.stroke.org/stroke-resources/stroke-support-groups

United Kingdom Stroke Association
http://www.stroke.org.uk/support/clubs-groups

Online Groups:
The Stroke Network
http://www.strokenetwork.org/

Stroke Net
http://www.strokeboard.net/

Caregiver Information and Services
Caregiver Action Network
2000 M St. NW, Suite 400
Washington, DC 20036
Phone: 202-772-5050
General e-mail: info@caregiveraction.org
http://www.caregiveraction.org/resources/agencies/

Care.com
http://www.care.com/

Family Caregiver Alliance
785 Market St., Suite 750
San Francisco, CA 94103
800 445-8106
https://www.caregiver.org/

Lotsa Helping Hands
34 Washington Street, Suite 310
Wellesley Hills, MA 02481
http://stroke.lotsahelpinghands.com/caregiving/home/

Medication Assistance Programs
NeedyMeds, Inc.
P.O. Box 219
Gloucester, MA 01931

HELPLINE
1-800-503-6897
http://www.needymeds.org/index.htm

Aphasia Resources
Aphasia Hope Foundation
P.O. Box 26304
Shawnee Mission, KS 66225
1 855-764-4673
http://www.aphasiahope.org/

National Aphasia Association
350 Seventh Ave. Suite 902
New York, NY 10001
212 267-2814 800 922-4622
http://www.aphasia.org/

REFERENCES

American Heart Association. (2013). *Understanding the financial costs of stroke caregiving.* Retrieved from https://yourethecure.org/aha/advocacy/details.aspx?BlogId=1&PostId=2106

American Health Care Association. (2011). *A comprehensive report on the quality of care in America's nursing homes and rehabilitation facilities.* Retrieved from http://www.ahcancal.org/quality_improvement/Documents/2011QualityReport.pdf

Boden-Albala, B., Litwak, E., Elkind, M., Rundek, T., & Sacco, R. (2005). Social isolation and outcomes post stroke. *Neurology, 64*(11), 1888–1892.

Brandon, I. L. (2013). Easing the burden on family caregivers. *Nursing, 43*(8), 36–42. doi: 10.1097/01.NURSE.0000432098.08196.8d

Calabro, R., & Bramanti, P. (2013). Post stroke sexual dysfunction: An overlooked and under-addressed problem. *Disability Rehabilitation, 36*(3), 263–264. doi:10.3109/09638288.2013.785603

Carod-Artal, F. (2010). Post-stroke depression: Can prediction help prevention? *Future Neurology, 5*(4), 569–580.

Clarke, D. J. (2013). The role of multidisciplinary team care in stroke rehabilitation. *Progress in Neurology and Psychiatry, 17*(4), 5–8. doi:10.1002/pnp.288

Duncan, P., Zorowitz, R., Bates, B., Choi, J., Glasberg, J., Graham, G., ... Reker, D. (2005). Management of adult stroke rehabilitation care: A clinical practice guideline. *Stroke, 36*, e100–e143. doi:10.1161/01.STR.0000180861.54180.FF

Family Caregiver Alliance. (2014). *Hospital discharge planning: A guide for families and caregivers.* Retrieved from https://caregiver.org/hospital-discharge-planning-guide-families-and-caregivers

Feigin, V. L., Forouzanfar, M. H., Krishnamurthi, R., Mensah, G. A., Connor, M., Bennett, D. A., . . . Murray, C. (2014). Global and regional burden of stroke during 1990-2010: Findings from the Global Burden of Disease Study 2010. *The Lancet, 383*(9913), 245–255. doi:10.1016/S2214-109X(13)70089-5

Flaster, M., Sharma, A., & Rao, M. (2013). Post stroke depression: A review emphasizing the role of prophylactic treatment and synergy with treatment for motor recovery. *Topics in Stroke Rehabilitation, 20*(2), 139–150. doi:10.1310/tsr2002-139

Group Health Cooperative. (2014). *Clinical review criteria: Hospice program.* Retrieved from http://www.ghc.org/all-sites/clinical/criteria/pdf/hospice.pdf

Johansson, B. (2011). Current trends in stroke rehabilitation. A review with focus on brain plasticity. *Acta Neurologica Scandinavica, 123,* 147–159. doi:10.1111/j.1600-0404.2010.01417.x

Jonsson, A., Lindgren, I., Hallstrom, B., Norring, B., & Lindgren, A. (2005). Determinants of quality of life in stroke survivors and their informed caregivers. *Stroke, 36,* 803–808. doi:10.1161/01.STR.0000160873.32791.20

Luengo-Fernandez, R., Gray, A. M., Bull, L., Welch, S., Cuthbertson, F., & Rothwell, P. M. (2013). Quality of life after TIA and stroke: Ten-year results of the Oxford Vascular Study. *Neurology, 81*(18), 1588–1595. doi:10.1212/WNL.0b013e3182a9f45f

Medicare. (2014). *Medicare coverage of skilled nursing facilities.* Retrieved from http://www.medicare.gov/Pubs/pdf/10153.pdf

Mosunmola, O., Adler, U., & Barrett, A. (2014). Strengthening synapses to achieve optimal outcomes. *Today's Geriatric Medicine, 7*(5), 12. Retrieved from http://www.todaysgeriatricmedicine.com/archive/0914p12.shtml

National Institute of Neurological Disorders and Stroke. (2014). *Stroke: Hope through research.* Retrieved from http://www.ninds.nih.gov/disorders/stroke/detail_stroke.htm#266231105

National Stroke Association. (2014a) *Living after stroke.* Retrieved from http://www.stroke.org/site/PageServer?pagename=living

National Stroke Association. (2014b). *Rehabilitation therapy after stroke.* Retrieved from http://www.stroke.org/site/PageServer?pagename=REHABT

Paolucci, S. (2008). Epidemiology and treatment of post-stroke depression. *Neuropsychiatric Disease and Treatment, 4*(1), 145–154.

Schultz, R., & Beach, S. (1999). Caregiving as a risk factor for mortality: The caregiver health effects study. *JAMA, 282*(23), 2215–2219.

Smith, J., Forster, A., House, A., Knapp, P., Wright, J., & Young, J. (2008). Information provision for stroke patients and their caregivers. *Cochrane Database of Systematic Reviews,* (2), CD001919. doi:10.1002/14651858.CD001919.pub2

Stroke Unit Trialists' Collaboration. (2013). Organised inpatient (stroke unit) care for stroke. *Cochrane Database of Systematic Reviews,* (9), CD000197. doi:10.1002/14651858.CD000197.pub3

The Joint Commission. (2013). *Advanced disease-specific care certification requirements for comprehensive stroke center (CSC).* Retrieved from http://www.jointcommission.org/assets/1/18/dsc_csc_chap.pdf

The Schwartz Center. (2010). *Patients, doctors strongly support compassionate healthcare.* Retrieved from http://http://www.theschwartzcenter.org/media/Patients-Doctors-Strongly-Support-Compassionate-Healthcare.pdf

Tsouna-Hadjis, E., Vemmos, K. N., Zakopoulos, N., & Stamatelopoulos, S. (2000). First-stroke recovery process: The role of family social support. *Archives of Physical Medicine and Rehabilitation, 81*(7), 881–887.

U.S. Department of Labor. (2014). *The family and medical leave act.* Retrieved from http://www.dol.gov/whd/regs/compliance/whdfs28.htm

Quality, Outcomes, and the Future of Stroke

CHAPTER 12

Quality, Outcomes, and Program Evaluation for Stroke

Joanne V. Hickey and Sarah L. Livesay

The national imperatives for quality and safety in health care have further enhanced the requirement for measuring and evaluating outcomes of health care. The most commonly cited definition of quality is from an Institute of Medicine [IOM] report which defines quality as "the degree to which health services for individuals and populations increase the likelihood of desired health outcomes and are consistent with current professional knowledge" (Lohr, 1990). The purpose of this chapter is to provide an overview of quality, outcomes, and program evaluation as it applies to stroke programs and clinical, population, and system outcomes. Quality and outcomes are connected in that quality is evidenced by measurable outcomes of achievements conducive with accepted standards of practice and care. This chapter is presented in two major parts. The first part of the chapter addresses the general background information and framework for quality, outcomes, and evaluation, whereas the second part of the chapter applies those concepts specifically to stroke care and stroke programs.

■■ BRIEF HISTORY OF OUTCOMES AND QUALITY

Although Florence Nightingale (1820 to 1910) is best known as the founder of modern nursing, she also made significant contributions as a social reformer and statistician. She collected data about the Crimean War and analyzed the data to support her request for resources to alleviate the deplorable conditions in the hospital. The statistical evidence from Nightingale's mortality rates in civilian and military hospitals showed the unsanitary living conditions leading to endemic diseases. The first reported systematic use of patient outcomes to evaluate health care is attributed to Nightingale who recorded and analyzed health care conditions and patient outcomes during the Crimean War of 1853 to 1856 (Lang & Marek, 1990; Mitchell, Heinrich, Moritz, & Hinshaw, 1997). Her carefully recorded details and analysis established her as the first statistician of her time and the first reformer for quality health care.

Ernest Codman, MD, (1869 to 1940) was a Boston surgeon who was a Harvard Medical School graduate, member of the surgical staff at Massachusetts General Hospital, and faculty member at Harvard. By 1905, Codman was carrying small cards, known as *end result ideas*, for all his patients/surgeries to which he added notes about how he might improve the care in the future by systematically following the progress of patients through recovery. His interest in quality led him to examine provider competency. In 1914, the hospital refused his request to evaluate surgeon competency, and his staff privileges were revoked. The notion that quality could be improved was heresy a century ago (Mallon, 2000). Without staff privileges, he had no place to practice. Coming from a family of wealth, Codman established his own hospital and published his own end results in a privately published book. With his fervent interest in health care quality, he was a leader in founding the American College of Surgeons and its Hospital Standardization Program, which eventually became Joint Commission on Accreditation of Healthcare Organizations, now called *The Joint Commission* (TJC). An advocate for hospital reform, he crusaded to have the Massachusetts Medical Society publish a summary of his end notes in their publication, the *New England Journal of Medicine*. The request was denied. The Codman Award, the prestigious annual award for quality and safety from TJC, bears his name. Codman's work is now recognized as the beginning of quality, transparency, patient centeredness, and outcomes management (Mallon, 2000).

Quality and outcomes in health care lay dormant for the next 50 years until Avedis Donabedian (1919 to 2000) assumed the gauntlet. Donabedian was a physician and researcher at the University of Michigan and founder of the study of quality in health care and medical outcomes research. In 1966, he developed a conceptual model that provides a framework for examining health services and evaluating the quality of care (Donabedian, 1966). According to his model, information about the quality of care can be drawn from the three categories of structure, process, and outcomes. *Structure* is defined as the settings in which health care takes place and the instrumentalities of which it is the product (Donabedian, 1980). It is the conditions under which care is provided including material resources, human resources, and organizational characteristics. *Process* refers to a set of activities that go on within and between practitioners and patients (Donabedian, 1980). It is the activities encompassing health care such as diagnosis, treatment, rehabilitation, and prevention as well as the interpersonal components such as education, counseling, decision making, and other aspects of communications. *Outcome* is defined as the consequences to the health and welfare of individuals and of society (Donabedian, 1980); it is a change in a patient's current and future health that can be attributed to some alteration in delivery of health care (**Table 12-1**). The level of analysis for outcomes can be at the individual patient, organization, system, or population/community level (**Table 12-2**). Donabedian (1982) classified outcomes into the categories of clinical, physiological-biochemical, physical, psychological (mental), social and psychological, integrative, and evaluative outcomes (**Table 12-3**). This comprehensive list of outcome categories can be applied at a variety of settings and levels of analysis. Although cost is listed in the Donabedian evaluative outcomes category, it is an area that has gained major prominence because the cost of health care has escalated and is out of control; thus, economic outcomes merit further discussion in this chapter. The Donabedian model continues to be the dominant framework and paradigm for assessing quality of health care.

Outcomes at the system level of health care are also described. The Institute of Medicine (IOM) report, *Crossing the Quality Chasm: A New Health System for the 21st Century* (IOM, 2001), called for a fundamental reform of health care to ensure that

TABLE 12-1 The Structure-Process-Outcomes Trilogy

	Structure	Process	Outcomes
Definition	The setting in which health care takes place and the instrumentalities of which it is the product (Donabedian, 1966)	A set of activities that go on within and between practitioner and patients (Donabedian, 1980)	Consequences to the health and welfare of individuals and of society (Donabedian, 1980)
Components	System, material resources, provider characteristics, patient characteristics	Technical and interpersonal	Clinical end points, health-related quality of life (HRQL), satisfaction with care
Examples of Components	**System**: type of organization, specialty mix of providers, workloads of providers, model of practice and care, access and convenience for patients **Material resources**: physical space, equipment, urban versus rural setting **Provider**: specialty training and certification, preferences, job satisfaction **Patient**: diagnosis or condition, severity, comorbidity, health beliefs/habits, socioeconomic characteristics	**Technical**: encounters with practitioner, medications, therapies and treatment, diagnostics, hospitalization, rehabilitation, prevention **Interpersonal**: practitioner's communication skills, empathic counseling, interpersonal skill, patient/family education, decision making	**Clinical end points**: signs and symptoms, laboratory values, death **Signs/symptoms**: blood pressure in acceptable range, urinary output, intact gag reflex **Laboratory data**: INR, BUN/creatinine, platelet count, serum osmolality, WBC **Other**: morbidity, mortality **HRQL**: physical, mental, social, and roles; Barthel Index; MMSE; Rankin score; NIHSS **Satisfaction with care**: convenience; access; quality; general satisfaction with overall care, medical care, and nursing care; focused satisfaction with educational information, symptom relief, pain management, control of adverse treatment effects

INR, international normalized ratio; BUN, blood urea nitrogen; WBC, white blood cell; MMSE, Mini-Mental State Examination; NIHSS, National Institutes of Health Stroke Scale.

all Americans receive care that is safe, effective, patient-centered, timely, efficient, and equitable. These six aims are designed to improve the delivery of care and improve patient outcomes (**Table 12-4**). The report further notes that care should be based on the strongest clinical evidence and be provided in a technically and culturally competent manner with good communication and shared decision making (IOM, 2001). The six aims are often cited as outcome criteria for quality of health care.

Another systems framework often mentioned as criteria for evaluating outcomes of health care is the "Triple Aim" model (Berwick, Nolan, & Whittington, 2008). The Triple Aim model is a framework developed by the Institute for Healthcare Improvement (IHI) that describes an approach to optimizing health system performance. The

	Patient	Institution	System	Population/Community
TABLE 12-2 Level of Analysis for Outcomes				
Level of analysis	Clinical level; focus is on treatment of a specific patient	Organizational entity such as a hospital or clinic	Health care system as a whole; includes all of its parts in the entire region or country	Population as a whole (e.g., ischemic stroke population) or a specific community with a high incidence of stroke
Risk and illness adjustment	**General**: NIHSS **Specific**: disease staging (e.g., Hunt-Hess scale)	Severity of illness, readmission rates, percent of Medicare patients	Age, gender, comorbidity	Demographics (age, gender, education, income level)
Examples	Particular outcomes for a patient with an ischemic stroke	Number of stroke patients admitted annually	Comorbidities of stroke patients admitted to the system annually	Prevalence of stroke in community

NIHSS, National Institutes of Health Stroke Scale.

IHI believes that new models must be developed to simultaneously pursue these three dimensions, called the *Triple Aim*, which includes improving the patient's experience of care (including quality and satisfaction), improving the health of populations, and reducing the per capita cost of health care (Berwick et al., 2008). This framework has become the organizing framework for the National Quality Strategy of the U.S. Department of Health and Human Services (HHS) and for strategies of other public and private health organization such as the Centers for Medicare and Medicaid Services (CMS), Premier, and the Commonwealth Fund (Stiefel & Nolan, 2012). The IHI has worked on finding ways to operationalize and measure these outcomes. The *Guide to Measuring the Triple Aim: Population Health, Experience of Care, and Per Capita Cost* (Stiefel & Nolan, 2012) is available for those interested in learning more about measuring outcomes at the system level.

■■ MEASURES AND MEASUREMENT

The terminology used to discuss measures and measurement is confusing in that terms such as *measure*, *indicator*, *metric*, and *outcome* are used interchangeably. A *measure* (noun) is an instrument, tool, or discrete entity (e.g., age, gender) used for measuring, recording, or monitoring some form of information; for setting a standard as a basis for comparison; and as an indicator of performance, that is, a reference point against which another something can be evaluated. To measure (verb) is to bring into comparison against a standard (National Quality Forum [NQF], n.d.-b). An *indicator* is observable and measurable evidence of the effect of some intervention or action on the recipient (Ingersoll, 2009). It is a device, instrument, or other entity for measuring, recording, and monitoring some type of information, that is, a measurement tool. An indicator may be further defined by terms such as *quality indicator*, *clinical indicator*, and *economic*

TABLE 12-3 Classification of Outcomes

Category of Outcomes	Description	Examples
Clinical	• Symptoms of clinical significance • Diagnostic categories that correlates with morbidity • Disease staging that affects functionality and prognosis • Reliability of diagnostics in confirming or ruling out diagnosis	• Symptoms such as transient blindness, new onset of word finding difficulty, hemiparesis • High NIHSS score • NYHA class IV for health failure • Transcranial Doppler to determine carotid stenosis
Physiological-biochemical	• Abnormal findings of physiology or diagnostic findings • Loss of function • Level of function during test situations under various degrees of stress	• INR of 4.0 indicative of over anticoagulation • Loss of pain and heat perception in a limb • Inability to walk 50 ft on an incline
Physical	• Loss or impairment of structural form or integrity	• Abnormalities of structure such as muscle atrophy • Defects such as impaired swallowing • Disfigurement such as contracture of a limb
Psychological, mental	• Feelings • Health beliefs and values • Knowledge relevant to healthy living, health care, and coping with illness • Impairments of psychological or mental functions under circumstances of daily living and under test conditions (with various degrees of stress)	• Pain, anxiety, fear; high level of stress • Lack of information or inaccurate information • Inability to make decisions
Social and psychological	• Coping with current illness or future health includes adherence to treatment plans and changes in health-related habits • Impact on role performance (e.g., marital, familial, occupational, interpersonal) • Performance under test conditions involving varying degrees of stress	• Inability to cope and adherence to treatment plan • Inability to maintain usual roles • Altered independence in activities of daily living (ADLs) and instrumental ADLs
Integrative	• Mortality • Longevity • Longevity with adjustments for impairments of physical, psychological, or psychosocial functions • Monetary impact on longevity	• Impact of illness on life expectancy • Years of life with disabilities that limit ADLs and IADLs • Burden of cost associated with managing a disease and impact on finances
Evaluative	• Patient satisfaction with care including accessibility, continuity, thoroughness, being informed, effectiveness, and cost	• Press-Ganey patient satisfaction score • SF-36 or SF-12

NIHSS, National Institutes of Health Stroke Scale; NYHA, New York Heart Association; INR, international normalized ratio; IADLs, instrumental activities of daily living; SF-36, Short Form 36-item Health Survey Questionnaire; SF-12, Short Form 12-item Health Survey Questionnaire.
From Donabedian, A. (1982). *Explorations in quality assessment and monitoring: Vol. II. The criteria and standards of quality.* Ann Arbor, MI: Health Administration Press.

indicator for greater specificity. Although the word *metric* is more expansive than the terms *measure* and *indicator*, the terms are often used interchangeably in health care measurement.

National organizations have developed sets of quality indicators. For example, the quality indicators developed and maintained by the Agency for Healthcare Research and Quality (AHRQ) respond to the need for multidimensional and accessible quality

TABLE 12-4 Institute of Medicine Six Aims for Improved Health Care

Aim	Description
Safe	Avoiding injuries to patients from the care that is intended to help
Effective	Providing services based on scientific knowledge to all who could benefit and refraining from providing services to those not likely to benefit (avoid underuse and overuse of services respectively)
Patient-centered	Providing care that is respectful of and responsive to individual patient preferences, needs, and values and ensuring that patient values guide all clinical decisions
Timely	Reducing waits and sometimes harmful delays for both those who receive and those who give care
Efficient	Avoiding waste, including waste of equipment, supplies, ideas, and energy
Equitable	Providing care that does not vary in quality because of personal characteristics such as gender, ethnicity, geographic location, and socioeconomic status

Data from Institute of Medicine. (2001). *Crossing the quality chasm: A new health system for the 21st century.* Washington, DC: National Academies Press.

measures that can be used to gage performance in health care. These quality indicators are evidence-based and can be used to identify variations in the quality of care provided by both inpatient and outpatient facilities. These measures are currently organized as four modules: the prevention quality indicators (PQIs), the inpatient quality indicators (IQIs), the patient safety indicators (PSIs), and the pediatric quality indicators (PDIs). They are available at the AHRQ website (Quality initiatives, n.d.). According to Donabedian (1966), an *outcome* is the end point, result, or consequence of care. Some authors use terms such as *structural outcomes* or *process outcomes*; however, these are structural measures and process measures. The term *outcome* is reserved to reflect the intent of the Donabedian (1966) definition. A further discussion of measure outcomes is provided in the following text.

Types of Measures

All measures are reflective of some level of performance. *Performance measures* include measures of health care processes, patient outcomes, patient perceptions of care, and organizational structure and systems associated with the ability to provide high-quality care. *Standardized performance measures* are those measures with detailed specification (e.g., definitions of the numerator and denominator, sampling strategy, if appropriate) that allow for comparison of like data. Collected data sometimes requires risk adjustment or stratification of results across key subgroups for better interpretation of data. *Risk adjustment* is a process that modifies the analysis of performance measurement results by those element of the patient population that affect results, but are out of the control of providers, and are likely to be common and not randomly distributed (IOM, 2006). In practice, variance in outcomes across settings is common and may require risk adjustment.

Some measures have a narrow focus examining discrete performance in conducting specific tasks such as beginning antithrombotic drug therapy within 48 hours of an ischemic stroke. Other measures provide a broader view over time such as change in mobility as a result of a 3-month physical therapy program after acute care discharge. Still, other measures have a comprehensive and integrated view such as perceived quality of life. Measures can be at the patient, provider, organization, or system level and can be patient related, system related, practitioner or performance related, and cost/financial related.

Classification of Measures

Some common classes of measures include structural, process, outcome, disease specific, economic, and composite. *Structural measures* examine fixed aspects of health care delivery such as the physical plant and human resources of the facility, board certification of providers, availability of multidisciplinary team members, diagnostics testing, and interventions. *Process measures* address observable behaviors or actions that a provider undertakes to deliver care including both technical and interpersonal components. Examples are checking to see if a patient smokes and providing smoking cessation information to smokers. A process measure can be as simple as determining if an item in the process of care has or has not been completed. Process measures are useful for internal quality improvement efforts. *Outcome measures* represent health care delivery end points or results of care and are of interest to the provider and/or patient. They comprise both beneficial and adverse impacts on health care such as survival, complications, functional status, and both general and specific quality of life aspects. Outcomes are the most complex measures to collect and interpret. Improvement in outcomes is the focus of most clinical trials and evidence-based guidelines. Outcome measures are useful both for internal and external comparisons and improvement activities.

Disease-specific measures are available for a multitude of disease entities. For example, in measuring impact of specific disease processes for individual patients with back pain, the Oswestry Low Back Disability Questionnaire is useful. The Karnofsky Performance Status Measure is used to assess functional performance and independence in patients with cancer. The National Institutes of Health Stroke Scale (NIHSS) is specific for assessing neurological functional performance for stroke patients. There are also measures of overall quality of a disease-specific program. TJC has disease-specific care certification performance measurement programs for both heart failure and stroke.

The *economics measures* of health care are more complicated. *Cost* is the amount of resources used to produce or purchase an item or service. *Charges* are the amount of money an institution bills for an item or service. In health care, charges can be deceptive in that they are often discounted, making it difficult to arrive at the bottom line for health care services. There are three analyses frequently used to arrive at useful economic measures: cost–benefit analysis, cost-effectiveness analysis, and cost–utility analysis. *Cost–benefit analysis* is a type of analysis that compares the financial costs with the benefits of two or more health care treatments or programs. Health care interventions that have the same or better benefit at a lower cost are better values than treatments or programs that are more expensive. A cost–benefit analysis can help in identifying differences. *Cost-effectiveness analysis* (n.d.) is a type of analysis that is similar to a cost–benefit analysis but is applicable when the benefits cannot be measured in financial terms or dollars. For example, it is not possible to calculate a dollar value for an extra year of life (Cost-effectiveness analysis, n.d.). Measures such as quality-adjusted life years (QALYs) and disability-adjusted life years (DALYs) are used to measure impact on life. *Cost–utility analysis* is a comparison evaluation of two or more interventions in which costs are calculated in dollars and end points are calculated in quality of life units (Brosnan & Swint, 2012; Drummond, Sculpher, Torrance, O'Briend, & Stoddart, 2005). These economic analyses provide helpful information when making decisions about treatment options and expected value of care options including cost.

A new approach to examining cost of health care is Time-Driven Activity-Based Costing (TDABC), a model developed by Kaplan and Anderson (2007) for the business world, which is now being adapted to health care to improve quality and reduce costs. TDABC model requires estimates of only two parameters: (1) the unit cost of supplying capacity and (2) the time required to perform a transaction or an activity (Kaplan & Anderson, 2007). For example, in examining a patient health care encounter for an outpatient surgery, the patient can be followed from the time he or she enters the facility's door until discharge. Following the patient every step of the way can be captured on a process map to which is added the time spent in each activity as well as what personnel interacted with the patient and any material resources used. The amount of time each provider spends with the patient can be used to calculate the cost of that service (e.g., salary/hour $\times$ amount of time spent). In addition, the cost of any materials or equipment used must be calculated. The process map can be easily assembled using a number of software packages. Once the process map and costs are assembled, the team of providers who provide the services and other stakeholders can analyze the map to identify inefficiencies and waste and reconfigure a new more efficient and cost-effective process map for implementation. By comparing calculated time and costs for the before and after process maps, improved efficiency and cost saving can be calculated. The TDABC approach offers a new model for improving the efficiency and quality of care from the perspective of patients and providers while reducing cost of care, a win-win scenario for all stakeholders.

Finally, *composite measures* of overall health-related quality of life (HRQL) are available. For example, the EuroQol and the Short Form 12-item Health Survey Questionnaire (SF-12) are generic measures that provide an overall assessment of multidimensional concepts such as HRQL. Other examples of composite multidimensional measures are patient satisfaction surveys such as the Press Ganey survey and measures of functional assessment such as the Functional Independence Measure (FIM) and the Barthel Index.

Value in Health Care

Michael Porter, a recognized leader for business management, has proposed transforming health care from one of cost control to one with a focus on value creation. He notes that achieving high value for patients must become the overarching goal of health care delivery. What is important to patients should be what is important to providers and become the mutual goal of all involved in the delivery of health care, thus supporting patient centeredness. *Value* is defined as the health outcomes achieved per dollar spent (Porter & Teisberg, 2006). Porter (2010) describes value as an equation in which outcome is the numerator (e.g., condition specific and multidimensional) and cost is the denominator (e.g., total costs of a *full cycle* of care for the patient's medical condition).

In *Redefining Health Care: Creating Value-Based Competition on Results* (Porter & Teisberg, 2006), the authors summarize their observations about the current health system and their vision of an efficient, high-value system. According to Porter and Teisberg (2006), value in health care is a function of the health outcomes achieved and the health-related costs incurred *over time* for an individual. Value is not simply based on minimizing costs. Rather, it is based on maximizing outcomes and minimizing costs *over time* for persons with discrete health needs. The health outcomes realized by individuals are not dichotomous (alive or dead) but multidimensional. Health outcomes or health can be categorized into three major categories: health risk status, disease status, and functional health status (e.g., physical, mental, and social domains). The cost incurred by individuals or payers are not limited to a single event such as a surgical procedure, a hospitalization, or a clinic visit but rather include the costs of a full set of services used during a full "care cycle" for a particular health problem or condition (Nelson, Batalden, Godfrey, & Lazar, 2011).

Porter and Teisberg (2006) underscore the notion that value is created by frontline integrated practice units (e.g., interprofessional teams) who provide care to individuals with discrete health needs (e.g., cardiac disease, diabetes mellitus, colon cancer). To measure value, one must track key multidimensional outcomes of individuals and subpopulations with a given health condition during the care cycle while simultaneously tracking the dollars expended by or on behalf of those individuals. The current U.S. payment systems do not reward high-value providers. Thus, their major recommendation for the transformation of the health care system is to build an environment for value-based competition in health care. Because value is in the eyes of the beholder, the work of measuring value is challenging but making progress as the science of quality improvement and measurement mature.

MEASUREMENT

Measurement is important because it drives quality improvement; informs providers, consumers, and policy makers; and influences payment (NQF, n.d.-b). According to the NQF, measures are the only way one can really know if care is safe, efficient, effective, and patient-centered. An often used cliché about measurement is, "if you can't count (measure) it, you can't control it." Therefore, the possibility of improving outcomes is based on valid and reliable measurement techniques and data. Because many aspects of health care can be measured, how do we choose what to measure, and how do we identify the most appropriate tool for measuring the desired phenomenon? The answer to what to measure depends on what is considered the critical elements or indicators that influence quality outcomes. National organizations such as AHRQ, NQF, and TJC have created portfolios of evidence-based measures for multiple health care conditions and settings (**Box 12-1**). Other organizations have created disease-specific measures. Choosing the right tool is the second step for consideration. One searches for the most

---

Box 12-1 National Quality Forum

National Quality Forum (NQF) is a not-for-profit, nonpartisan, membership-based organization that works to catalyze improvements in health care. The NQF endorsement is considered a gold standard for health care quality. NQF-endorsed measures are evidence-based and valid and in tandem with the delivery of care and payment reform. NQF has a portfolio of endorsed performance measures that can be used to measure and quantify health care processes, outcomes, patient perceptions, and organizational structure and/or systems associated with high-quality care. Once a measure is endorsed by NQF, it can be used by hospitals, health care systems, and government agencies such as the Centers for Medicare and Medicaid Services (CMS) for public reporting and quality improvement (NQF, n.d.-a). In fact, CMS use of NQF measures is tied to reimbursement for services.

appropriate valid and reliable measure to collect the desired information. For example, to measure blood pressure, a thermometer would be useless. However, a thermometer is appropriate for measuring temperature.

Characteristics of Measures and Indicators

In choosing any measure, indicator, or tool, there are several attributes important for consideration. These attributes include that the measure/indicator is (1) based on a clear operational definition, (2) specific and sensitive to the phenomenon of interest, (3) valid and reliable, (4) one that discriminates well, (5) related to the clearly identifiable interest of the user (e.g., if meant for the provider, it is relevant to providers' practice), (6) one that permits useful comparison, and (7) evidence-based. Each measure/indicator must be clearly defined and must provide sufficient data specifications so that it can be accurately collected, analyzed, and interpreted for the intended purpose (Mainz, 2003a, 2003b).

The basic principles of measurement include addressing validity, reliability, and bias. *Validity* is the degree to which the indicator measures what it is intended to measure (i.e., the indicator accurately captures the true state of the phenomenon being measured). As applied to health care quality, a valid indicator discriminates between care that meets accepted standards and care that does not. The indicator also concurs with other measures designed to measure the same dimension of quality (Mainz, 2003a). *Reliability* is the extent to which repeated measurements of a stable phenomenon by different data collectors, judges, or instruments, at different times and places, provide similar results. In order to make comparisons among or within groups or populations over time, the characteristic of reproducibility and consistency are critical characteristic of reliability (Mainz, 2003a). There can be variations in validity and reliability of indicators, so the user must be aware of these factors. Bias is another consideration in use of measures/indicators. *Bias* is any factor, recognized or not, that distorts the findings of a study. In research studies, bias can influence the observations, results, and conclusions of the study and make results less accurate, thus threatening validity and reliability (Cost-effectiveness analysis, n.d.). For example, the origin of the bias can come from selection of patients for inclusion, the evaluator, data collection process, analytic techniques, or interpretation of results. It is clear from this brief discussion that the selection of quality measures/indicators is critical for addressing quality and outcomes in health care.

Comparing Measures and Outcomes

Information gathered from the use of measures and indicators is important to inform quality improvement work for both internal and external comparisons and benchmarking. A *benchmark* in health care refers to an attribute or achievement that serves as a standard; it may be used for other providers or institutions to emulate. Benchmarks differ from other standard care goals in that benchmarks are derived from empirical data (e.g., performance or outcomes data). For example, a statewide survey might produce risk-adjusted 30-day rates for death or other major adverse outcomes from stroke. After adjusting for relevant clinical factors, the top 10% performer hospitals can be identified based on particular outcome measures. These institutions would then provide benchmark data about these outcomes (Patient safety, n.d.). Maintaining a robust database or registry is the basis for benchmarking. Benchmarking individual results to high-performance outcomes help individuals and groups (teams) to gain a realistic picture about their current performance and gaps in quality, and it helps them to set targets for the future. Performance data are being reported using mechanisms such as scorecards, dashboards, and report cards to provide a visual snapshot of achievement on specific outcomes. These formats of comprehensive information can be the basis for informed decision making about current and future goals for practice and care. It also provides information for program evaluation.

INTERPROFESSIONAL TEAMS

What is the relevance of quality, measurement, and outcomes for the interprofessional health care team? Quality, and its inherent component of safety, is a national priority for a transformed health care system. Quality is multidimensional, and those dimensions can be measured using a variety of measures and indicators which can discriminate between best evidence-based practices and outcomes and those that are not. In order to provide the best care, thus high-quality care, interprofessional teams must integrate responsibility and accountability for outcomes management into the work of delivering care. Ellwood (1988), considered the founder of outcomes management, defined *outcomes management* as "a technology of patient experience designed to help patients, payers, and providers make rational medical care–related choices based on better insight into the effect of these choices on the patient's life." Further, he notes that this technology "consists of a common patient-understood language of health outcomes; a national database containing information and analysis on clinical, financial, and health outcomes that estimates, as best we can, the relation between medical interventions and health outcomes, as well as the relation between health outcomes and money; and an opportunity for each decision-maker to have access to the analyses that are relevant to the choices they must make." (Ellwood, 1988, p.) This description sets a framework for the work of all members of the interprofessional team and includes the following: (1) commitment, as an individual and as a team, to the mutual goal of ongoing quality management and improvement and accept responsibility and accountability for outcomes; (2) knowledge of what the key evidence-based measures or quality indicators are related to your patient population and practice; (3) understanding of how data are collected, recorded, and analyzed to appreciate the influence of validity, reliability, and bias; (4) monitoring key selected outcomes on a regular basis and over time to see trends; (5) presentation of the data in a concise format such as a scorecard for all stakeholders to easily see and understand; (6) basing of practice and care decisions on data; and (7) benchmarking with national organizations to gauge your performance. Ongoing attention to quality improvement and decreasing the cost of care are critical to transforming the current health care system into one that is value driven and patient-centered.

QUALITY AND OUTCOMES SPECIFIC TO STROKE

Part one of this chapter has addressed quality measures, indicators, outcomes, and measurement in health care as foundational information for discussion specific to stroke care and stroke programs. Part two addresses the role of quality and outcome measurement in a hospital or program focused on the care of patients with stroke. Stroke quality and outcome measurement has evolved over the past decade, as the greater health care system has turned its attention to improving care and measuring the outcome of care. The development of stroke program quality measures and outcome assessment is rooted in the development of stroke systems of care through third-party certification. External certification-guided stroke program performance improvement and measurement of outcomes has evolved to a large extent since 2003. Stroke quality and outcome measurement has also been influenced by the ongoing development of national quality programs through the CMS, commonly called *core measures*. Therefore, this section will first provide an overview of the development of national stroke quality measures influenced by TJC and CMS. Finally, current controversies complicating the measurement of stroke care quality and reporting will also be discussed.

Quality and Outcomes in Stroke Programs

Certification Standards

Disease-specific certification (DSC) is a voluntary third-party certification of a program of care within an accredited hospital. Although TJC is not the only organization providing external disease program certification, they were the first to do so and remain the largest organization in the country offering this service (TJC, 2014). The TJC also has a formal relationship with American Heart Association/American Stroke Association (AHA/ASA) and develops and revises certification requirements in conjunction with thought leaders from the AHA/ASA. Therefore, the certification remains influential nationally and is guiding the development of a stroke system of care in the United States.

The DSC certification requirements consist of a set of standards and performance measures. The first DSC certification program was offered by TJC for stroke programs in 2003, and stroke certification continues to be the largest DSC program for the organization (TJC, 2003, 2014). The DSC standards and metrics provide a health care program management infrastructure for all programs, regardless of the disease process reviewed. The standards are written with the framework of Donabedian's health care model of structure, process, and outcome. The standards, coupled with the TJC published performance metrics (a separate document), address all three areas of health care program evaluation. Many standards are general and apply to all programs regardless of the disease population managed. Standards are minimum criteria within the program that must be met. Some standards are then expanded to include elements specific to the disease managed. For example, all DSC programs must have a performance improvement program where staff monitors quality within the program and intervenes when quality or processes are compromised. Additional specificity is then provided to stroke programs by stating certain elements of the program must be monitored, such as the process and outcomes of intravenous fibrinolysis for ischemic stroke and endovascular therapies.

For stroke program certification, TJC standards are developed in conjunction with the AHA/ASA's technical advisory panel. The technical advisory panel is composed of a physician, a nurse, and other interprofessional leaders in the stroke field who provide input into TJC standards ⊙. The TJC DSC standards are revised to reflect current practice and national clinical practice guidelines every 18 to 24 months. The standards have included a performance measurement chapter since the inception of the program, establishing program quality monitoring and outcome measurement as a hallmark of certified stroke programs. With each revision, performance measurement has remained a central focus of program certification. Current standards state a program must have the following:

- An organized, comprehensive approach to performance improvement
- Develop a performance improvement plan
- Trend and compare data to evaluate processes and outcomes

- Use information garnered from measurement data to improve or validate clinical practice
- Use patient-specific, care-related data
- Evaluate the patient's perception of the quality of care
- Maintain data quality and integrity (TJC, 2014)

This attention to performance measurement and improvement in the DSC standards cemented quality and outcome measurement as a cornerstone of hospital-based stroke program over the past decade.

Certification Performance Measures

The TJC also maintains DSC performance measures in addition to minimum program standards. The performance measurements analyze either processes of care or patient outcome, whereas program standards generally address the structure of care delivered. Similar to the process for standard development, performance metrics are developed in conjunction with the AHA/ASA and reviewed every 18 to 24 months. The performance measures have evolved over the years, as clinical practice has changed based on evidence and as the technical advisory panel evaluated the metrics. With the initial stroke DSC certification in 2003, 10 performance measures were launched (**Table 12-5**) (TJC, 2008). The initial measures were all assessments of process of care, evaluating the initial emergency room treatment of the patient with ischemic stroke and the in-hospital treatment of patients with transient ischemic attack (TIA), ischemic stroke, intracerebral hemorrhage (ICH), and subarachnoid hemorrhage (SAH). Although the definitions of the numerators and denominators changed over the years between 2003 and 2009, the measures remained relatively constant. Until the late 2000s, only hospitals pursuing stroke certification were required to monitor these measures and certified centers had to report their performance to TJC. However, public reporting was not required. This changed in 2009 when the TJC stroke measures were evaluated by CMS and the NQF and became a part of the CMS Inpatient Quality Reporting program, commonly called *core measures*.

TABLE 12-5 The Joint Commission Primary Stroke Center Performance Measures: A Comparison of 2003 and 2014 Measures

2003 TJC PSC Performance Measures	2014 TJC PSC Performance Measures
STK1 Deep vein thrombosis (DVT) prophylaxis	STK1 Deep vein thrombosis (DVT) prophylaxis
STK 2 Discharged on antithrombotic therapy	STK 2 Discharged on antithrombotic therapy
STK 3 Patients with atrial fibrillation/flutter receive anticoagulation therapy	STK 3 Patients with atrial fibrillation/flutter receive anticoagulation therapy
STK 4 Thrombotic therapy administered	STK 4 Thrombotic therapy administered
STK 5 Antithrombotic therapy by end of hospital day 2	STK 5 Antithrombotic therapy by end of hospital day 2
STK 6 Discharged on statin medication	STK 6 Discharged on statin medication
STK 7 Dysphagia screening	Dropped
STK 8 Stroke education	STK 8 Stroke education
STK 9 Smoking cessation, advice, counselling	Dropped
STK 10 Assessed for rehabilitation	STK 10 Assessed for rehabilitation

TJC, The Joint Commission; PSC, primary stroke center.
From The Joint Commission. (2014). *Disease-specific care certification program: Comprehensive stroke performance measurement implementation guide.* Retrieved from http://www.jointcommission.org/assets/1/6/CSTK_Manual.pdf

Centers for Medicare and Medicaid Services Core Measures

The TJC core measure reporting program began in 1999 as an attempt to collect quality performance data from hospitals accredited by TJC. The initiative was conceptualized in the 1987 TJC's *The Agenda for Change*, an overhaul of their hospital accreditation processes (TJC, 2014). In 1995, TJC appointed the Advisory Council on Performance Measurement to evaluate a process to develop hospital performance measures. Hospitals began reporting initial performance measurement information to TJC in 1999. The initial program allowed hospitals the flexibility to select from over 100 measures, and the reported data were used for hospital accreditation purposes. This flexibility hindered comparisons of quality between hospital organizations and between providers (Goodrich, Garcia, & Conway, 2012).

Between 1999 and 2001, the national advisory panel continued to identify disease focus areas and developed a standardized measurement set to assess the quality of care provided by hospitals. Through a process of advisory panel statements, calls for public comment, and review by the national stakeholders, a set of measures were identified within three specific disease processes (acute myocardial infarction, heart failure, and community-acquired pneumonia). Once the initial measures were identified, 83 hospitals in nine states piloted the measures. A large majority of the measures were process-related, with a single measure addressing inpatient hospital mortality in one disease process. Throughout the 2000s, the measures continued to be refined. Although TJC-accredited hospitals were required to report performance data to the organization since the inception of the performance measurement program, reporting was not initially linked to reimbursement for care.

The CMS developed the Inpatient Quality Reporting (IQR) program in the early 2000s. The IQR program was initially conceptualized and mandated by the Medicare Prescription Drug, Improvement, and Modernization Act of 2003 and was meant to interface with the performance measure program in development by TJC (CMS, 2014). The IQR program collected core measure from hospitals, initially through a voluntary submission process, and eventually moving toward an incentivized submission structure. Hospitals who chose not to report receive a percentage reduction of reimbursement. Initially, hospitals received 0.4% less reimbursement in 2003. This was increased to 2% in 2005, a sizable financial penalty for hospitals that do not report their outcomes (CMS, 2014). By the mid-2000s, hospitals were required to report performance using measures that were consistent and comparable between organizations. Therefore, organizations were incentivized to use performance improvement methodology to improve performance measures and not lose CMS reimbursement.

Adoption of Stroke as a Centers for Medicare and Medicaid Services Core Measure

The stroke quality measures initially developed by TJC were only mandatory for hospitals certified by the program and were only reported to TJC between 2003 and 2009 (CMS, 2014). However, in 2009, the stroke measures were reviewed by CMS and NQF and proposed for formal adoption into the CMS IQR program (TJC, 2014). The stroke quality measures underwent moderate revision in definitions of numerators and denominators, and the measures for dysphagia screening were not endorsed by NQF. This reflected the lack of evidence, at the time, to guide programs in appropriate dysphagia screening. The organizations involved in metric review reiterated that dysphagia screening was a priority for patients with stroke. However, more evidence was necessary before screening was endorsed as a reportable metric for all hospitals across the country (**Table 12-5**). In 2010, the revised stroke metrics became a reportable core measure for hospitals across the country, regardless of certification status as a stroke center. Hospital performance on the stroke core measures were also directly linked to CMS reimbursement as a result of the measures being endorsed as CMS IQR core measures.

Addition of Comprehensive Stroke Programs

In 2012, TJC launched a second DSC certification program for comprehensive stroke centers (CSCs). CSC certification was developed for centers with the highest surgical sophistication to treat the most complicated patients with ischemic stroke, ICH, and SAH. The CSC certification was the next step in moving toward a stroke system of care in the United States (for more information on certification programs, please refer to Chapter 2, Development of Stroke Systems of Care). The CSC certification continues to move the field of stroke program outcome measurement forward. In the year prior to TJC's CSC program launch, the AHA/ASA published a 30-page analysis of possible measures of outcome and quality in a CSC (Leifer et al., 2011). One major criticism of the primary stroke center (PSC) metrics by clinicians was the focus on process measures and the lack of patient outcome measures. The AHA/ASA analysis include 26 possible focus areas for CSC quality outcome measures and included both process and patient outcome measures for each focus area. This document provided a framework for the development of the AHA/ASA and TJC's final metrics for CSC centers (**Table 12-6**).

The TJC CSC metrics were beta-tested and refined prior to finalization in 2014. The eight final metrics remain largely focused on process, with a few that directly address patient outcome after treatment (**Table 12-7**) (TJC, 2014). Additionally, the CSC standards mandate additional internal collection and analysis of patient outcome measures, including mortality and complications after procedures commonly performed at CSCs. All TJC CSC certified programs are required to submit CSC metrics to the TJC on a quarterly basis as of January 2015. As with the PSC metrics initially published in 2013, it is expected the TJC metrics will undergo continued analysis and refinement as the field responds to the metrics in public forums as well as through research and publication.

A large majority of the stroke certifications nationwide are completed by TJC. Less than 5% of programs are currently certified by Det Norske Veritas (DNV) nationally. Outcome metrics for PSC-certified organizations through DNV is similar to TJC, and the performance metrics are now endorsed at a national level by NQF and CMS. The DNV does require certified CSC programs to collect and analyze performance data and used the published analysis from AHA/ASA to guide their standard development. DNV CSC programs are required to demonstrate on annual review that they are collecting the outcome data and using performance improvement methodologies to address any areas where performance is lacking. However, DNV CSC centers are not required to report performance back to DNV at this time (DNV GL Healthcare, 2014).

Impact of Certification Standards and Metrics

The TJC and DNV certification standards and TJC metrics for performance-guided outcome measurement in stroke care in the United States over the past decade has grown. At a population level, there is evidence that the organization's care and the focus on

TABLE 12-6 AHA/ASA Summary of Metrics for Comprehensive Stroke Centers

Metric	Core Metric	Ischemic Stroke, TIA, or Asymptomatic Cerebrovascular Stenosis	SAH and Nonruptured Aneurysm	ICH and AVM (With or Without Hemorrhage)
Metric 1: Percentage of patients who have an ischemic stroke or who have a TIA with a deficit at the time of the initial admitting note or neurology consultation note for whom an NIHSS score is documented.	Yes	Ischemic stroke, TIA	...	...
Metric 2: Percentage of ischemic stroke patients eligible for intravenous thrombolysis who receive it within the appropriate time window.	Yes	Ischemic stroke seen within 4.5 h of patient last being seen at baseline	...	...
Metric 3: Percentage of patients who are treated for acute ischemic stroke with intravenous thrombolysis whose treatment is started ≤60 minutes after arrival.	Yes	Ischemic stroke treated with intravenous thrombolysis	...	...
Metric 4: Median time from arrival to start of multimodal CT or MR brain and vascular imaging (MRI/MRA or CT/CTA) for ischemic stroke patients arriving within 6 hours of the time that they were last known to be at baseline, if 1 of these studies is ordered.	Yes	Ischemic stroke seen within 6 h of patient last being known to be at baseline	...	...
Metric 5: Percentage of ischemic stroke patients seen within 6 hours of the time they were last known to be at baseline who have documentation that an endovascular recanalization procedure either was performed or was considered and deemed not to be appropriate or possible. A reason should be documented if an endovascular procedure was not performed.	No	Ischemic stroke seen within 6 h of patient last being known to be at baseline	...	...
Metric 6: Median time from arrival to start of treatment for acute ischemic stroke patients undergoing an endovascular intervention.	No	Ischemic stroke treated with endovascular intervention	...	...
Metric 7: Percentage of patients treated with intravenous thrombolysis who have symptomatic intracranial hemorrhage within 36 hours of treatment.	Yes	Ischemic stroke treated with intravenous thrombolysis	...	...
Metric 8: Percentage of acute ischemic stroke patients treated with endovascular interventions who develop significant intracranial hemorrhage within 36 hours of treatment.	Yes	Ischemic stroke treated with endovascular intervention	...	...
Metric 9: Percentage of acute ischemic stroke patients who are treated with intravenous thrombolysis or who undergo endovascular interventions for whom there is documentation of a 90-day mRS score.	Yes	Ischemic stroke treated with intravenous thrombolysis or endovascular procedure	...	...
Metric 10: Percentage of patients undergoing CEA, or carotid angioplasty or stenting, with stroke or death within 30 days of the procedure.	No	CEA or stenting	...	...

(continued)

343

TABLE 12-6 AHA/ASA Summary of Metrics for Comprehensive Stroke Centers *(continued)*

Metric	Core Metric	Ischemic Stroke, TIA, or Asymptomatic Cerebrovascular Stenosis	SAH and Nonruptured Aneurysm	ICH and AVM (With or Without Hemorrhage)
Metric 11: Percentage of patients undergoing intracranial angioplasty and/or stenting for atherosclerotic disease with stroke or death within 30 days of the procedure.	No	Intracranial angioplasty and/or stenting	…	…
Metric 12: Percentage of SAH, ICH, and AVM patients for whom initial severity measures are documented.	Yes	…	Hunt and Hess scale if SAH	ICH score if ICH (whether or not AVM); Spetzler-Martin for all AVM
Metric 13: Median time from admission to start of procedure intended to obliterate a ruptured aneurysm by surgical clipping or endovascular coiling for patients who arrive within 48 hours of the hemorrhage that led directly to admission.	Yes	…	SAH	…
Metric 14: Percentage of patients with aneurysmal SAH arriving within 48 hours of hemorrhage for whom a coiling or clipping procedure was not started within 36 hours of arrival who have a documented reason for not having undergone coiling or clipping within 36 hours of arrival.	No	…	SAH	…
Metric 15: Percentage of patients with documented aneurysmal SAH for whom nimodipine treatment (60 mg every 4 hours or 30 mg every 2 hours) is stared within 24 hours of diagnosis and for whom such treatment is continued until 21 days after the hemorrhage or until discharge if they are discharge <21 days after the SAH.	Yes	…	SAH	…
Metric 16: Percentage of SAH patients with diminished level of consciousness and ventriculomegaly who are treated with EVD.	No	…	SAH	…
Metric 17: Median frequency of noninvasive monitoring performed for surveillance for vasospasm in patients with aneurysmal SAH during the period between 3 days after SAH.	No	…	…	…
Metric 18: Complication rates for aneurysm coiling and clipping.	No	…	All	…
Metric 19: Median time from arrival to start of treatment to reverse the INR with a procoagulant preparation (eg, fresh frozen plasma, recombinant factor VIIa, prothrombin complex concentrates) for patients with warfarin-associated ICH and an elevated INR (INR >1.4).	Yes	…	…	ICH (if warfarin-associated)

Metric				...	...	AVM
Metric 20: Percentage of patients undergoing surgical or endovascular treatment of an AVM with stroke or death within 30 days of the procedure.	No					
Metric 21: Percentage of patients with ischemic or hemorrhagic stroke or TIA transferred from another hospital to the CSC with documentation of the time from the first call from the transferring hospital to the CSC (to a member of a stroke program or to a centralized transfer center) to arrival time at the CSC.	No		All patients transferred from another hospital		All patients transferred from another hospital	All patients transferred from another hospital
Metric 22: Percentage of patients admitted to each type of unit to which patients with ischemic or hemorrhagic stroke or TIA are initially admitted (eg, neurological/neurosurgical ICU, medical ICU, surgical ICU, general ICU, coronary care unit, burn ICU, stroke unit, other intermediate-level-of-care unit, neurology floor, or other floor). A separate percentage should be calculated for each type of unit.	No		All		All	All
Metric 23: Percentage of patients with stroke or death within 24 hours of diagnostic neuroangiography.	Yes		If diagnostic angiogram is performed		If diagnostic angiogram is performed	If diagnostic angiogram is perfromed
Metric 24: Percentage of patients who have a diagnosis of ischemic or hemorrhagic stroke who undergo EVD and then develop ventriculitis.	No		If patient has EVD		If patient has EVD	If patient has EVD
Metric 25: Median number of days from admission to completion of evaluations for physical therapy, occupational therapy, speech-language pathology, and rehabilitation medicine, unless there is documentation on admission that some or all of these evaluations are not needed or that the patient cannot tolerate them because of medical instability.	No		All		All	All
Metric 26: Percentage of patients admitted with diagnoses of ischemic stroke, SAH, intracranial hemorrhage, extracranial cervical stenosis, intracranial stenosis, or TIA who are enrolled in a clinical research study.	No		All		All	All

AHA, American Heart Association; ASA, American Stroke Association; TIA, transient ischemic attack; SAH, subarachnoid hemorrhage; ICH, intracerebral hemorrhage; AVM, arteriovenous malformation; NIHSS, National Institutes of Health Stroke Scale; CT, computed tomography; MR, magnetic resonance; MRI, magnetic resonance imaging; MRA, magnetic resonance angiography; CTA, computed tomography angiography; mRS, modified Rankin Scale; CEA, carotid endarterectomy; EVD, external ventricular drain; INR, international normalized ratio; CSC, comprehensive stroke center; ICU, intensive care unit.

From Leifer, D., Bravata, D. M., Connors, J. J., III, Hinchey, J. A., Jauch, E. C., Johnston, S. C., . . . Zorowitz, R. (2011). Metrics for measuring quality of care in comprehensive stroke centers: Detailed follow-up to Brain Attack Coalition comprehensive stroke center recommendations: A statement for healthcare professionals from the American Heart Association/American Stroke Association. *Stroke, 42*(3), 849–877. doi:10.1161 /STR.0b013e318208eb99

TABLE 12-7 The Joint Commission 2014 Comprehensive Stroke Center Performance Measures

National Institutes of Health Stroke Scale (NIHSS) performed for ischemic stroke patients
Modified Rankin Score (mRS at 90 days)
Severity measurement performed for patients with SAH and ICH
Procoagulant reversal agent initiation for ICH
Hemorrhagic transformation after intravenous thrombolysis or endovascular treatment
Nimodipine treatment administered in SAH
Median time to endovascular revascularization
Thrombolysis in cerebral infarction measured by TICI reperfusion grade

SAH, subarachnoid hemorrhage; ICH, intracerebral hemorrhage; TICI, thrombolysis in cerebral infarction.
From The Joint Commission. (2014). *Disease-specific care certification program: Comprehensive stroke performance measurement implementation guide.* Retrieved from http://www.jointcommission.org/assets/1/6/CSTK_Manual.pdf

outcome measurement and performance improvement at an organizational level have impacted national stroke demographics. This impact is measured through both access to care, delivery of care, and patient outcomes. Over the past decade since stroke DSC certification began, a larger number of patients have access to organized stroke care nationally. As of 2010, over half of the residents in the United States live in counties where emergency medical services personnel are trained to recognize stroke and route the patient to a certified stroke center (Gorelick, 2013).

As a result of certification and DSC performance metrics, more patients are receiving organized stroke care and certification is associated with improved performance outcomes. A 2009 analysis of the *Get with the Guidelines-Stroke* (GWTG-S) database demonstrated significant improvement in hospital performance of stroke-related care between 2003 and 2009 (**Fig. 12-1**) (Schwamm et al., 2009). The study analyzed 322,847 in-hospital stroke records entered into the database. Improvement was noted in all PSC stroke metrics over the 6-year reporting period. For example, hospitals reporting administration of thrombolysis for appropriate patients with ischemic stroke improved from 42% in 2003 to 73% in 2009. This analysis was conducted before the CMS IQR adoption of the stroke measures as core measures. Therefore, it is reasonable to expect performance in these metric areas has only continued to improve. However, analysis will need to be conducted in the coming years to evaluate the impact of CMS IQR adoption of the stroke measures as core measures.

Improvement in stroke care processes has also been noted in the past several years with the development of CSC quality programs and CSC program certification, although evaluation is ongoing. The development of national metrics, in conjunction with organized care and program certification, is associated with the improvement of time to treatment for intravenous thrombolysis and timeliness of endovascular services as well (Gorelick, 2013). The development of performance metrics with certification standards emphasizing the role of performance improvement in stroke programs has clearly driven the measurement of outcomes in stroke programs throughout the United States (Gorelick, 2013).

Databases

In 2005, the AHA/ASA set forth an agenda to create a U.S. stroke system of care. The care model included the development of a national registry for patients with stroke

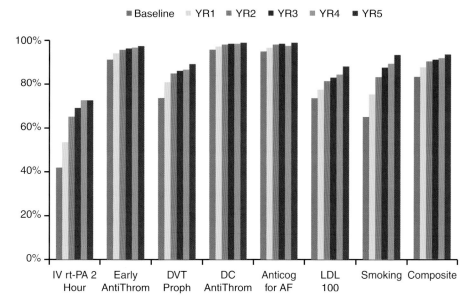

FIGURE 12-1 Sustained stroke performance improvement, 2003–2009. Improvement over time in GWTG-Stroke displayed as the percentage of eligible patients who received each evidence-based measure per program year. Composite measure was defined as the total number of interventions provided in eligible patients divided by the total number of possible interventions in eligible patients. *IV*, intravenous; *rt-PA*, recombinant tissue plasminogen activator; *antithrom*, antithrombotics; *DVT*, deep vein thrombosis; *proph*, prophylaxis; *DC*, discharge; *anticog*, anticoagulation; *AF*, atrial fibrillation; *LDL*, low-density lipoprotein. *(Schwamm, L. H., Fonarow, G. C., Reeves, M. J., Pan, W., Frankel, M. R., Smith, E. E., . . . Labresh, K. A. (2009). Get with the guidelines --Stroke is associated with sustained improvement in care for patients hospitalized with acute stroke or transient ischemic attack. Circulation, 119(1), 107 -115. doi:10.1161/CIRCULATIONAHA.108.783688)*

(Schwamm et al., 2005). Programs during the initial years of stroke certification largely used an internally developed database to track stroke performance metrics. As the patient populations grew and the stroke performance metric numerator, denominator, and patient population grew more complicated, many organizations began purchasing database access from third-party vendors. The largest stroke database available to track outcomes is the AHA/ASA GWTG-S database. Over 1,700 hospitals currently participate in GWTG-S and represent over 2.5 million patient encounters as of May 2013 (AHA & ASA, 2013). Participating hospitals include academic and nonacademic facilities from both rural and urban geographical locations. The GWTG-S registry has provided the platform for multiple database research studies evaluating the impact of stroke program development on patient outcomes as well as the geographic distribution and disparities of stroke and stroke care across the nation (Allen et al., 2011; Fonarow et al., 2011; Schwamm et al., 2009).

The second largest stroke database available to organizations is the Paul Coverdell National Acute Stroke Registry. The database started as a state registry for Georgia developed in 2001 in memory of Senator Paul Coverdell who died of a stroke the year before. The Coverdell registry is funded by the Centers for Disease Control and Prevention (CDC). After funding a 3-year pilot period in Georgia, the Coverdell registry was expanded to 11 states and continues to be primarily funded through the CDC. The registry serves as a model for the development of state-based stroke databases to help measure quality and performance and also to guide the development of regional stroke systems of care (CDC, 2009). The New Jersey disease registry Myocardial Infarction Data Acquisition System (MIDAS) has also been expanded to include stroke disease performance database elements and is used at some facilities across the nation (Robert Wood Johnson Medical School, 2014).

◼◼ STROKE PERFORMANCE AND QUALITY CONTROVERSIES

Quality and outcome measurement in the United States has been largely influenced by external program certification by organizations such as TJC and DNV and the subsequent development of performance metrics. Although this has positively influenced stroke care, the current state of stroke quality, outcome, and program evaluation is both incomplete and controversial. Although an organized performance improvement and program evaluation is required for certified stroke programs, only approximately 36% of hospitals in the United States are certified. Therefore, a majority of hospitals are not mandated to have an organized approach to evaluation of outcomes for patients with stroke. There are also concerns that although progress has been made in the evaluation of stroke outcomes, the current system across the nation is incomplete.

Performance Measures and Patient Outcomes

Although the TJC and CMS performance measures for stroke are tested for validity and reliability across multiple centers, some continue to question if the measures are accurate reflections of both program performance and the care delivered to the individual stroke patient (Poisson & Josephson, 2011). Overall, national mortality for stroke has declined. The reasons for the decline are multifactorial, and the organization of care at the hospital level is thought to be a major contributor. However, linking performance measured by the metrics to improved patient outcome within a single hospital is difficult using the PSC performance measures. The link between performance measures and improved patient outcomes may be more evident with the CSC measures that include patient outcome measures in addition to process outcome measures. However, more time is needed to adequately assess the impact of the CSC performance measures.

A major concern in measuring stroke program and patient outcomes is that improvements in hospital processes may or may not improve the actual patient outcomes (Parker, Schwamm, Fonarow, Smith, & Reeves, 2012). Even studies that demonstrate a positive association between improved process measure compliance and patient outcomes advise caution regarding overinterpreting results (Parker et al., 2012). For example, screening a patient for a swallow dysfunction is an evaluation of program process and structure. However, it does not necessarily reflect the patient outcome. The patient outcome would be best measured by monitoring aspiration pneumonia rates in the same patient population. Coupling the process measure with the patient outcome gives a more accurate picture of the quality of the program as it relates to swallow assessment. But most programs are not monitoring both the assessment of the process as well as the patient outcome. This leads to the concern that programs are not able to assess the end impact of their processes. Although the CSC performance measures include several patient outcome measures, the process-based measures have yet to be analyzed to determine if improvement in process yields improvement in patient outcomes.

Public Reporting

Overall, efforts to improve transparency and access to health care quality data are gaining traction nationally (Kelly, Thompson, Tuttle, Benesch, & Holloway, 2008). Given the concern that current national stroke process measures may not accurately reflect the quality of care delivered by a program or the actual impact on patient outcome, there has been resistance to public reporting of stroke metrics (Parker et al., 2012). Studies evaluating the outcome data available for stroke program structure, process, outcome, finances, and usage suggest that available data is fraught with inaccuracy and variability (Kelly et al., 2008). Definitions are often either inaccurate or poorly defined, leading to difficulty when comparing organizations. Therefore, moving quickly to allow the general public access to much of the data currently collected and reported on stroke care in programs and patient outcomes after stroke may have unintended consequences (Kelly et al., 2008). This is of concern particularly if the definitions and mechanism for reporting isn't regulated and is used as a marketing tool by stroke programs motivated to shift the local market share.

Risk Adjustment and In-Hospital Mortality

The CMS has attempted to include in-hospital mortality and readmission rates as reportable measures as a part of the CMS IQR system (CMS, 2013). This has been met with considerable opposition by stroke clinicians due to concern that the proposed measures lacked a methodology to risk-adjust the report. Centers caring for the most acutely ill stroke patients, such as CSCs, would likely have a higher mortality rate due to the higher acuity. Without risk adjustment, CSCs would bear a higher financial penalty for having higher mortality. The role of in-hospital mortality as an outcome measure for clinical trials as well as reimbursement has been questioned by many clinicians in the stroke field (Parker et al., 2012). Currently, CMS is slated to begin collecting in-hospital mortality and readmission rates in 2016. How the rates will reflect patient acuity remains to be seen.

Centers for Medicare and Medicaid Services Hospital-Acquired Events

As CMS has evaluated compromised safety and quality events in the hospital setting, they developed a list of hospital-acquired events (HAEs) or conditions that are considered avoidable and should never occur. The HAE span diseases and care settings within the hospital and include operative events such as wrong-site surgery and postoperative respiratory failure, infection from indwelling catheters or sepsis, as well as in-hospital falls and skin breakdown or pressure sores. The list is commonly referred to as *never events*. After a period of monitoring, CMS now withholds reimbursement in certain circumstances if these events occur during a hospitalization. However, determining risk at a disease-specific level for HAEs is both difficult and controversial (Rahman, Neal, Fargen, & Hoh, 2013). Many organizations choose to address HAE at a hospital level rather than at a disease-specific level. Recent analyses demonstrate that stroke patients are at higher risk for specific HAEs, including fall and stage III and IV pressure ulcer development (Rahman et al., 2013). Given the natural disease course for stroke, the risk of fall from cognitive impairment and disability and pressure ulcer formation from immobility appear appropriate. However, stroke programs are not routinely monitoring and reporting these outcomes, and these HAEs are not often included in DSC program review. As the CMS HAE program continues to develop, stroke programs may reasonably be required to monitor these rates and lead performance improvement projects in these areas when appropriate.

Incomplete Quality Assessment

Perhaps of greatest concern in the overall discussion of measuring quality, outcomes, and stroke program evaluation is the lack of a comprehensive approach to measuring performance and outcomes. A comprehensive assessment of stroke care quality and outcomes include evaluation of the structure of care, processes of care, patient-level outcomes, and economic outcomes at the program level as well as regionally and nationally. The current state of stroke quality and outcome assessment at the program and national level is incomplete, representing only pieces of a comprehensive analysis. Assessment of stroke quality and outcomes will become increasingly complex as additional national initiatives aimed at cost containment are implementing such as the meaningful use initiative for electronic health records (EHRs) and CMS's value-based purchasing initiative. To date, the largest driver of stroke program quality improvement and performance measurement has been external certification. A broader approach to program evaluation and patient outcome assessment would provide a more accurate picture of quality and outcome.

SUMMARY

Although the national imperatives for quality and safety in health care have driven enhanced measurement and evaluation of health care outcomes, the full implementation of this goal within stroke care has yet to be achieved. A long-rooted history of health care quality and outcome measurement, coupled with more recent attention to the shortcomings of hospital safety and quality, has driven forward the national agenda for monitoring and improving hospital quality. External certification of stroke has provided significant influence on the current state of program evaluation and outcome measurement. The addition of CSC centers and additional external forces including health care reform and an incomplete system for assessing quality and outcome in stroke care will continue to shape program development and evaluation in the years to come.

REFERENCES

Allen, L. A., Hernandez, A. F., Peterson, E. D., Curtis, L. H., Dai, D., Masoudi, F. A., . . . Fonarow, G. C. (2011). Discharge to a skilled nursing facility and subsequent clinical outcomes among older patients hospitalized for heart failure. *Circulation Heart Failure, 4*(3), 293–300. doi:10.1161/CIRCHEARTFAILURE.110.959171

American Heart Association & American Stroke Association. (2013). *Get with the guidelines—stroke registry.* Retrieved from http://www.heart.org/idc/groups/heart-public/@wcm/@adv/documents/downloadable /ucm_438049.pdf

Berwick, D. M., Nolan, T. W., & Whittington, J. (2008). The triple aim: Care, cost, and quality. *Health Affairs, 27*(3), 759–769.

Brosnan, C. A., & Swint, M. (2012). Economic evaluation. In J. V. Hickey & C. A. Brosnan (Eds.), *Evaluation of health care quality in advanced practice nursing* (pp. 73–96). New York, NY: Springer Publishing.

Centers for Disease Control and Prevention. (2009). *Paul Coverdell National Acute Stroke Registry: Strategies from the field.* Retrieved from http://www.cdc.gov/dhdsp/docs/coverdell_strategies_from_the_field.pdf

Centers for Medicare and Medicaid Services. (2013). *Fact sheets: CMS final rule to improve quality of care during hospital inpatient stays*. Retrieved from http://www.cms.gov/newsroom/mediareleasedatabase /fact-sheets/2013-fact-sheets-items/2013-08-02-3.html

Centers for Medicare and Medicaid Services. (2014). *Hospital inpatient quality reporting program*. Retrieved from https://www.cms.gov/Medicare/Quality-Initiatives-Patient-Assessment-Instruments/HospitalQualityInits /HospitalRHQDAPU.html

Cost-effectiveness analysis. (n.d.). In *AHRQ effective health care program glossary of terms*. Retrieved from http://effectivehealthcare.ahrq.gov/glossary-of-terms/?filterletter=c

DNV GL Healthcare. (2014). *Comprehensive stroke center certification*. Retrieved from http://dnvglhealthcare .com/certifications/comprehensive-stroke-center-certification

Donabedian, A. (1966). Evaluating the quality of medical care. *The Milbank Memorial Fund Quarterly, 44*(Pt. 2), 166–206.

Donabedian, A. (1980). *Explorations in quality assessment and monitoring: Vol. 1. The definition of quality and approaches to its assessment*. Ann Arbor, MI: Health Administration Press.

Donabedian, A. (1982). *Explorations in quality assessment and monitoring: Vol. 2. The criteria and standards of quality*. Ann Arbor, MI: Health Administration Press.

Drummond, M. F., Sculpher, M. J., Torrance, G. W., O'Briend, B. J., & Stoddart, G. L. (2005). *Methods for the economic evaluation of health care programmes*. Oxford, United Kingdom: Oxford University Press.

Ellwood, P. M. (1988). Shattuck lecture—outcomes management. A technology of patient experience. *The New England Journal of Medicine, 318*, 1549–1556.

Fonarow, G. C., Smith, E. E., Reeves, M. J., Pan, W., Olson, D., Hernandez, A. F., . . . Schwamm, L. H. (2011). Hospital-level variation in mortality and rehospitalization for medicare beneficiaries with acute ischemic stroke. *Stroke, 42*(1), 159–166. doi:10.1161/STROKEAHA.110.601831

Goodrich, K., Garcia, E., & Conway, P. H. (2012). A history and vision for CMS quality measurement programs. *Joint Commission Journal on Quality and Patient Safety, 38*(11), 465–470.

Gorelick, P. B. (2013). Primary and comprehensive stroke centers: History, value and certification criteria. *Journal of Stroke, 15*(2), 78–89. doi:10.5853/jos.2013.15.2.78

Ingersoll, G. L. (2009). Outcome evaluation and performance: An integrative review of research on advanced practice nursing. In A. B., Hamric, J. A. Spross, & C. M. Hansen (Eds.), *Advanced practice nursing: An integrative approach* (4th ed.). St. Louis, MO: Saunders Elsevier.

Institute of Medicine. (2001). *Crossing the quality chasm: A new health system for the 21st century*. Washington, DC: National Academies Press.

Institute of Medicine. (2006). *Performance measurement: Accelerating improvement*. Washington, DC: National Academies Press.

Kaplan, R. S., & Anderson, S. R. (2007). *Time driven activity-based costing: A simpler and more powerful path to higher profits*. Boston, MA: Harvard Business School Press.

Kelly, A., Thompson, J. P., Tuttle, D., Benesch, C., & Holloway, R. G. (2008). Public reporting of quality data for stroke: Is it measuring quality? *Stroke, 39*(12), 3367–3371. doi:10.1161/STROKEAHA.108.518738

Lang, N. M., & Marek, K. D. (1990). The classification of patient outcomes. *Journal of Professional Nursing, 6*, 153–163.

Leifer, D., Bravata, D. M., Connors, J. J., III, Hinchey, J. A., Jauch, E. C., Johnston, S. C., . . . Zorowitz, R. (2011). Metrics for measuring quality of care in comprehensive stroke centers: Detailed follow-up to Brain Attack Coalition comprehensive stroke center recommendations: A statement for healthcare professionals from the American Heart Association/American Stroke Association. *Stroke, 42*(3), 849–877. doi:10.1161 /STR.0b013e318208eb99

Lohr, K. N. (Eds.). (1990). *Medicare: A strategy for quality assurance*. Washington, DC: The National Academies Press.

Mainz, J. (2003a). Defining and classifying clinical indicators for quality improvement. *International Journal for Quality in Health Care, 15*(6), 523–530.

Mainz, J. (2003b). Developing clinical indicators. *International Journal of Quality Health Care, 15*(Suppl. 1), i5–i11.

Mallon, W. J. (2000). *Ernest Amory Codman: The end result of a life in medicine*. Philadelphia, PA: Saunders.

Mitchell, P. H., Heinrich, J., Moritz, P., & Hinshaw, A. S. (Eds.). (1997). Outcome measures and care delivery systems conference. *Medical Care, 35*(11, Suppl.), NS1–NS5.

National Quality Forum. (n.d.-a). *Measuring performance*. Retrieved from http://www.qualityforum.org /Measuring_Performance/Measuring_Performance.aspx

National Quality Forum. (n.d.-b). *The ABCs of measurement*. Retrieved from http://www.qualityforum.org /Measuring_Performance/ABCs_of_Measurement.aspx

Nelson, E. C., Batalden, P. B., Godfrey, M. M., & Lazar, J. S. (Eds.). (2011). *Value by design: Developing clinical microsystems to achieve organizational excellent*. San Francisco, CA: Jossey-Bass.

Parker, C., Schwamm, L. H., Fonarow, G. C., Smith, E. E., & Reeves, M. J. (2012). Stroke quality metrics: Systematic reviews of the relationships to patient-centered outcomes and impact of public reporting. *Stroke, 43*(1), 155–162. doi:10.1161/STROKEAHA.111.635011

Patient safety. (n.d.). In *AHRQ patient safety network glossary*. Retrieved from http://psnet.ahrq.gov/glossary .aspx?indexLetter=P

Poisson, S. N., & Josephson, S. A. (2011). Quality measures in stroke. *Neurohospitalist, 1*(2), 71–77. doi:10.1177/1941875210392052

Porter, M. E. (2010). What is value in health care? *New England Journal of Medicine, 363*(26), 2477–2481.

Porter, M., & Teisberg, E. O. (2006). *Redefining health care: Creating value-based competition on results.* Boston, MA: Harvard Business School Press.

Quality initiatives. (n.d.) In *AHRQ quality indicator glossary*. Retrieved from http://www.qualityindicators .ahrq.gov/

Rahman, M., Neal, D., Fargen, K. M., & Hoh, B. L. (2013). Establishing standard performance measures for adult stroke patients: A nationwide inpatient sample database study. *World Neurosurg, 80*(6), 699.e2–708. e2. doi:10.1016/j.wneu.2013.08.024

Robert Wood Johnson Medical School. (2014). *MIDAS—Myocardial Infarction Data Acquisition System.* Retrieved from http://rwjms.rutgers.edu/cvinj/Research/MIDAS_1.html

Schwamm, L. H., Fonarow, G. C., Reeves, M. J., Pan, W., Frankel, M. R., Smith, E. E., . . . Labresh, K. A. (2009). Get with the guidelines—Stroke is associated with sustained improvement in care for patients hospitalized with acute stroke or transient ischemic attack. *Circulation, 119*(1), 107–115. doi:10.1161 /CIRCULATIONAHA.108.783688

Schwamm, L. H., Pancioli, A., Acker, J. E., III, Goldstein, L. B., Zorowitz, R. D., Shephard, T. J., . . . Adams, R. J. (2005). Recommendations for the establishment of stroke systems of care: Recommendations from the American Stroke Association's Task Force on the Development of Stroke Systems. *Circulation, 111*(8), 1078–1091. doi:10.1161/01.CIR.0000154252.62394.1E

Stiefel, M., & Nolan, K. (2012). *A guide to measuring the triple aim: Population health, experience of care, and per capita cost.* Cambridge, MA: Institute for Healthcare Improvement. Retrieved from http://www .ihi.org/resources/Pages/IHIWhitePapers/AGuidetoMeasuringTripleAim.aspx

The Joint Commission. (2003). *A comprehensive review of development and testing for national implementation of hospital core measures.* Retrieved from http://www.jointcommission.org/assets/1/18/A_Comprehensive _Review_of_Development_for_Core_Measures.pdf

The Joint Commission. (2008). *Disease-specific care certification program: Stroke performance measurement implementation guide* (2nd ed., Version 2.a). Retrieved from http://www.jointcommission.org/assets/1/18 /stroke_pm_implementation_guide_ver_2a.pdf

The Joint Commission. (2014). *Disease-specific care certification program: Comprehensive stroke performance measurement implementation guide.* Retrieved from http://www.jointcommission.org/assets/1/6/CSTK_Manual.pdf

CHAPTER 13

The Future of Stroke Care

Sarah L. Livesay and Joanne V. Hickey

◼ INTRODUCTION

As stroke care has changed rapidly over the last several decades, we continue to progress and are on the precipice of major change both in stroke care as well as health care. Several looming developments will impact the care of stroke patients in the short term, including clinical research, technological advances both in health care and other industries, and health care reform in the United States. Beyond the more immediate impact of developments in progress, the rapid pace of technological development and its adaptation to health care will undoubtedly impact the future of stroke patient management. This chapter will review the rapid evolution of stroke care over the past decades, the projected stroke patient population of the future, and the current and anticipated developments in the understanding and management of stroke at the individual and population levels.

Rapid Evolution of Stroke Care

The scientific and empirical bases for understanding stroke pathophysiology, treatment, and recovery have evolved at an astounding pace over the past three decades. As thrombolysis changed the entire paradigm of ischemic stroke treatment in the late 1990s, and intra-arterial treatment options for ischemic stroke and subarachnoid hemorrhage (SAH) evolved in the 2000s, stroke researchers and practitioners are expected to continue to rapidly produce research to guide individual and population-level interventions to improve outcomes for patients after stroke. Stroke caregivers and program leaders must work to remain current in their understanding of the science of stroke care and integrate new knowledge and best practices into the evidence-based care that supports optimal patient and population outcomes.

Clinical practice guidelines (CPGs) published and used throughout the world play a critical role in synthesizing current evidence and best practice and serve to guide stroke program organization and individual clinical care. A discerning caregiver should review CPGs with a critical eye. A review and recommendations on CPG trustworthiness conducted by the Institute of Medicine (IOM) in 2011 observed that the adoption of evidence-based medicine has resulted in over 3,700 guidelines from more than 39 countries (IOM, 2011). However, not all guidelines are created using the same degree of rigor. The trustworthiness of CPGs may be hindered by lack of transparency in the goal and methodology of guideline preparation and undisclosed real or potential biases or conflicts of interest from authors. Several tools are available to help evaluate the quality of a CPG, including the IOM guideline review tool, the Appraisal of Guidelines for Research and Evaluation (AGREE), the Cluzeau Appraisal Instrument, and Shaneyfelt Methodological Standards Tool (IOM, 2011).

Guidelines should be evaluated for their trustworthiness and applicability to clinical practice. Recommendations from the 2011 IOM Committee on Standards for Developing Clinical Practice Guidelines advise that guidelines should (IOM, 2011):

- Be based on a systematic review of the existing evidence
- Be developed by a knowledgeable, multidisciplinary panel of experts and representatives from key affected groups
- Consider important patient subgroups and patient preferences, as appropriate;
- Be based on an explicit and transparent process that minimizes distortions, bias, and conflicts of interest
- Provide a clear explanation of the logical relationships between alternative care options and health outcomes
- Provide ratings of both the quality of evidence and the strength of the recommendation
- Be reconsidered and revised, as appropriate, when important new evidence warrants modifications of recommendations.

In addition to disease-specific CPGs, other forms of recommendations provided by credible sources influence practice by addressing preventive services. For example, the U.S. Preventive Services Task Force (USPSTF) recently published a recommendation on screening for asymptomatic carotid artery stenosis. The USPSTF recommends against screening for asymptomatic carotid artery stenosis in the general adult population (LeFevre, 2014). It based its recommendation on the evidence of both the benefits and harm of the service and an assessment of the balance; it does not consider the cost of the service. The USPSTF uses a five-level grading scale from A to D, with A representing recommendation of the service and that there is high certainty that the net benefit is substantial. The grade of D represents a recommendation against the service and the statement that there is moderate or high certainty that the service has no net benefit or that the harms outweigh the benefits (LeFevre, 2014). The scale also includes an "I statement" which says that the USPSTF concludes that the current evidence is insufficient to assess the balance of benefits and harm. The recommendation against screening for asymptomatic carotid artery stenosis was a grade D recommendation. Practitioners should monitor guidelines in their area of practice to say abreast of changes in recommendations.

FORECASTING THE FUTURE OF STROKE

Global Burden of Stroke

A recent review of over 20 years of publications addressing the global burden of stroke revealed the startling impact of stroke beyond the United States. Whereas stroke is the fourth leading cause of death in the United States, stroke is the second leading cause of death and the leading cause of disability worldwide (Mukherjee & Patil, 2011). Although compiling epidemiological statistics for stroke spanning the globe is difficult, statistics from the World Health Organization (WHO) estimate that stroke accounts for more than 5.5 million deaths each year (Mukherjee & Patil, 2011). This number is expected to rise significantly by 2030, with an estimated 7.8 million deaths attributed to stroke.

Global stroke-related mortality reveals fluctuating outcomes according to a country's income and prosperity. Projected stroke death rates in well-developed countries such as the United States and western European countries are similar and expected to remain relatively flat or even decline slightly over the next several decades (Mukherjee & Patil, 2011). However, stroke-related mortality rates in low- and middle-income countries are expected to increase significantly. For stroke in all age groups worldwide, approximately 85% of current global deaths from stroke occur in low- and middle-income countries. The number climbs to over 90% for stroke victims older than the age of 70 years.

The factors contributing to the tremendous global impact of stroke and disproportionate mortality burden seen in low- and middle-income countries are multifactorial and complex (Mukherjee & Patil, 2011; Ovbiagele et al., 2013). The lack of primary and secondary prevention strategies to address risk factors as well as the lack of organized stroke care is thought to be major factors impacting global stroke mortality. The global aging population also contributes to the overall stroke prevalence. Low- and middle-income countries often lack the primary care infrastructure to detect and treat hypertension, smoking, and diabetes mellitus, significant risk factors that contribute to the development of stroke.

Additionally, when stroke occurs, these countries lack the emergency medical service (EMS) response infrastructure to identify and facilitate timely treatment (Mukherjee & Patil, 2011). Even once stroke is identified, current best practice for stroke dictate the administration of thrombolytics for ischemic stroke and neurosurgical intervention for conditions in all stroke types. Thrombolysis for ischemic stroke is costly and requires specialist care. Most low- and middle-income countries lack a structure for administering thrombolytics as well as the neurosurgical and critical care infrastructure to care for stroke patients. Low- and middle-income countries often do not have neurology or neurosurgical subspecialty–trained practitioners.

Researchers postulate that primary care and prevention may be more sustainable and cost-effective as an initial initiative in low- and middle-income countries than building a treatment EMS infrastructure (Ovbiagele et al., 2013). Although this is a reasonable recommendation for policy planning, several countries such as India, China, Brazil, and Argentina have demonstrated positive steps to address both prevention and acute emergency response. As the United States and the more developed countries in Western Europe continue to develop new interventions to treat patients with stroke and new systems of care to improve overall stroke outcomes, the feasibility and sustainability of such efforts on a global scale must be considered.

United States Burden of Stroke

Stroke Statistics and Disparities

A recent analysis by the American Stroke Association projects the U.S. prevalence of stroke to increase to 3.4 million individuals in 2030 compared to 2012 statistics (Ovbiagele et al., 2013). The aging population in the United States plays a key role in this growth, as overall stroke incidence and mortality has declined in recent years. However, stroke is a disease primarily of the aged, and as the baby boomer generation ages into the 60s, the overall prevalence of stroke is expected to increase. An estimated 4% of the U.S. population will have survived a stroke in the year 2030, a statistic largely impacted by the falling mortality and improved stroke survival outcomes seen in recent years. This increase in stroke survivorship is expected to significantly impact the U.S. health care system and economy.

Further analysis of the U.S. statistics reveals the nation is experiencing its own disparities, and not all populations experience the decreased mortality and increased stroke survivorship seen at a national level (Ovbiagele et al., 2013). Stroke-related mortality is higher for the very old (>80 years of age) experiencing stroke, due in part to what appears to be a caregiver bias. Studies reveal that lifesaving interventions are often withheld in the very old experiencing stroke. Additionally, the very old appear to receive less stroke prevention interventions.

Stroke is a disease that disproportionally affects African Americans and Latino Americans in the United States. Although overall stroke incidence has decreased nationwide, the decrease is primarily in the Caucasian population. Stroke incidence continues to increase in African Americans and Latino Americans (Ovbiagele et al., 2013). When these groups experience stroke, their survival rates are also lower than those of Caucasians. Much like the global burden of stroke, these statistics are reflective of a multifaceted and complex problem. Access to primary care, acute stroke treatment, secondary prevention of stroke, as well as geographic and socioeconomic disparities likely all impact the higher stroke incidence and mortality experienced by African and Latino Americans. Additionally, there is some evidence that African Americans are less aware of stroke signs and symptoms than other races or ethnicities and less likely to call EMS when experiencing new stroke symptoms, resulting in delays in care (Ovbiagele et al., 2013). Furthermore, studies suggest that African Americans are less likely to receive standard stroke treatment once they arrive at the hospital with stroke signs and symptoms (Ovbiagele et al., 2013). These findings serve to further reinforce that stroke is not experienced in the same way by all races and ethnicities in the United States. Although national stroke incidence and mortality statistics are encouraging, additional research and initiatives are needed to ensure all Americans experience less strokes and receive the best treatments if they do experience a stroke.

Studies suggest that access to primary care as well as organized stroke care at the time of an acute event varies according to geographic region, with decreased access in regions with lower socioeconomic status (Ovbiagele et al., 2013). The stroke belt, a region in the southeastern United States in which stroke incidence and mortality is significantly higher than the rest of the nation, has been recognized for several decades in the stroke community. People experiencing a stroke in the stroke belt states have a 20% to 40% higher mortality rate compared to the rest of the nation. The exact cause for this significant disparity remains elusive, particularly as studies suggest that those who are born in the stroke belt states, but move to another area of the United States, are still at higher risk for stroke and death from stroke. The stroke belt is likely a confluence of factors including decreased access to primary care for management of stroke risk factors and decreased access to EMS care and stroke systems of care. Additional research and initiatives to address these disparities are needed.

Changing Causes of Stroke

As health care evolves and the burden of chronic disease such as heart disease, diabetes, and other risk factors for stroke evolve in coming decades, the causes of stroke are expected to shift (Ovbiagele et al., 2013). Some of the decrease in U.S. stroke incidence is attributed to improved primary prevention and control of risk factors such as hypertension and hyperglycemia. Although primary care of patients with hypertension has improved measurably, the rapid rise in obesity poses a significant risk for increasing the incidence of stroke in coming decades. Obesity is strongly associated with stroke risk factors, including hypertension, diabetes mellitus, dyslipidemia, and cardiovascular disease. The true impact of the obesity crisis has yet to be fully understood. Chronic obesity may contribute to increased stroke frequency and at a younger age.

With the aging population, chronic heart disease is expected to lead to an increased prevalence of heart failure and atrial fibrillation. Atrial fibrillation is a significant risk factor for ischemic stroke, and stroke prevention necessitates chronic anticoagulation. However, chronic anticoagulation is also a risk factor for hemorrhagic stroke. Therefore, the increase in heart failure and atrial fibrillation over the next several decades may result in an increase in both ischemic and hemorrhagic stroke.

▮▮ THE CHANGING STROKE LANDSCAPE

Several factors are expected to contribute to a changing stroke landscape over the next several decades. These factors build on significant work conducted thus far in the areas of clinical research, stroke systems of care, as well as health care structure and payment reform in the United States and internationally. The future of stroke care is expected to be molded by continued bench- and patient-focused clinical research as well as industry and technological developments at the level of the individual patient as well as population level.

National and International Advocacy

Several organizations support ongoing initiatives to measure and improve outcomes for stroke victims. At an international level, the WHO has supported epidemiological studies to measure the global impact of stroke and to build basic care infrastructures to improve stroke care infrastructure and outcomes. In the United States, the American Heart Association (AHA) established the American Stroke Association (ASA) in the late 1990s with the goal of decreasing disability and death due to stroke and reducing stroke death by 25% (Schwamm et al., 2010). The AHA/ASA has accomplished this mission through several initiatives including research, the development of stroke systems of care, and the development of a national database to measure the impact and outcome of stroke. The AHA/ASA has also worked in recent years to impact national and state legislation and set priorities for health care reform focused on stroke care and stroke recovery. The Brain Attack Coalition (BAC) and the National Institute for of Neurological Disorders and Stroke (NINDS) are two additional national organizations influencing stroke research, policy, and clinical care.

Research

Basic stroke research is uncovering the influence of genetics as a risk factor for stroke and biochemical genetic markers for stroke. For example, in a recent press release from the National Institutes of Health (NIH, 2014), the caption says, "Researchers Discover Underlying Genetics, Marker for Stroke." Reporting on a study by Williams et al. (2014), the researchers studied the genomes of nearly 5,000 people and pinpointed a genetic variant tied to an increased risk of stroke. They also found that circulating homocysteine (tHcy), a product of the folate one-carbon metabolism pathway (FOCM) through the demethylation of methionine, is heritable and is associated with an increased risk of stroke, cardiovascular disease, cancer, and dementia. These findings may provide new clues to understanding the underlying genetic and biochemical influences in the development of stroke and cardiovascular disease and may also help lead to new treatment strategies (NIH, 2014). Although the translation from "bench to bedside" is a long road, this is a recent example of the kind of research that will lead to new knowledge and a better understanding of stroke. This research serves as a springboard for other research that will eventually lead to efficacy studies, clinical trials for effectiveness, and finally, translation into CPGs for better patient outcomes.

Another important area of research is pharmacogenomics, the study of the role of genetics in drug response. The goal of pharmacogenomics is to develop rational means to optimize drug therapy, with respect to the patients' genotype, to ensure maximum efficacy with minimal adverse effects (Becquemont, 2009). This approach is tied to the development of "personalized medicine" in which drugs and drug combinations are optimized for each individual's unique genetic makeup (Squassina et al., 2010). Clopidogrel (Plavix) is a thienopyridine-class antiplatelet agent used to inhibit blood clot formation in coronary artery disease and cerebrovascular disease. It is frequently prescribed for patients after stroke or stent placement. In 2010, the U.S. Food and Drug Administration (2010) announced a warning about Plavix to inform prescribers that the drug may not be effective in patients who carry a particular gene variant. About 30% of people cannot metabolize Plavix to convert it to an active drug. Without the intact functioning gene, the liver cells responsible for metabolism, known as *cytochrome 2C19* (or CYP2C19), Plavix does not adequately suppress the platelets or prevent blood clots. The patient is placed unknowingly at risk. Without the knowledge of a person's genetics, this drug could be prescribed to a patient with this genetic so-called loss-of-function allele (Topol, 2012).

The discussion of Plavix helps to frame a discussion of personalized medicine or personalized health care. With the recognition of genetic variability in an individual's response to drug and other therapies, the need to tailor treatment according to the individual genetic profile of the patient is apparent. This challenge is overcome with individual patient genomics profiles generated by a growing number of high-throughput molecular platforms (Oracle Health Sciences, 2014). Personalized medicine focuses on delivering preventive and therapeutic treatments to those persons who will most likely benefit while sparing the expense and the side effects for those who will not benefit. Whole genome sequencing is a laboratory process that determines the complete DNA sequence of an organism's genome at a single time (Harbron & Rapley, 2004). It includes gene sequencing at the single nucleotide polymorphisms (SNPs) level, enables scientists to pinpoint functional variants from association studies, and improves the knowledge available to researchers or predicting disease susceptibility and drug response (Li, Kadura, Fu, & Watson, 2004). The cost of whole genome sequencing is dropping significantly so that, in the future, it will be available to the general public as a tool to personalize and individualize health care. Are we there yet? The answer is no, but it is on the horizon. Biotechnology continues to make monumental strides in developing the methodology for clinical use.

Technology

New and innovative uses of technology are having a tremendous impact on stroke care now and will have in the future. The following briefly discusses a technology-rich future for stroke care.

Perhaps one of the most profound changes in the future will be with physiological monitoring in relationship to use of smart phones in association with new downloadable applications (apps) and other forms of wireless monitoring. In the past, a few physiological parameters such as blood pressure, pulse, respirations, and temperature were monitored with discrete measurements occurring over time. With available wireless technology and smart phones, the vital sign parameters plus many other parameters will be amenable to monitor on a continuous basis. Not only will the monitoring be continuous, but there will also be the ability to analyze the data continuously without having to download it to another program. Continuous monitoring of cerebral electrical activity with an ongoing electroencephalogram (EEG) will provide a mechanism to discern seizure activity and be able to associate it with activities in which the person is engaged. Monitoring a physiological parameter continuously around the clock has the advantage of being able to capture data through variations in real-life situations such as stress and sleep.

Although current intensive care unit (ICU) standard of care includes continuous monitoring of heart rate, heart rhythm, respiratory rate, and oxygen saturation, neurological assessment parameters such as monitoring of intracranial pressure (ICP) and EEG are generally collected in single discrete time samples hourly or less frequently. New bedside clinical care technology is attempting to integrate neurological physiology parameters such as ICP, EEG, and brain tissue oxygenation and adding cerebral microdialysis sampling of excitatory neurotransmitters such as glutamate to allow continuous monitoring of cellular cerebral function. Companies such as Moberg Research and Integra LifeSciences have recently launched neuromonitoring technologies aimed at continuous monitoring of these parameters (Integra LifeSciences, 2014; Moberg Research, 2014). The future ICU care for a stroke patient could include continuous multimodal neuromonitoring in addition to standard cardiopulmonary monitoring.

In the United States, the chronic disease burden largely results from a short list of risk factors including tobacco use, poor diet and physical inactivity (both strongly associated with obesity), excessive alcohol consumption, uncontrolled high blood pressure, and hyperlipidemia, all of which can be effectively addressed (Bauer, Briss, Goodman, & Bowman, 2014). All of these risk factors are also risk factors for stroke and need to be addressed simultaneously to prevent stroke or recurrent stroke in a patient who has had a previous stroke. Monitoring for these risk factors via smart phone and biosensor technology could help with immediate alerts both to the patient and health care provider. There could also be educational interventions that could be sent to the patient once a risk factor was identified. For stroke patients, in addition to the parameters already mentioned, sleep, blood coagulation, blood glucose, cardiac rate and rhythm for evidence of atrial fibrillation, and numerous other areas of interest can be monitored in a variety of settings across the continuum of care including home.

The medical appointment of the future may very well be a virtual appointment in which the health care provider will review data from these various sources with the patient and interaction with a real-time video presence. It remains to be seen if health policy, reimbursement, and the technology will support this possible future. Part of the criteria to measure quality may be to determine if care is safe, equitable, effective, efficient, timely, and patient-centered, as described by the IOM (2001).

Biotechnology

Biotechnology is defined as the manipulation (as through genetic engineering) of living organisms or their components to produce useful usually commercial products such as novel pharmaceuticals (Biotechnology, n.d.). It merges biological information with computer technology and includes nanotechnology. The size of technology is becoming smaller and portable. For example, the Vscan is a mobile echocardiogram unit that fits into the pocket of a laboratory coat. It is easy to use, provides reliable data, and allows the health care provider to give real-time feedback to patients about their cardiac function. One point to make about the technology for an echocardiogram is that it does not require ionizing radiation like an x-ray, computed tomography scan, fluoroscopy, or nuclear scans. The need for ionizing radiation is a limiting factor for making these diagnostics as small and mobile as the echocardiogram (Topol, 2012).

Nanotechnology is science, engineering, and technology conducted at the nanoscale, which is about 1 to 100 nanometers (nanometers = one billionth of a meter). A nanometer is 40,000 smaller than the thickness of human hair. Nanotechnology is the study and application of extremely small things and can be used across all the other science fields, such as chemistry, biology, physics, engineering, and medicine (National Nanotechnology Initiative, 2014). When applied to medicine, nanotechnology is the medical applications of nanomaterials, nanoelectronic biosensors, and even possible future applications of molecular nanotechnology. The possibilities of wireless sensors and genomics for targeted therapies are incredible. Nanotechnology is expected to revolutionize drug delivery, gene therapy, diagnostics, and many areas of research, development, and clinical application. Nanotechnology is being used for targeted drug therapies with more effective drug delivery systems leading to fewer side effects. It is in the early stage of developing scaffolding in nerve regeneration research which could someday lead to replacement of the brain tissue injured by stroke (Project on Emerging Nanotechnologies, 2014). The possibilities for stroke prevention and treatment are huge.

Robotics

Robotics is the use of computer-controlled robots to perform manual tasks. In medicine, robotics is used for surgery, patient care, and rehabilitation. It is frequently used after stroke, traumatic brain injury, spinal cord injury, or other nervous system conditions related to loss of function. For stroke patients, robotics could be used for surgical complexity and precision procedures such as hematoma removal. In stroke rehabilitation, robotics are being used to assist with cognitive disorders, communication deficits, sensorimotor training of paralyzed or paretic limbs, balance retraining, and other stroke-related deficits (Fasoli, Krebs, & Hogan, 2004; Volpe et al., 2000). For example, robot-based technologies such as the Lokomat (Sensory-Motor Systems Lab) are designed to combine medical and engineering approaches to help patients regain mobility faster, with less pain. The Lokomat uses a robot to automate treadmill training, affording patients longer and more frequent sessions and resulting in a faster and improved return to mobility. The robot intelligently adapts its behavior to the patient's individual capabilities. Improved pelvis and hip actuation and control can make walking with the Lokomat more natural, and virtual training environments can increase patients' motivation and engagement (Diana, 2011). Although robotics is not new to stroke rehabilitation, its use will expand and become a standard practice in stroke rehabilitation.

The integration of technology on the future of stroke care and management is sure to have a huge impact on both the prevention and treatment of stroke. The previous discussion is but a quick glimpse on what the future holds.

Improved Clinical Care

The current U.S. health care system disproportionality focuses on acute care rather than primary care and secondary prevention efforts. Improved primary prevention focused on mitigating stroke risk factors will have a clear impact on stroke incidence and stroke recovery. The Affordable Care Act (ACA), enacted in 2010, promises an increased focus on primary care and disease prevention. The act is still in the early phases of implementation, and the full impact of health care reform on primary care and the future of stroke remains to be seen. The potential impact of the ACA is discussed in more detail in the following text.

Related to recognition of stroke risk and prevention, current efforts are underway to develop electronic tools to calculate risk of stroke. One can envision a future where all people have the ability and accountability for measuring their future stroke risk using such tools. With the significant focus on the cost of health care and the individual's role in risk reduction, one can envision a future where all individuals have calculate their risk for disease and will be held accountable for risk factor reduction. Although controversial, population-level interventions aimed at targeting high-risk health behavior using taxation, reporting, and adjustment of health premiums has been successful to change. Behaviors such as smoking, obesity, uncontrolled diabetes, and uncontrolled hypertension are all risk factors for stroke that the individual may be increasingly responsible for reporting and held accountable for behavior change.

Clinical care at a population level has been greatly impacted by the development of stroke systems of care. The past decade has seen the development of two stroke program certifications, primary stroke center (PSC) and comprehensive stroke center (CSC) certification offered by several regulatory safety and quality agencies. To date, approximately 1,400 of the 5,700 national hospitals are certified as PSCs, and 69 facilities are certified as CSCs (American Hospital Association, 2014). Additionally, nearly half of the states in the United States have enacted legislation guiding the development of stroke systems of care, generally supporting hospital stroke certification and prehospital bypass of non–stroke-certified facilities. Some states have developed registries and require health care organizations to submit outcomes to the state, in addition to national and regulatory reporting.

Although stroke certification levels have developed and gained popularity over the past decade, a full stroke system that allows all U.S. residents access to expert stroke care is yet to be realized. Currently, it is unclear how PSC and CSCs work together to ensure all people in the nation have access to organized stroke care. Furthermore, much of the rural United States remains more than 60 minutes away from a PSC or CSC. Although many states have enacted stroke system of care legislation, states vary in their level and stage of implementation and sophistication. The AHA/ASA recently outlined a series of national, state, and EMS policy priorities to further improve stroke systems of care in the United States. **Table 13-1** shows a comprehensive list of ASA/AHA policy initiatives (Ovbiagele et al., 2013).

TABLE 13-1   American Heart Association Policy Strategies to Address Stroke Systems of Care

Stroke Systems of Care	Advocacy/Policy Strategies
Prevention	**Federal** • Incorporate measures of physical activity levels into electronic medical records and counsel in the healthcare environment • Advocate for regular revision and update of the "Physical Activity Guidelines for Americans" • Obesity counseling and treatment coverage in the healthcare environment • Robust surveillance and monitoring of obesity • Partner with US Department of Health and Human Services to promote the Million Hearts campaign • Work to eliminate food deserts and improve access to and affordability of healthy foods • Reduce sodium in the food supply • Implement the Institute of Medicine's recommendations to reduce sodium in the food supply • Improve food labeling to increase consumer understanding of sodium levels in packaged foods • Advocate for robust sodium limits in procurement standards, nutrition standards in schools, and other government feeding programs **State** • Increase sports, recreational opportunities, parks, and green spaces in the community • Support efforts to design workplaces, communities, and schools around active living and integrate physical activity opportunities throughout the day • Support the use of zoning policy to increase access to safe places for recreation • Create and maintain comprehensive worksite wellness programs • Advocate for adequate prevention, diagnosis, and treatment of overweight and obesity in the healthcare environment • Advocate for continued funding for obesity prevention research and work to ensure a strong evaluation component is a part of the implementation of new laws and programs • Include sodium information through the use of warnings on the menu as allowed by federal law and support strategies that reduce sodium in the flood supply • Support the elimination of food deserts through policies that increase the availability of fruits, vegetables, and water in underserved neighborhoods • Support the use of zoning policy to increase access to healthy foods and decrease access to unhealthy foods • Support the establishment of food procurement policies that meet AHA guidelines for government offices • Support policies that change relative pieces of healthy vs unhealthy food items • Support policies designed to encourage retailers to increase access to healthy foods while decreasing access to unhealthy foods • Increase funding for programs that eliminate health disparities • Promote public funding for heart disease and stroke programs • Support policies that ensure the availability of evidence-based stroke prevention benefits in private insurance and public health programs that are consistent with the AHA position statement, "Recommended Model Benefits Package: Preventive Cardiovascular Services" and the US Preventive Services Task Force recommendations for preventive health services. Support policies that eliminate cost sharing (including copays and deductibles) associated with these stroke-related preventive services. Oppose policies that establish punitive measures within health plans for those with CVD risk factors such as tobacco use, being overweight or obese, hypertension, and high cholesterol.

TABLE 13-1 American Heart Association Policy Strategies to Address Stroke Systems of Care *(continued)*	
Stroke Systems of Care	**Advocacy/Policy Strategies**
EMS transport	Federal/state • Support public policy and sustainable appropriations initiatives and other activities that promote increased quality and timely use of 9-1-1 systems. This includes the ability of current and future generations of telecommunication technology to supply enhanced 9-1-1 (E9-1-1) capabilities to their customers. • Promote the use of sustainable funding for nationally recognized emergency medical dispatch protocols and appropriate quality improvement programs among 9-1-1 dispatch agencies to ensure that bystanders promptly receive effective coaching and support and that dispatch personnel provide prearrival medical instructions • Support public policy, sustainable appropriations, and other initiatives that promote a strong, well-trained, data-driven, quality EMS system that improves collaboration, responsiveness, and effectiveness • Strengthen EMS systems by supporting efforts that will eliminate geographic, racial, ethnic, sex, and socioeconomic disparities in EMS care • Using current AHA/ASA guidelines for stroke care, promote within EMSs statewide standardization and implementation of stroke training, assessment, treatment, and transportation protocols

AHA, American Heart Association; CVD, cardiovascular disease; EMS, emergency medical service; ASA, American Stroke Association.
For AHA/ASA advocacy resources including fact sheets, policy briefs, published papers, and position statements, go to: http://www.heart.org/HEARTORG/Advocate/PolicyResources/Policy-Resources_UCM_001135_SubHomePage.jsp.
From Ovbiagele, B., Goldstein, L. B., Higashida, R. T., Howard, V. J., Johnston, S. C., Khavjou, O. A., . . . Trogdon, J. G. (2013). Forecasting the future of stroke in the United States: A policy statement from the American Heart Association and American Stroke Association. *Stroke, 44*(8), 2361–2375. doi:10.1161/STR.0b013e31829734f2

With the growth of national database monitoring, the care of patients with stroke such as *Get With The Guidelines*, one can envision a future where high-quality population-level research may reveal interventions and care priorities for subsets of patients, such as certain ethnicities and age groups. Such databases may be helpful in determining regional variations in care and outcomes and help with planning stroke systems of care. Finally, with extensive national databases, the future may allow for matching individual patient characteristics with national databases to determine care and prevention priorities.

Health Care Reform

The ACA, passed by the U.S. Congress in 2010, has the potential to improve stroke care and outcomes through a number of initiatives. The legislation is complex, with many aspects of the bill still being developed and implemented across the nation. Fundamentally, the ACA is expected to improve all American's access to affordable health care coverage. This is expected to translate to improved primary prevention and risk factor reduction for stroke avoidance that is expected to result in a measured impact on incidence and mortality from stroke. Aspects of the ACA are also expected to improve poststroke care for survivors by improving access and quality of rehabilitation. This may greatly impact stroke outcomes, as studies demonstrate that stroke survivors without stroke insurance have higher mortality rates than patients with insurance (Ovbiagele et al., 2013).

The ACA may impact stroke risk factors in a positive way by building preventive care benefits and incentives into the health care system. This includes financial and other rewards for healthy behaviors as well as funding for population-level projects seeking to implement wide-reaching primary preventions strategies (Ovbiagele et al., 2013). Improved preventive care aimed at addressing risk factors such as obesity, hypertension, diabetes, and hyperlipidemia should translate to less stroke events in later life.

The ACA legislation is expected to promote high-quality care through a number of initiatives, including building systems of care, prioritizing research to address disparities in care, and supporting outcome-focused research. These initiatives may incentivize the continued development of stroke systems of care through external certification and state-based legislation as well as possible reform of poststroke rehabilitation policies by offering more extensive rehabilitation care. Additional support for research funding was enacted through the Patient-Centered Outcomes Research Institute (PCORI), with an emphasis on outcome-based research. Again, the expected gains in stroke research as well as stroke outcomes as a result of the ACA initiatives will depend on program implementation and will take time to measure.

FUTURE STROKE CAREGIVERS

A final critical element expected to impact the future of stroke care is the shortage of stroke caregivers and the projected future of a health care workforce with stroke specialty education and training. Stroke care has generally been under the expertise of neurology and with a more recent addition of the neurovascular neurology subspecialty of medicine (Freeman & Vatz, 2010). Much like nursing, medicine is experiencing an aging workforce. According to an American Academy of Neurology survey conducted in 2004, 34% of neurologists practicing at that time were between the ages of 50 and 60 years. This is compared to an expected projected 28.6% each decade if evenly distributed, indicating an aging neurology workforce without younger trainees to take the place of retiring neurologists. Given current neurology residency enrollment, the attrition of neurologists is expected to exceed the rate of neurologists completing residency and entering practice. The need for subspecialty neurologists is expected to continue to increase in coming decades, and current models suggest the demand for neurologists in coming years will far exceed demand. This need may be particularly pronounced in stroke and neurocritical care inpatient specialties, particularly in rural and underserved communities (Freeman & Vatz, 2010).

To address the shortage of physicians who are stroke specialists, the stroke field has witnessed an increasing role of telehealth to manage both the shortage of neurologists as well as geographic disparities (Freeman & Vatz, 2010). Telemedicine, or telestroke, allows a stroke caregiver to examine and provide expert consultation using telephone or audiovisual computer connection with the stroke victim regardless of geographic location (Schwamm, Holloway, et al., 2009). Telestroke, as a means to further develop a national stroke system of care and provide stroke treatment to geographically underserved areas, is endorsed by the AHA/ASA (Schwamm, Audebert, et al., 2009). Telestroke programs are expected to continue to grow in the coming years. As stroke and inpatient acute neurological care grows in complexity, two inpatient neurology subspecialties have evolved. The neurology hospitalist and the neurointensivist both represent neurology-trained physicians with a focused specialty in the inpatient emergent and acute care of the patient with stroke. This represents a departure from the traditional model of the neurology specialty, where the neurologist was primarily outpatient focused and provided inpatient consultation as needed. The impact of widespread use of neurohospitalists and neurointensivist remains to be measured.

Physician shortage surveys also demonstrate an increased number of nonphysician advanced practice providers, such as advanced practice nurse practitioners and clinical nurse specialists, as well as physician assistants employed by physician and hospital practices to provide specialty stroke care (Freeman & Vatz, 2010). The 2012 CSC standards published by The Joint Commission (2014) mandates that to become a certified program, the stroke center must employ advanced practice nurses (APNs) with stroke expertise. Additionally, several small studies demonstrate that APNs provide expert, safe care in the hyperacute, acute, and telestroke care settings (Demaerschalk & Kiernan, 2010).

Interprofessional Teams of the Future

It is well known that interprofessional team care leads to the best outcomes for patients and the safest care. In the future, movement toward team care will accelerate driven by evidence-based practice guidelines and reimbursement tied to achievement of outcomes. Students entering the health care professions will be educated and prepared with the competencies to practice effectively in teams. Those currently in practice will need to be retooled with the competencies of interprofessional team care. What will change will be the nature of teams. The stable team in which the same health care providers work together on a regular basis will decrease (Hackman, 2002). Instead, health care providers will come together as a team for a focused short-term purpose and disband; this process will be repeated with new team members as the need arises over and over again. What this means for health professionals is that they will have to have the flexibility, communications skills, and focus to work comfortably to deliver safe and effective care in this short-term and less structured model (Edmondson, 2012). The enhanced focus on an engaged patient as an equal partner in decision making about his or her care is also the future. This model will be the model in which stroke care will be delivered, and health professionals will need to be competent in this revised model of care. See Chapter 3 for further discussion on interprofessional team care.

S U M M A R Y

Stroke care has changed rapidly over the past three decades, spurred in large part by significant gains in understanding of the mechanism and treatment of the disease through clinical research. Significant efforts to develop a system of care in which all U.S. and global citizens have access to evidence-based stroke care are underway. Additionally, the demographics of stroke incidence, prevalence, and outcomes are changing and expected to continue to change in coming years. The future of stroke care is exciting and daunting. Clinical research, technological advances both in health care and other industries, and improved stroke care delivery infrastructure are expected to transform stroke care in ways known and unknown for individuals and populations. The interprofessional team, working together to prevent stroke, intervene when acute stroke occurs, and care for stroke survivors as they integrate back into their community, hold the power to change the future of stroke for individuals. Similar efforts at the population level should lead to healthy communities and achievement of national health goals.

REFERENCES

American Hospital Association. (2014). *Fast facts on US hospitals.* Retrieved from http://www.aha.org/research/rc/stat-studies/fast-facts.shtml

Bauer, U. E., Briss, P. A., Goodman, R. A., & Bowman, B. A. (2014). Prevention of chronic disease in the 21st century: Elimination of the leading preventable causes of premature death and disability in the USA. *Lancet, 348,* 45–52.

Becquemont, L. (2009). Pharmacogenomics of adverse drug reactions: Practical applications and perspectives. *Pharmacogenomics, 10*(6), 961–969. doi:10.2217/pgs.09.37

Biotechnology. (n.d.). In *Merriam-Webster's online dictionary* (11th ed.). Retrieved from http://www.merriam-webster.com/dictionary/biotechnology

Demaerschalk, B. M., & Kiernan, T. J. (2010). Vascular neurology nurse practitioner provision of telemedicine consultations. *International Journal of Telemedicine and Applications.* Advance online publication. doi:10.1155/2010/507071

Diana, A. (2011). 12 Advances in medical robotics. *InformationWeek: Connecting the Business Technology Community.* Retrieved from http://www.informationweek.com/healthcare/patient-tools/12-advances-in-medical-robotics/d/d-id/1095720?

Edmondson, A. C. (2012). *Teaming: How organizations learn, innovate, and compete in the knowledge economy.* San Francisco, CA: Jossey-Bass.

Fasoli, S. E., Krebs, H. I., & Hogan, N. (2004). Robotic technology and stroke rehabilitation: Translating research into practice. *Topics in Stroke Rehabilitation, 11*(4), 11–19. doi:10.1310/G8XB-VM23-1TK7-PWQU

Freeman, W. D., & Vatz, K. A. (2010). The future of neurology. *Neurologic Clinics, 28*(2), 537–561. doi:10.1016/j.ncl.2009.11.006

Hackman, J. R. (2002). *Leading teams: Setting the stage for great performances.* Boston, MA: Harvard Business School Press.

Harbron, S., & Rapley, R. (Eds.). (2004). *Molecular analysis and genome discovery.* London, United Kingdom: John Wiley & Sons.

Institute of Medicine. (2001). *Crossing the quality chasm: A new health system for the 21st century.* Washington, DC: National Academy Press.

Institute of Medicine. (2011). *Clinical practice guidelines we can trust.* Washington, DC: National Academy Press.

Integra LifeSciences. (2014). *Integra products.* Retrieved from http://integralife.com/index.aspx?redir=products

LeFevre, M. L. (2014). Screening for asymptomatic carotid artery stenosis: U.S. Preventive Services Task Force recommendation statement. *Annals of Internal Medicine, 161*(5), 356–362. doi:10.7326/M14-1333

Li, B., Kadura, I., Fu, D. J., & Watson, D. E. (2004). Genotyping with TaqMAMA. *Genomics, 83*(2), 311–320. doi:10.1016/j.ygeno.2003.08.005

Moberg Research. (2014). *Neuromonitoring.* Retrieved from http://mobergresearch.com/products-services/neuromonitoring

Mukherjee, D., & Patil, C. G. (2011). Epidemiology and the global burden of stroke. *World Neurosurgery, 76*(6, Suppl.), S85–S90. doi:10.1016/j.wneu.2011.07.023

National Institutes of Health. (2014). *Researchers discover underlying genetics, marker for stroke, cardiovascular disease.* Retrieved from http://www.nih.gov/news/health/mar2014/nhgri-20.htm

National Nanotechnology Initiative. (2014). *What is nanotechnology?* Retrieved from http://www.nano.gov/nanotech-101/what/definition

Oracle Health Sciences. (2014). *Personalized medicine: Informatics challenges on the road to the clinic.* Retrieved from http://www.oracle.com/webapps/dialogue/ns/dlgwelcome.jsp?p_ext=Y&p_dlg_id=15727918&src=7878597&Act=17&sckw=WWHS13049178MPP001

Ovbiagele, B., Goldstein, L. B., Higashida, R. T., Howard, V. J., Johnston, S. C., Khavjou, O. A., . . . Trogdon, J. G. (2013). Forecasting the future of stroke in the United States: A policy statement from the American Heart Association and American Stroke Association. *Stroke, 44*(8), 2361–2375. doi:10.1161/STR.0b013e31829734f2

Project on Emerging Nanotechnologies. (2014). *Nanotechnology and medicine.* Retrieved from http://www.nanotechproject.org/inventories/medicine/

Schwamm, L. H., Audebert, H. J., Amarenco, P., Chumbler, N. R., Frankel, M. R., George, M. G., . . . White, C. J. (2009). Recommendations for the implementation of telemedicine within stroke systems of care: A policy statement from the American Heart Association. *Stroke, 40*(7), 2635–2660. doi:10.1161/STROKEAHA.109.192361

Schwamm, L., Fayad, P., Acker, J. E., III, Duncan, P., Fonarow, G. C., Girgus, M., . . . Yancy, C. W. (2010). Translating evidence into practice: A decade of efforts by the American Heart Association/American Stroke Association to reduce death and disability due to stroke: A presidential advisory from the American Heart Association/American Stroke Association. *Stroke, 41*(5), 1051–1065. doi:10.1161/STR.0b013e3181d2da7d

Schwamm, L. H., Holloway, R. G., Amarenco, P., Audebert, H. J., Bakas, T., Chumbler, N. R., . . . Wechsler, L. R. (2009). A review of the evidence for the use of telemedicine within stroke systems of care: A scientific statement from the American Heart Association/American Stroke Association. *Stroke, 40*(7), 2616–2634. doi:10.1161/STROKEAHA.109.192360

Squassina, A., Manchia, M., Manolopoulos, V. G., Artac, M., Lappa-Manakou, C., Karkabouna, S., . . . Patrinos, G. P. (2010). Realities and expectations of pharmacogenomics and personalized medicine: Impact of translating genetic knowledge into clinical practice. *Pharmacogenomics, 11*(8), 1149–1167.

The Joint Commission. (2014). *Advanced certification comprehensive stroke centers.* Retrieved from http://www.jointcommission.org/certification/advanced_certification_comprehensive_stroke_centers.aspx

Topol, E. (2012). *The creative destruction of medicine: How the digital revolution will create better health care.* New York, NY: Basic Books.

U.S. Food and Drug Administration. (2010). *FDA announces new boxed warning on Plavix: Alerts patients, health care professionals to potential for reduced effectiveness.* Retrieved from http://www.fda.gov/NewsEvents/Newsroom/PressAnnouncements/ucm204253.htm

Volpe, B. T., Krebs, H. I., Hogan, N., Edelstein, L., Diels, C., & Aisen, M. (2000). A novel approach to stroke rehabilitation: Robot-aided sensorimotor stimulation. *Neurology, 54*(10), 1938–1944. doi:10.1212/WNL.54.10.1938

Williams, S. R., Yang, Q., Chen, F., Liu, X, Keene, K. L., Jacques, P., . . . Sales, M. M. (2014). Genome-wide meta-analysis of homocysteine and methionine metabolism identifies five one carbon metabolism loci and a novel association of ADLH1L1 with ischemic stroke. *PLoS Genetics, 10*(3), 1–13, e1004214.

Acronyms Used in Book

AAPM&R	American Academy of Physical Medicine and Rehabilitation
ABCs	Airway, breathing, circulation
ACA	Affordable Care Act
ACA	Anterior cerebral artery
ACO	Accountable care organization
ADA	Americans with Disabilities Act
ADC	Apparent diffusion coefficient
ADH	Antidiuretic hormone
ADL	Activities of daily living
AED	Antiepileptic drug
AF	Atrial fibrillation
AHA	American Heart Association
AHRQ	Agency for Healthcare Research and Quality
ALOS	Average length of stay
ALS	Advanced life support
AOTA	American Occupational Therapy Association
APN	Advanced practice nurse
ApoE	Apolipoprotein E
App	Application
APTA	American Physical Therapy Association
ARDS	Acute respiratory distress syndrome
ARF	Acute rehabilitation facility
ARN	Association of Rehabilitation Nurses
ASA	American Stroke Association
ASA	Aspirin
ASCVD	Atherosclerotic cardiovascular disease
ASHA	American Speech-Language-Hearing Association
AST	Acute stroke team
AT	Antithrombotic therapy
ATP	Adenosine triphosphate
ATRA	American Therapeutic Recreation Association
aSAH	Aneurysmal subarachnoid hemorrhage
AVM	Arteriovenous malformation
BAC	Brain Attack Coalition
BiPAP	Bilevel positive airway pressure
BLS	Basic life support
BNP	Brain natriuretic peptide
BP	Blood pressure
BPH	Benign prostatic hypertrophy
CAA	Cerebral amyloid angiopathy
CAD	Coronary artery disease
CAM-ICU	Confusion assessment method for theintensive care unit
CARF	Commission on Accreditation of Rehabilitation Facilities
CAS	Carotid angioplasty and stenting
CAUTI	Catheter-associated urinary tract infection
CCAC	Continuing Care Accreditation Commission
CCB	Calcium channel blocker
CDC	Centers for Disease Control and Prevention
CE	Contrast enhanced
CEA	Carotid endarterectomy
CHF	Congestive heart failure
CIMT	Constraint-induced movement therapy
CLABSI	Central line–associated bloodstream infection
CLRD	Chronic lower respiratory disease
CME	Continuing medical education
CMG	Case-Mix Group
CMS	Centers for Medicare and Medicaid Services

CN	Cranial nerve
CNS	Central nervous system
CoP	Conditions of participation
COPD	Chronic obstructive pulmonary disease
CPAP	Continuous positive airway pressure
CPG	Clinical practice guideline
CPP	Cerebral perfusion pressure
CPR	Cardiopulmonary resuscitation
CPSP	Central poststroke pain
CRP	C-reactive protein
CSC	Comprehensive stroke center
CSF	Cerebrospinal fluid
CSW	Cerebral salt wasting
CT	Computed tomography
CTA	Computed tomography angiography
CTP	Computed tomography perfusion
CUS	Concern, uncomfortable, stopping
CVA	Cerebrovascular accident
CVST	Cerebral venous sinus thrombosis
DAD	Discharge Abstract Database
DALYs	Disability-adjusted life years
DBP	Diastolic blood pressure
DCI	Delayed cerebral ischemia
DHHS	U.S. Department of Health and Human Services
DIND	Delayed ischemic neurological
DM	Diabetes mellitus
DMEPOS	Durable Medical Equipment, Prosthetics, Orthotics, and Supplies
DNR	Do not resuscitate
DNV	Det Norske Veritas
DSC	Disease-specific certification
DVT	Deep vein thrombosis
DWI	Diffusion-weighted imaging
EBI	Early brain injury
EBP	Evidence-based practice
ECA	Emergency care attendant
ED	Emergency department
EEG	Electroencephalography
EF	Ejection fraction
EMG	Electromyography
EMR	Electronic medical record
EMS	Emergency medical services
EMSS	Emergency medical services system
ET-A	Endothelin antagonists
ETT	Endotracheal tube
EVD	External ventricular drain
FDA	U.S. Food and Drug Administration
FEES	Fiberoptic endoscopic evaluation of swallowing
FIM	Functional Independence Measure
FIRDA	Frontal intermittent delta activity
FLAIR	Fluid attenuated inversion recovery
FOCM	Folate one-carbon metabolism
GBD	Global Burden of Diseases, Injuries, and Risk Factors Study
GCS	Glasgow Coma Scale
GOS	Glasgow Outcome Scale
GRE	Gradient recalled echo
GU	Genitourinary
GWTG	Get with the Guidelines
HACs	Hospital-acquired conditions
HAPU	Hospital-acquired pressure ulcer
HCP	Hydrocephalus
HFAP	Healthcare Facilities Accreditation Program
HHA	Home health agency
HIT	Heparin-induced thrombocytopenia
HOB	Head of bed
HRQL	Health-related quality of life
HSP	Hemiplegic shoulder pain
IA	Intracranial aneurysm
IABP	Intra-aortic balloon pump
IADL	Independent activities of daily living
ICD	International Classification of Diseases
ICH	Intracerebral hemorrhage
ICP	Intracranial pressure
ICU	Intensive care unit
IHI	Institute for Healthcare Improvement
IL	Interleukin
INR	International normalized ratio
IOM	Institute of Medicine
IPC	Intermittent pneumatic compression
IQIs	Inpatient quality indicators
IQR	Inpatient Quality Reporting
IRF	Inpatient rehabilitation facility
IRF-PAI	Inpatient Rehabilitation Facility Patient Assessment Instrument

IRF PPS	Inpatient Rehabilitation Facility Prospective Payment System		PED	Pipeline Embolization Device
IV	Intravenous		PEG	Percutaneous endoscopic gastrostomy
IVH	Intraventricular hemorrhage		PFO	Patent foramen ovale
JNC	Joint National Committee		PICA	Posterior inferior cerebellar artery
KSA	Knowledge, skills, and actions		PICC	Peripherally inserted central catheter
LDL	Low-density lipoprotein			
LMWH	Low-molecular-weight heparin		PLED	Periodic lateralizing epileptiform discharge
LP	Lumbar puncture			
LTAC	Long-term acute care		PNF	Proprioceptive neuromuscular facilitation
MAP	Mean arterial pressure			
MBS	Modified barium swallow		PO	Orally
MCA	Middle cerebral artery		POD	Postoperative delirium
MI	Myocardial infarction		PPV	Pars plana vitrectomy
MICU	Mobile intensive care unit		PQIs	Prevention quality indicators
MRA	Magnetic resonance angiography		PRN	As needed
			PSC	Primary stroke center
MRI	Magnetic resonance imaging		PSD	Poststroke depression
mRS	Modified Rankin Scale		PSIs	Patient safety indicators
MRV	Magnetic resonance venography		PSS	Poststroke spasticity
			PT	Physical therapy
NDNQI	National Database of Nursing Quality Indicators		PT	Prothrombin time
			PTT	Partial thromboplastin time
NDT	Neurodevelopmental treatment		PVR	Postvoid residual
NHSN	National Healthcare Safety Network		PWI	Perfusion-weighted imaging
			QALYs	Quality-adjusted life years
NICU	Neuroscience intensive care unit		QRP	Quality Reporting Program
NIH	National Institutes of Health		REM	Rapid eye movement
NIHSS	National Institutes of Health Stroke Scale		RHQDAPU	Reporting hospital quality data for annual payment update
NINDS	National Institute of Neurological Disorders and Stroke		RICs	Rehabilitation Impairment Categories
			RN	Registered nurse
NIS	National Inpatient Sample		RSI	Rapid-sequence intubation
NMES	Neuromuscular electrical stimulation		RT	Respiratory therapist
			rTMS	Repetitive transcranial magnetic stimulation
NQF	National Quality Forum			
NSA	National Stroke Association		rtPA	Recombinant tissue plasminogen activator
NSTEMI	Non-ST-segment elevation myocardial infarction		SAH	Subarachnoid hemorrhage
OAT	Oral anticoagulation therapy		SBAR	Situation, background, assessment, recommendation
OSA	Obstructive sleep apnea			
OT	Occupational therapy		SBP	Systolic blood pressure
PA	Physician assistant		SIADH	Syndrome of inappropriate secretion of antidiuretic hormone
PA	Pulmonary artery			
PACU	Postanesthesia care unit			
PCCs	Prothrombin complex concentrates		SLP	Speech and language pathologist
PCORI	Patient-Centered Outcomes Research Institute		SNF	Skilled nursing facility
			SNP	Single nucleotide polymorphism
PCP	Primary care provider		SSCM	Stroke systems of care model
PDIs	Pediatric quality indicators			
PE	Pulmonary embolism		SSI	Social Security Income

SSNRI	Selective serotonin–norepinephrine reuptake inhibitors	TMS	Transcranial magnetic stimulation
SSRIs	Selective serotonin reuptake inhibitors	TTE	Transthoracic echocardiogram
		UE	Upper extremity
ST	Speech therapy	UFH	Unfractionated heparin
STEMI	ST-segment elevation myocardial infarction	UI	Urinary incontinence
		UP	Universal Protocol
STEP	Status of the patient, team members, environment, and progress	USPSTF	U.S. Preventive Services Task Force
		UTI	Urinary tract infection
SW	Social worker	VA	Vertebral artery
SWI	Susceptibility-weighted imaging	VA	U.S. Department of Veterans Affairs
		VAEs	Ventilator-associated events
TCA	Tricyclic antidepressant	VAP	Ventilator-associated pneumonia
TCD	Transcranial Doppler		
TEE	Transesophageal echocardiogram	VBP	Value-based purchasing
		VEP	Visual evoked potential
TEFRA	Tax Equity and Fiscal Responsibility Act	VTE	Venous thromboembolism
		WBC	White blood cell
tHcy	Homocysteine	WFNS	World Federation of Neurological Surgeons
TIA	Transient ischemic attack		
TJC	The Joint Commission	WHO	World Health Organization

Index

Note: Page numbers followed by t denote tables; f denotes figures; b denotes boxes.